# HEART TRANSPLANTATION

## *Collected Reprints (1993–2022)*

By

William C. Roberts, MD

and

Colleagues

ISBN: 979-8-88680-083-8
Printed in the United States of America on acid-free paper.

# Preface

Heart transplantation (HT) became a predictably successful procedure in the early 1980s. Since that time, HT has brought new life to thousands of patients. Early in my career, the autopsy was the source of most of the cases for my publications. Subsequently, the autopsy rate in most hospitals worldwide has dropped dramatically and the frequency of HT has risen dramatically. In my laboratory, more studies by a considerable margin now come from native hearts removed at HT rather than at autopsy.

With a few exceptions, HT is performed because of severe heart failure due to a variety of causes, most commonly ischemic cardiomyopathy and idiopathic dilated cardiomyopathy. At Baylor University Medical Center, we have a program where the explanted native heart is shown to the recipient of the HT. We now have shown the native heart to approximately 190 HT recipients. Baylor University Medical Center has provided the cardiac pathology unit with a storage facility such that HT recipients can be shown their native heart many years after the HT procedure. During that session, I try to explain to patients the importance of caring for their new heart and to emphasize how lucky they are to have a second chance. The USA has a population of approximately 330 million, about 240 million of whom are >20 years of age. About 6 million have chronic heart failure, and about 3000 of the 6 million have a HT in the USA each year. Thus, the recipients of HT are the lucky ones. Few of the HT recipients pay for their own HT, an extremely expensive procedure paid for mainly by the non-HT community. Of course, HT has brought much new information on heart disease, which can provide hope to many of the non-HT recipients.

*—William C. Roberts, MD*

# Table of Contents

*Articles are numbered based on WCR's CV.

# Clinicopathologic Features of Hypertrophic Cardiomyopathy Managed by Cardiac Transplantation

Jamshid Shirani, MD,* Barry J. Maron, MD,† Richard O. Cannon III, MD, Sheyda Shahin, and William C. Roberts, MD‡

**Clinical records, electrocardiographic, echocardiographic, hemodynamic and radionuclide data, and the operatively excised hearts were reviewed in 10 patients (aged 19 to 46 years, mean 35) who had cardiac transplantation for hypertrophic cardiomyopathy. Severe congestive heart failure unassociated with outflow obstruction was the indication for transplantation in 9 patients. During a pretransplantation period ranging from 45 to 312 months (mean 137) in these 9 patients, pulmonary artery wedge pressure increased from 19 ± 9 to 27 ± 7 mm Hg, left ventricular ejection fraction decreased from 51 ± 11% to 41 ± 1%, left ventricular end-diastolic dimension increased from 42 ± 6 to 48 ± 4 mm, and total 12-lead QRS voltage decreased from 209 ± 50 to 156 ± 41 mm. In these 9 patients, the explanted hearts had dilated left ventricular cavities, and 8 had left ventricular scars without significant narrowing of the epicardial coronary arteries. The tenth patient had a nondilated left ventricular cavity and had transplantation because of recurrent, refractory syncope. Of the 10 patients, 3 died within the first month, and another died 8 months after transplantation. The remaining 6 patients have survived 20 to 54 months (mean 39) after transplantation and are in functional class I or II.**

**(Am J Cardiol 1993;72:434–440)**

From the Pathology and Cardiology Branches, National Heart, Lung, and Blood Institute, National Institutes of Health, Bethesda, Maryland.
Manuscript received and accepted March 9, 1993.

*Division of Cardiology, Department of Medicine, Medical College of Virginia, Richmond, Virginia 23298.

†Cardiovascular Research Division, Minneapolis Heart Institute Foundation, Minneapolis, Minnesota 55407.

‡Baylor Cardiovascular Institute, Baylor University Medical Center, Dallas, Texas 75246.

Approximately 3,000 cardiac-transplantations were performed worldwide in 1990.[1] In adults, idiopathic dilated cardiomyopathy is the most common indication for cardiac transplantation, closely followed by atherosclerotic coronary artery disease. Only 1 report describing clinicopathologic features in 2 patients having cardiac transplantation for hypertrophic cardiomyopathy (HC) has appeared.[2] During the last 15 years, 12 patients with HC studied at the National Heart, Lung, and Blood Institute have had cardiac transplantation, and in 10 of them, the explanted hearts have been examined by us. This report describes clinicopathologic findings in the latter 10 patients.

## METHODS

**Study patients:** The files of the Pathology Branch of the National Heart, Lung, and Blood Institute were searched for cases coded as having "idiopathic hypertrophic subarotic stenosis" or "hypertrophic cardiomyopathy." Of the 229 cases so coded between the years 1975 and 1992, 10 had heart transplantation and are the subjects of this report.

**Sources of the data:** Although patients were studied clinically in the Cardiology Branch of the National Heart, Lung, and Blood Institute, the transplantation procedures were performed at medical centers other than the National Institutes of Health. The hearts in the 10 patients, however, were submitted to the Pathology Branch of the National Heart, Lung, and Blood Institute for study. The hearts, which came from 10 different medical centers, were initially examined by WCR and subsequently by JS. The clinical records, electrocardiograms, echocardiograms, hemodynamic data, photographs of the explanted hearts, and microscopic slides of the hearts were reviewed in all 10 patients. Follow up data were obtained by contacting the centers where the cardiac transplantation operations were performed.

**Statistical analysis:** Data are expressed as mean ± SD. Differences between means were determined using the unpaired or paired Student *t* test where appropriate.

## RESULTS

**Clinical observations:** AGE, SYMPTOMS AND TREATMENT: Pertinent clinical findings in the 10 patients are summarized in Table I. The age at onset of symptoms of cardiac dysfunction ranged from 12 to 32 years (mean 22); the estimated age at the onset of left ventricular dilatation, which occurred in 9 patients, ranged from 18 to 45 years (mean 29), and cardiac transplantation was performed at ages 19 to 46 years (mean 35), a mean of 15 years from the onset of symptoms of cardiac dysfunction

**TABLE I** Clinical, Hemodynamic and Ventriculographic Findings in 10 Patients with Cardiac Transplantation for Hypertrophic Cardiomyopathy

| | Age at: | | | | | | | | | | | | | | | | LV-SA Psg | | | | | Radionuclide Ventriculography | |
|---|---|---|---|---|---|---|---|---|---|---|---|---|---|---|---|---|---|---|---|---|---|---|---|
| Pt. | Onset of Symptoms | Diagnosis | Estimated Onset of Left Ventricular Enlargement | Cardiac Transplant | Sex | FH of HC | AP | CHF | Sy | Interval Study to Transplant (mos) | RA (mean) | RV (s/d) | PA (s/d) | PAW (mean) | LV (s/d) | SA (s/d) | At Rest | With Provocation | CI (L/min/m²) | MR (1–3+) | Dilated LV | Interval to Transplant (mos) | LVEF (%) |
| 1 | 12 | 12 | 18 | 19 | M | + | + | + | 0 | 24 | 18 | 51/— | 60/30 | 32 | 117/15 | 116/85 | 0 | — | 2.0 | + | 0 | 9 | 48 |
| | | | | | | | | | | 9 | 22 | 50/20 | 50/30 | 28 | 108/24 | 120/76 | 0 | — | 1.8 | ++ | + | — | — |
| 2 | 18 | 21 | — | 24 | F | 0 | 0 | + | + | 34 | 5 | 22/2 | 13/5 | 5 | 100/10 | 120/65 | 0 | 14 | 3.3 | 0 | 0 | 33 | 72 |
| | | | | | | | | | | 8 | 3 | 22/6 | 22/8 | 9 | 110/12 | 105/59 | 20 | 64 | 3.4 | + | 0 | 30 | 65 |
| 3 | 16 | 16 | 22 | 27 | M | 0 | 0 | + | 0 | 89 | — | — | — | — | 108/20 | 108/65 | 0 | 0 | — | 0 | 0 | 68 | 66 |
| | | | | | | | | | | 3 | 22 | 45/20 | 45/35 | 29 | — | 110/70 | — | — | 2.6 | — | — | 63 | 64 |
| 4 | 17 | 17 | 31 | 33 | F | 0 | 0 | + | 0 | 156 | 3 | 36/4 | 27/12 | 13 | 84/12 | 96/54 | 0 | — | 3.4 | 0 | 0 | — | — |
| | | | | | | | | | | 27 | 7 | 50/9 | 50/19 | 28 | 95/23 | 95/68 | 0 | — | 2.0 | — | + | — | — |
| 5 | 23 | 23 | 33 | 36 | M | + | + | + | + | 120 | 3 | 32/5 | 34/14 | 15 | 105/18 | 100/60 | 0 | 60 | 1.9 | 0 | 0 | 37 | 67 |
| | | | | | | | | | | 34 | — | 45/23 | 55/26 | 30 | — | — | — | — | — | — | — | — | — |
| 6 | 19 | 22 | 36 | 37 | F | 0 | 0 | + | + | 175 | 6 | 50/15 | 50/21 | 24 | 105/17 | 105/70 | 0 | 0 | 2.8 | + | 0 | 4 | 40 |
| | | | | | | | | | | 4 | 6 | 47/8 | 44/20 | 32 | 110/17 | 120/60 | 0 | 10 | 2.9 | ++ | + | 2 | 41 |
| 7 | 32 | 36 | 36 | 40 | M | + | 0 | + | 0 | 48 | 12 | 60/16 | 65/30 | 20 | 110/28 | 110/80 | 0 | — | 1.3 | 0 | + | 35 | 38 |
| | | | | | | | | | | — | — | — | — | — | — | — | — | — | — | — | — | 7 | 30 |
| 8 | 29 | 17 | 39 | 42 | M | + | + | + | 0 | 312 | 3 | 20/3 | 20/9 | 8 | 145/15 | 95/55 | 50 | 110 | 2.5 | 0 | 0 | 66 | 53 |
| | | | | | | | | | | 151 | 4 | 36/12 | 28/10 | 12 | 160/27 | 110/60 | 50 | 85 | 3.3 | 0 | 0 | 11 | 39 |
| 9 | 20 | 36 | 41 | 45 | F | + | + | + | 0 | — | — | — | — | — | — | — | — | — | — | — | — | 67 | 53 |
| | | | | | | | | | | 25 | 16 | 70/21 | 70/35 | 36 | 140/21 | 155/88 | 0 | — | 1.8 | — | — | 4 | 44 |
| 10 | 16 | 19 | 45 | 46 | M | + | + | + | 0 | 276 | — | — | — | — | — | — | 60 | — | — | 0 | 0 | 38 | 43 |
| | | | | | | | | | | 2 | 4 | 48/4 | 44/22 | 23 | 96/24 | 110/60 | 0 | 0 | 2.8 | + | + | 3 | 29 |
| Totals | 12–32 | 12–36 | 18–45 | 19–46 | Men = 6/10 | 6/10 | 5/10 | 10/10 | 3/10 | I = 137 | 7 ± 6 | 39/8† | 38/17 | 17 ± 9† | 109/17 | 106/67 | — | — | 2.5 ± 0.8 | 2/9 | 1/9 | 40 | 53 ± 12† |
| | (20 ± 6) | (22 ± 8) | (28 ± 8) | (35 ± 9) | | | | | * | vs | vs | vs | vs | vs | vs | vs | | | vs | vs | vs | vs | vs |
| | | | | | | | | | | II = 29 | 11 ± 8 | 45/14 | 45/22 | 25 ± 9 | 117/21 | 115/67 | | | 2.6 ± 0.6 | 4/5 | 4/6 | 17 | 45 ± 15 |

*I (upper row) and II (lower row) represent the mean values for the first and second studies, respectively.
†$p < 0.05$.
AP = angina pectoris; CHF = congestive heart failure; CI = cardiac index; F = female; FH = family history; HC = hypertrophic cardiomyopathy; LV = left ventricle; LVEF = left ventricular ejection fraction; M = male; MR = mitral regurgitation; PA = pulmonary artery; PAW = pulmonary artery wedge; Psg = peak systolic gradient; RA = right atrium; RV = right ventricle; SA = systemic artery; s/d = systolic/diastolic; Sy = syncope.

**TABLE II** Electrocardiographic Findings in 10 Patients with Cardiac Transplantation for Hypertrophic Cardiomyopathy

| Pt. | Interval Study to Transplant (months) | Rhythm | Rate (beats/min) | Intervals (ms) PR | QRS | QTc | QRS Voltage (mm) I | II | III | aVR | aVL | aVF | $V_1$ | $V_2$ | $V_3$ | $V_4$ | $V_5$ | $V_6$ | Total 12-lead | Conduction Abnormality |
|---|---|---|---|---|---|---|---|---|---|---|---|---|---|---|---|---|---|---|---|---|
| 1 | 45 | S | 60 | 16 | 8 | 42 | 8 | 24 | 21 | 16 | 12 | 21 | 17 | 22 | 35 | 44 | 44 | 27 | 291 | 0 |
| | 10 | AF | 63 | — | 12 | — | 12 | 12 | 17 | 18 | 12 | 14 | 13 | 8 | 9 | 14 | 15 | 12 | 146 | RBBB, LPFB |
| 2 | 57 | S | 88 | 18 | 8 | 44 | 18 | 21 | 12 | 23 | 10 | 18 | 22 | 33 | 45 | 51 | 34 | 26 | 313 | 0 |
| | 39 | S | 72 | 19 | 8 | 40 | 23 | 34 | 15 | 27 | 11 | 23 | 29 | 44 | 46 | 44 | 41 | 41 | 378 | 0 |
| 3 | 68 | AF | 100 | — | 8 | — | 12 | 14 | 7 | 12 | 8 | 8 | 5 | 14 | 16 | 23 | 20 | 10 | 149 | 0 |
| | 4 | AF | 70 | — | 16 | — | 10 | 11 | 15 | 4 | 10 | 13 | 3 | 8 | 13 | 13 | 14 | 7 | 121 | Pacemaker |
| 4 | 23 | S | 54 | 24 | 16 | 34 | 20 | 33 | 7 | 21 | 33 | 16 | 7 | 8 | 5 | 10 | 14 | 12 | 186 | IVCD |
| | — | AF | — | — | — | — | — | — | — | — | — | — | — | — | — | — | — | — | — | — |
| 5 | 33 | S | 50 | 26 | 16 | 39 | 5 | 13 | 18 | 7 | 11 | 14 | 9 | 17 | 23 | 42 | 24 | 34 | 219 | LBBB |
| | 15 | AF | 80 | — | 9 | — | 6 | 5 | 11 | 2 | 8 | 8 | 7 | 5 | 12 | 12 | 21 | 12 | 109 | 0 |
| 6 | 89 | AF | 70 | — | 14 | — | 19 | 21 | 7 | 19 | 9 | 12 | 8 | 23 | 22 | 15 | 7 | 6 | 168 | Pacemaker |
| | 24 | AF | 70 | — | 15 | — | 12 | 14 | 14 | 12 | 12 | 12 | 10 | 19 | 26 | 24 | 9 | 8 | 172 | Pacemaker |
| 7 | 48 | S | 65 | 26 | 12 | 44 | 5 | 12 | 11 | 6 | 7 | 11 | 12 | 21 | 26 | 18 | 27 | 21 | 177 | IVCD |
| | 23 | S | 61 | 29 | 15 | 50 | 3 | 10 | 9 | 5 | 5 | 8 | 10 | 22 | 21 | 13 | 21 | 18 | 145 | IVCD |
| 8 | 169 | S | 80 | 14 | 12 | 51 | 11 | 22 | 28 | 7 | 20 | 24 | 14 | 31 | 27 | 9 | 11 | 10 | 214 | IVCD |
| | 125 | AF | 70 | — | 14 | — | 6 | 18 | 20 | 5 | 13 | 16 | 13 | 29 | 28 | 24 | 17 | 12 | 201 | IVCD |
| 9 | 78 | S | 60 | 20 | 8 | 39 | 12 | 19 | 24 | 10 | 17 | 19 | 23 | 41 | 33 | 32 | 23 | 18 | 271 | 0 |
| | 40 | S | 64 | 22 | 9 | 36 | 7 | 17 | 19 | 9 | 12 | 16 | 24 | 46 | 27 | 23 | 15 | 12 | 227 | 0 |
| 10 | — | S | — | — | — | — | — | — | — | — | — | — | — | — | — | — | — | — | — | — |
| | 2 | S | 60 | 30 | 22 | 54 | 5 | 7 | 8 | 5 | 6 | 7 | 13 | 25 | 19 | 12 | 11 | 12 | 130 | IVCD |
| Totals | I = 66 | S = 8/10 | 70 ± 16 | 21 | 11 | 42 | 13 | 20 | 15 | 13 | 14 | 16 | 13 | 25 | 26 | 27 | 23 | 18 | 221 ± 58† | |
| * | vs | vs | vs | vs | vs | vs | vs | vs | vs | vs | vs | vs | vs | vs | vs | vs | vs | vs | vs | |
| | II = 31 | 4/10 | 68 ± 6 | 25 | 14 | 45 | 9 | 14 | 14 | 10 | 10 | 13 | 14 | 23 | 22 | 20 | 18 | 15 | 181 ± 83 | |

*I (upper row) and II (lower row) represent the mean values for the first and second 12-lead electrocardiograms, respectively.
†$p < 0.05$.
AF = atrial fibrillation; IVCD = interventricular conduction delay; LBBB = left bundle branch block; LPFB = left posterior fascicular block; RBBB = right bundle branch block; S = sinus.

**TABLE III** Echocardiographic and Cardiac Morphologic Findings in 10 Patients with Cardiac Transplantation for Hypertrophic Cardiomyopathy

| Pt. | Interval Study to Transplant (months) | Dimensions (mm) | | | | Thickness (mm) | | | Heart Weight (g) | Thickness (mm) | | Dilatation (1–3+) | | LVOT Plaque | Thickened AML | Epi-cardial CAD | Gross Fibrosis (1–3+) | | Myofiber Disarray in VS | Thickened IMCA | Follow-Up | | |
|---|---|---|---|---|---|---|---|---|---|---|---|---|---|---|---|---|---|---|---|---|---|---|---|
| | | LA | LVDd | LVDs | FS (%) | VS | LVFW | SAM | | VS | LVFW | LV | RV | | | | VS | LVFW | | | Year Transplant Performed | Months After Trans-plant | Outcome |
| 1 | 41 | 39 | 36 | 27 | 25 | 15 | 15 | 0 | 385 | 20 | 15 | + | + | 0 | 0 | 0 | 0 | 0 | + | + | 1988 | 43 | FC I |
| | 21 | 55 | 45 | 33 | 27 | 13 | 13 | 0 | | | | | | | | | | | | | | | |
| 2 | 34 | 37 | 30 | 15 | 50 | 29 | 30 | 0 | 650 | 34 | 32 | 0 | 0 | 0 | 0 | 0 | 0 | 0 | + | + | 1988 | 52 | FC I–II |
| | 8 | 44 | 31 | 16 | 48 | 31 | 35 | + | | | | | | | | | | | | | | | |
| 3 | 57 | 50 | 32 | 22 | 31 | 22 | 13 | 0 | 340 | 20 | 20 | + | + | 0 | 0 | 0 | + | + | + | + | 1985 | <1 | Died (rejection) |
| | 14 | 54 | 42 | 29 | 31 | 20 | 10 | 0 | | | | | | | | | | | | | | | |
| 4 | — | — | — | — | — | — | — | — | 340 | 15 | 14 | + | + | 0 | 0 | 0 | +++ | +++ | + | + | 1977 | 1 | Died (toxo-plasmosis) |
| | 27 | — | — | — | — | 15 | 11 | 0 | | | | | | | | | | | | | | | |
| 5 | 37 | 38 | 44 | 24 | 45 | 19 | 13 | + | 390 | 17 | 11 | + | + | 0 | 0 | 0 | +++ | +++ | + | + | 1979 | <1 | Died (rejection) |
| | 11 | 50 | 48 | 27 | 44 | 16 | 10 | + | | | | | | | | | | | | | | | |
| 6 | 95 | 54 | 40 | 26 | 35 | 14 | 11 | 0 | 290 | 17 | 13 | + | + | 0 | 0 | 0 | + | + | + | + | 1988 | 54 | FC II |
| | 4 | 54 | 45 | 34 | 24 | 14 | 10 | 0 | | | | | | | | | | | | | | | |
| 7 | 48 | 52 | 52 | 43 | 17 | 17 | 9 | 0 | 310 | 19 | 11 | + | + | 0 | 0 | 0 | +++ | +++ | + | + | 1987 | 8 | Died (rejection) |
| | 4 | 56 | 53 | 45 | 15 | 14 | 8 | 0 | | | | | | | | | | | | | | | |
| 8 | 143 | 43 | 42 | 28 | 33 | 22 | 12 | + | 455 | 18 | 13 | +++ | +++ | + | + | 0 | +++ | ++ | + | + | 1990 | 20 | FC I |
| | 126 | 44 | 45 | 30 | 33 | 17 | 11 | + | | | | | | | | | | | | | | | |
| 9 | 89 | 30 | 48 | 38 | 21 | 15 | 11 | — | 350 | 15 | 11 | + | + | 0 | 0 | 0 | + | + | + | + | 1989 | 39 | FC I–II |
| | 40 | 56 | 48 | 40 | 17 | 12 | 10 | 0 | | | | | | | | | | | | | | | |
| 10 | 58 | 52 | 43 | 34 | 21 | 23 | 15 | 0 | 480 | 18 | 18 | +++ | +++ | + | + | 0 | +++ | ++ | + | + | 1985 | 27 | FC I |
| | 2 | 58 | 55 | 38 | 31 | 17 | 10 | 0 | | | | | | | | | | | | | | | |
| Totals * | I = 67 vs II = 28 | 44 ± 8† vs 52 ± 5 | 41 ± 7 vs 46 ± 7 | 29 ± 9 vs 32 ± 8 | 31 ± 11 vs 30 ± 11 | 20 ± 5 vs 17 ± 5 | 14 ± 6 vs 12 ± 8 | 2/10 vs 3/10 | 290–650 (400 ± 110) | 19 ± 5 (19 ± 7) | 16 ± 6 (16 ± 9) | 9/10 | 9/10 | 2/10 | 2/10 | 0/10 | 8/10 | 8/10 | 10/10 | 10/10 | | | |

*I (upper row) and II (lower row) represent mean values for the first and second echocardiograms, respectively.
AML = anterior mitral leaflet; CAD = atherosclerotic coronary artery disease; FC = New York Heart Association functional class; FS = fractional shortening; IMCA = intramural coronary arteries; LA = left atrial; LV = left ventricular; LVD (d and s) = left ventricular dimension (in diastole and systole); LVFW = left ventricular free wall; LVOT = left ventricular outflow tract; RV = right ventricular; SAM = systolic anterior motion of the anterior mitral leaflet; VS = ventricular septal.

and 13 years from the diagnosis of HC. All patients had signs and symptoms of left ventricular failure, and 9 had cardiac failure refractory to medical therapy. Patient 2 (Table I) had cardiac transplantation for recurrent syncope. In 4 patients (nos. 2, 3, 6 and 10), a permanent pacemaker had been placed, and 2 (nos. 5 and 8) had undergone ventricular septal myotomy and myectomy.

CARDIAC CATHETERIZATION (TABLE I): Only 1 patient (no. 2) had normal right-sided pressures. In 3 patients (nos. 2, 8 and 10), a pressure gradient was present be-

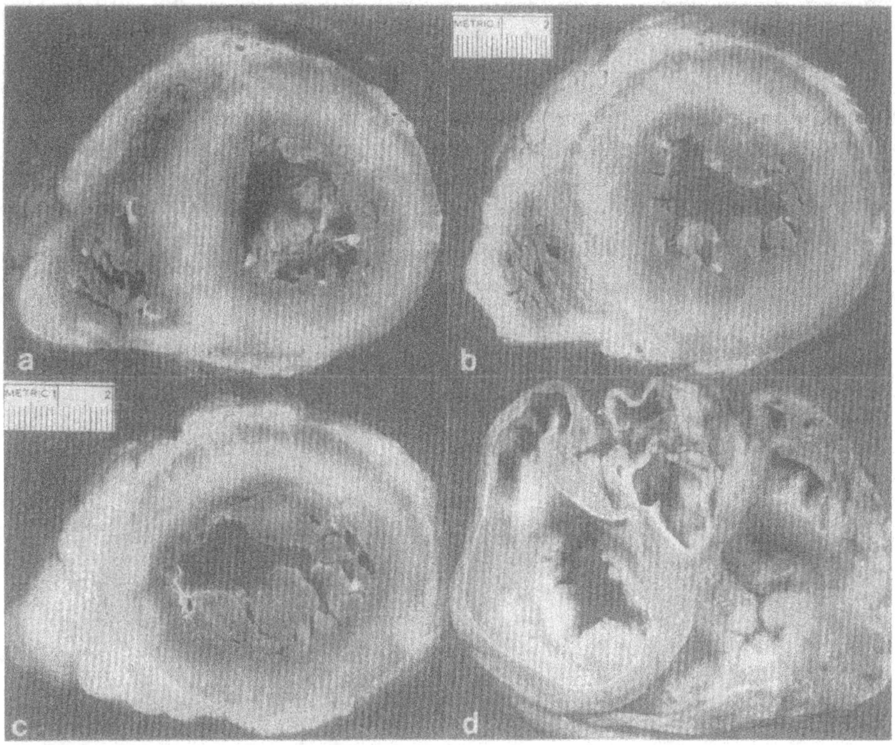

**FIGURE 1. Heart of a 40-year-old man (pt. 7) with hypertrophic cardiomyopathy who had cardiac transplantation for refractory congestive heart failure. *a*, *b*, and *c*, views of the cardiac ventricles at different levels, showing a dilated left ventricle and grossly visible scars in the ventricular septum and the left ventricular free wall. *d*, view of the cardiac atria from above, showing dilated cavities and thickened walls.**

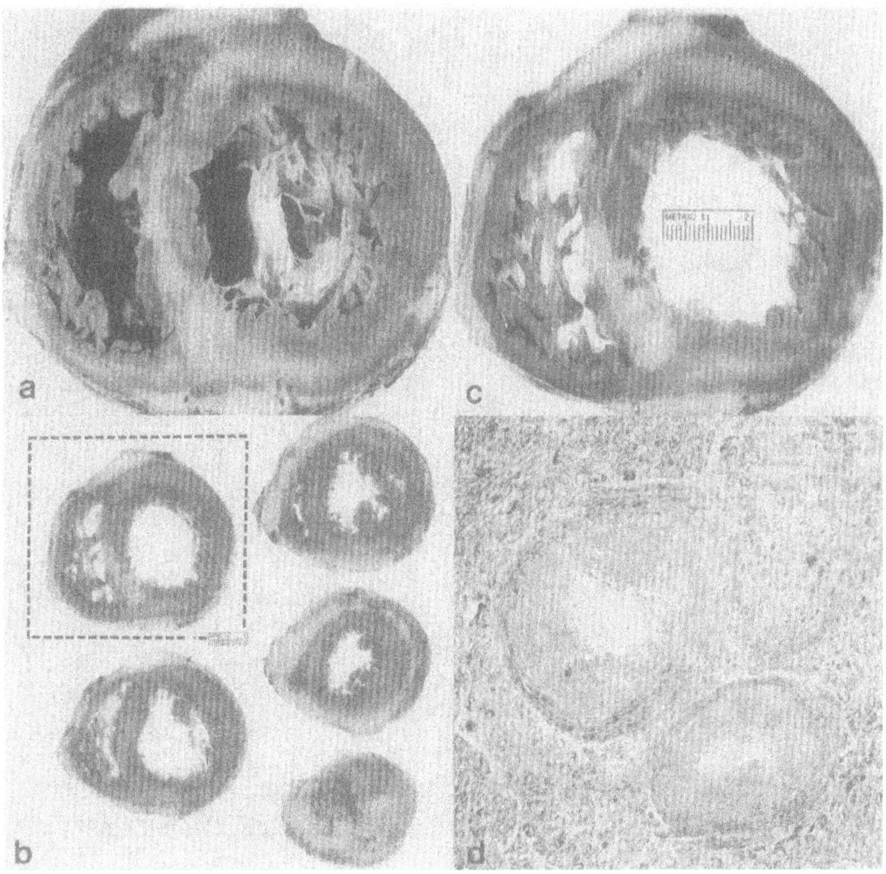

**FIGURE 2. Heart of a 42-year-old man (pt. 8) with hypertrophic cardiomyopathy and progressive systolic dysfunction. *a*, view of the basal portion of the cardiac ventricles. *b*, transverse section of the cardiac ventricles. A close-up of the section *in brackets* is shown in *c*. The ventricular cavities are dilated, and the septum and portions of the left and right ventricular walls are scarred. *d*, photomicrograph of intramural coronary arteries in the ventricular septum showing thickened walls and narrowed lumens. Movat stain × 100; reduced by 24%.**

tween the left ventricle and ascending aorta during peak systole; this gradient was 50 and 60 mm Hg in patients 8 and 10, respectively. In patient 10, myotomy and myectomy were performed, and in patient 8, the peak systolic gradient was absent at the second cardiac catheterization when the left ventricle was markedly dilated, and the left ventricular ejection fraction was 29%. In 8 patients in whom the results of a second cardiac catheterization were available, the right atrial, right ventricular, pulmonary arterial and pulmonary artery wedge pressures had increased compared with the results at the first study over a mean time span of 108 months. The cardiac index did not change significantly between the 2 studies. More patients had mitral regurgitation at the second left ventricular cineangiogram than at the first (2 of 9 vs 4 of 5). The left ventricular cavity was dilated in 1 of 9 patients at the first study and in 4 of 6 at the second.

RADIONUCLIDE VENTRICULOGRAPHY (TABLE I): The left ventricular ejection fraction, assessed by radionuclide ventriculography, decreased from a mean of 53 to 45% ($p \leq 0.05$) in 2 studies performed a mean of 40 and 17 months, respectively, before transplantation in 7 patients.

ELECTROCARDIOGRAPHIC FINDINGS (TABLE II): Comparison of the 12-lead electrocardiographic recordings obtained at a mean of 66 and 31 months before transplantation showed an increase in the prevalence of atrial fibrillation (from 2 of 10 to 6 of 10 patients, respectively), and a significant decrease in the total 12-lead QRS voltage (from a mean of 221 to 181 mm, respectively; $p < 0.05$).

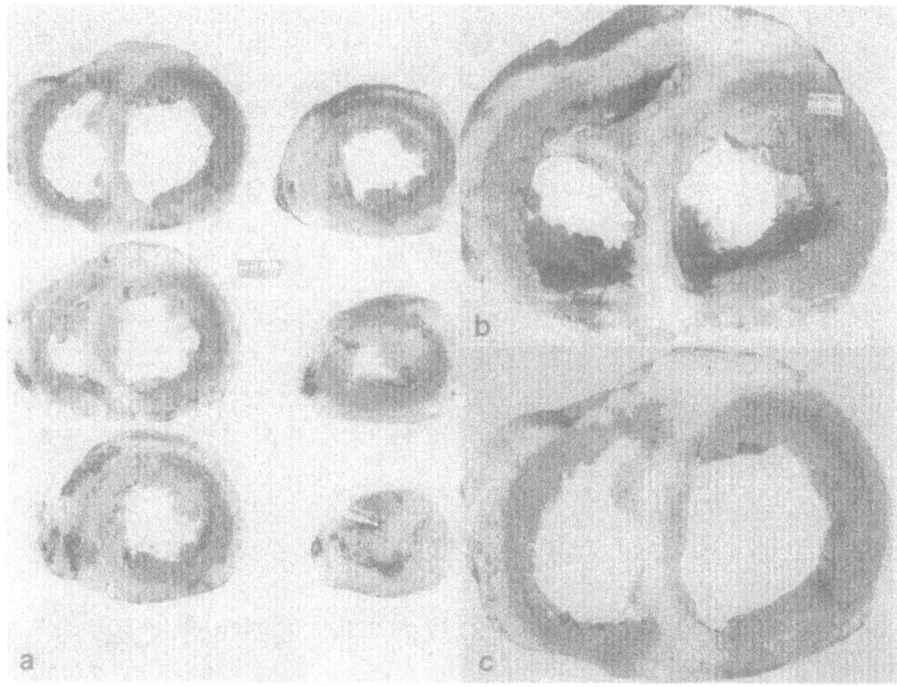

**FIGURE 3. Heart of a 46-year-old man (pt. 10) with hypertrophic cardiomyopathy, progressive congestive heart failure, systolic dysfunction (left ventricular ejection fraction 29%) and total 12-lead QRS voltage of 130 mm. Views of the cardiac ventricles *(a, b, and c)* showing markedly dilated cavities and extensive scars, which involve the ventricular septum more than the left and right ventricular free walls.**

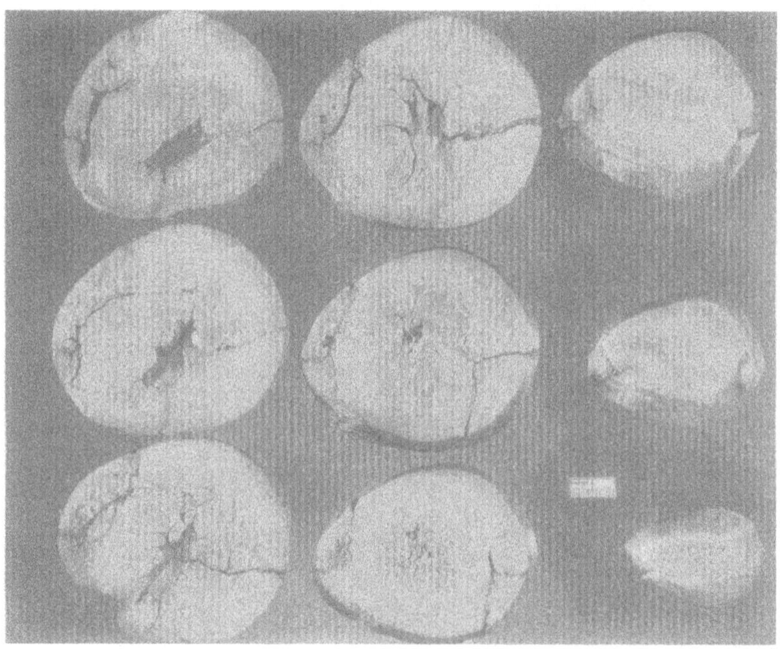

**FIGURE 4. Heart of a 24-year-old woman (pt. 2) with hypertrophic cardiomyopathy and recurrent, refractory syncope. Transverse sections of cardiac ventricles show no cavity dilatation, and greatly thickened walls. The myocardium is free of grossly visible lesions.**

ECHOCARDIOGRAPHIC FINDINGS (TABLE III): The left atrial, and left ventricular systolic and diastolic dimensions increased from a mean of 44, 29 and 41 mm to 52, 32 and 46 mm, respectively, in a mean interval of 39 months before transplantation. In the same period, the thickness of the ventricular septum decreased from a mean of 20 to 17 mm, and that of the left ventricular free wall from 14 to 12 mm.

OUTCOME OF TRANSPLANTATION (TABLE III): Three of 10 patients died within the first month after transplantation: 2 because of rejection of the implanted homograft, and 1 of infection due to *Toxoplasma gondii*. Another patient died 8 months after transplantation, because of rejection. The remaining 6 patients have survived 20 to 54 months (mean 39) after transplantation and are in New York Heart Association functional class I or II.

**Morphologic observations:** The weight of the explanted hearts ranged from 290 to 650 g (mean 400). (This weight excludes portions of the atria, ascending aorta and pulmonary trunk.) The maximal thickness of the ventricular septum and left ventricular free wall ranged from 15 to 34 mm (mean 19) and 11 to 32 mm (mean 16), respectively. Both right and left ventricular cavities were dilated by gross inspection in 9 patients (Figure 1): mild to moderate in 7 and severe in 2 (Figures 2 and 3). In 1 heart, both left and right ventricular cavities were small (Figure 4). Grossly visible scars were present in the ventricular septa and left ventricular free walls in 8 patients (Figures 1 to 3), and they were extensive in 5. Histologically, myocardial replacement and interstitial fibrosis were present in all 10 hearts. No major epicardial coronary artery in any patient was significantly narrowed. In 2 hearts, the anterior mitral valve leaflet was thickened, and a fibrous plaque was present on the mural endocardium of the ventricular septum in apposition to this leaflet. Histologic sections of the ventricular septum in all 10 patients showed marked myofiber disorganization and thickening of the walls of the intramural coronary arteries (Figure 2).

## DISCUSSION

**Indications for transplantation:** Of the 10 patients, 9 had transplantation because of refractory congestive heart failure. In each of these patients, the left ventricular cavities dilated during the pretransplantation period (left ventricular end-diastolic dimension from 42 ± 6 to 48 ± 4 mm; $p < 0.05$), left ventricular ejection fraction decreased (from 51 ± 11% to 41 ± 13%; $p < 0.05$), total 12-lead QRS voltage decreased (from 209 ± 50 to 156 ± 40 mm; $p < 0.05$), the ventricular septa thinned (from 18 ± 4 to 15 ± 2 mm; $p < 0.01$), and the left ventricular free wall thinned (from 12 ± 2 to 10 ± 1 mm; $p < 0.05$). The remaining patient (no. 2), a 24-year-old woman, had transplantation for recurring syncope that began at age 19. The syncope was refractory to antiarrhythmic medications and placement of a cardiac pacemaker, but was eliminated by transplantation. In the last 8 months before transplantation, she had daily syncope. She was the only patient among the 10 with a nondilated ventricular cavity, without progressive ventricular wall thinning, without progressive decrease in total 12-lead QRS voltage and, with one other exception (no. 1), without ventricular wall scarring.

**Left ventricular dilatation and wall thinning:** In adults with HC, the occurrence of severe heart failure in the absence of outflow obstruction is often marked by an increase in the left ventricular end-diastolic dimension, and thinning of the ventricular septum and left ventricular free wall.[3–7] The prognosis for such patients is poor.[8] In 7 of our patients, the left ventricular diastolic dimension, as measured by M-mode echocardiography, increased by 1 to 12 mm (mean 6). The largest increase in left ventricular cavity size occurred in the 2 patients with the most severe myocardial scarring (nos. 8 and 10). The left ventricular end-diastolic dimension was >52 mm (upper limit of normal for adults) in 2 patients. The thickness of the ventricular septum decreased by 2 to 6 mm (mean 3) in 7 patients, and that of the left ventricular wall by 1 to 5 mm (mean 2) in 8 patients. The ventricular septal thickness decreased the most (5 and 6 mm) in the 2 patients (nos. 8 and 10, respectively) with the most scarring.

**Electrocardiographic findings:** In a study by Dollar and Roberts,[9] the mean total 12-lead QRS voltage in 57 patients with HC was 205 and 155 mm for those without and with transmural left ventricular scars, respectively. Those values are comparable to those of our 9 patients before and after the onset of left ventricular enlargement (209 and 156 mm, respectively). The decrease in total 12-lead QRS voltage in our patients was, for the most part, proportional to the severity of left ventricular scarring.


**1.** Kriett JM, Kaye MP. The registry of the international society of heart and lung transplantation: eight official report-1991. *J Heart Lung Transplant* 1991;10:491–498.

**2.** Warren SE, Cohen LH, Schoen FJ, Mudge GH, Lorell BH. Advanced diastolic heart failure in familial hypertrophic cardiomyopathy managed with cardiac transplantation. *J Applied Cardiol* 1988;3:415–422.

**3.** ten Cate FJ, Roelandt J. Progression of the left ventricular dilatation in patients with obstructive hypertrophic cardiomyopathy. *Am Heart J* 1979;97:762–765.

**4.** Fujiwara H, Onodera T, Tanaka M, Shirane H, Kato H, Yoshikawa J, Osakada S, Sasayama S, Kawai C. Progression from hypertrophic obstructive cardiomyopathy to typical dilated cardiomyopathy-like features in the end stage. *Jpn Circ J* 1984;48:1210–1214.

**5.** Funakoshi M, Imamura M, Sasaki J, Fujimo M, Kawano T, Sasaki Y, Nakashima Y, Motooka T, Fukuda F, Imagawa M, Hiroki T, Arakawa K. Seventeen year follow-up of a patient with hypertrophic cardiomyopathy which progressed to dilated cardiomyopathy. *Jpn Heart J* 1984;25:805–809.

**6.** Spirito P, Maron BJ. Absence of progression of left ventricular hypertrophy in adult patients with hypertrophic cardiomyopathy. *J Am Coll Cardiol* 1987;9:1013–1017.

**7.** Spirito P, Maron BJ, Bonow RO, Epstein SE. Severe functional limitation in patients with hypertrophic cardiomyopathy and only mild localized left ventricular hypertrophy. *J Am Coll Cardiol* 1986;8:537–544.

**8.** Spirito P, Maron BJ, Bonow RO, Epstein SE. Occurrence and significance of progressive left ventricular wall thinning and relative cavity dilatation in hypertrophic cardiomyopathy. *Am J Cardiol* 1987;60:123–129.

**9.** Dollar AL, Roberts WC. Usefulness of total 12-lead QRS voltage compared with other criteria for determining left ventricular hypertrophy in hypertrophic cardiomyopathy: analysis of 57 patients studied at necropsy. *Am J Med* 1989;87:377–381.

# Frequency and Characteristics of Coronary Thrombosis in the Epicardial Coronary Arteries After Cardiac Transplantation

Eloisa Arbustini, MD, Barbara Dal Bello, MD, Patrizia Morbini, MD, Maurizia Grasso, PhD, Marta Diegoli, ScD, Roberta Fasani, ScD, Andrea Pilotto, ScD, Ornella Bellini, ScD, Carlo Pellegrini, MD, Luigi Martinelli, MD, Carlo Campana, MD, Antonello Gavazzi, MD, Giuseppe Specchia, MD, Mario Viganò, MD, and William C. Roberts, MD

**We investigated at autopsy or at retransplantation the frequency and characteristics of coronary thrombosis in 76 cardiac allografts: 37 in place for ≤2 months (early) and 39 in place >2 to 99 months (late). The 76 allografts were inserted in 69 patients: a single 1 in 56 patients and 2 allografts in 13 patients, 7 of whom subsequently died and had an autopsy. An average of 140 sections from 70 5-mm-long segments of 8 epicardial coronary arteries were examined from each of the 76 allografts with both hematoxylin-eosin and Movat pentachrome stains. Thrombus was found in only 1 coronary artery (3%) (the right one) of the 37 early allografts, and in 24 of 39 late allografts (61%). Of the latter 39 grafts, 29 (79%) had allograft vascular disease (AVD) and 24 (83%) of them had coronary thrombosis. Of the 312 epicardial coronary arteries (4 major and 4 minor) examined in the 39 late cases, 66 arteries (21%) contained thrombus. Of the 24 late cases with thrombus in at least 1 artery, thrombus was present in 66 (34%) of the 192 epicardial coronary arteries examined: in 6 of the 8 arteries in 3 patients; in 5 arteries in 2 patients; in 4 arteries in 1 patient; in 3 arteries in 5 patients; in 2 arteries in 6 patients, and in a single artery in 7 patients. In all 66 arteries with thrombus (24 patients) the thrombus was longer than 5 mm. The thrombus in the late cases was entirely nonocclusive (mural) in 51 (77%) of the 66 epicardial coronary arteries containing thrombus and entirely occlusive in 10 arteries (15%). It consisted exclusively of multiluminal channels in 6 arteries (9%) and combinations in 1 artery (2%). Acute myocardial infarcts were present in 3 patients, all of whom had occlusive thrombi. In all 10 arteries with occlusive thrombi, the thrombus was larger than the underlying plaque and no occlusive thrombi were located over ulcerated plaques. These observations demonstrate that thrombus is common in epicardial coronary arteries >2 months after cardiac transplantation.**

**(Am J Cardiol 1996;78:795–800)**

Allograft vascular disease (AVD) is a major cause of late failure of transplanted hearts.[1] The hallmarks of AVD include smooth muscle cell neointimal proliferation, extracellular matrix deposition, and mononuclear cells infiltration.[2–9] Coronary thrombus was not described in any of the 106 cases reported by Billingham[3] in 1987, or by Foerster[10] in 1992, or by several other authors.[2,4–10] In 1993, Rose et al[11] described 13 recent and 3 revascularized thrombi in the epicardial coronary arteries of 43 transplanted hearts. In an angiographic and morphologic study, Johnson et al[12] described fresh or organized thrombi in 21 of 67 type A lesions (31%) and in 1 of 14 type B lesions (7%) according to Gao et al.[13] Recently, however, Billingham observed that "it is not unusual to see mural thrombi in these hearts."[14] Most reported morphologic studies, however, have been based on examining only random sections of the coronary arteries from each case. Since our first cardiac transplantation in Pavia, Italy, in 1985, we have examined histologically at least 1 section from each 5-mm-long segment of each of the 4 major (right, left main, left anterior, left circumflex) epicardial coronary arteries, and from 4 minor (posterolateral, posterior descending, first diagonal, obtuse marginal) epicardial coronary arteries in patients dying after cardiac transplantation or having a second transplantation, irrespective of the cause of death or of graft failure. In the present study, we report the frequency and characteristics of coronary thrombi in 76 consecutive cardiac allografts in 69 patients.

From the Pathologic Anatomy Institute, Cardiac Surgery Department, Cardiology Department, IRCCS-Policlinico San Matteo, University of Pavia, Pavia, Italy, and Baylor Cardiovascular Institute, Baylor University Medical Center, Dallas, Texas. This study was supported by grants "Trapianto Cardiaco," "Trapianto Cuore-Polmoni," and "Rigetto cronico nel cuore trapiantato" from Health Ministry to IRCCS Policlinico San Matteo, Pavia, Italy—Ricerche Finalizzate 1989 to 1990, 1991 to 1993, and 1993 to 1995. Manuscript received March 15, 1996; revised manuscript received and accepted June 14, 1996.

Address for reprints: Eloisa Arbustini, MD, Istituto di Anatomia Patologica, Viale Forlanini 16, 27100 Pavia, Italy.

## METHODS

The 69 patients included 65 men and 4 women aged 9 to 65 years (mean 50 ± 10) who underwent cardiac transplantation and then died or underwent repeat transplantation at the Cardiac Surgery Department of Policlinico San Matteo–Pavia from No-

**TABLE 1** Clinical and Morphologic Data on 39 Patients Who Underwent Cardiac Transplantation and Survived >2 Months

| Patient | Recipient Age (yr) & Sex | Diagnosis | Donor Age (yr) & Sex | Duration (mo) Allograft in Place | Cause of Allograft Failure | AVD Severity (0–4+) | Thrombus in any Coronary Artery | Thrombus in Coronary Artery: LM | LAD | LC | Right | FD | LOM | PD | PL | Myocardial Infarct |
|---|---|---|---|---|---|---|---|---|---|---|---|---|---|---|---|---|
| 1 | 43 M | IC | 17 M | 3 | AR | 0 | 0 | 0 | 0 | 0 | 0 | 0 | 0 | 0 | 0 | 0 |
| 2* | 52 M | IC | 28 F | 3 | Graft failure | 0 | 0 | 0 | 0 | 0 | 0 | 0 | 0 | 0 | 0 | 0 |
| 3 | 56 M | IC | 36 M | 3 | M-O F | + | + (3) | 0 | +‡ | + | + | 0 | 0 | 0 | 0 | 0 |
| 4 | 64 M | IC | 14 M | 3 | Infection | 0 | 0 | 0 | 0 | 0 | 0 | 0 | 0 | 0 | 0 | 0 |
| 5 | 39 F | IDC | 45 F | 4 | PE | ++ | + (2) | 0 | + | + | 0 | 0 | 0 | 0 | 0 | 0 |
| 6 | 60 M | IDC | 46 F | 5 | Infection | ++ | + (1) | 0 | 0 | 0 | + | 0 | 0 | 0 | 0 | 0 |
| 7 | 57 M | IC | 39 F | 6 | Infection | 0 | 0 | 0 | 0 | 0 | 0 | 0 | 0 | 0 | 0 | 0 |
| 8 | 60 M | IC | 24 F | 6 | M-O F | 0 | 0 | 0 | 0 | 0 | 0 | 0 | 0 | 0 | 0 | 0 |
| 9 | 44 M | IDC | 18 M | 7 | Mediastinitis | 0 | 0 | 0 | 0 | 0 | 0 | 0 | 0 | 0 | 0 | 0 |
| 10 | 47 M | IC | 22 M | 7 | AVD | +++ | + (1) | 0 | 0 | 0 | + | 0 | 0 | 0 | 0 | 0 |
| 11 | 23 M | IDC | 19 M | 8 | Poisoning | 0 | 0 | 0 | 0 | 0 | 0 | 0 | 0 | 0 | 0 | 0 |
| 12 | 47 M | IDC | 36 M | 8 | AVD | +++ | + (1) | 0 | 0 | 0 | + | 0 | 0 | 0 | 0 | 0 |
| 13* | 48 M | IDC | 44 M | 11 | AVD | +++ | + (6) | 0 | + | + | + | + (Oc) | + | + | 0 | 0 |
| 14 | 53 M | IC | 25 M | 11 | Aortic rupture | 0 | 0 | 0 | 0 | 0 | 0 | 0 | 0 | 0 | 0 | 0 |
| 15 | 54 M | IC | 25 M | 12 | Neoplasm | ++ | + (1) | 0 | + | 0 | 0 | 0 | 0 | 0 | 0 | 0 |
| 16 | 58 M | IDC | 26 M | 12 | AVD | +++ | + (2) | 0 | + (Oc) | 0 | 0 | + (Oc) | 0 | 0 | 0 | + (Acute) |
| 17 | 45 M | IDC | 33 M | 13 | AVD | +++ | + (1) | 0 | 0 | 0 | + | 0 | 0 | 0 | 0 | 0 |
| 18 | 60 M | VHD | 56 M | 14 | Neoplasm | +++ | + (2) | 0 | + (MLC) | 0 | + (MLC) | 0 | 0 | 0 | 0 | 0 |
| 19 | 46 M | IDC | 34 M | 15 | Neoplasm | ++ | 0 | 0 | 0 | 0 | 0 | 0 | 0 | 0 | 0 | 0 |
| 20 | 49 M | IDC | 18 M | 15 | Infection | 0 | 0 | 0 | 0 | 0 | 0 | 0 | 0 | 0 | 0 | 0 |
| 21 | 43 M | IC | 43 F | 16 | AVD | +++ | + (3) | 0 | + (Oc§) | 0 | + (Oc) | 0 | 0 | + | 0 | + (Acute) |
| 22 | 61 M | IC | 19 M | 16 | Neoplasm | ++ | 0 | 0 | 0 | 0 | 0 | 0 | 0 | 0 | 0 | 0 |
| 23 | 50 M | VHD | 14 M | 21 | AVD | +++ | + (3) | 0 | + (Oc) | 0 | 0 | + (Oc) | + (Oc) | 0 | 0 | + (Acute) |
| 24 | 54 M | IC | 19 M | 22 | Neoplasm | 0 | 0 | 0 | 0 | 0 | 0 | 0 | 0 | 0 | 0 | 0 |
| 25 | 53 M | Amyloid | 44 M | 25 | AVD | +++ | 0 | 0 | 0 | 0 | 0 | 0 | 0 | 0 | 0 | 0 |
| 26 | 35 M | IDC | 17 M | 33 | PE | +++ | + (5) | + | + | + | + | 0 | 0 | 0 | + | 0 |
| 27 | 47 M | IDC | 20 F | 34 | Neoplasm | ++ | + (2) | 0 | + | + | 0 | 0 | 0 | 0 | 0 | 0 |
| 28* | 28 M | IDC | 34 M | 40 | AVD | +++ | + (5) | 0 | + | + | + | 0 | 0 | + | + | 0 |
| 29* | 45 M | IC | 22 M | 48 | AVD | +++ | + (6) | + | + | + (MLC§) | + (MLC) | + | 0 | + (Oc) | 0 | 0 |
| 30 | 39 M | IC | 32 M | 55 | AVD | +++ | + (2) | 0 | + | 0 | + | 0 | 0 | 0 | 0 | + (Healed) |
| 31 | 56 M | IDC | 53 M | 58 | Infection | ++ | 0 | 0 | 0 | 0 | 0 | 0 | 0 | 0 | 0 | 0 |
| 32 | 39 M | IC | 14 F | 60 | Cirrhosis | +++ | + (3) | 0 | 0 | + | + | 0 | 0 | + (Oc) | 0 | + (Healed) |
| 33 | 41 M | IC | 15 F | 70 | AVD | +++ | + (2) | 0 | + | 0 | + (MLC) | 0 | 0 | 0 | 0 | + (Healed) |
| 34 | 44 M | VHD | 35 M | 70 | PE | ++ | + (4) | + | + | + | + | 0 | 0 | 0 | 0 | 0 |
| 35* | 49 M | IC | 46 M | 72 | AVD | +++ | + (6) | + | + (MLC) | + | 0 | + (MLC) | + | 0 | + | 0 |
| 36† | 44 M | IDC | 18 F | 83 | M-O F | +++ | + (1) | 0 | + | 0 | 0 | 0 | 0 | 0 | 0 | 0 |
| 37 | 46 M | IDC | 8 M | 91 | Aortic rupture | +++ | + (3) | 0 | + | 0 | + | + | 0 | 0 | 0 | 0 |
| 38* | 53 M | IC | 35 M | 93 | AVD | +++ | + (1) | 0 | 0 | 0 | + | 0 | 0 | 0 | 0 | 0 |
| 39 | 42 M | HC | 26 F | 99 | Neoplasm | ++ | 0 | 0 | 0 | 0 | 0 | 0 | 0 | 0 | 0 | 0 |
| TOTALS | 38 M<br>1 F | IC = 18<br>IDC = 16<br>VHD = 3<br>HC = 1<br>Amyloid = 1 | 28 M<br>11 F | | AVD = 14<br>Infection = 5<br>Neoplasm = 7<br>Misc. = 12<br>AR = 1 | 29 | 24 (66) | 4 | 18 | 10 | 17 | 6 | 3 | 5 | 3 | 3 Acute<br>3 Healed |

*Heart obtained at retransplantation; † Heart obtained at necropsy from patients previously retransplanted; ‡ The + sign indicates mural thrombus only unless otherwise stated; § Also mural thrombus.

AVD = allograft vascular disease; AR = acute rejection; F = female; FD = first diagonal; HC = hypertrophic cardiomyopathy; IC = ischemic cardiomyopathy; IDC = idiopathic dilated cardiomyopathy; LAD = left anterior descending; LC = left circumflex; LM = left main; LOM = left obtuse marginal; M = male; MLC = multiluminal channels; MOF = multiorgan failure; Oc = occlusive; PD = posterior descending; PE = pulmonary embolism; PL = posterolateral; VHD = valvular heart disease.

vember 1985 to November 1995. Of the 69 patients, 56 had a single transplant and each died at varying intervals thereafter. The other 13 patients had 2 cardiac transplants: 6 of these patients are still alive and thus 6 allografts were available to be studied; the other 7 patients died from 3 days to 83 months after the second transplant, and therefore, 14 allografts were available to be studied in them. Of the 76 hearts studied, 63 were obtained at autopsy and 13 at retransplantation. The interval from first transplantation to death or to the second transplantation ranged from 4 hours to 99 months (mean 16 ± 26 months). The indications for heart transplantation were: idiopathic dilated cardiomyopathy in 30 patients, ischemic cardiomyopathy in 32, valvular heart disease in 4, hypertrophic cardiomyopathy in 1, cardiac amyloidosis in 1, and granulomatous myocarditis in 1. The indications for heart retransplantation were: graft failure in 4 cases, myocarditis in 1, persistent acute rejection in 1, hyperacute rejections in 2, and AVD in 5. One of the retransplanted patients had coronary artery bypass grafting for AVD of the first graft; analysis of the 2 aortocoronary bypass conduits in this patient is not included in this report. Twenty-five heart donors were women and 51 were men; their ages ranged from 6 to 61 years (mean 33 ± 15).

The major epicardial coronary arteries were dissected from either formalin-fixed or unfixed allograft hearts, according to previously described methods.[15,16] The left main, left anterior descending, left circumflex, and right coronary arteries were excised intact with attached closely adherent tissues and the latter 3 arteries were divided into proximal, middle, and distal portions. In all cases, the first diagonal, obtuse marginals, posterolateral, and posterior descending branches also were excised and also divided into 5-mm segments. Usually the tissues surrounding the coronary arteries were included in the tissues to be processed for histologic study. These techniques provided approximately 70 five-mm-long segments of the epicardial coronary arteries and 140 sections from each heart. Coronary artery samples were fixed in 10% buffered formalin solution, dehydrated, and then embedded in paraffin. Each paraffin block was sectioned at 5-$\mu$m intervals and the resulting 5-$\mu$m thick section was stained with hematoxylin-eosin and another with Masson's trichrome (3 cases) or Movat pentachrome (73 cases). Except for a few early cases with donor atherosclerosis, decalcification procedures were unnecessary in early and in all late cases. Three full thickness samples extending from endocardium to epicardium of the walls of both right and left ventricles were prepared for histologic study from each heart.

## RESULTS

**Early cases:** Of all 76 allografts, 37 had been in place for ≤2 months (early) and 39 for >2 months (late) (Table I). The 37 early allografts had a mean follow-up of 17 ± 21 days. The causes of failure were: hyperacute rejection in 2 cases; acute rejections in 2 cases; graft failure in 13 cases; sepsis in 10 cases; multiorgan failure in 5; cerebrovascular events in 4; and eosinophilic myocarditis in 1 case. Seven hearts had been obtained during retransplantation for acute graft failure; 5 patients then died: 1 of graft failure, 1 of multiorgan failure, 1 of sepsis, 1 of acute rejection, and 1 of multiorgan failure with AVD. One heart had been obtained at autopsy from a patient who died 2 months after retransplantation for AVD (his first graft had a follow-up of 8 years); the cause of death had been graft failure. Twenty-three heart donors were men and 14 were women, aged 9 to 64 years (mean 37 ± 16).

In 11 of the 37 early allografts (30%) atherosclerosis of the native coronary arteries was found: in 3 the atherosclerosis caused critical stenosis (≥75% cross-sectional area narrowing) of 1 major epicardial coronary artery (donor ages were 47, 48, 56 years, respectively, and donor cause of death was trauma in 1 and cerebral hemorrhage in 2).

In only 1 of the 37 patients (3%) surviving <2 months was thrombus found in a coronary artery. The thrombus was located at 2 sites in the right coronary artery, it was nonocclusive (i.e., mural) and the patient lived only 3 days after transplantation.

**Late cases:** Of the 39 late allografts, 6 were obtained at retransplantation (the indication was AVD in 5 cases and graft failure in 1) and 33 at autopsy. Findings in these 39 cases are tabulated in Table I. These 39 late grafts had been in place a mean of 32 ± 30 months. Four of the 5 patients retransplanted for AVD are alive; 1 died of acute graft failure 2 months later. The coronary bypass allograft patient survived 24 months after revascularization; then the patient underwent retransplantation and is alive 14 months after retransplantation. Of the 39 late grafts, 29 (74%) had AVD and 24 (83%) of them had coronary thrombus.

Of the 39 late allografts, thrombus was found in 1 or more epicardial coronary arteries in 24 (62%). Of the 312 epicardial coronary arteries (4 major, 4 minor) examined in the 39 late cases, 66 arteries (21%) contained thrombus. Of the 24 late cases with thrombus in at least 1 artery, thrombus was present in 66 (34%) of the 192 epicardial coronary arteries examined: in 6 of 8 arteries in 3 patients; in 5 arteries in 2 patients; in 4 arteries in 1 patient; in 3 arteries in 5 patients; in 2 arteries in 6 patients, and in a single artery in 7 patients. All thrombi in the 66 epicardial coronary arteries involved more than one 5-mm-long segment.

The thrombi in the right, left anterior descending, and left circumflex coronary arteries involved the proximal, middle, and distal portions of these 3 arteries or only 1 or 2 portions of these arteries. Thrombi were present in 18 left anterior descending arteries, involving the artery's proximal third in 16 allografts, the middle third in 9, and the distal third in 6. Thrombus was present in the left circumflex artery in 10 allografts: proximal portion in 6, middle portion in 6, and distal portion in 1. Thrombi involved the right coronary artery in 17 allografts:

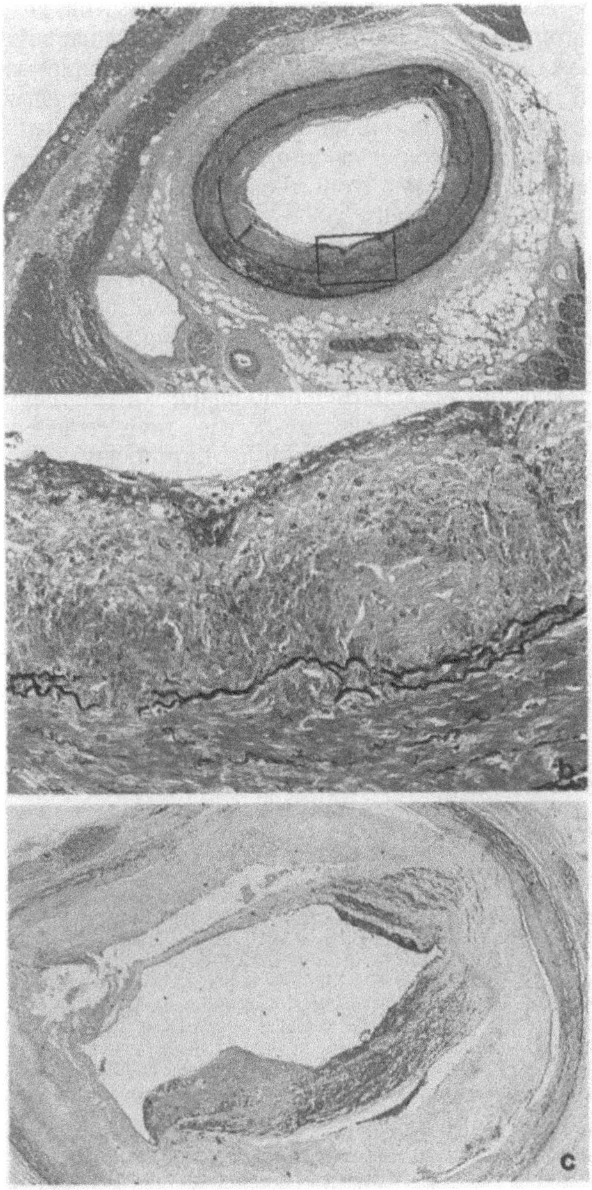

**FIGURE 1.** *A* **and** *B*, **mural thrombus in the proximal tract of the first obtuse marginal branch from the allograft of a 44-year-old man who died 70 months after transplantation for postembolic lung infarctions.** *C*, **luminal nonocclusive thrombus partly incorporated into the plaque in the proximal portions of the right coronary artery from the same patient of** *A* **and** *B*. **(Movat pentachrome stain:** *A*, **×102;** *B*, **×280;** *C*, **×102 [reduced by 55%].)**

proximal portion in 12, middle portion in 8, and distal portion in 6.

The thrombi were entirely nonocclusive (mural) in 51 (77%) of the 66 epicardial coronary arteries containing thrombus (Figure 1); entirely occlusive in 10 arteries (15%) (Figure 2); it consisted exclusively of multiluminal channels in 6 arteries (9%) (Figure 3); and combinations in 1 artery (2%). Of the 6 patients with 1 or more occlusive thrombi, 3 had acute myocardial infarcts, and 1 had a healed myocardial infarct.

In addition to the luminal thrombi, fibrin deposits occurred within fibrous plaques in 15 patients. These fibrin deposits occurred only in the superficial layers of the fibrous plaques (Figure 4). The superficial intramural thrombi were of 2 patterns: (1) focal, so that only a portion of the arterial circumferential surface was covered by thrombotic material; and (2) diffuse along the entire internal lumen circumference. Multiple and large foci of endothelial cell denudation were commonly seen in the affected vessels.

## DISCUSSION

These results indicate that coronary thrombosis is a frequent finding in the coronary arteries of transplanted hearts surviving >2 months after transplantation. Thrombus was found in 83% of late explanted hearts with AVD and in none of the late hearts without AVD. The frequency of coronary thrombus in our patients was much higher than reported previously.[2–12,14] Every 5-mm segment of 8 epicardial cor-

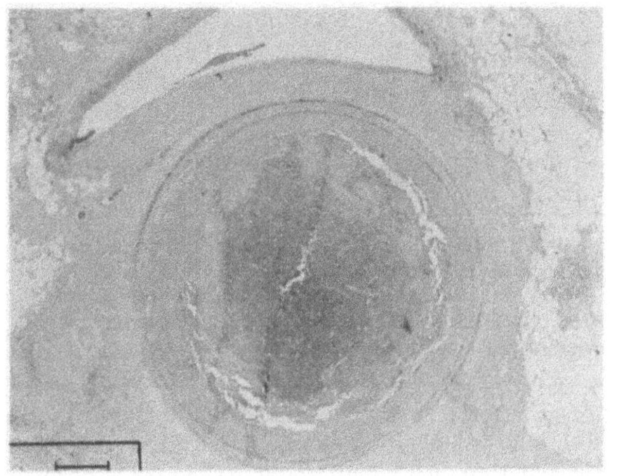

**FIGURE 2. Endoluminal occlusive thrombus in the proximal portions of the left anterior descending coronary artery of a 50-year-old man who died from allograft vascular disease 21 months after transplantation. (Movat pentachrome stain, ×102 [reduced by 59%].)**

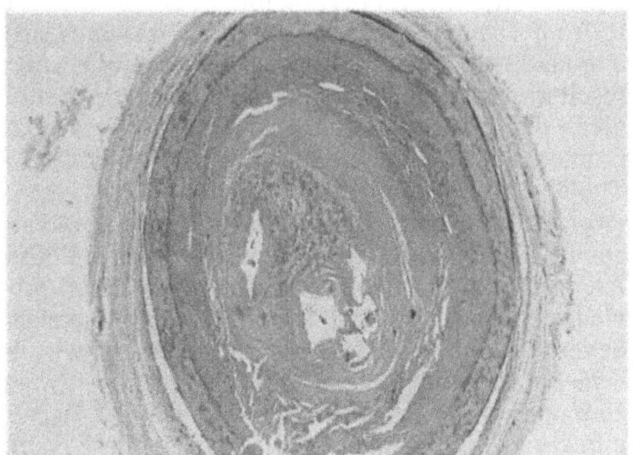

**FIGURE 3. Multichannel pattern in the mid-left anterior descending coronary artery of an explanted graft that survived 72 months after transplantation. The patient, a 49-year-old man, is doing well 14 months after second transplantation. (Movat pentachrome stain, ×102 [reduced by 59%].)**

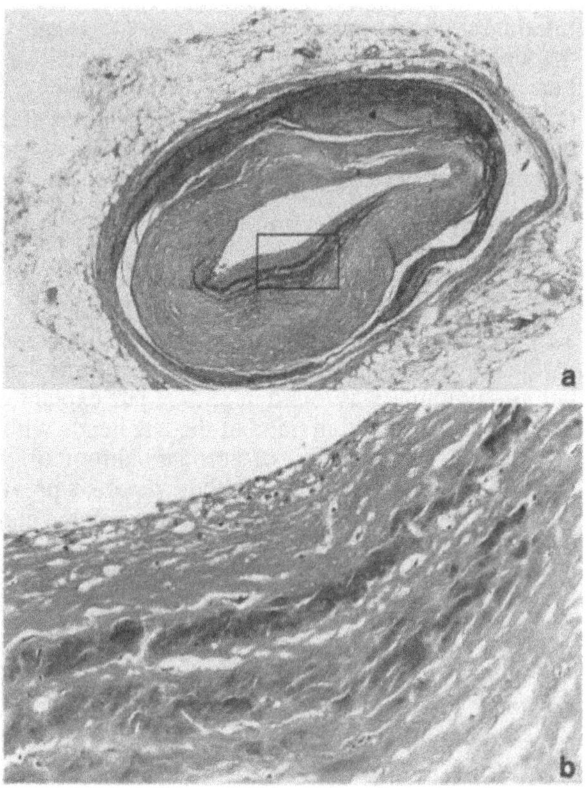

**FIGURE 4. Fibrin deposits embedded within the superficial plaque layers in the posterolateral branch of a graft explanted 72 months after first transplantation (same patient as Figure 3). (Movat pentachrome stain: (a) ×102 and (b) high magnification view of the squared area ×340.)**

onary arteries was examined in our 76 allografts, and this type of detailed examination has not been reported previously. Only random sections of coronary arteries have been studied histologically in nearly all previously reported studies.[5,9–11]

The occurrence of coronary thrombosis in a large percent (83%) of the late grafts with AVD and their absence in the late grafts without AVD suggest that coronary thrombosis plays a role in the progression of AVD. The neointimal hyperplasia, which usually dominates the morphologic picture of AVD[14] may result in part from the organization of these thrombi, given that platelets contain growth factors that may promote or favor smooth muscle cell proliferation.[17] The absence of continuous endothelial cell layer in most affected coronary arteries is a prothrombotic condition because of the exposure of the subendothelial collagen to blood flow. Intimal denudation provides an ideal substrate for adhesion of platelets. Several factors may cause endothelial cell injury and detachment: immunologic[18–22] or infectious[23,24] or common risk factors for atherosclerosis.[25,26] Recent intravascular ultrasound studies have emphasized the role of endothelial cell dysfunction in the pathogenesis of the AVD.[27]

Although thrombus has not specifically been dealt with in previous reports dealing with AVD in cardiac allografts, several observations support the concept that thrombosis may play a role in the progression of AVD: (1) the perturbed hemostasis with prothrombotic changes of heart transplanted patients, described by Hunt et al[28] in 1993; (2) the depletion of tissue plasminogen activator[29]; and 3) the early loss of the antithrombin component (of the heparin sulphate proteoglycan antithombin natural anticoagulant pathway) from the intima and vascular smooth muscle cells.[30]

Occlusive thrombi in our patients (also described by Johnson et al[12]) occurred over noncritically narrowed chronic lesions, and they did not form over ulcerated plaques. The AVD lesions underlying occlusive thrombosis clearly are different from those of spontaneous atherosclerotic plaques.[14] This study shows that in AVD patients there is a high frequency of coronary thrombosis, and that thrombosis probably accelerates the progression of AVD.


1. Hosenpud JD, Novick RJ, Breen TJ, Keck B, Daily P. The Registry of the International Society for Heart and Lung Transplantation: Twelfth Official Report. *J Heart Lung Transplant* 1995;14:805–815.
2. Kosek JC, Bibier CP, Lower RR. Heart graft arteriosclerosis. *Transplant Proc* 1974;3:512–514.
3. Billingham ME. Cardiac transplantation atherosclerosis. *Transplant Proc* 1987;19:19–25.
4. Billingham ME. Graft coronary disease: the lesions and the patients. *Transplant Proc* 1989;21:3665–3666.
5. Johnson DE, Gao SZ, Schroeder JS, DeCampli WM, Billingham ME. The spectrum of coronary artery pathology in human cardiac allografts. *J Heart Transplant* 1989;8:349–359.
6. Billingham ME. Histopathology of graft coronary disease. *J Heart Transplant* 1992;11:S38–S44.
7. Gravanis MB. Allograft heart accelerated atherosclerosis: evidence for cell-mediated immunity in pathogenesis. *Modern Pathol* 1989;2:495–505.
8. Pucci AM, Forbes RDC, Billingham ME. Pathologic features in long-term cardiac allografts. *J Heart Transplant* 1990;9:339–345.
9. Symmans WF, Nielsen H, Dell R, Rose E, Marboe CC. Cardiac allograft pathology: a clinicopathologic correlation. *Cardiovasc Pathol* 1994;3:249–256.
10. Foerster A. Vascular rejection in cardiac transplantation. A morphological study of 25 human cardiac allografts. *APMIS* 1992;100:367–376.
11. Rose AG, Viviers L, Odell JA. Pathology of chronic cardiac rejection: an analysis of the epicardial and intramyocardial coronary arteries and myocardial alterations in 43 human allografts. *Cardiovasc Pathol* 1993;2:7–19.
12. Johnson DE, Alderman EL, Schroeder JS, Gao SZ, Hunt S, DeCampli WM, Stinson E, Billingham ME. Transplant coronary artery disease: histopathologic correlations with angiographic morphology. *J Am Coll Cardiol* 1991;17:449–457.
13. Gao SZ, Alderman EL, Schroeder JS, Silverman JF, Hunt SA. Accelerated coronary vascular disease in the heart transplant patient: coronary arteriographic findings. *J Am Coll Cardiol* 1988;12:334–340.
14. Billingham ME. Pathology of graft vascular disease after heart and heart-lung transplantation and its relationship to obliterative bronchiolitis. *Transplant Proc* 1995;27:2013–2016.
15. Arbustini E, Grasso M, Diegoli M, Morbini P, Aguzzi A, Fasani R, Specchia G. Coronary thrombosis in non-cardiac death. *Coronary Artery Disease* 1993;4:751–759.
16. Arbustini E, Grasso M, Diegoli M, Pucci A, Bramerio M, Ardissino D, Angoli L, DeServi S, Bramucci E, Mussini A, Minzioni G, Viganò M, Specchia G. Coronary atherosclerotic plaques with and without thrombus in ischemic heart syndromes: A morphologic, immunohistochemical, and biochemical study. *Am J Cardiol* 1991;68:36B–50B.
17. Hayry P, Yilmaz S. Role of growth factors in graft vessel disease. *Transplant Proc* 1995;27:2066–2067.
18. Costanzo-Nordin MR. Cardiac allograft vasculopathy: relationship with acute cellular rejection and histocompatibility. *J Heart Lung Transplant* 1992;11:S90–103.
19. Paavonen T, Mennander A, Lautenschlager I, Mattile S, Hayry P. Endothelialitis and accelerated arteriosclerosis in human heart transplant coronaries. *J Heart Lung Transplant* 1993;12:117–122.
20. Hammond EH, Yowell RL, Price GD, Menlove RL, Olsen SL, O'Connell JB, Bristow MR, Doty DB, Millar RC, Karwande SV, Jones KW, Gay WA, Renlund DG. Vascular rejection and its relationship to allograft coronary artery disease. *J Heart Lung Transplant* 1992;11:S111–119.
21. Lowry RP, Takeuchi T, Cremesi H, Conieczny B, Someren A. Chronic rejection of organ allografts may arise from injuries sustained in recurring foci of acute rejection that resolve spontaneously. *Transplant Proc* 1993;25:2103–2105.
22. Hengstenberg C, Rose ML, Page C, Taylor PM, Yacoub MH. Immunocy-

tochemical changes suggestive of damage to endothelial cells during rejection of human cardiac allografts. *Transplantation* 1990;49:895–899.
**23.** Grattan MT, Moreno-Cabral CE, Starnes VA, Oyer PE, Stinson EB, Shumway NE. Cytomegalovirus infection is associated with cardiac rejection and atherosclerosis. *JAMA* 1989;261:3561–3566.
**24.** Loebe M, Schuler S, Zais O, Warnecke H, Fleck E, Hetzer R. Role of cytomegalovirus infection in the development of coronary artery disease in the transplanted heart. *J Heart Transplant* 1990;9:707–711.
**25.** Johnson MR. Transplant coronary disease: nonimmunologic risk factor. *J Heart Lung Transplant* 1992;11:S124–132.
**26.** Hess ML, Hastillo A, Thompson JA, Sansonetti DJ, Szentpetery S, Barnhart G, Lower RR. Lipid mediators in organ transplantation: does cyclosporine accelerate coronary atherosclerosis? *Transplant Proc* 1987;19:71–73.
**27.** Davis SF, Yeung AC, Meredith IT, Charbonneau F, Ganz P, Selwyn AP, Anderson TJ. Early endothelial dysfunction predicts the development of transplant coronary artery disease at 1 year posttransplantation. *Circulation* 1996;93:457–462.
**28.** Hunt BJ, Segal H, Yacoub M. Hemostatic changes in heart transplant recipients and their relationship to accelerated coronary sclerosis. *Transplantation* 1993;55:309–315.
**29.** Labarrere CA, Pitts D, Nelson DR, Faulk WP. Coronary artery disease in cardiac allografts: association with depleted arteriolar tissue plasminogen activator. *Transplant Proc* 1995;27:1941–1943.
**30.** Faulk WP, Labarrere CA, Nelson DR, Pitts D. Coronary artery disease in cardiac allografts: association with arterial antithrombin. *Transplant Proc* 1995;27:1944–1946.

# Morphologic Observations in the Epicardial Coronary Arteries and Their Surroundings Late After Cardiac Transplantation (Allograft Vascular Disease)

Eloisa Arbustini, MD, and William Clifford Roberts, MD

Although a number of publications have appeared describing various features of the coronary arteries at diverse times after cardiac transplantation, most reports have been based on histopathologic study of relatively small portions of the coronary trees.[1-3] For several years, we have histologically examined a section from each 5-mm-long segment of each of the 4 major (right, left main, left anterior descending, and left circumflex) epicardial coronary arteries and from each of the 4 minor (posterolateral, posterior descending, first diagonal, obtuse marginal) coronary arteries in patients dying after cardiac transplantation or having retransplantation because of early or late graft failure. This technique provides approximately 70 5-mm-long segments of the epicardial coronary arteries and therefore 140 sections, 1 stained by hematoxylin-eosin and 1 by the Movat method,[4] from each case. This review is based on study of 76 hearts from 69 patients, 63 at necropsy and 13 after retransplantation. The 69 patients underwent cardiac transplantation from November 1985 to November 1995 in Pavia, Italy, and died or had retransplantation 4 hours to 99 months later. A total of 5,320 hematoxylin-eosin stained cross sections and 5,320 Movat stained cross sections of coronary artery were examined histologically from the 76 allografts, 39 of which survived from >2 to 99 months (mean 32 ± 30).

**Intimal lesions in coronary arteries:** Two different types of intimal lesions were seen in the allograft epicardial coronary arteries: (1) the pretransplant intimal lesions, and (2) the post-transplant intimal lesions (Figure 1, Figure 2, and Table I). Generally, by age 20 years, in most nontransplanted human hearts, the thickness of the intima is roughly the same as the media and the thickening is uniform around the entire inner circumference of the epicardial arteries. This intimal lesion consists primarily of cellular fibrous tissue and elastic lamellae arranged roughly parallel to the internal elastic membrane. This intimal lesion occurs in all populations and appears to be the normal arterial response to the intra-arterial pressure. Thus, this intimal lesion can be observed in most transplanted hearts when the age of the donor is ≥20 years.

Unfortunately, other unexpected pretransplant intimal lesions are also often observed. Whenever large quantities of intimal plaque are observed in the epicardial coronary arteries of donor hearts in which the graft survived ≤2 months (37 of the 76 hearts of our series: 30 at autopsy and 7 retransplant), it is reasonable to assume that the intimal plaque had been present in the donor heart at the time of transplantation. These pretransplantation plaques (donor plaques) are similar to nontransplanted coronary plaques and consist primarily of cellular and acellular fibrous tissue, pultaceous debris (extracellular lipid) including cholesterol clefts, occasional foam cells, and calcific deposits (in 8 of 37 grafts ≤2 months). Some of these plaques are quite large with resulting luminal narrowing, at times of severe degree (Figure 2). In 2 of the 76 grafts the pretransplant intimal plaques were so large that the resulting luminal narrowing appeared to have played a role in the patients' early graft failure and death.

The post-transplant intimal lesions occur in all transplanted hearts; they are diffuse in that they occur in all 5-mm segments of each of the 4 major and 4 minor coronary arteries. They involve, with rare exception, the entire intimal circumference and they usually are relatively uniform. The uniformity or homogenicity of the intimal lesions is the most characteristic feature of the post-transplant intimal lesions. The lesions consist primarily of cellular and acellular fibrous tissue and the thickness of the intimal lesion (i.e., the distance from the lining of the lumen to the internal elastic membrane) is roughly similar at all points in the circumference of the artery (Figure 3). Because these distances are similar, the lumen is usually centrally located (Figure 3).

The post-transplant intimal lesions, however, do not remain uniform. Approximately 5 years after cardiac transplantation the intimal lesions may transform into lesions similar to those in nontransplanted coronary arteries, with considerable amounts of pultaceous debris, calcific deposits, cholesterol clefts, etc.[3]

From the Department of Pathologic Anatomy, Istituto di Ricovero e Cura a Carattere Scientifico, IRCCS Policlinico S. Matteo, Pavia, Italy, and the Baylor Cardiovascular Institute, Baylor University Medical Center, Dallas, Texas, USA. This report was supported by Grant "Chronic Allograft Rejection" (1992) from the Health Ministry to IRCCS Policlinico San Matteo of Pavia, Pavia, Italy. Manuscript received March 15, 1996; revised manuscript received and accepted June 14, 1996.

Address for reprints: Eloisa Arbustini, MD, Istituto di Anatomia Patologica, Via Forlanini 16, 27100 Pavia, Italy.

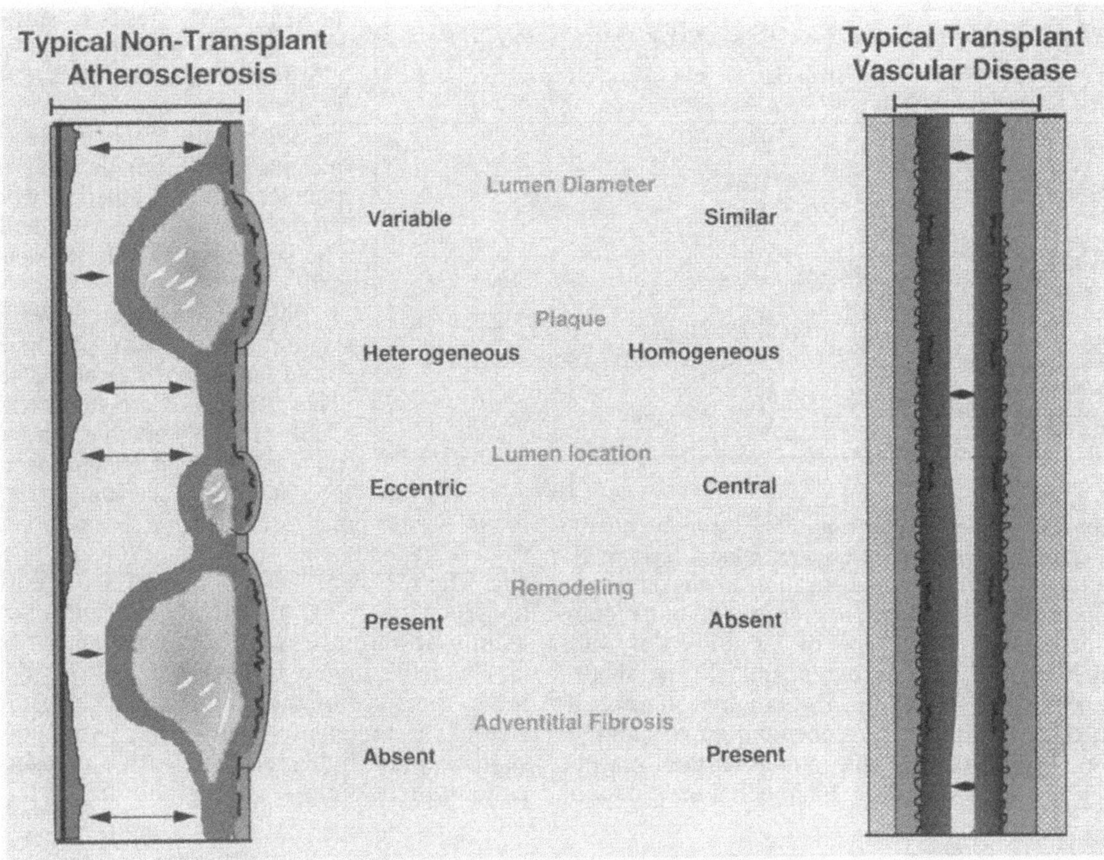


**FIGURE 1. Diagram of differences between natural atherosclerosis and post-transplant vascular disease.**

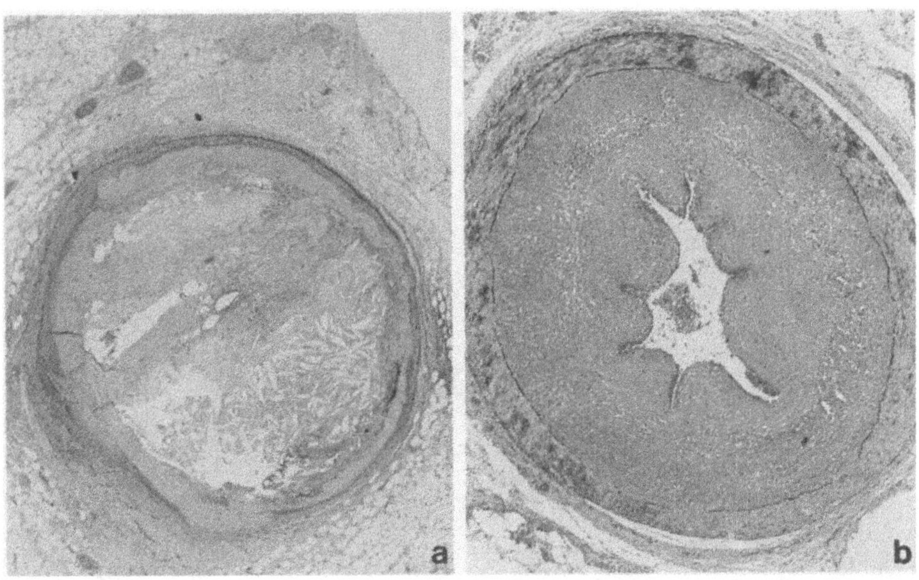


**FIGURE 2. Two photomicrographs of typical spontaneous atherosclerosis *(a)* and allograft *(b)* vascular disease. *a,* Spontaneous coronary atherosclerosis of the left anterior descending coronary artery in a male patient who survived 30 days after transplantation; the donor was a 38-year-old male who died from cerebral hemorrhage. The recipient died from cerebrovascular event, but the graft functioned poorly for the survival interval. (Movat pentachrome stain, ×102.) *b,* Allograft vascular disease: diffuse, concentric neointimal hyperplasia with severely narrowed vessel lumen in the distal left anterior descending coronary artery of a graft that failed 93 months after transplantation for allograft vascular disease. (Movat pentachrome stain, ×160 [reduced by 63%].)**

**TABLE I** Comparison of Composition of Donor and Recipients Coronary Lesions

| Intimal Material | Pretransplant "Plaque" (spontaneous) (donor plaque) | Post-transplant "Lesions" (recipient lesions) |
|---|---|---|
| Fibrous tissue | ++ | ++++ |
| Mesenchymal cells | ++ | + |
| Pultaceous debris | + | 0 |
| Foam cells | + | + |
| Calcium | + | 0 |
| Mucoid material | + | 0 |
| Endothelial cells | + | 0 |
| Inflammatory cells | ± | + |
| Giant cells | + | 0 |
| Fibrin (also in lumen) | + | + |
| Platelet aggregates | + | + |
| Revascularized channels | +++ | + |
| Elastic fibers | + | 0 |

**Luminal shapes in post-transplant coronary arteries with absent or small pretransplant intimal lesions:** As mentioned previously, the location of the lumen in the post-transplant coronary artery is most commonly central. The shape of the lumen is variable. It may be circular, ovoid, spiked (star-shaped or spasm-like), slit or linear, triangular, dumbbell-shaped, foliated, or have a bow-and-arrow configuration, among others. The intimal surface may be either smooth or irregular. Endothelial cells may be present on the lesion's surface or they may be absent. In the precyclosporin era, one of us (WCR) observed the surface of the plaque to be lined uniformly by layers of plasma cells. Fibrin deposits and/or platelet aggregates also may be seen on the luminal surface of the lesion and sometimes within the lesion itself.

**Difference between pretransplant (donor plaques) and post-transplant (recipient lesions) coronary lesions:** The differences are summarized in Table I. To reiterate, the donor plaques are usually heterogeneous, eccentrically located, and contain fibrous tissue, pultaceous debris, cholesterol clefts, calcific deposits, and the lumen typically is eccentric. The recipient lesions, in contrast, are usually homogeneous, symmetrically located, consist mainly of fibrous tissue (both cellular and acellular) and the lumen typically is central. Furthermore, the sizes of the plaques, and therefore, the size of the lumens in each of the 5-mm coronary segments are highly variable in the pretransplant patient; therefore, the angiogram often detects fo-

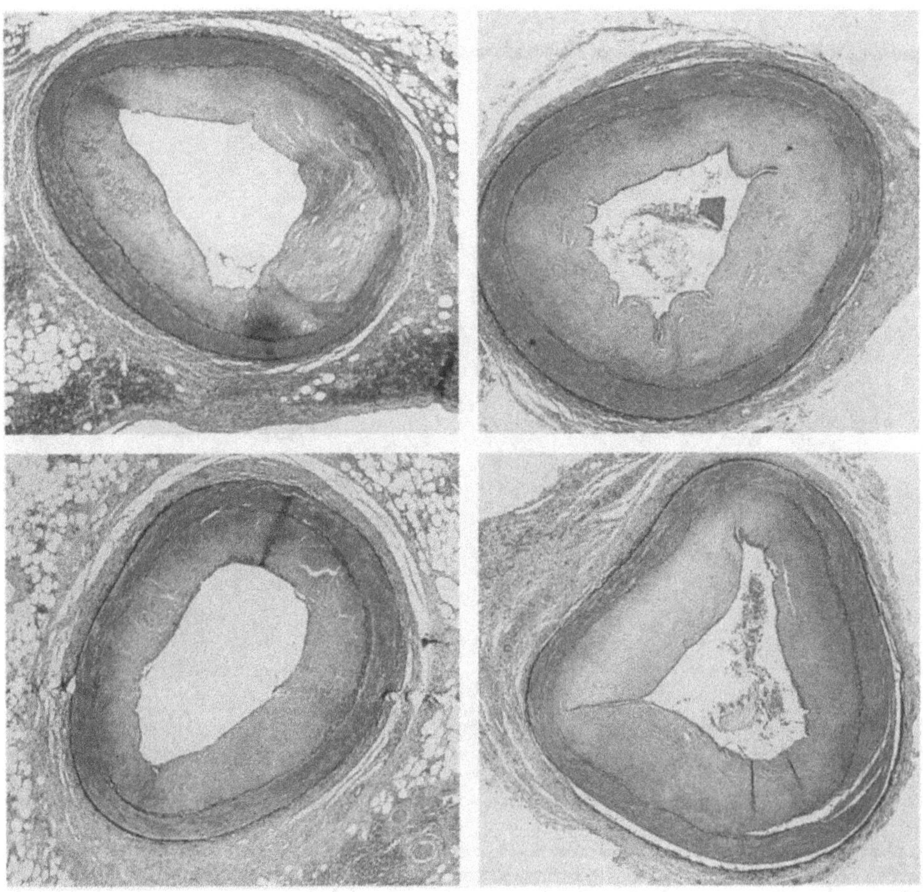

**FIGURE 3. Four photomicrographs of transplant coronary arteries showing homogenicity of the intimal lesions and central orifices. Multiple segments of the right coronary artery from the allograft of a 35-year-old male recipient who died 17 months after transplantation from allograft vascular disease. (Movat pentachrome stain, ×102 [reduced by 63%].)**

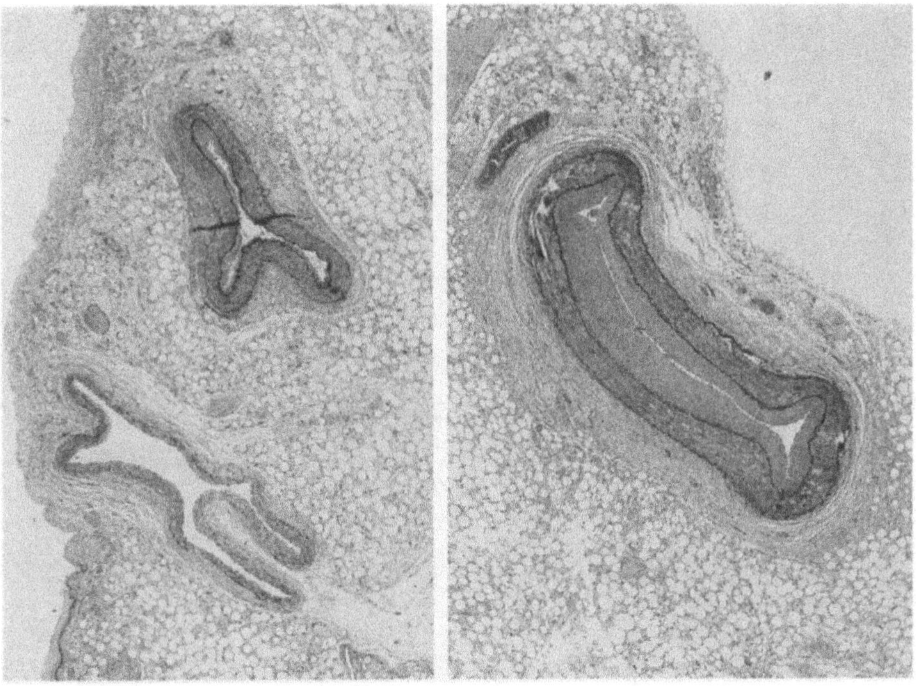

**FIGURE 4. Photomicrographs of epicardial coronary arteries showing distorted lumen, probably the result of constriction from adventitial fibrous tissue. Distal left circumflex *(left)* and proximal *(right)* from the allograft of a 56-year-old male recipient who died 6 months after transplantation from multiorgan failure. (Movat pentachrome stain, ×102 [reduced by 72%].) Note the epicardial fat inflammatory infiltrates, which produce steatonecrosis.**

cal narrowings. The size of the lumen in each 5-mm coronary segment is quite regular in the post-transplant patient; thus, the angiogram detects focal narrowings less often (Figure 1).

**Intraluminal and intralesion thrombus:** In 26 of the 39 allografts surviving >2 months, thrombus was observed in ≥1 of the epicardial coronary arteries. The thrombus was small and nonocclusive in 18 allografts, and both occlusive and nonocclusive in 4 allografts (Figure 5). Three of the latter 4 patients had acute myocardial infarcts. In addition to the intraluminal thrombus, small thrombi, mainly fibrin, were observed within the lesion itself in several patients.These intralesion fibrin deposits suggest that thrombus was playing a role in the progression of the lesion itself.[5–7]

Finally, many patients had coronary lesions with ≥1 luminal channel. If thrombi are injected into systemic veins in nonhuman animals, the thrombi migrate to the intrapulmonary arteries, and there they often organize into lesions containing multiluminal channels.[6] Thus, the presence of multiluminal channels in lesions, a finding observed in some coronary segments after cardiac transplantation, is evidence that organization of thrombi plays a role in progression of at least some coronary lesions after cardiac transplantation.

**Medial lesions in coronary arteries:** This section discusses changes in the internal elastic membrane, the media itself, and the external elastic membrane. Although some earlier articles[2,8] indicated that the post-transplant internal elastic membrane was usually intact, our experience varies with this earlier observation. Most commonly the internal elastic membrane is focally disrupted such that portions of it are absent. In 1 patient, who was studied 6 years after transplantation, the internal elastic membrane was completely absent in most 5-mm segments of the major coronary arteries. Occasionally, the internal elastic membrane is replicated such that 2 or 3 or more parallel membranes are observed.

The media may be normal; focally thinned; uniformly or focally thickened; focally lysed (lysis of smooth muscle cells); infiltrated or invaded focally by inflammatory cells or foam cells (mediolysis), or vascular channels; and/or replaced focally by fibrous tissue, foam cells or mucopolysaccharide material. Focal thinning of the media after transplantation is relatively infrequent, particularly so in contrast with the focal thinning (erosion) which is commonly observed in the coronary arteries containing large plaques in nontransplanted patients (Figure 1).

Similar to the internal elastic membrane, the external elastic membrane may be intact or it may be focally absent or replicated. Disruption of the external elastic membrane, however, is far less common than disruption or focal absence of the internal elastic membrane. Whenever inflammatory cells are present in the media, the external elastic membrane is disrupted, an observation suggesting that loss of the integrity of this membrane is required for invasion of the media by inflammatory cells. The internal elastic membrane is usually disrupted when foam cells and/or lymphocytes are present in the media.

**Adventitia of epicardial coronary arteries:** The adventitia of the epicardial coronary arteries is ab-

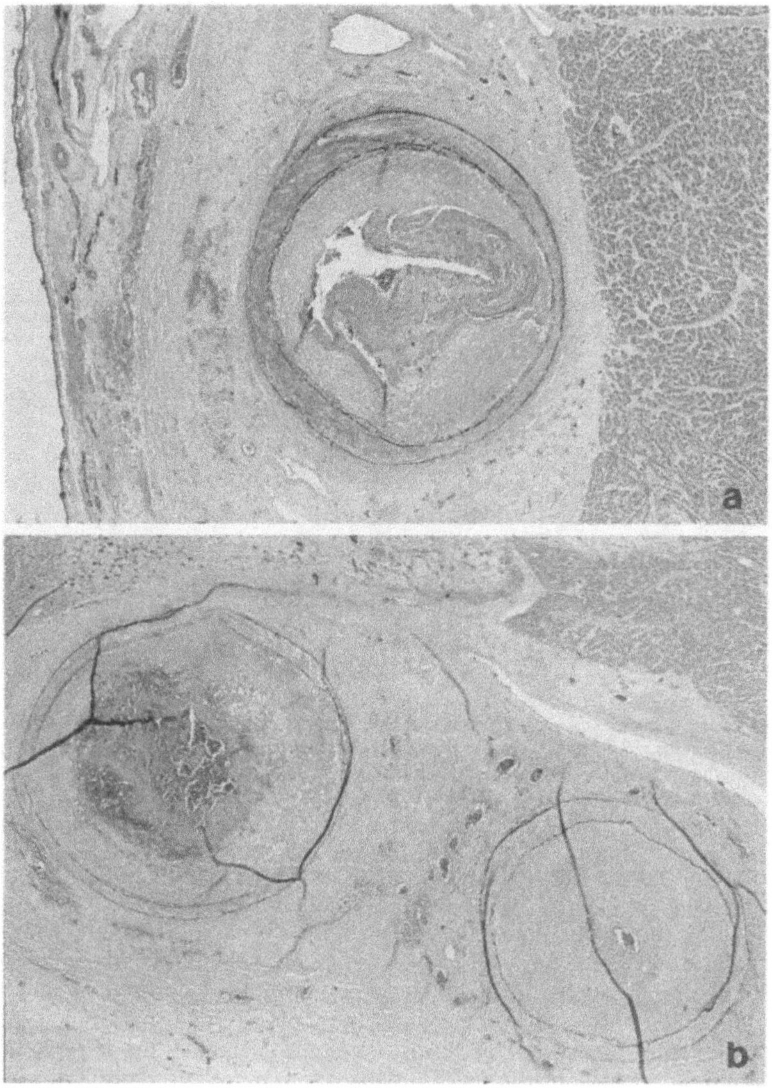

**FIGURE 5. Photomicrographs showing thrombus in the lumen *(a)* and incorporated into lesion *(b)*. Left anterior descending coronary artery from the allograft of a 43-year-old male recipient who died 16 months after transplantation for allograft vascular disease: *a*, lumen thrombus incorporated into lesion with surrounding fibrous tissue in the first segment of the left anterior descending artery; *b*, occlusive, more recent thrombus in the left anterior descending segments between proximal and middle tract. (Movat pentachrome stain, ×102 [reduced by 73%].)**

normal in most post-transplantation epicardial coronary arteries (Figure 4 and Figure 5). The most common abnormality is the presence of fibrous tissue, usually quite dense, about the entire circumference of the arteries. The adventitial fibrosis makes dissection or isolation of the individual coronary arteries quite difficult at necropsy late after transplantation and likewise makes coronary artery bypass grafting late after transplantation a particularly arduous procedure. The thick and dense circumferential adventitial fibrous tissue appears at times to constrict or restrict expansion and remodeling of the epicardial coronary arteries, and the shape of the artery's lumen may be deformed by the external constricting fibrous tissue (Figure 4). Often clusters of inflammatory cells, mainly lymphocytes and plasma cells, are present in the adventitial fibrous tissue, and these cells may invade the artery's media after first destroying portions of the external elastic membrane (Figure 6).

Adventitial fibrosis is also characteristically observed in the epicardial coronary arteries in radiation heart disease, but the intraluminal plaques in radiation heart disease resemble those of naturally occurring atherosclerosis rather than that following cardiac transplantation.[9,10]

**Coronary arterial size and cardiac size after transplantation:** In general, the size of the major epicardial coronary arteries is proportional to myocardial mass.[11] Thus, hearts enlarged from systemic hypertension, aortic valve stenosis, aortic regurgitation, or hypertrophic cardiomyopathy, for example, have epicardial coronary arteries much larger than those observed in hearts of normal weight. Most donor hearts at the time of transplantation are presumably of normal or near-normal weight and the size of the

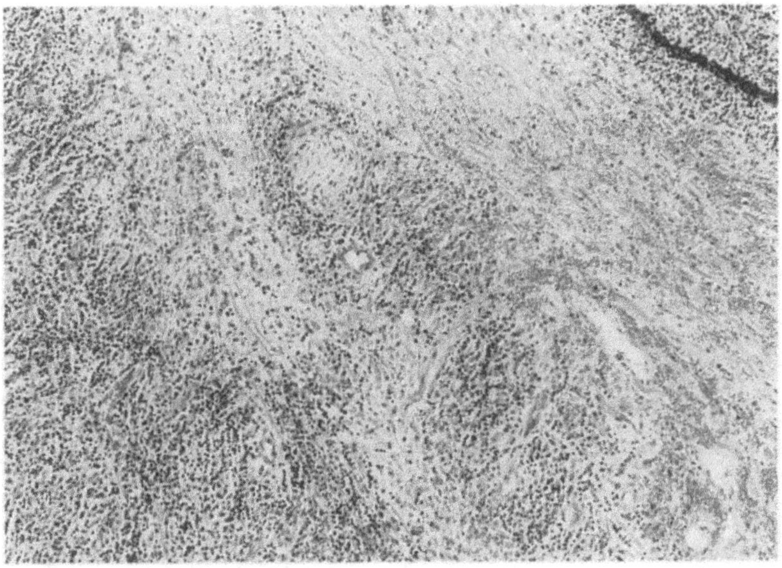

FIGURE 6. Inflammatory infiltrates in subepicardial adipose tissue.

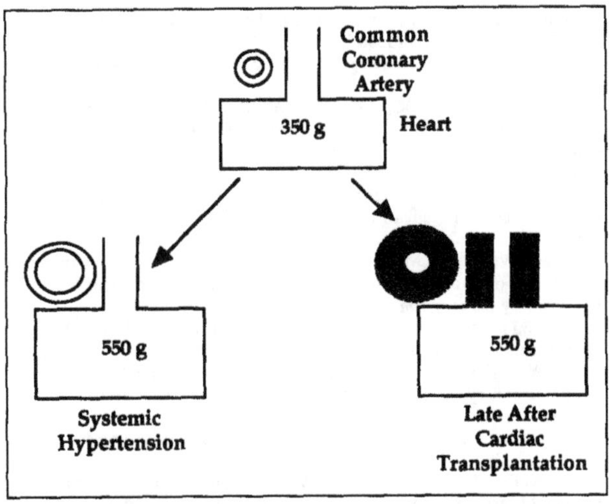


FIGURE 7. Diagram showing that the coronary arteries late after cardiac transplantation may be smaller in exterior dimension than at the time of transplantation even though myocardial mass may actually increase after cardiac transplantation.

coronary arteries presumably is proportional to that weight. What happens to the weight of the donor heart late after transplantation has not been determined, mainly because the weight of the donor heart at the time of transplantation is rarely determined. It is our belief that myocardial mass increases late after cardiac transplantation in many patients. It is also our impression that the size of the epicardial coronary arteries does not increase late after cardiac transplantation, and indeed that the opposite is the case (i.e., that the size of the coronary arteries actually decreases late after cardiac transplantation) (Figure 7). The reason for this suspected size reduction may be related to the extensive perivascular fibrosis and the heavy infiltration of the subepicardial adipose tissue by fibrous tissue, which not only may prevent dilation or expansion (remodeling) of the epicardial coronary arteries, but may actually restrict or constrict them, making them appear smaller than might be expected (Figure 7).

**Epicardium and subepicardial tissues:** Thus far, this review has concentrated entirely on alterations in the epicardial coronary arteries. The focus of this section now moves to changes in the epicardium and subepicardial tissues. The parietal pericardium is incised, of course, at the time of cardiac transplantation, and thereafter it becomes adherent to the epicardium (visceral pericardium) diffusely, usually obliterating the pericardial cavity. Early after cardiac transplantation, the epicardium is covered by fibrin and its organization causes the parietal and visceral pericardia to adhere to one another. As a consequence, the epicardium is thickened by fibrous tissue, similar to that observed in other postsurgery nontransplanted hearts; the thickening, however, is uneven, some areas being thicker than others.

The major components of the subepicardial tissues are fat, coronary arteries, coronary veins, lymphatics, and nerves. The coronary changes have been discussed. Some changes also occur in the coronary veins (Figure 4). Their walls may be focally replaced by fibrous tissue and occasionally inflammatory cells may invade their walls. Luminal obstruction of coronary veins by thrombus or other material was observed in 1 of our cases. The lumina of the veins may be compressed by the subepicardial fibrous tissue. Lymphatics in the subepicardium are difficult to discern late after transplantation. The nerves in the subepicardium are usually normal but we have observed focal invasion of them by inflammatory cells (lymphocytes) (Figure 6).

A major tissue in the subepicardium is adipose tissue and the quantity of adipose tissue in this region may be enormous in part owing to the corticosteroid therapy transplant patients receive. The quantity of fat in the heart late after transplantation may be so excessive that the heart floats in water.[12,13] Early after transplantation, inflammatory cells, mainly lymphocytes and plasmacytes, enter the subepicardium. The inflammatory cells are observed in the tissue between the lipocytes. The inflammatory cell invasion of the lipocytes and their resulting necrosis produces a true panniculitis. These inflamed and steatonecrotic tissues later are replaced by fibrous tissue, which can become so extensive that some interference to ventricular filling may result as described by an echocardiogram.[14] Even when the subepicardial tissues are replaced later by fibrous tissue, the parietal pericardium, which is diffusely adherent to the epicardium, is not thickened. Within the subepicardial fibrous tissue, large focal collections of inflammatory cells are evidence of allogenic reaction and they are present far more frequently than inflammatory cells in the myocardial interstitium. In other words, the rejection "war" appears to take place primarily in the epicardial fat, not in the myocardium. The myocardium can be safely biopsied; the subepicardium tissues, of course, cannot be safely biopsied. The fibrous tissue in the subepicardium often extends into the epicardial half of the left ventricular wall within the myocardial interstitium, often causing perivascular fibrosis of the intramural coronary arteries. The inflammatory cells, which are typically seen in the subepicardial fat, are less commonly seen in the myocardial wall late after transplantation. When observed again, they are most common in the epicardial half of the myocardial wall. The intramural coronary arteries in the epicardial half of the myocardial wall may have changes similar to those affecting these arteries in the subepicardium, a finding not observed in coronary atherosclerosis and not associated with cardiac transplantation.

**Clinical implications:** Because the degree of luminal narrowing tends to be uniform in most coronary segments late after cardiac transplantation, coronary angiography may not be as helpful in detecting the amount of coronary narrowing as in nontransplanted patients who have considerably more variability in lesion size, and therefore, resulting luminal size.

Because there is evidence of recent (intraluminal and intralesion thrombus) and old (multiluminal channels in lesions) thrombus formation in the epicardial coronary arteries late after cardiac transplantation, aspirin or warfarin therapy (or both) may have a beneficial role in some of these patients. Although the cause of coronary allograft disease still is uncertain, lipid-lowering drug therapy has been demonstrated to be useful in retarding coronary lesion development after cardiac transplantation.[15]

**Summary:** Conclusions from this review, based primarily on study of 39 cardiac allografts in place for >2 months, but also on a study of 37 grafts in place for ≤2 months, might include the following: (1) allograft vascular disease affects all layers of the epicardial coronary arteries and usually the intramural coronary arteries in the outer one-half of the left ventricular wall; (2) the resulting intimal lesion is relatively uniform, consisting mainly of cellular and acellular fibrous tissue; it is diffuse, affecting all segments of the major and minor epicardial coronary arteries; (3) the degree of resulting luminal narrowing is similar in most 5-mm coronary segments, making coronary angiography hazardous in reliably predicting accurately the degree of luminal narrowing; (4) the extensive adventitial fibrosis and the extensive fibrous tissue infiltration of the subepicardial tissues probably inhibit dilation and remodeling of the epicardial coronary arteries and indeed may constrict them; (5) luminal narrowing of the epicardial coronary arteries after transplantation may be the consequence of both intraluminal lesions and exterior compression from the surrounding fibrous tissue; (6) intraluminal and intralesion thrombus is commonly observed as are multiluminal channels in coronary plaques, suggesting that organization of thrombi plays some role in the progression of post-transplant epicardial coronary disease; (7) the coronary lesions developing after cardiac transplantation are morphologically quite different in composition than those occurring in natural (nontransplantation) atherosclerosis; and (8) inflammatory cellular infiltrates are often extensive in the subepicardial tissues and the infiltrates in this area may be extensive even when interstitial myocardial inflammatory infiltrates are minimal or absent.


1. Billingham ME. Graft coronary disease: the lesions and the patients. *Transplant Proc* 1989;21:3665–3666.
2. Billingham ME. Histopathology of graft coronary disease. *J Heart Transplant* 1992; 11:S38–S44.
3. Pucci AM, Forbes RDC, Billingham ME. Pathologic features in long-term cardiac allografts. *J Heart Transplant* 1990;9:339–345.
4. Movat HZ. Demonstration of all connective tissue elements in a single section. *Arch Pathol* 1955;60:289–295.
5. Roberts WC. Does thrombosis play a major role in the development of symptom-producing atherosclerotic plaque? *Circulation* 1973;48:1161–1166.
6. Roberts WC, Buja LM. The frequency and significance of coronary arterial thrombi and other observations in fatal acute myocardial infarction. A study of 107 necropsy patients. *Am J Med* 1972;52:425–443.
7. Arbustini E, Dal Bello B, Morbini P, Grasso M, Diegoli M, Fasani R, Bellini O, Pellegrini C, Martinelli L, Campana C, Gavazzi A, Specchia G, Viganò M, Roberts WC. Frequency and characteristics of coronary thrombosis in the epicardial coronary arteries after cardiac transplantation. *Am J Cardiol* 1996;78:795–800
8. Billingham ME. Cardiac transplantation atherosclerosis. *Transplant Proc* 1987;19:19–25.
9. Brosius FC III, Waller BF, Roberts WC. Radiation heart disease: analysis of 16 young (aged 15–33 years) necropsy patients who received over 3500 rads to the heart. *Am J Med* 1981;70:519–530.
10. Harvey LAC, DeMaio SJ, Roberts WC. Radiation-induced cardiovascular disease including stenosis of coronary ostium, coronary and carotid arteries, and aortic valve. *Baylor University Medical Center Proceedings* 1994;7:33–36.
11. Roberts CS, Roberts WC. Cross-sectional area of the maximal portions of the three major epicardial coronary arteries in 98 necropsy patients with different coronary events: relationship to heart weight, age, and sex. *Circulation* 1980;62:953–959.
12. Roberts WC, Roberts JD. The floating heart or the heart too fat to sink. Analysis of 55 necropsy patients. *Am J Cardiol* 1983;52:1286–1289.
13. Shirani J, Berezowsky K, Roberts WC. Quantitative measurement of normal and excessive (cor adiposum) subepicardial adipose tissue, its clinical significance, and its effect on electrocardiographic QRS voltage. *Am J Cardiol* 1995;76:414–416.
14. Valantine HA, Appleton CP, Hatle LK, Hunt SA, Billingham ME, Shumway NE, Stinson EB, Popp RL. A hemodynamic and Doppler echocardiographic study of ventricular function in long-term cardiac allograft recipients. Etiology and prognosis of restrictive-constrictive physiology. *Circulation* 1989;79:66–75.
15. Kobashigawa JA, Katznelson S, Laks H, Johnson JA, Yeatman L, Wang XM, Chia D, Terasaki PI, Sabad A, Cogert GA, Trosian K, Hamilton MA, Moriguchi JD, Kawata N, Hage A, Drinkwater DC, Stevenson LW. Effect of pravastatin on outcomes after cardiac transplantation. *N Engl J Med* 1995;333:621–627.

# Effectiveness of Cardiac Transplantation for Primary (AL) Cardiac Amyloidosis

Frank Pelosi, Jr., MD, John Capehart, MD, and William C. Roberts, MD

From 1968 to April 1996, according to the United Network for Organ Sharing, cardiac transplantation (CT) was performed in nearly 36,000 persons. Although most patients underwent this procedure because of ischemic cardiomyopathy or idiopathic dilated cardiomyopathy, at least 44 had CT because of cardiac amyloidosis. Follow-up information on these 44 patients, however, is not available to us. At least 7 patients having CT for cardiac amyloidosis and followed to death have been reported (Table I).[1–6] The present report was prompted by studying a patient who also had CT for cardiac AL amyloidosis and survived 69 months without again developing cardiac dysfunction. This report describes the latter patient and summarizes findings in those previously reported patients having CT for cardiac amyloidosis. The question asked is: Is CT worthwhile in patients with life-threatening cardiac dysfunction from cardiac amyloidosis?

• • •

A.C., a 66-year-old white man who was born on September 14, 1928, and died on July 3, 1995, had been well until June 1985 (51 months before CT) when he noted pedal edema. In January 1987, he noted the onset of exertional dyspnea which progressively worsened. Evaluation in June 1987 disclosed his blood pressure to be 135/85 mm Hg (Figure 1). Pitting ankle edema was present. No abdominal organs were palpable. The electrocardiogram disclosed complete left bundle branch block. Cardiac catheterization was performed and the data are tabulated in Table II.

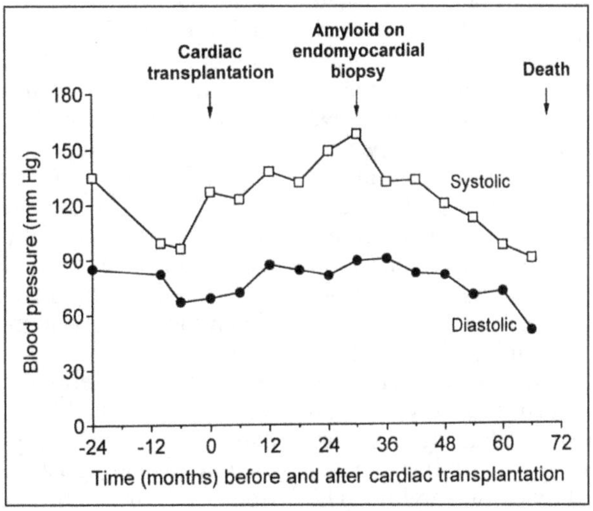


**FIGURE 1. Indirect systemic arterial systolic and diastolic blood pressures before and after cardiac transplantation.**

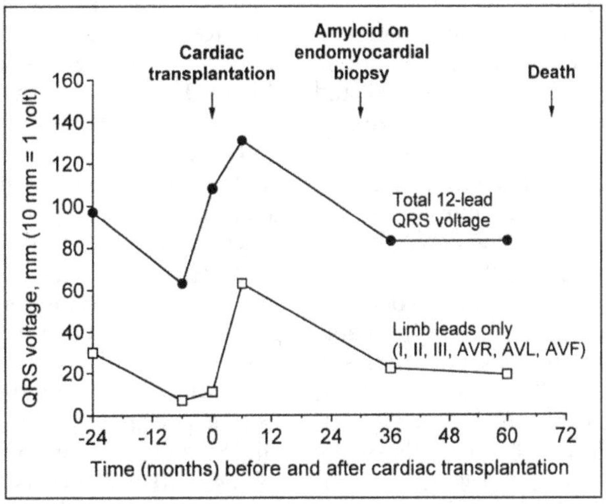


**FIGURE 2. Total and limb-lead QRS voltage at various time periods before and after cardiac transplantations in patient A.C.**

In May 1989, he was hospitalized again because of worsening congestive cardiac failure. Blood pressure was 95/65 mm Hg, heart rate 120 beats/min, and respiratory rate, 26 breaths/min. He now had diminished heart sounds, an $S_3$ gallop, diffuse pulmonary rales, hepatosplenomegaly, ascites, and massive subcutaneous pitting edema. With diuretic therapy, he lost 26 pounds. M-mode and 2-dimensional echocardiograms revealed normal-sized ventricular chambers, and decreased ventricular wall motion. Endomyocardial biopsy revealed amyloid. Monoclonal gammopathy was absent by serum and urine protein electrophoresis, and plasma cell dyscrasia was absent on bone marrow biopsy. Liver biopsy showed no amyloid. Orthotopic CT was performed on October 7, 1989; the donor was a 32-year-old man. The

From the Departments of Medicine (Cardiology Division), Cardiothoracic Surgery and Pathology, Baylor University Medical Center, Dallas, Texas. Dr. Roberts' address is: Baylor Cardiovascular Institute, Baylor University Medical Center, 3500 Gaston Avenue, Dallas, Texas 75246. Manuscript received July 31, 1996; revised manuscript received and accepted September 17, 1996.

explanted heart (excludes most of the atrial walls) weighed 485 g and extensive amyloid was present in the intramyocardial blood vessels without amyloid in the myocardial interstitium. After CT, evidence of heart failure vanished. Posttransplant cardiac catheterizations (Table I) and biopsies were performed and disclosed no abnormalities until April 1992 when endomyocardial biopsy revealed amyloid by light microscopy. Bence-Jones protein also was found in the urine protein electrophoresis. After onset of dysphagia in August 1992, esophageal and pre-pyloric biopsies showed amyloid. Two-dimensional and Doppler echocardiography in April 1995 revealed no evidence of cardiac dysfunction. Renal biopsy for declining renal function showed no amyloid. The serum albumin was 2.7 g/dl. He died suddenly at home while watching television on July 3, 1995, 69 months after CT.

At necropsy, the heart weighed 505 g. Comparison of the cardiac amyloid findings in the native and donor hearts are summarized in Table III. Amyloid was present in large and roughly equal amounts in the walls of the intramural and small epicardial vessels in the native heart and in the donor heart, and was absent from myocardial interstitium in both. Amyloid also was present in the small arteries in the liver (1,000 g) and kidney but, as in the native and donor hearts, it was limited to the walls of the small vessels. Furthermore, although amyloid was found in the tongue, pancreas, stomach, colon, spleen (275 g), skin, and adrenal glands, the deposits were limited to the the small vessels in these structures. In the lung the deposits also were present primarily in the small vessels but some deposits were found in alveolar septa. Amyloid deposits were present in large quantities in the interstitium, as well as in the walls of the small blood vessels, in the esophagus.

• • •

The hitherto described patient had CT for extensive primary cardiac amyloidosis and died suddenly at home 69 months later. During the post-CT period, he never developed evidence of cardiac dysfunction even though amyloid was found in a myocardial biopsy 3 years before his death.

The presently described patient is the only one with cardiac amyloid among 179 CT recipients at Baylor University Medical Center. Follow-up information from CT to death is available in at least 7 previously reported patients (Table I) who had CT for cardiac amyloidosis. Connor and associates[1] first reported CT for cardiac amyloidosis, and their 48-year-old man lived 46 months after CT. Valentine and Billingham's[2] 30-year-old woman died 13 months after CT. Hosenpud and colleagues[3] described 2 patients who had CT for cardiac amyloidosis: 1 died in the early postoperative period and the other lived 30 months. Deng and colleagues[4] described a 53-year-old woman who died 6 months after CT (from infection). The longest survivor is Dr. Reginald Hall who, in a unique report,[5] described his own illness. He underwent CT for cardiac amyloidosis and reported the first 112 months of his post-CT course. At 36 months after CT, endomyocardial biopsy disclosed amyloid and chemotherapy was instituted. The quantity of amyloid at myocardial biopsy appeared to be reduced by this therapy. We have recently learned that Dr. Hall died 118 months after CT from sepsis and that he never had clinical evidence of cardiac amyloidosis after CT (personal communication, P.N. Hawkins, MD, July 22, 1996). Dubrey et al[6] described a 54-year-old woman who survived 47 months after CT. If the patient who died early postoperatively is eliminated, the other 6 survived 6 to 118 months (median 46) after CT: 4 died from consequences of noncardiac amyloidosis and 2 from superimposed infection. In addition to the reported data and that from our patient, Dubrey (personal communication, July 11, 1996) has informed us that CT has been performed for cardiac amyloidosis in at least 4 other patients followed in his amyloid clinic: 3 died at 10,

**TABLE I** Certain Data in Seven Previously Reported Patients Having Cardiac Transplantation for Cardiac Amyloidosis and Follow-Up to Death Plus Our Presently Described Patient

| Case | Publication Year | First Author (reference) | Age (yr) at CT | Gender | Duration (mo) Symptoms Before CT | Interval CT to Death (mo) | Extracardiac Amyloid Before CT | Signs of Cardiac Dysfunction After CT | Amyloid Found in Transplanted Heart After CT (mo) | Death Secondary to CHF | Death Secondary to Noncardiac Amyloid | Chemotherapy Before or After CT | Weight of Transplanted Heart (g) |
|---|---|---|---|---|---|---|---|---|---|---|---|---|---|
| 1. | 1988 | Conner[1] | 48 | M | 48 | 46 | + | 0 | 0 | 0 | + | 0 | — |
| 2. | 1989 | Valentine[2] | 30 | F | 4 | 13 | + | + | + | 0 | + | 0 | — |
| 3. | 1991 | Hosenpud[3] | — | — | — | <1 | — | 0 | — | 0 | 0 | 0 | — |
| 4. | — | — | — | — | — | 30 | — | — | — | — | — | — | — |
| 5. | 1992 | Deng[4] | 53 | F | 24 | 6 | 0 | 0 | + (6) | 0 | 0 | 0 | — |
| 6. | 1994 | Hall[5] | 53 | M | 72 | 118 | 0 | + | + (36) | 0 | 0 | + | — |
| 7. | 1995 | Dubrey[6] | 54 | F | 13 | 47 | 0 | + | + (36) | + | 0 | + | 540 |
| 8. | 1997 | Pelosi | 60 | M | 52 | 69 | 0 | 0 | + (30) | 0* | 0 | 0 | 504 |

* Death was sudden at home, but congestive heart failure was never present after cardiac transplantation.
+ = present or positive; 0 = absent or negative; — = no information available.
CHF = congestive heart failure; CT = cardiac transplantation.

| **TABLE II** Cardiac Catheterization Findings in the Patient Described | | | | | | | | |
|---|---|---|---|---|---|---|---|---|
| Interval (mo) Before (−) and After (+) CT | RA* (mean) | RV* (s/d) | PA* (s/d) | PAW* (mean) | LV* (s/d) | Aorta* (s/d) | CO (L/min) | Amyloid in Myocardial Biopsy |
| −24 | 15 | 36/8 | 42/20 | 20 | 100/6 | 110/60 | 3.4 | − |
| −4 | 18 | 43/8 | 45/25 | 26 | 97/30 | 97/68 | 2.7 | +† |
| | | | CARDIAC TRANSPLANT OCTOBER 1989 | | | | | |
| +12 | 7 | 25/7 | 28/9 | 8 | 99/11 | 101/61 | 5 | 0 |
| +24 | 3 | 30/8 | 32/10 | 12 | 119/9 | 118/67 | 4.3 | 0 |
| +30 | − | −/− | −/− | − | −/− | −/− | − | +† |
| +66 | 7 | 27/7 | 30/14 | 13 | −/− | −/− | − | +† |
| +69 | | | DIED SUDDENLY AT HOME JULY 1995 | | | | | |

* In mm Hg.
† In walls of intramural vessels and their lumens only.
CO = cardiac output; CT = cardiac transplantation; LV = left ventricle; PA = pulmonary artery; PAW = pulmonary artery wedge; RA = right atrium; RV = right ventricle; s/d = peak systole/end-diastole; − = not done; + = present or positive; 0 = absent or negative.

| **TABLE III** Morphologic Cardiac Findings | | |
|---|---|---|
| Location of Amyloid by Light Microscopy | Native Heart | Donor Heart |
| Myocardial Interstitium (0–4+) | 0 | 0 |
| Intramural coronary arteries (0–4+) | | |
| Walls | ++++ | ++++ |
| Lumens | +++ | +++ |
| Epicardium (0–4+) | | |
| Walls of small coronary vessels | ++++ | ++++ |
| Lumens of small coronary vessels | + | + |
| Perivascular regions | +++ | +++ |
| Parietal pericardium | − | +++* |

* Of native heart.

14, and 15 months, respectively, after CT of noncardiac amyloidosis and 1 is still alive 49 months after CT.

Our patient had amyloid in both native and donor hearts limited to the walls of intramural coronary vessels often narrowing their lumens without amyloid deposits in myocardial interstitium. Nevertheless, there was evidence of cardiac dysfunction, i.e., heart failure before the CT but never afterwards. Our patient never had evidence of angina pectoris, something that has been observed with cardiac amyloidosis limited to intramyocardial vessels,[7] but he did die suddenly at home with documented ventricular fibrillation. At necropsy, none of the lumens of the major epicardial coronary arteries were significantly narrowed. It therefore appears reasonable to attribute his sudden unexpected death to the focal but extensive luminal narrowing by amyloid of numerous intramural coronary arteries.

Cardiac transplantation in cardiac amyloidosis, of course, provides the opportunity to compare cardiac function both before and after heart replacement (Table II). His indirect systemic arterial blood pressure fell progressively before CT, rose immediately thereafter, and fell again approximately at a time corresponding to cardiac endomyocardial biopsies showing amyloid in the walls of intramural coronary vessels (Figure 1). Furthermore, total 12-lead QRS voltage[8] fell to 63 mm (10 mm = 1 mV) just before CT, rose shortly after CT to a peak of 130 mm (>100% increase) and fell after amyloid was again found in endomyocardial biopsy, to 84 mm (Figure 2).

Now to the question posed in the introduction: Is CT worthwhile in patients with cardiac amyloidosis causing severe cardiac dysfunction? At the moment, the answer remains uncertain. Some persons benefit enormously, Dr. Hall, our patient, for example. Dr. Hall, who lived 118 months after CT, developed angina pectoris during his last several years of life. Our patient, who lived 69 months after CT, died suddenly without significant epicardial coronary artery disease. Our patient, however, had severe narrowing of numerous intramural coronary arteries and Dr. Hall did as well (personal communication, P.N. Hawkins, MD, July 30, 1996): neither had amyloid in the myocardial interstitium. It may be that CT will prove to be worthwhile if cardiac amyloid deposits are limited to the walls and lumina of intramural coronary arteries, but not worthwhile if myocardial interstitium is the major location of the amyloid deposits.

**In summary, a patient is described who developed severe cardiac dysfunction from amyloid deposited entirely in the walls and lumens of intramural coronary arteries, underwent CT, survived another 69 months, died suddenly, and at necropsy had amyloid again limited to the walls and lumens of the intramyocardial coronary arteries in the donor heart. The rather lengthy survival in this patient and the 118-month survival in a similar previously reported patient suggests that CT may be an appropriate procedure for some patients with cardiac amyloidosis.**

1. Conner R, Hosenpud JD, Norman DJ, Pantely GA, Cobanoglu MA, Starr A. Heart transplantation

for cardiac amyloidosis: successful one-year outcome despite recurrence of the disease. *J Heart Transplant* 1988;7:165–167.

**2.** Valentine HA, Billingham ME. Recurrence of amyloid in a cardiac allograft four months after transplantation. *J Heart Transplant* 1989;8:337–341.

**3.** Hosenpud JD, DeMarco T, Frazier H, Griffith BP, Uretsky BF, Menkis AH, O'Connell JB, Olivari M-T, Valentine HA. Progression of systemic disease and reduced long-term survival in patients with cardiac amyloidosis undergoing heart transplantation: follow-up results of a multicenter survey. *Circulation* 1991;84(suppl III):III-338–III-343.

**4.** Deng M, Park J-W, Roy-Chowdury R, Knieriem H-J, Reinhard U, Heinrich KW. Heart transplantation for restrictive cardiomyopathy: development of cardiac amyloidosis in preexisting monoclonal gammopathy. *J Heart Lung Transplant* 1992; 11:139–141.

**5.** Hall R, Hawkins PN. Cardiac transplantation for AL amyloidosis. *Br Med J* 1994;309:1135–1137.

**6.** Dubrey S, Simms RW, Skinner M, Falk RH. Recurrence of primary (AL) amyloidosis in a transplanted heart with four-year survival. *Am J Cardiol* 1995;76:739–741.

**7.** Saffitz JE, Sazama K, Roberts WC. Amyloidosis limited to small arteries causing angina pectoris and sudden death. *Am J Cardiol* 1983;51:1234–1235.

**8.** Roberts WC, Waller BF. Cardiac amyloidosis causing cardiac dysfunction: analysis of 54 necropsy patients. *Am J Cardiol* 1983; 52:137–146.

# Cardiac Transplantation in Adults With Small Hearts

Thomas A. Waller, MD, John E. Capehart, MD, and William C. Roberts, MD

Most persons with symptomatic heart disease have hearts of increased mass. A study of nearly 900 patients with fatal coronary artery disease showed that 80% had hearts of increased weight (≥350 g in women; ≥400 g in men).[1] In patients with valvular heart disease, cardiomyopathy and congenital heart disease, well over 90% have hearts of increased weight.[2–7] In a recent study of 100 native hearts explanted at the time of cardiac transplantation, 91 had hearts weighing >300 g (most of the atrial walls are not included in hearts explanted for cardiac transplantation). This report briefly describes findings in the 9 patients whose explanted heart at cardiac transplantation weighed <300 g.

• • •

Pertinent clinical and morphologic features in the 9 patients are summarized in Table I. Their ages ranged from 24 to 65 years (mean 42); 5 were women and 4 were men. Two had ischemic cardiomyopathy, 2 had hypertrophic cardiomyopathy, 3 had idiopathic dilated cardiomyopathy, 1 had adriamycin toxicity, and 1 had sarcoidosis involving both lung and heart with severe pulmonary hypertension. All but 1 patient (case #8) had dilated right and left ventricular (>4 cm maximal internal diameter) cavities. Four patients (#1 to #4) had large transmural scars of the left ventricular free wall with or without similar scarring of the ventricular septum, 1 (case #4) had transmural left ventricular necrosis (acute myocardial infarction), none had intracardiac thrombi, and 2 (cases #3 and 4) had severe (>75% cross-sectional area) narrowing of ≥1 major epicardial coronary artery and each had 3 major arteries so narrowed. Except for 1 patient (#2), who was studied >1 year before cardiac transplantation, all had left ventricular ejection fractions ≤40%. Eight had right ventricular peak systolic pressures >30 mm Hg, and 7 had pulmonary arterial wedge pressures and left ventricular end-diastolic pressures >12 mm Hg. Seven of 8 had total 12-lead QRS voltage <175 mm (1 mV = 10 mm).[8] Four (cases #1, 5, 8, and 9) had atrial fibrillation and 1 (case #3) had runs of ventricular tachycardia. All had PR intervals ≤0.20 second. One patient (case #5) had complete bundle branch block (left).

• • •

The heretofore described patients all had excised recipient hearts at the time of cardiac transplantation weighing <300 g. Little published information is available on weights of individual native hearts excised at the time of cardiac transplantation, and much less information on explanted hearts weighing <300 g. Were the weights of the left and right atrial walls included in the explanted heart weights, most or all still would have weighed <350 g.

From the Departments of Medicine (Division of Cardiology), Cardiothoracic Surgery, and Pathology and the Baylor Cardiovascular Institute, Baylor University Medical Center, Dallas, Texas. Dr. Roberts' address is: Baylor Cardiovascular Institute, Baylor University Medical Center, 3500 Gaston Avenue, Dallas, Texas 75246. Manuscript received April 1, 1997; revised manuscript received and accepted May 4, 1997.

**TABLE I** Comparison of Explanted Native Hearts Weighing ≤300 g

| Pt. No. | Etiology | Age (yr) | G | Interval (mo) S → CT | HW (g) | BW (kg) | LVMD (cm) | H (%) | TC (mg/dl) | TG (mg/dl) | LVEDD (cm) | LVESD (cm) | LAD (cm) | VSW (cm) | LVFW (cm) | MR (0–4) | TR (0–4) | LVEF (%) | ECG Total QRS Voltage (mm) | SA (s/d) | LV (s/d) | RV (s/d) | RA (mean) | PAW (mean) | CI (L/min/m²) |
|---|---|---|---|---|---|---|---|---|---|---|---|---|---|---|---|---|---|---|---|---|---|---|---|---|---|
| | Patient Demographics | | | | Morphology | | | Laboratory | | | Echocardiogram | | | | | | | | ECG | Pressures (mm Hg) | | | | | |
| 1 | HC* | 37 | F | 216 | 290 | — | — | — | — | — | 4.5 | 3.4 | 5.4 | 1.4 | 1.0 | 2 | — | 40 | 172 | 120/60 | 110/17 | 47/8 | 6 | 32 | 2.9 |
| 2 | HC* | 43 | F | 36 | 220 | 60 | 5 | 39 | 183 | 98 | 3.7 | 2.5 | 5.0 | 1.8 | 1.3 | 2 | 2 | 60 | 287 | 100/60 | — | 41/17 | 15 | 27 | 1.3 |
| 3 | IC† | 53 | M | 6 | 260 | — | — | 33 | 260 | 658 | 4.3 | 2.9 | 3.3 | — | 1.0 | 0 | 0 | — | 91 | 125/60 | 125/40 | — | 12 | 24 | 2.4 |
| 4 | IC† | 65 | M | 1 | 280 | — | 5 | — | — | — | — | — | — | — | — | — | — | 30 | 97 | 140/80 | 140/40 | 45/14 | 10 | 30 | — |
| 5 | IDC‡ | 28 | F | 3 | 280 | 62 | 5 | 39 | 180 | 200 | 6.0 | — | 3.0 | — | — | 0 | 2 | 15 | 121 | 128/60 | — | 16/6 | 0 | 3 | 2.5 |
| 6 | IDC‡ | 36 | F | 42 | 290 | 57 | 6 | 31 | 138 | 57 | 5.7 | 4.8 | — | — | — | 3 | 3 | 37 | 217 | 100/86 | 98/11 | 34/5 | 4 | 14 | 3.4 |
| 7 | IDC‡ | 51 | M | 25 | 285 | 92 | 4 | 27 | 121 | 70 | 6.2 | 5.0 | 4.7 | 0.7 | 0.8 | 2 | 4 | 25 | 60 | 100/65 | — | 27/16 | 23 | 24 | 2.0 |
| 8 | Adriamycin | 24 | M | 24 | 275 | 38 | — | 33 | 142 | 110 | — | — | — | — | — | 4 | 4 | 17 | — | 86/60 | — | 34/5 | 5 | 10 | 2.1 |
| 9 | Sarcoid | 42 | F | 48 | 300 | 81 | — | 45 | 129 | 133 | 5.5 | 3.0 | 3.7 | 1.2 | 0.8 | 2 | 3 | 30 | 175 | 136/90 | 125/7 | 77/14 | 14 | 15 | 1.4 |

*Among a total of 10 patients with dilated hypertrophic cardiomyopathy.
†Among 47 patients with ischemic cardiomyopathy.
‡Among 35 patients with idiopathic dilated cardiomyopathy.
BW = body weight; CI = cardiac index; CT = cardiac transplantation; G = gender; H = hematocrit; HC = hypertrophic cardiomyopathy; HW = heart weight; IC = ischemic cardiomyopathy; IDC = idiopathic dilated cardiomyopathy; LAD = left atrial diameter; LV = left ventricle; LVEDD = left ventricular end-diastolic diameter; LVEF = left ventricular ejection fraction; LVESD = left ventricular end-systolic diameter; LVMD = left ventricular maximum diameter; LVFW = left ventricular free wall; mo = months; MR = mitral regurgitation; PAW = pulmonary artery wedge; RA = right atrium; RV = right ventricle; S = symptoms; SA = systemic arterial; S/D = peak systole/end diastole; TC = total cholesterol; TG = triglyceride; TR = tricuspid regurgitation; VSW = ventricular septal width.

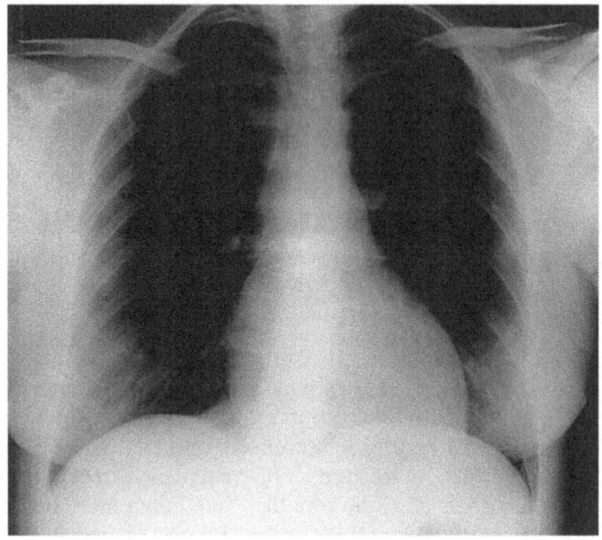

**FIGURE 1. Anteroposterior chest radiograph just before cardiac transplantation in patient 5 demonstrating a normal-sized cardiac silhouette.**

Why were the heart weights in these 9 patients small or at least not increased in mass? Several factors may be responsible: (1) *Gender:* Five of the 9 patients were women and, in general, women have smaller hearts than men. (2) *Small people:* Small adults tend to have smaller hearts than large adults. Seven of the 9 patients weighed <65 kg (<140 lbs) including 1 patient (#5) who weighed only 39 kg. (3) *Extensive left ventricular scarring:* Scarred left ventricular walls weigh less than nonscarred left ventricular walls. Four of the 9 patients had extensive left ventricular wall scarring and a fifth patient (#8) had a small left ventricular scar. (4) *Unusual kind of heart disease:* One patient (case #9) had pulmonary sarcoidosis and underwent combined heart and lung transplantation primarily because of severe pulmonary hypertension. (The fact that the patient had sarcoidosis as the cause of the pulmonary hypertension was not diagnosed until both the heart and lungs had been excised at the time of transplantation. The excised heart also had small sarcoid implants.) However, pulmonary hypertension, although, it increases the weight of the right ventricular wall, the overall weight of the heart increases only a small amount. One patient (case #8) had adriamycin toxicity and this condition may not cause an increase in cardiac mass. Of 12 reported patients ≥18 years of age with clinical evidence of anthracycline toxicity, the hearts ranged in weight from 240 to 500 g (mean 335).[9]

**In summary, cardiac transplantation is performed in some adults having cardiac conditions causing considerable cardiac dysfunction in the absence of an increase in cardiac mass.**

1. Roberts WC, Potkin BN, Solus DE, Reddy SG. Mode of death, frequency of healed and acute myocardial infarction, number of major epicardial coronary arteries severely narrowed by atherosclerotic plaque, and heart weight in fatal

atherosclerotic coronary artery disease: Analysis of 889 patients studied at necropsy. *J Am Coll Cardiol* 1990;15:196–203.
2. Roberts WC. The congenitally bicuspid aortic valve. A study of 85 autopsy cases. *Am J Cardiol* 1970;49:151–159.
3. Roberts WC. Anatomically isolated aortic valvular disease. The case against its being of rheumatic etiology. *Am J Med* 1970;49:151–159.
4. Roberts WC, Perloff JK, Costantino T. Severe valvular aortic stenosis in patients over 65 years of age. A clinicopathologic study. *Am J Cardiol* 1971;27:497–506.
5. Roberts WC, Waller BF. Cardiac amyloidosis causing cardiac dysfunction: analysis of 54 necropsy patients. *Am J Cardiol* 1983;52:137–147.
6. Roberts WC, Siegel RJ, McManus BM. Idiopathic dilated cardiomyopathy. Analysis of 152 necropsy patients. *Am J Cardiol* 1987;60:1340–1355.
7. Roberts CS, Roberts WC. Morphologic features (of hypertrophic cardiomyopathy). *Prog Cardiol* 1989;2/2:3–32.
8. Siegel RJ, Roberts WC. Electrocardiographic observations in severe aortic valve stenosis: correlative necropsy study to clinical, hemodynamic, and ECG variables demonstrating relation of 12-lead QRS amplitude to peak systolic transaortic pressure gradient. *Am Heart J* 1982;103:210–221.
9. Isner JM, Ferrans VJ, Cohen SR, Witkind BG, Virmani R, Gottdiener JS, Beck JR, Roberts WC. Clinical and morphologic cardiac findings after anthracycline chemotherapy. Analysis of 64 patients studied at necropsy. *Am J Cardiol* 1983;51:1167–1174.

# Comparison of Clinical and Morphologic Cardiac Findings in Patients Having Cardiac Transplantation for Ischemic Cardiomyopathy, Idiopathic Dilated Cardiomyopathy, and Dilated Hypertrophic Cardiomyopathy

Thomas A. Waller, MD,* William L. Hiser, MD,† John E. Capehart, MD, and William C. Roberts, MD

**This article compares intergroup and intragroup clinical and morphologic findings in patients with ischemic cardiomyopathy (IC), idiopathic dilated cardiomyopathy (IDC), and dilated hypertrophic cardiomyopathy (HC) undergoing cardiac transplantation (CT). Few previous publications have described findings in native hearts explanted at the time of CT. The explanted heart in 92 patients having CT was examined in uniform manner with particular attention to the sizes of the ventricular cavities and the presence of and extent of ventricular scarring. Of the 92 hearts examined, 47 had IC, 35 had IDC, and 10 had dilated HC. Although considerable degrees of intragroup variation occurred, the mean degree of left ventricular dilatation was similar among the patients with IC, IDC, and dilated HC. All patients with IC had left ventricular free wall scarring more extensive than that involving the ventricular septum, but the intragroup variation in the amounts of scarring was considerable. Nine of the 10 patients with dilated HC also had ventricular wall scarring, but it was more extensive in the ventricular septum than in the left ventricular free wall and involvement of the right ventricular wall also was present. Eight (23%) of the 35 IDC patients also had grossly visible ventricular scars but they were small and only 1 of the 8 had coronary narrowing and that was not in the distribution of the scarring. Narrowing of 1 or more epicardial coronary arteries >75% in cross-sectional area by plaque was present in all 47 IC patients, in 8 of the 35 IDC patients (7 had no ventricular scars), and in none of the 10 dilated HC patients. Coronary angiography was the major clinical tool allowing separation of the IC, IDC, and HC patients. Coronary angiography did not detect narrowing in any of the 8 patients with IDC who were found to have coronary narrowing on anatomic study. Thus, among patients with IC, IDC, and dilated HC having CT, distinctive anatomic features allow separation of patients with IC, IDC, and dilated HC, but within each group considerable variation in left ventricular cavity size and extent of ventricular scarring occurs.** ©1998 by Excerpta Medica, Inc.

**(Am J Cardiol 1998;81:884–894)**

Cardiac transplantation (CT) has become a recognized therapy for the treatment of patients with irreversible and intractable heart failure. Each year approximately 3,000 patients have CT worldwide.[1] We have studied in uniform fashion the recipient's native explanted heart in 92 patients having CT for 1 of 3 different conditions: ischemic cardiomyopathy (IC), idiopathic dilated cardiomyopathy (IDC), and dilated hypertrophic cardiomyopathy (HC). Review of previously published articles on CT surprisingly have provided few details of native hearts excised at the time of CT. This report describes various morphologic features in these hearts explanted for these 3 conditions and correlates electrocardiographic, echocardiographic, and hemodynamic findings with the morphologic changes.

## PATIENTS STUDIED AND METHODS

**Sources of cases:** Of the 92 patients, the cardiac transplant operation was performed at Baylor University Medical Center in 58 (63%) from March 1, 1993, until June 2, 1997. Each heart was examined, weighed (each on the same accurate scales), and described initially by WCR. Most were reexamined by TAW and WLH. The remaining 34 recipient hearts (37%) were submitted to the Pathology Branch of the National Heart, Lung, and Blood Institute in Bethesda, Maryland, from 1977 until 1993. The submitting institutions were Fairfax Hos-

From the Departments of Medicine, Cardiothoracic Surgery, and Pathology, and the Baylor Cardiovascular Institute, Baylor University Medical Center, Dallas, Texas. Manuscript received November 18, 1997; revised manuscript received and accepted January 6, 1998.

Address for reprints: William C. Roberts, MD, Baylor Cardiovascular Institute, Baylor University Medical Center, 3500 Gaston Avenue, Dallas, Texas 75246.

*Present address: 1600 Coit Road, Suite 301, Plano, Texas 75075.

†Present address: Section of Cardiology, Department of Medicine, University of Nebraska Medical Center, Omaha, Nebraska 68198.

**TABLE I** Clinical and Morphologic Findings in the 47 Patients With Ischemic Cardiomyopathy

| Patient Demographics | | | | Morphology | | | | | | Laboratory | | | Echocardiogram | |
|---|---|---|---|---|---|---|---|---|---|---|---|---|---|---|
| Pt. No. | Age (yr) | Sex | Interval (mo) S→CT | HW (g) | BW (kg) | T | CABG (grafts) | CA >75% ↓ | LVMD (cm) | H (%) | TC (mg/dl) | TG (mg/dl) | LVEDD (cm) | LVESD (cm) |
| 1 | 42 | M | 12 | 325 | 70 | 0 | 0 | 4 | 5.5 | 44 | 308 | 138 | — | — |
| 2 | 43 | M | 5 | 380 | 64 | 0 | 0 | 3 | 7.0 | 23 | 241 | 286 | — | — |
| 3 | 43 | M | 60 | 450 | — | +(LV) | 0 | 1 | 5.5 | — | 308 | — | — | — |
| 4 | 43 | M | 6 | — | — | 0 | 0 | 2 | — | — | — | — | — | — |
| 5 | 45 | M | 8 | 475 | 76 | 0 | 0 | 1 | 6.5 | 30 | 135 | 50 | 7.4 | 6.4 |
| 6 | 45 | M | — | 305 | — | 0 | +(4) | 4 | 4.0 | — | — | — | — | — |
| 7 | 46 | F | 4 | 365 | 73 | 0 | +(4) | 3 | — | 41 | 126 | 243 | 5.0 | 4.0 |
| 8 | 46 | M | 14 | — | 74 | 0 | +(1) | 3 | — | 50 | 168 | — | — | — |
| 9 | 49 | M | 8 | 351 | 58 | 0 | +(3) | 4 | 5.0 | 38 | 252 | 74 | 6.2 | 5.5 |
| 10 | 49 | M | 24 | 490 | 72 | 0 | 0 | 3 | 6.5 | 39 | 167 | 188 | 8.0 | — |
| 11 | 50 | M | 15 | 345 | 91 | 0 | 0 | 1 | 5.0 | 43 | 162 | 316 | 6.2 | 4.8 |
| 12 | 50 | M | 84 | 570 | 89 | 0 | +(1) | 3 | 6.0 | 42 | 125 | 115 | 6.5 | 5.8 |
| 13 | 50 | M | 30 | 395 | 78 | 0 | 0 | 3 | 6.5 | 30 | 180 | 97 | 5.5 | 4.8 |
| 14 | 51 | M | 11 | 440 | 73 | 0 | +(2) | 4 | — | 34 | 247 | 278 | 6.9 | 6.3 |
| 15 | 51 | M | 30 | 565 | 71 | +(LV) | 0 | 3 | 5.0 | 40 | 242 | 115 | — | — |
| 16 | 51 | M | 36 | 503 | 72 | 0 | +(3) | 3 | 5.0 | 46 | 155 | 54 | 7.0 | 6.0 |
| 17 | 51 | M | 7 | 450 | 70 | 0 | 0 | 2 | 5.5 | 32 | 194 | 90 | — | — |
| 18 | 52 | M | 41 | 510 | 75 | 0 | +(2) | 3 | 4.0 | 32 | 334 | 296 | 8.0 | 7.0 |
| 19 | 52 | M | 24 | 565 | — | 0 | +(3) | 3 | 5.0 | — | 240 | — | — | — |
| 20 | 53 | M | 6 | 260 | — | 0 | 0 | 3 | — | 33 | 260 | 658 | 4.3 | 2.9 |
| 21 | 53 | M | 11 | 535 | 96 | 0 | +(4) | 3 | 6.3 | 42 | 264 | — | — | — |
| 22 | 54 | M | 1 | 500 | — | 0 | 0 | 3 | — | — | 226 | — | — | — |
| 23 | 55 | M | 108 | 490 | 74 | 0 | +(3) | 4 | 5.5 | 37 | 158 | 156 | 6.0 | 5.5 |
| 24 | 55 | M | — | 430 | — | 0 | +(3) | 3 | — | — | — | — | — | — |
| 25 | 56 | M | 240 | 520 | 85 | 0 | +(3) | 2 | 6.0 | 43 | 204 | 180 | 6.5 | — |
| 26 | 56 | M | 15 | 430 | 82 | 0 | 0 | 4 | 6.0 | 39 | 280 | 501 | — | — |
| 27 | 56 | F | 60 | 385 | 50 | 0 | 0 | 3 | 6.0 | 30 | 219 | 168 | 6.2 | 5.7 |
| 28 | 56 | M | 33 | 720 | 103 | 0 | 0 | 2 | 7.9 | 31 | 240 | 123 | 7.4 | 6.2 |
| 29 | 56 | M | 36 | — | — | 0 | +(4) | 4 | — | — | — | — | — | — |
| 30 | 57 | M | 24 | 415 | 77 | 0 | 0 | 3 | 5.5 | 37 | 183 | 96 | 6.5 | 5.0 |
| 31 | 57 | M | 144 | 535 | 90 | 0 | +(2) | 3 | 6.5 | 34 | 227 | 147 | 8.0 | — |
| 32 | 57 | M | 4 | — | — | 0 | +(4) | 3 | — | 31 | 174 | — | — | — |
| 33 | 57 | M | 1 | — | — | 0 | 0 | 1 | — | — | — | — | — | — |
| 34 | 58 | M | 11 | 352 | 75 | 0 | +(4) | 4 | — | 35 | 281 | 147 | 4.3 | 3.8 |
| 35 | 58 | M | 56 | 580 | 99 | 0 | +(4) | 1 | 3.5 | 38 | 267 | 170 | — | — |
| 36 | 58 | M | 12 | 590 | 70 | 0 | +(4) | 4 | 6.6 | 37 | 132 | — | — | — |
| 37 | 59 | M | 8 | 390 | — | 0 | 0 | 1 | 5.5 | — | — | — | 7.0 | 6.5 |
| 38 | 59 | M | 13 | 490 | 88 | 0 | +(3) | 3 | 5.3 | 35 | 105 | 65 | 6.5 | 5.1 |
| 39 | 60 | M | 21 | 365 | 72 | +(LV) | 0 | 2 | 6.0 | 42 | 146 | 69 | 7.5 | 6.0 |
| 40 | 60 | M | 31 | 610 | 74 | 0 | 0 | 2 | 6.0 | 30 | 131 | 106 | 6.0 | — |
| 41 | 61 | M | 12 | 690 | 94 | 0 | +(4) | 3 | 6.5 | 39 | 198 | 147 | 5.7 | 4.2 |
| 42 | 61 | M | 47 | 385 | 77 | 0 | +(4) | 3 | 6.7 | 36 | 202 | 73 | 6.4 | 6.1 |
| 43 | 62 | F | 120 | 480 | 66 | 0 | 0 | 3 | 6.5 | 35 | 161 | 232 | 7.8 | 7.1 |
| 44 | 62 | M | 24 | 503 | 68 | 0 | 0 | 2 | 6.5 | 40 | 217 | — | 8.8 | 7.2 |
| 45 | 63 | M | 13 | 450 | 84 | 0 | +(3) | 3 | 4.5 | 33 | 209 | 83 | 6.0 | 4.8 |
| 46 | 63 | M | 36 | 750 | 80 | 0 | 0 | 3 | 6.3 | 42 | — | — | — | — |
| 47 | 65 | M | 1 | 280 | — | 0 | 0 | 3 | 5.0 | — | — | — | — | — |

*When not in atrial fibrillation.

AF = atrial fibrillation; BBB = bundle branch block; BW = body weight; CABG = coronary artery bypass graft; CHB = complete heart block; CI = cardiac index; CT = cardiac transplantation; H = hematocrit; HW = heart weight; L = left; LAD = left atrial diameter; LV = left ventricle; LVEDD = left ventricular end-diastolic diameter; LVEF = left ventricular ejection fraction; LVESD = left ventricular end systolic diameter; LVFW = left ventricular free wall; LVMD = left ventricular maximum diameter; MR = mitral regurgitation; PAW = pulmonary artery wedge; R = right; RA = right atrium; RV = right ventricle; S = symptoms; SA = systemic arterial; s/d = peak systole/end diastole; T = thrombus; TC = total cholesterol; TG = triglyceride; TR = tricuspid regurgitation; VSW = ventricular septal width; VT = ventricular tachycardia; + = positive or present; 0 = negative or absent; — = no information available.

pital, Fairfax, Virginia; Medical College of Virginia, Richmond, Virginia; Georgetown University Medical Center, George Washington University Medical Center, and Washington Hospital Center, all in Washington, DC. During this time WCR was Chief of the Pathology Branch and he examined each heart and also histologic sections of the heart prepared in the same manner as the cases studied at Baylor University Medical Center. Nine of the 10 cases having dilated HC have been reported previously elsewhere.[2]

**Methods of examining the recipient hearts:** The hearts in each of the 92 patients were examined and described initially by WCR. The cardiac ven-

**TABLE I** (Continued)

| Echocardiogram | | | | | | | Electrocardiogram | | | | Pressures (mm Hg) | | | | | | | |
|---|---|---|---|---|---|---|---|---|---|---|---|---|---|---|---|---|---|---|
| LAD (cm) | VSW (cm) | LVFW (cm) | MR (0–4) | TR (0–4) | LVEF (%) | BBB | Total QRS Voltage (mm) | AF | VT | PR (>200 ms) | SA (s/d) | LV (s/d) | RV (s/d) | PA (s/d) | RA (mean) | PAW (mean) | CI (L/min/m²) |
| — | — | — | 2 | 2 | 15 | 0 | 120 | 0 | 0 | 0 | 106/70 | — | 36/3 | 36/14 | 0 | 19 | 2.7 |
| — | — | — | — | — | 28 | +(L) | 129 | 0 | 0 | 0 | 121/60 | — | 29/2 | 25/14 | 1 | 10 | — |
| — | — | — | — | — | 8 | — | — | — | — | — | — | — | — | — | — | — | — |
| — | — | — | — | — | 10 | 0 | — | 0 | 0 | 0 | — | — | — | — | — | — | — |
| 5.0 | 1.2 | 1.3 | 2 | 2 | 20 | 0 | 101 | + | + | AF | 100/60 | — | 47/15 | 46/23 | 5 | 27 | 2.4 |
| — | — | — | — | — | — | — | — | — | — | — | — | — | — | — | — | — | — |
| 4.0 | 1.2 | 1.1 | — | — | 23 | 0 | 131 | 0 | + | 0 | 146/79 | 115/24 | 31/3 | 35/10 | 3 | 7 | 3.1 |
| — | — | — | — | — | 30 | +(L) | 83 | 0 | + | 0 | 120/80 | 130/28 | — | — | — | — | — |
| 4.6 | 0.5 | 1.0 | 4 | 4 | 15 | 0 | 188 | 0 | 0 | 0 | 100/78 | 92/3 | 30/10 | 33/13 | 3 | 10 | 2.1 |
| 4.5 | — | — | 3 | 2 | 20 | 0 | 220 | 0 | 0 | 0 | 142/80 | — | 58/9 | 48/21 | 4 | 27 | 1.8 |
| 5.2 | 0.7 | 0.7 | 4 | 1 | 37 | 0 | 97 | + | + | +* | 118/94 | — | 39/9 | 39/17 | 4 | 19 | 2.2 |
| 3.0 | 1.0 | 1.0 | 1 | 1 | 25 | +(L) | 120 | 0 | 0 | + | 100/60 | — | 34/1 | 34/19 | 8 | 14 | 1.5 |
| 4.0 | — | — | — | 0 | 20 | 0 | 87 | 0 | + | 0 | 118/76 | — | 21/7 | 25/8 | 2 | 7 | 1.9 |
| 4.2 | 0.8 | 0.9 | 0 | 0 | 22 | +(L) | 201 | 0 | + | 0 | 114/76 | 117/25 | 52/6 | 42/23 | 3 | 26 | — |
| — | — | — | — | — | 15 | 0 | 180 | 0 | 0 | 0 | 100/70 | 93/13 | 31/6 | 26/ | 3 | 5 | 3.3 |
| 4.5 | 0.8 | 1.0 | 2 | 0 | 25 | 0 | 74 | + | 0 | AF | 92/60 | — | 46/11 | 39/24 | 8 | 22 | 2.9 |
| — | — | — | 3 | — | — | 0 | 86 | 0 | 0 | 0 | 84/66 | 77/23 | 65/14 | 67/32 | 13 | 24 | 1.2 |
| 4.5 | 0.9 | 0.9 | 3 | 0 | 15 | 0 | 138 | + | 0 | 0* | 121/52 | — | 25/1 | 23/8 | 3 | 8 | — |
| — | — | — | — | — | 15 | +(R) | — | 0 | — | — | — | — | — | 55/30 | — | 27 | — |
| 3.3 | — | 1.0 | 0 | 0 | — | 0 | 91 | 0 | + | 0 | 125/60 | 125/40 | — | 64/22 | 12 | 24 | 2.4 |
| — | — | — | — | — | 11 | — | — | — | — | — | 140/90 | — | — | — | — | — | — |
| — | — | — | — | — | 15 | — | — | — | — | — | — | — | — | — | 12 | 12 | — |
| 4.0 | 1.0 | 1.0 | 2 | 0 | 20 | +(R) | 152 | 0 | 0 | 0 | 116/74 | 112/39 | — | 34/15 | — | 12 | 2.0 |
| — | — | — | — | — | — | — | — | — | — | — | — | — | — | — | — | — | — |
| 5.0 | — | — | 3 | 3 | 25 | 0 | 133 | 0 | 0 | + | 100/60 | — | 58/15 | 55/26 | 15 | 30 | 2.0 |
| — | — | — | — | — | 20 | 0 | 184 | 0 | 0 | 0 | 116/57 | — | 32/11 | 28/13 | 5 | 9 | 2.5 |
| — | — | — | 4 | 2 | 13 | 0 | 159 | 0 | 0 | + | 100/56 | — | — | 35/20 | — | 14 | 2.7 |
| 5.3 | 1.3 | 1.3 | 3 | 3 | 20 | 0 | 97 | + | + | +* | 97/56 | — | 59/4 | 61/25 | 3 | 19 | 2.6 |
| — | — | — | — | — | — | — | — | — | — | — | — | — | — | — | — | — | — |
| 4.5 | 1.0 | 1.0 | 1 | 0 | 28 | 0 | 86 | 0 | 0 | 0 | 110/60 | 98/7 | 41/6 | 30/2 | 0 | 5 | 2.5 |
| 5.0 | 0.8 | 0.8 | 3 | 2 | 25 | 0 | 234 | 0 | + | + | 95/60 | — | 34/7 | 33/10 | 5 | 7 | 2.2 |
| — | — | — | — | — | — | 0 | 108 | 0 | 0 | 0 | 120/60 | 120/25 | 37/8 | 38/20 | — | 7 | — |
| — | — | — | — | — | — | — | — | — | + | — | — | — | — | — | — | — | — |
| 4.1 | 1.4 | 1.6 | — | — | 40 | 0 | 115 | 0 | 0 | 0 | — | — | 21/8 | 19/7 | 6 | 7 | 2.2 |
| 5.0 | — | — | 2 | 2 | 30 | 0 | 154 | 0 | 0 | 0 | 120/80 | — | 22/7 | 47/7 | 1 | 9 | 2.4 |
| — | — | — | — | — | 10 | — | — | — | — | — | 100/60 | — | 47/14 | 47/28 | 15 | 27 | 2.0 |
| — | — | — | 2 | — | 15 | — | — | 0 | + | — | 98/70 | — | — | 25/12 | 3 | 8 | — |
| 5.1 | 1.2 | 1.1 | 3 | 1 | 19 | — | — | — | — | — | 103/70 | — | 60/14 | 56/33 | 12 | 26 | 1.9 |
| 4.5 | 1.0 | 1.0 | 2 | 0 | 20 | +(R) | 70 | 0 | 0 | + | 112/82 | — | 50/11 | 46/24 | 13 | 28 | 1.8 |
| 5.0 | 1.1 | 1.1 | 4 | 3 | 15 | 0 | 128 | + | + | AF | 105/62 | — | — | 50/29 | 9 | 30 | 2.5 |
| 4.1 | 1.0 | 1.0 | — | — | 25 | +(L) | 132 | 0 | + | + | 138/55 | — | 28/5 | 20/6 | 2 | 4 | — |
| 4.4 | 0.8 | 0.7 | 3 | 3 | 15 | 0 | 98 | + | + | +* | 94/62 | 95/14 | 32/9 | 32/13 | 5 | 12 | 1.7 |
| 4.8 | 0.7 | 0.9 | 1 | 0 | 15 | +(L) | 172 | 0 | 0 | 0 | 110/59 | 106/10 | 30/5 | 23/11 | 2 | 10 | 2.7 |
| 4.1 | 1 | 1.1 | 4 | 2 | 8 | +(L) | — | 0 | — | — | 90/60 | 90/26 | — | 40/16 | — | 18 | 2.5 |
| 4.6 | 1.2 | 1.2 | 0 | 0 | 20 | +(CHB) | 94 | + | 0 | CHB | 100/60 | — | 43/12 | 44/19 | 13 | 22 | 2.8 |
| — | — | — | — | 3 | — | — | — | — | — | — | 160/90 | 160/44 | 50/10 | 50/30 | 7 | 24 | 2.4 |
| — | — | — | — | — | 30 | 0 | 97 | 0 | 0 | + | 140/80 | 140/40 | 45/14 | 45/28 | 10 | 30 | — |

*When not in atrial fibrillation.

AF = atrial fibrillation; BBB = bundle branch block; BW = body weight; CABG = coronary artery bypass graft; CHB = complete heart block; CI = cardiac index; CT = cardiac transplantation; H = hematocrit; HW = heart weight; L = left; LAD = left atrial diameter; LV = left ventricle; LVEDD = left ventricular end-diastolic diameter; LVEF = left ventricular ejection fraction; LVESD = left ventricular end systolic diameter; LVFW = left ventricular free wall; LVMD = left ventricular maximum diameter; MR = mitral regurgitation; PAW = pulmonary artery wedge; R = right; RA = right atrium; RV = right ventricle; S = symptoms; SA = systemic arterial; s/d = peak systole/end diastole; T = thrombus; TC = total cholesterol; TG = triglyceride; TR = tricuspid regurgitation; VSW = ventricular septal width; VT = ventricular tachycardia; + = positive or present; 0 = negative or absent; — = no information available.

tricles were cut into transverse slices about 1 cm in width beginning at the cardiac apex and extending to about 2 cm caudal to the posterior atrioventricular sulcus. The cuts were made parallel to the posterior atrioventricular sulcus. The maximum internal diameter of the left ventricular cavity, either left to right or anterior to posterior, was determined and recorded. The specimen was weighed after removing any intracavity blood or thrombus and any noncardiac epicardial attachments. The heart weight included only portions of the atrial walls and atrial septum. The major epicardial coronary arteries were incised transversely at varying intervals, usually 5-mm ones, throughout their courses. At least 4

**TABLE II** Clinical and Morphologic Findings in the 35 Patients With Idiopathic Dilated Cardiomyopathy

| Patient Demographics | | | | Morphology | | | | | | Laboratory | | | Echocardiogram | |
|---|---|---|---|---|---|---|---|---|---|---|---|---|---|---|
| Pt. No. | Age (yr) | Sex | Interval (mo) S→CT | HW (g) | BW (kg) | F | T | CA >75%↓ | LVMD (cm) | H (%) | TC (mg/dl) | TG (mg/dl) | LVEDD (cm) | LVESD (cm) |
| 1 | 14 | M | 5 | 355 | 66 | 0 | 0 | 0 | — | 33 | 111 | 85 | 8.5 | 7.5 |
| 2* | 25 | M | 4 | 480 | — | 0 | 0 | 0 | — | 31 | 116 | 70 | 7.7 | 7.4 |
| 3† | 25 | F | 1 | — | 81 | 0 | 0 | 0 | 6.5 | — | — | — | — | — |
| 4 | 26 | M | 2 | 401 | 68 | 0 | +(LV) | 0 | 5.0 | 33 | 157 | 107 | 6.9 | 6.7 |
| 5 | 26 | M | — | 890 | — | + | 0 | 0 | — | — | — | — | — | — |
| 6 | 28 | F | 23 | 371 | 84 | 0 | 0 | 0 | 5.5 | 40 | 203 | 170 | 7.5 | 6.0 |
| 7 | 28 | F | 3 | 280 | 62 | 0 | 0 | 0 | 5.0 | 39 | 180 | 200 | 6.0 | — |
| 8 | 28 | F | 7 | 385 | 56 | 0 | 0 | 0 | 7.0 | 33 | 151 | 62 | 6.8 | 6.4 |
| 9 | 32 | M | — | 501 | 75 | 0 | 0 | 0 | — | — | — | — | — | — |
| 10 | 36 | F | 42 | 290 | 57 | 0 | 0 | 0 | 6.3 | 31 | 138 | 57 | 5.7 | 4.8 |
| 11 | 45 | F | 132 | 380 | 77 | 0 | 0 | 0 | 5.0 | 40 | 140 | 105 | 7.0 | 6.5 |
| 12 | 46 | M | — | 525 | — | 0 | 0 | 1 | — | — | — | — | — | — |
| 13 | 47 | M | 21 | 605 | 78 | + | 0 | 0 | 7.0 | 33 | 143 | 95 | 8.1 | 7.4 |
| 14 | 48 | F | 168 | 320 | 64 | 0 | 0 | 0 | 3.5 | 34 | 154 | 177 | — | — |
| 15 | 48 | M | 12 | 450 | 82 | 0 | 0 | 1 | 4.5 | 42 | 252 | 183 | 6.0 | — |
| 16 | 50 | F | 48 | 450 | 79 | 0 | 0 | 0 | 4.5 | 41 | 146 | 306 | — | — |
| 17 | 51 | M | 25 | 285 | 92 | + | 0 | 0 | 4.0 | 27 | 121 | 70 | 6.2 | 5.0 |
| 18 | 53 | F | 11 | 425 | 64 | 0 | 0 | 1 | — | 42 | 125 | 110 | — | — |
| 19 | 53 | F | 276 | 505 | 67 | + | 0 | 0 | 6.0 | 35 | 158 | 223 | 7.2 | 6.2 |
| 20 | 53 | M | 47 | 630 | 78 | 0 | 0 | 0 | 6.8 | 31 | 135 | 121 | 6.1 | — |
| 21 | 54 | F | 37 | 625 | 56 | + | 0 | 0 | 7.6 | 37 | 179 | 104 | 9.7 | 8.3 |
| 22 | 55 | F | 22 | 325 | 67 | 0 | 0 | 0 | 6.0 | 41 | 213 | 172 | 6.0 | 4.9 |
| 23 | 55 | M | 11 | 455 | — | 0 | 0 | 2 | — | — | 200 | — | 7.3 | — |
| 24 | 57 | F | 28 | 580 | 68 | + | 0 | 0 | 6.0 | 38 | 213 | 108 | 7.1 | 6.7 |
| 25 | 57 | F | 92 | 485 | 53 | 0 | 0 | 0 | 6.0 | 36 | 245 | 198 | 7.0 | 6.0 |
| 26 | 58 | F | 10 | 330 | 59 | 0 | 0 | 0 | — | 40 | — | — | — | — |
| 27 | 59 | F | 59 | 550 | 66 | 0 | 0 | 0 | 5.5 | 40 | 207 | 156 | 6.5 | — |
| 28 | 61 | M | 24 | 545 | 94 | 0 | 0 | 0 | 6.5 | 39 | 192 | 187 | 6.0 | — |
| 29 | 61 | M | 9 | 435 | 73 | 0 | 0 | 2 | 5.5 | 48 | 165 | 236 | 6.9 | 6.0 |
| 30§ | 62 | M | 20 | 450 | 74 | 0 | 0 | 0 | 6.0 | 40 | 181 | 109 | — | — |
| 31 | 62 | F | 24 | 425 | — | 0 | 0 | 0 | 5.9 | 39 | 155 | 100 | — | — |
| 32 | 63 | F | 86 | 475 | 45 | + | 0 | 0 | 6.0 | 36 | 137 | 67 | 7.0 | 6.0 |
| 33 | 64 | F | 55 | 325 | 51 | + | 0 | 2 | 5.5 | 33 | 192 | 397 | 6.1 | 5.7 |
| 34 | 64 | F | 22 | 310 | 78 | 0 | 0 | 0 | 3.5 | 39 | 179 | 183 | 7.0 | 6.0 |
| 35 | 66 | F | 300 | 515 | 51 | 0 | 0 | 3 | 5.0 | 35 | 207 | 61 | 7.0 | — |

*This patient had a history of androgen use and was a weightlifter.
†This patient developed symptoms of IDC during her third trimester of pregnancy.
‡When not in atrial fibrillation.
§This patient had hyperthyroidism.
CA = coronary arteries; F = fibrosis; G = gender; other abbreviations as in Table I.

hematoxylin-eosin stained sections of left ventricular myocardium (including ventricular septum) were prepared from the heart of each patient and examined with a microscope.

**Other cases studied during the same time period:** In the time period during which the heretofore mentioned 92 recipient hearts were studied, an additional 8 others also were examined and studied morphologically in similar fashion. Of these 8 other patients, 4 had valvular heart disease necessitating valve replacement, including 1 with associated atherosclerotic coronary artery disease and previous myocardial infarction. All 4 had dilated ventricles. One patient had combined heart/lung transplant because of severe pulmonary hypertension from sarcoidosis and she also had dilated ventricular cavities. One patient had significant narrowing of 3 major coronary arteries but no grossly visible myocardial scars and normal-sized ventricular cavities despite poor left ventricular function clinically. This patient also had recurring ventricular arrhythmias. One patient was treated with adriamycin for sarcoma and subsequently developed a dilated cardiomyopathy. The final patient had HC but nondilated ventricular cavities and nonscarred ventricular walls; she had CT because of severe recurring ventricular arrhythmias despite the presence of an implantable cardiac defibrillator. Of these 8 cases, 5 were studied in the Pathology Branch of the National Heart, Lung, and Blood Institute, and the other 3 at Baylor University Medical Center. These 8 patients with "other cardiac conditions" will not be further discussed in this article.

**Methods of collecting clinical data:** The hospital records were reviewed in each of the 92 patients. Most of the echocardiographic data were taken from the echocardiographic reports in the hospital charts.

**TABLE II** (Continued)

| Echocardiogram | | | | | | Electrocardiogram | | | | | Pressures (mm Hg) | | | | | | |
|---|---|---|---|---|---|---|---|---|---|---|---|---|---|---|---|---|---|
| LAD (cm) | VS (cm) | LVFW (cm) | MR (0–4) | TR (0–4) | LVEF (%) | BBB | Total QRS Voltage (mm) | AF | VT | PR (>200 ms) | SA (s/d) | LV (s/d) | RV (s/d) | PA (s/d) | RA (mean) | PAW (mean) | CI (L/min/m²) |
| — | — | — | — | — | 10 | 0 | 207 | 0 | 0 | 0 | 78/57 | 87/29 | 30/10 | 34/22 | 8 | 23 | 1.4 |
| 5.8 | 0.8 | 0.8 | — | — | 10 | 0 | 130 | 0 | 0 | 0 | 100/80 | 112/11 | 46/2 | 42/23 | — | 17 | — |
| — | — | — | — | — | — | +(R) | — | 0 | — | 0 | — | — | — | — | — | — | — |
| 5.0 | 0.9 | 1.0 | 4 | 4 | 25 | 0 | 130 | + | + | 0† | 88/57 | 87/20 | 41/7 | 41/20 | 3 | 17 | 2.9 |
| — | — | — | — | — | — | — | — | — | — | — | — | — | — | — | — | — | — |
| 5.0 | 0.8 | 0.8 | 2 | 0 | 25 | +(L) | 173 | 0 | + | 0 | 130/80 | — | 38/3 | 37/6 | 2 | 16 | — |
| 3.0 | — | — | 0 | 2 | 15 | +(L) | 121 | 0 | 0 | 0 | 128/60 | — | 16/6 | 13/ | 0 | 3 | 2.5 |
| 4.2 | 0.8 | 1.0 | 3 | 3 | 26 | +(L) | 146 | 0 | 0 | 0 | 102/66 | — | — | 38/24 | 9 | 20 | 2.0 |
| — | — | — | 2 | — | — | — | — | — | — | — | — | — | — | — | — | — | — |
| — | — | — | 3 | 3 | 37 | 0 | 217 | 0 | 0 | 0 | 100/86 | 98/11 | 34/5 | 34/14 | 4 | 14 | 3.4 |
| 5.2 | 0.8 | 0.9 | 1 | 2 | 20 | 0 | 64 | 0 | 0 | 0 | 90/60 | — | 28/0 | 28/10 | 3 | 6 | 2.7 |
| — | — | — | — | — | 9 | — | — | — | + | — | — | — | — | 69/34 | 32 | 46 | — |
| 5.8 | 0.7 | 1.0 | 3 | 3 | 15 | 0 | 307 | + | 0 | AF | 111/70 | — | 78/20 | 76/26 | 11 | 38 | 3.0 |
| — | — | — | 2 | 0 | 28 | 0 | 142 | 0 | 0 | 0 | 106/58 | 101/2 | 32/5 | 22/13 | 5 | 8 | 2.8 |
| 4.7 | 1.0 | 1.0 | — | — | 40 | 0 | 81 | + | 0 | AF | 96/78 | 93/16 | 51/17 | 53/34 | 16 | 31 | 2.5 |
| — | — | — | 3 | 2 | 16 | 0 | — | 0 | 0 | 0 | 90/65 | — | 55/10 | 45/22 | 10 | 22 | 2.4 |
| 4.7 | 0.7 | 0.8 | 2 | 4 | 25 | 0 | 60 | + | 0 | AF | 100/65 | — | 27/16 | 34/22 | 23 | 24 | 2.0 |
| — | — | — | 3 | — | 20 | +(L) | 164 | 0 | 0 | 0 | 114/75 | 110/25 | 43/13 | 39/21 | 9 | 30 | 1.6 |
| 5.3 | 1.2 | 1.2 | 2 | 1 | 13 | +(L) | 203 | 0 | 0 | 0 | 112/80 | 103/24 | 24/7 | 39/13 | 3 | 18 | 2.3 |
| 4.5 | 1.0 | 1.0 | 4 | 3 | 15 | +(R) | 53 | 0 | + | 0 | 92/55 | 104/43 | 42/6 | 51/29 | 15 | 31 | 1.3 |
| 5.3 | 0.8 | 1.0 | 4 | 3 | 20 | +(L) | 160 | + | + | 0‡ | 85/60 | — | 43/15 | 45/31 | 9 | 28 | 1.6 |
| 4.1 | 0.8 | 0.9 | 2 | 0 | 20 | 0 | 153 | 0 | 0 | 0 | 90/70 | 88/21 | 33/7 | 23/18 | 1 | 11 | 2.5 |
| — | — | — | 3 | — | 14 | +(L) | 149 | 0 | 0 | 0 | 80/56 | 80/25 | 45/15 | 40/22 | 10 | 25 | 1.5 |
| 4.3 | 1.0 | 1.0 | 2 | 0 | 14 | +(L) | 166 | 0 | 0 | 0 | 112/82 | — | 47/7 | 47/17 | 13 | 17 | 1.7 |
| 4.5 | 1.0 | 1.0 | 2 | 1 | 20 | +(L) | 236 | 0 | 0 | + | 118/80 | — | 49/7 | 50/28 | 5 | 32 | 2.0 |
| — | — | — | 4 | — | 25 | 0 | — | 0 | + | + | 128/50 | 128/12 | 55/4 | 55/23 | 4 | 27 | 3.7 |
| 4.8 | — | — | 0 | 0 | 23 | +(R) | 121 | 0 | 0 | 0 | 104/56 | 103/15 | 42/5 | 42/12 | 4 | 19 | 3.0 |
| 5.0 | — | — | 2 | 2 | 30 | 0 | 86 | + | + | AF | 92/60 | 90/19 | 52/5 | 54/25 | 11 | 30 | 1.8 |
| 6.2 | 0.8 | 0.8 | 2 | 3 | 15 | 0 | 201 | 0 | 0 | 0 | 150/80 | 126/29 | 30/5 | 28/12 | 3 | 15 | 3.2 |
| — | — | 2 | 3 | 20 | 0 | 0 | 86 | 0 | 0 | 0 | 114/64 | 108/24 | 37/3 | 37/11 | 4 | 18 | 3.3 |
| — | — | — | 3 | 3 | 19 | +(L) | — | 0 | 0 | 0 | — | — | 11/6 | — | 2 | 4 | 1.8 |
| 4.5 | 1.0 | 1.0 | 1 | 0 | 10 | +(CHB) | 168 | 0 | 0 | CHB | 120/62 | — | 30/9 | 36/15 | 2 | 11 | 2.8 |
| 4.1 | 1.1 | 1.2 | 2 | 0 | 10 | +(L) | 223 | + | + | 0‡ | 95/58 | — | 39/3 | 39/9 | 0 | 11 | 2.9 |
| 4.0 | 1.1 | 1.0 | 1 | 1 | 25 | 0 | 109 | 0 | 0 | 0 | 110/74 | 132/16 | 23/5 | 21/9 | 3 | 5 | 3.1 |
| 6.0 | — | — | 4 | 3 | 15 | 0 | 120 | + | 0 | AF | 96/60 | — | 35/15 | 42/25 | — | 22 | — |

*This patient had a history of androgen use and was a weightlifter.

†This patient developed symptoms of IDC during her third trimester of pregnancy.

‡When not in atrial fibrillation.

§This patient had hyperthyroidism.

CA = coronary arteries; F = fibrosis; G = gender; other abbreviations as in Table I.

When certain items were missing or unclear, the last echocardiogram before CT was reviewed by TAW. Each of the electrocardiograms were reviewed by TAW and the total 12-lead QRS voltage was measured by a method described elsewhere,[3] and other electrocardiographic findings also were recorded. Most data derived at cardiac catheterization were those present in the final cardiac catheterization record in the hospital chart. Where data were missing the original pressure tracings were reviewed. The interval from initial onset of symptoms of cardiac dysfunction or myocardial ischemia to CT was determined from first onset of angina or acute myocardial infarction in the case of IC, and from onset usually of evidence of heart failure or a ventricular arrhythmia in the case of IDC or dilated HC.

**Statistical analysis:** Differences between groups were determined by 2-tailed Student's *t* test or chi-square analysis (SPSS for MS Windows, version 6.1). Because the 3 groups differed in size, the Levine technique was used to test for nonhomogeneity of variances. When the degree of heterogeneity was not significant ($p > 0.05$), 1-way analysis of variance was performed to determine the differences in groups. When the Levine test was significant, Kruskal Wallis 1-way analysis of variance was used. Significance was defined as $p < 0.05$. When the results were significant, Fisher's LSD post hoc analysis was employed to determine which of the differences in group means accounted for the significance. The Tamhane's T2 post hoc analysis was used after finding a significance with Kruskal Wallis. Chi square was used to determine differences in groups when the dependent variable was measured at the nominal level (e.g., gender).

**TABLE III** Clinical and Morphologic Data in the 10 Patients With Dilated Hypertrophic Cardiomyopathy

| Demographics | | | | Morphology | | | Echocardiogram | | | | | | | | Electrocardiogram | | | | Pressures (mm Hg) | | | | | |
|---|---|---|---|---|---|---|---|---|---|---|---|---|---|---|---|---|---|---|---|---|---|---|---|---|
| Pt No. | Age (yr) | Sex | Interval (mo) S→CT | HW (g) | F | LVMD (cm) | LVEDD (cm) | LVESD (cm) | LAD (cm) | VSW (cm) | LVFW (cm) | MR (0–4) | TR (0–4) | LVEF (%) | BBB | Total QRS Voltage (mm) | AF | PR >200 ms | SA (s/d) | LV (s/d) | RV (s/d) | RA (mean) | PAW (mean) | CI (L/min/m²) |
| 1 | 19 | M | 84 | 385 | 0 | — | 4.5 | 3.3 | 5.5 | 1.3 | 1.3 | 3 | 0 | 48 | +(R) | 146 | + | AF | 120/76 | 108/24 | 50/20 | 22 | 28 | 1.8 |
| 2 | 27 | M | 132 | 340 | + | — | 4.2 | 2.9 | 5.4 | 2.0 | 1.0 | 0 | 0 | 64 | 0 | 121 | + | AF | 110/70 | 108/20 | 45/20 | 22 | 29 | 2.6 |
| 3 | 33 | F | 192 | 340 | + | — | — | — | — | 1.5 | 1.1 | 0 | 0 | — | — | — | 0 | — | 95/68 | 95/23 | 50/9 | 7 | 28 | 2.0 |
| 4 | 36 | M | 156 | 390 | + | — | 4.8 | 2.7 | 5.0 | 1.6 | 1.0 | 0 | 0 | 67 | 0 | 109 | + | AF | — | 105/18 | 45/23 | — | 30 | — |
| 5 | 37 | F | 216 | 290 | + | — | 4.5 | 3.4 | 5.4 | 1.4 | 1.0 | 3 | 0 | 41 | 0 | 172 | + | AF | 120/60 | 110/17 | 47/8 | 6 | 32 | 2.9 |
| 6 | 40 | M | 96 | 310 | + | 3.8 | 5.3 | 4.5 | 5.6 | 1.4 | 0.8 | 0 | 0 | 30 | 0 | 145 | + | +* | 110/80 | 110/28 | 60/16 | 12 | 20 | 1.3 |
| 7 | 42 | M | 156 | 455 | + | 4.5 | 4.5 | 3.0 | 4.4 | 1.7 | 1.1 | 0 | 0 | 39 | 0 | 201 | + | AF | 110/60 | 160/27 | 36/12 | 4 | 12 | 3.3 |
| 8 | 43 | F | 36 | 220 | + | 5.0 | 3.7 | 2.5 | 5.0 | 1.8 | 1.3 | 3 | 2 | 60 | 0 | 287 | 0 | 0 | 100/60 | — | 41/17 | 15 | 27 | 1.3 |
| 9 | 45 | F | 300 | 350 | + | — | 4.8 | 4.0 | 5.6 | 1.2 | 1.0 | — | 0 | 44 | 0 | 227 | 0 | + | 155/88 | 140/21 | 70/21 | 16 | 36 | 1.8 |
| 10 | 46 | M | 360 | 480 | + | 5.1 | 5.5 | 3.8 | 5.8 | 1.7 | 1.0 | 2 | 0 | 29 | 0 | 130 | 0 | + | 110/60 | 96/24 | 48/4 | 4 | 23 | 2.8 |

* When not in atrial fibrillation.
Abbreviations as in Tables I and II.

## DEFINITIONS

**Ischemic cardiomyopathy[4]:** These patients had hearts with dilated ventricular cavities, 1 or more grossly visible transmural scars in the left ventricular free wall with or without similar scars in the ventricular septum and right ventricular free wall, narrowing >75% in cross-sectional area by atherosclerotic plaque of 1 major (right, left anterior descending and left circumflex) epicardial coronary artery, normal or nearly normal cardiac valves, and absent inflammatory, giant, neoplastic cells or nonfibrous myocardial infiltrates (such as amyloid). The intramural coronary arteries were normal.

**Idiopathic dilated cardiomyopathy[5]:** These patients had dilated ventricular cavities, normal or nearly normal cardiac valves, normal epicardium, and no inflammatory, giant, or neoplastic cells or infiltrates (such as amyloid) in the cardiac walls. The epicardial coronary arteries were usually normal; a few patients had atherosclerotic plaques including some in whom the plaques narrowed the lumen >75% in cross-sectional areas in 1 or more major epicardial coronary arteries. The patients with associated coronary narrowing, however, either had no myocardial scars or (1 patient) a very small scar. The intramural coronary arteries were normal.

**Dilated hypertrophic cardiomyopathy[2]:** These patients had dilated ventricular cavities but past clinical evidence of nondilated cavities. Transmural scarring of the ventricular septum with or without scarring of the left and right ventricular free walls was present in all but 1 patient. The ventricular septum at sometime in the past or presently was thicker than the left ventricular free wall; typical myofiber disorganization was present in the ventricular septum, and the intramural coronary arteries were abnormal (on histologic study).[6]

## RESULTS

Of the 92 cases, 47 had IC (Table I), 35 had IDC (Table II), and 10 had dilated HC (Table III) (Figures 1 to 12). Various comparative findings in each of these 3 groups are summarized in Table IV. The mean ages of the 3 groups were different (IC = 54; IDC = 47, and HC = 37 years) ($p < 0.001$). The percentage of men in each of the 3 groups was different: IC 94% (44 of 47); IDC 40% (14 of 35); and dilated HC 60% (6 of 10) ($p < 0.001$). The mean intervals from onset of symptoms of cardiac dysfunction and/or myocardial ischemia to CT were significantly longer in the dilated HC group (173 months) than in the IC (24 months) and IDC (51 months) groups ($p < 0.001$). The mean heart weights of the IC and IDC groups were similar (467 and 455 g) and heavier than those in the HC group (351 g) ($p < 0.02$). The mean body weights of each of the 3 groups were different (77.2 vs 69.0 vs 59.5 kg) ($p < 0.03$). By definition, 100% of the 47 patients with IC had relatively large transmural left ventricular scars with or without ventricular septal scars, and 9 (90%) of the 10 HC patients had transmural ventricular septal scars with or without

**TABLE IV** Comparison of Findings in Patients With Ischemic Cardiomyopathy (IC), Idiopathic Dilated Cardiomyopathy (IDC), and Dilated Hypertrophic Cardiomyopathy (HC) Having Cardiac Transplantation (CT)

| | Etiology | | |
|---|---|---|---|
| | IC (n = 47) | IDC (n = 35) | HC (n = 10) |
| Morphology | | | |
| Age (yr) | 54 ± 6* | 47 ± 15** | 37 ± 9** |
| Men | 44 (94%)* | 14 (40%)* | 6 (60%)* |
| Women | 3 (6%)* | 21 (60%)* | 4 (40%)* |
| Duration of symptoms to CT (mos) | 34 ± 45** | 51 ± 73** | 173 ± 99* |
| Heart weight (g) (mean): men/women | 471/410** | 501/418** | 393/300* |
| Body weight (kg) (mean): men/women | 79/63 | 78/61 | 53/60 |
| LV or ventricular septal necrosis | 4 (9%) | 0 | 0 |
| LV or ventricular septal fibrosis | 47 (100%)* | 8 (23%)* | 9 (90%)* |
| LV or right ventricular thrombus | 3 (6%) | 1 (3%) | 0 |
| LV mural plaque | 31 (66%)* | 25 (74%)* | 2 (20%)* |
| Epicardial CAs narrowed >75% in CSA | 47 (100%)* | 7 (20%)* | 0* |
| LV diameter (cm) | 5.8 ± 0.9 | 5.6 ± 1.0 | 4.6 ± 0.6 |
| Laboratory | | | |
| Hematocrit | 37% ± 6% | 37% ± 4% | 41% ± 4% |
| Total cholesterol (mg/dl) | 207 ± 57* | 170 ± 37* | 141 ± 36* |
| Triglycerides (mg/dl) | 176 ± 132 | 146 ± 79 | 60 ± 34 |
| Electrocardiogram | | | |
| Interval study to CT (mo) | 3 ± 4** | 4 ± 4** | 28 ± 39* |
| Heart rate (beats/min) | 83 ± 17 | 96 ± 23*** | 68 ± 6*** |
| Bundle branch block | 11/36 (31%)* | 15/31 (48%)* | 1 (10%)* |
| Total 12-lead QRS voltage (mm) | 129 ± 43 | 149 ± 59 | 171 ± 58 |
| Atrial fibrillation | 8/37 (22%) | 8/32 (25%) | 6 (60%) |
| PR Interval >0.20 sec. | 10/30 (33%)* | 2/26 (8%)* | 3/4 (75%)* |
| Ventricular tachycardia | 14/36 (39%) | 7/31 (23%) | 3 (30%) |
| Echocardiogram | | | |
| Interval study to CT (mo) | 7.7 ± 6.3** | 9.1 ± 12.2** | 26.6 ± 37.3* |
| LV end-diastole (cm) | 6.6 ± 1.1** | 6.9 ± 0.9** | 4.6 ± 0.5* |
| LV end-systole (cm) | 5.5 ± 1.1* | 6.3 ± 0.9* | 3.3 ± 0.7* |
| LA cavity (cm) | 4.5 ± 0.6*** | 4.8 ± 0.8 | 5.3 ± 0.4*** |
| Ventricular septum (cm) | 1.0 ± 0.2** | 0.9 ± 0.3** | 1.6 ± 0.3* |
| LV free wall (cm) | 1.0 ± 0.2 | 0.9 ± 0.3 | 1.1 ± 0.2 |
| Mitral regurgitation 3+ or 4+/4+ | 13/26 (50%) | 12/29 (41%) | 3/9 (33%) |
| Tricuspid regurgitation 3+ or 4+/4+ | 6/26 (23%) | 11/25 (44%) | 0 |
| LV ejection fraction | 20% ± 7%** | 19% ± 8%** | 45% ± 14%* |
| Hemodynamics | | | |
| Interval study to CT (mo) | 3 ± 5 | 3 ± 3 | 31 ± 45 |
| Systemic artery (mm Hg) (s/d) | 113/68 | 104/67 | 114/69 |
| Left ventricle (mm Hg) (s/d) | 111/24 | 99/18 | 117/23 |
| Right ventricle (mm Hg) (s/d) | 40/8 | 38/8 | 49/14 |
| Pulmonary artery (mm Hg) (s/d) | 39/18 | 40/20 | 49/24 |
| Right Atrial mean (mm Hg) | 6 ± 5*** | 8 ± 7 | 12 ± 7*** |
| Pulmonary artery wedge (mm Hg) | 17 ± 9*** | 20 ± 10 | 26 ± 6*** |
| Cardiac index (L/min/m$^2$) (mean) | 2.3 ± 0.5 | 2.4 ± 0.7 | 2.2 ± 0.7 |
| Right ventricular end-diastole >6 mm Hg | 20/31 (65%) | 15/30 (50%) | 9 (90%) |
| Pulmonary artery peak systole >40 mm Hg | 15/38 (39%)* | 14/31 (45%)* | 9 (90%)* |
| Pulmonary artery wedge mean >12 mm Hg | 21/39 (54%)* | 26/32 (81%)* | 9 (90%)* |
| Cardiac index >2.5 L/min/m$^2$ | 8/30 (27%) | 13/28 (46%) | 4/9 (44%) |

*—* = all 3 numbers are significantly different ($p < 0.05$).
*—** = one (*) of the 3 numbers is significant different.
***—*** = 2 of the 3 numbers are significantly different.
CAs = coronary arteries; CSA = cross-sectional area; other abbreviations as in Table I.

left ventricular free wall scars; in contrast, 8 (23%) of the 35 IDC patients had left ventricular scars and in each they were small. Only 4 patients had left ventricular thrombi: 3 with IC and 1 with IDC. By definition, 1 or more major epicardial coronary arteries were narrowed >75% in cross-sectional area at some point by atherosclerotic plaque in 100% of the IC patients, but similar, much less extensive narrowing by plaque was present in 1 or more epicardial coronary arteries in 20% (7 of 35) of the IDC group; none of the dilated HC patients had significant narrowing of any of the epicardial coronary arteries. The mean maximal internal diameters of the left ventricular cavities in each of the 3 groups was similar (5.8 vs 5.6 vs 5.0 cm).

The IC group had higher average serum total cholesterol levels (207 mg/dl) than either the IDC (170 mg/dl) or the HC (183 mg/dl) group ($p <0.02$). The average serum triglyceride levels were insignificantly different among the 3 groups.

On their last electrocardiogram or Holter monitoring before CT, the frequency of atrial fibrillation and runs of ventricular tachycardia were similar in the 3 groups. The frequency of prolonged (>0.20 second) PR intervals was higher in the HC group (75%) than in either the IDC (8%) or IC (33%) group ($p = 0.03$).

By echocardiogram, the left ventricular end-diastolic and peak systolic cavity sizes were similar in the IC and IDC groups (6.6 and 5.5 cm; 6.9 and 6.3 cm, respectively) and smaller in the HC group (4.6 and 3.3 cm) ($p <0.001$). The mean left atrial cavity size was significantly smaller in the IC group (4.5 cm), and larger in the HC group (5.3 cm) ($p <0.001$). The mean thickness of the ventricular septum was similar to that of the left ventricular free wall in both the IC and IDC groups (1.0 and 0.9 cm), but the septum was thicker than the free wall (1.6 vs 1.1 cm) in the HC group and significantly thicker than the ventricular septum of the IC and IDC groups ($p <0.001$). The mean ejection fraction was similar in the IC and IDC groups (20% and 19%) but significantly higher in the HC group (45%) ($p <0.001$).

By cardiac catheterization, the right atrial mean pressure was significantly less in the IC group (6

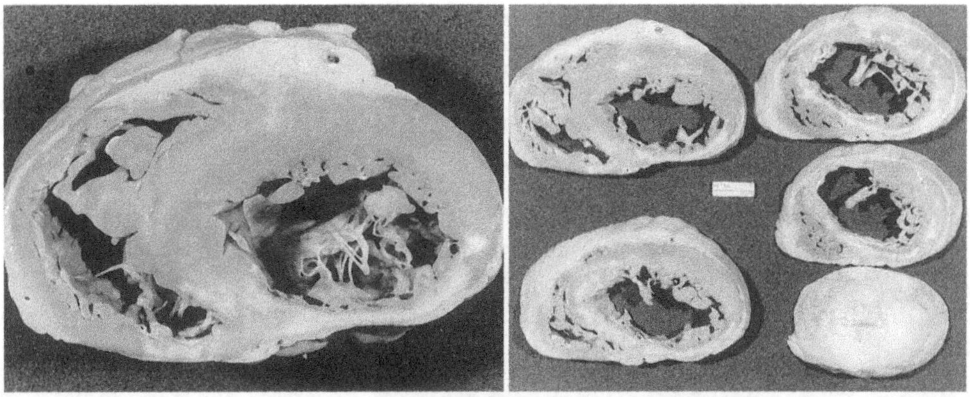

FIGURE 1. Patient #13, Table I. Transverse section exposing the cephalad portion of the heart (*left*) and 1-cm-thick slices of the caudal portion of the heart (*right*) in a 50-year-old man (BUMC #S96-674) with IC. The posterior portion of the left ventricle, ventricular septum, and right ventricle are scarred and thinned basally and apically and also apically the anterior, lateral, and septal walls are scarred.

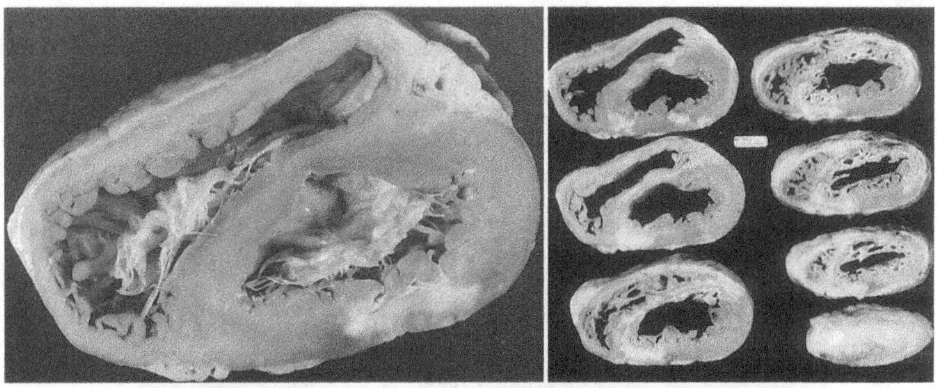

FIGURE 2. Patient #17, Table I. Transverse section exposing the cephalad portion (*left*) and caudal slices (*right*) of the heart in a 51-year-old man (BUMC #S96-10318) with IC. A distant posterior scar is present basally and the scarring apically is circumferential and associated with extensive wall thinning.

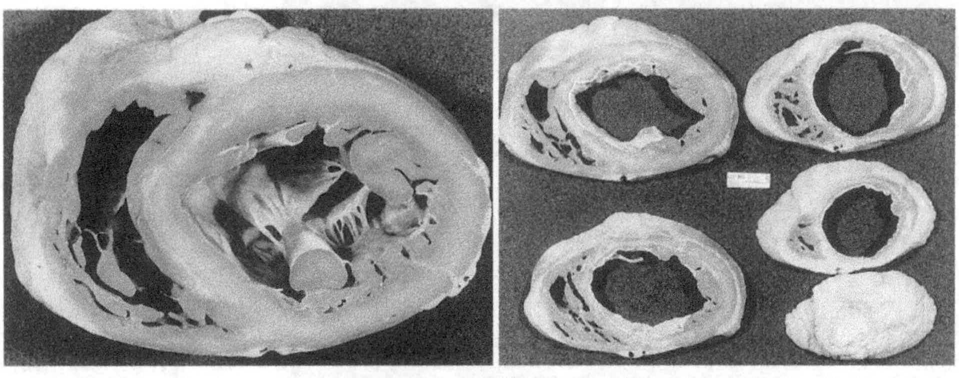

FIGURE 3. Patient #27, Table I. Transverse section exposing the cephalad portion (*left*) and caudal slices (*right*) of the heart in a 56-year-old woman (BUMC #S 95-9546) with IC. Some scarring is present in the central portion of the ventricular septum (left) and circumferentially in the more apical portions (right), which are also severely thinned.

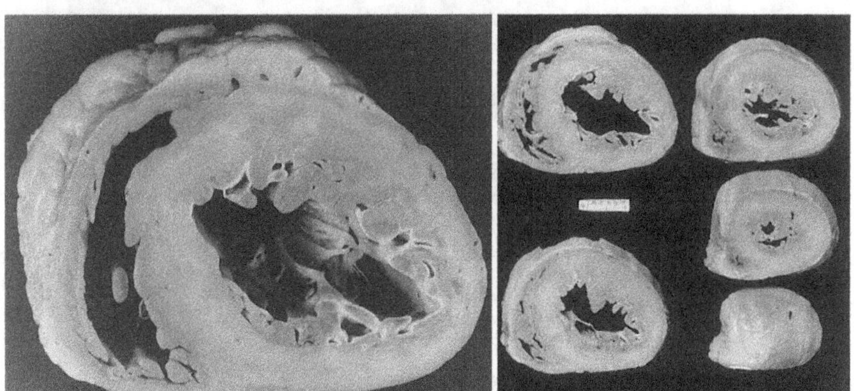

FIGURE 4. Patient #26, Table I. Transverse section exposing the basal portion (*left*) and caudal slices (*right*) of the heart in a 56-year-old man (BUMC #S95-274) with IC. Scarring and thinning is mainly localized to the lateral wall.

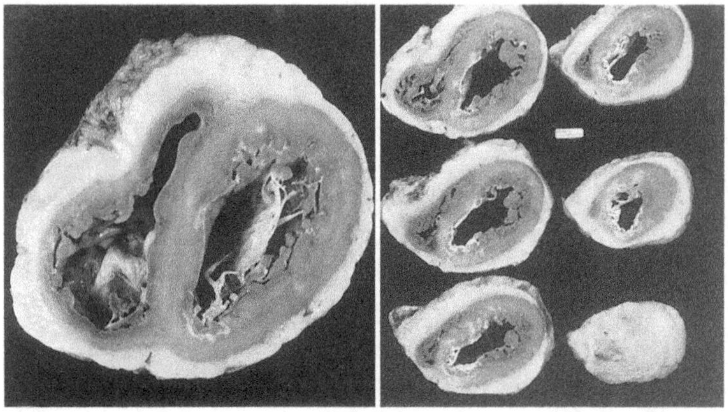

FIGURE 5. Patient #41, Table I. Transverse section exposing the cephalad portion (*left*) and transverse slices of caudal portion (*right*) in a 61-year-old man (BUMC #S96-12855) with IC. A small posterior wall scar is seen basally and more apically the scar extends into the ventricular septum and anterior free wall.

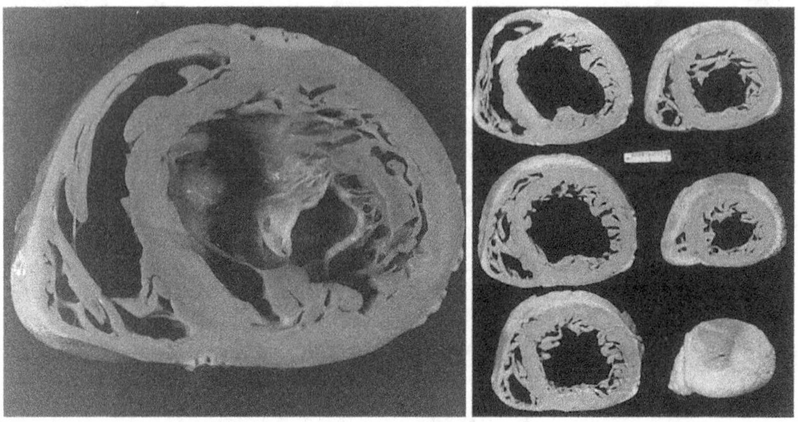

FIGURE 6. Patient #10, Table II. Transverse section exposing the cephalad portion (*left*) and transverse slices of the caudal portion (*right*) of the heart in a 36-year-old woman (BUMC #S95-15071) with IDC. Both ventricular cavities are enormously dilated and the walls are free of scars.

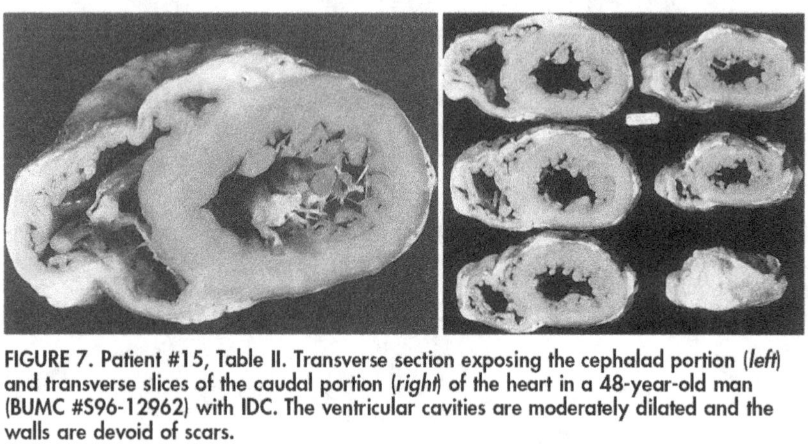

FIGURE 7. Patient #15, Table II. Transverse section exposing the cephalad portion (*left*) and transverse slices of the caudal portion (*right*) of the heart in a 48-year-old man (BUMC #S96-12962) with IDC. The ventricular cavities are moderately dilated and the walls are devoid of scars.

mm Hg) than in the dilated HC group (12 mm Hg) (p = 0.04). Similarly, the pulmonary artery wedge pressure was significantly less in the IC group (17 mm Hg) than in the dilated HC group (26 mm Hg) (p = 0.01). The percentage of patients with pulmonary artery peak systolic pressures >40 mm Hg and pulmonary artery wedge pressures >12 mm Hg was smallest in the IC group (39% and 54%), intermediate in the IDC group (45% and 81%), and highest in the dilated HC group (90%) (p <0.05).

## DISCUSSION

Although numerous reports have appeared describing cardiac morphologic findings *after* CT (i.e., those in the donor heart),[7,8] few reports have appeared describing morphologic findings in the native heart (i.e., the one excised at the time of CT). Indeed, we found only 7 publications[2,9–14] that described in any detail features of the operatively excised native heart, and in only 2 of these publications[2,9] was 1 or more gross photographs of a native heart presented. In 4 reports,[9,10,12–14] photomicrographs of certain features in the native hearts were presented.

The present study compares cardiac morphologic and clinical findings in operatively excised native hearts in 3 different conditions. Although the hearts in each of the 3 conditions were distinctly different morphologically and these differences were readily discernible from examination of the operatively excised heart, considerable intragroup morphologic variation occurred. The intragroup amounts of scarring in the left ventricular free wall and ventricular septum, for example, varied considerably among patients in the IC group and also within the dilated HC group. Furthermore, the amounts of intragroup ventricular cavity dilatation varied considerably.

Despite the clear intergroup anatomic differences among the 3 groups of patients, clinically there were considerably fewer differences in clinical characteristics. The clinical presentation, electrocardiographic, echocardiographic, and hemodynamic features usually were not specific in separating patients in one group from another group. Coronary angiography was the key clinical tool separating patients in one group from another. Although 7 patients in the IDC group had narrowing of 1 or more major epicardial coronary

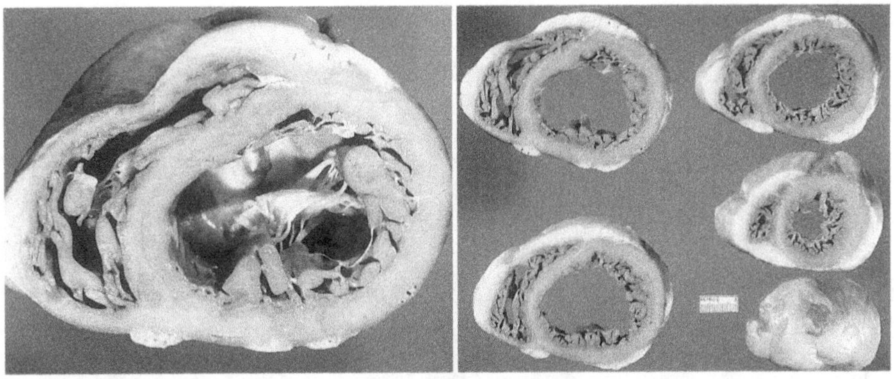

FIGURE 8. Patient #16, Table II. Transverse section exposing the cephalad portion (*left*) and transverse slices of the caudal portion (*right*) of heart in a 50-year-old woman (87S-8929) with IDC. Both ventricular cavities are severely dilated and the walls are devoid of scars.

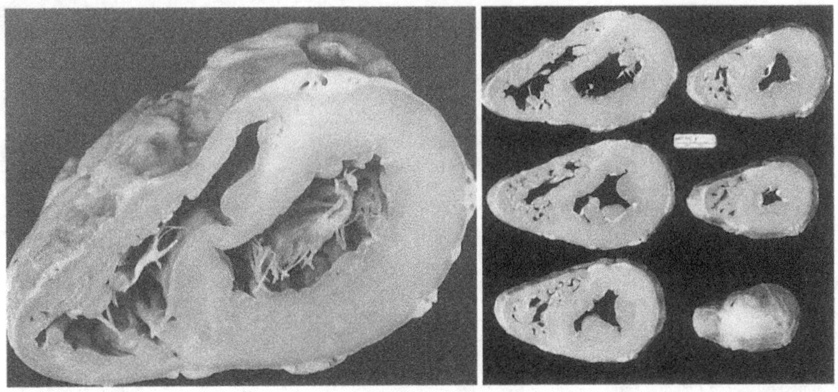

FIGURE 9. Patient #17, Table II. Transverse section exposing the cephalad portion (*left*) and slices of the caudal portion (*right*) in a 51-year-old man (BUMC #S96-05417) with IDC. A small scar is present in the anterior wall (*left*). The ventricles are moderately dilated.

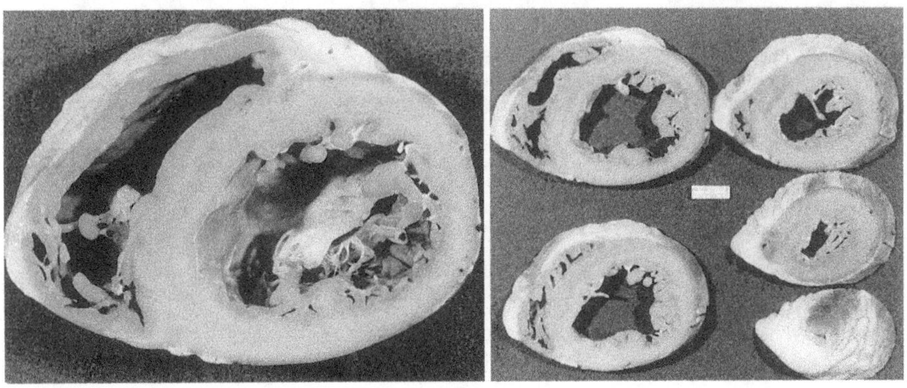

FIGURE 10. Patient #29, Table II. Transverse cut exposing the cephalad portion (*left*) and slices of the caudal portion (*right*) of the heart in a 61-year-old man (BUMC #S95-07656) with IDC. This patient also had narrowing >75% in cross-sectional area of 2 of the 3 major epicardial coronary arteries. Angiographically, however, before CT, no coronary narrowing of significance was noted. No ventricular scars are present.

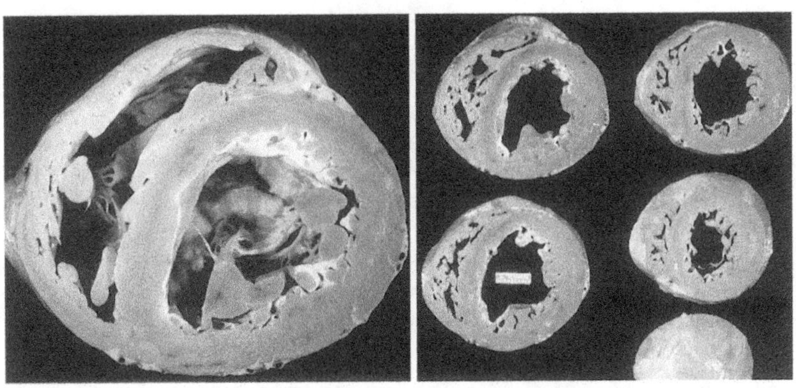

FIGURE 11. Patient #31, Table II. Transverse section exposing the cephalad portion (*left*) and transverse slices of the caudal portion (*right*) of heart in a 62-year-old woman (#91S-11353) with IDC. The ventricles are severely dilated and the walls are free of scars. The left ventricular endocardium is focally thickened by fibrous tissue, probably the result of organization of intracardiac thrombi.

arteries on anatomic examination, coronary angiography before CT had not detected such narrowings. In contrast, all 47 patients with IC had angiographic documentation of severe narrowings in 1 or more major epicardial coronary arteries before CT.

**Acknowledgment:** We are indebted to J. Carolyn Bank, PhD, for providing statistical support, John F. Dixon, MSN, RN, for creating a patient database program for analyzing data, Bonnie Martinez for photographic support, and Linda B. Maddox for secretarial support.

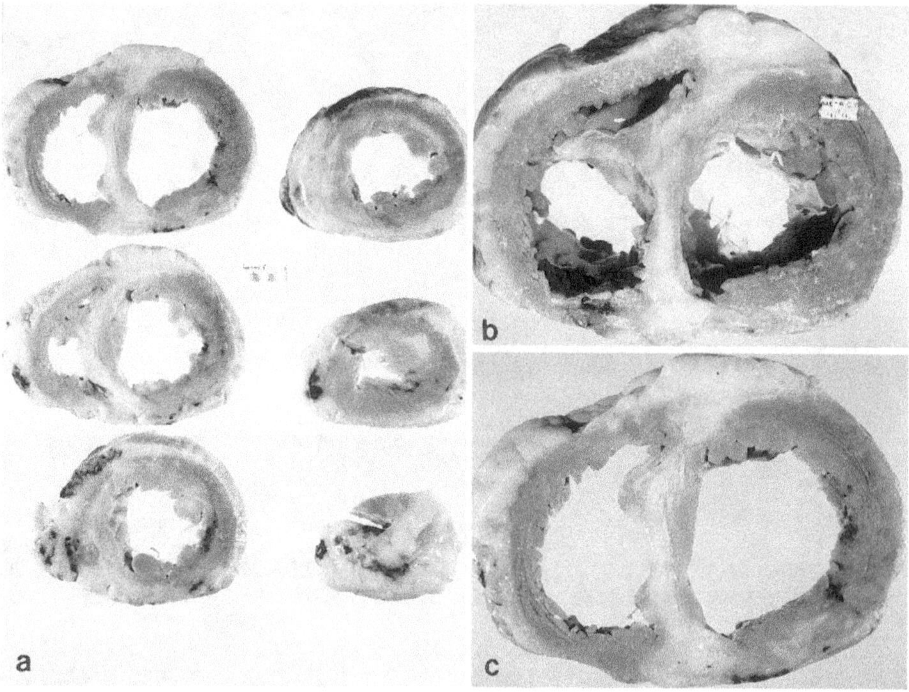


**FIGURE 12. Patient #10, Table III. Transverse cuts exposing the caudal portions (*a*) and cephalad portions (*b,c*) of the heart in a 46-year-old man with dilated HC. The ventricular cavities are severely dilated, the ventricular septum is severely scarred and thinned. Small scars are present in the posterior walls of both right and left ventricles. The major epicardial coronary arteries were not significantly narrowed. (Reproduced with permission from reference 4).**

**1.** Hosenpud JD, Novick RJ, Bennett LE, Keck BM, Fiol B, Daily OP. The registry of the International Society for Heart and Lung Transplantation: Thirteenth Official report-1996. *J Heart Lung Transplant* 1996;15:661–674.

**2.** Shirani J, Maron BJ, Cannon RO III, Shahin S, Roberts WC. Clinicopathologic features of hypertrophic cardiomyopathy managed by cardiac transplantation. *Am J Cardiol* 1993;72:434–440.

**3.** Siegel RJ, Roberts WC. Electrocardiographic observations in severe aortic valve stenosis: correlative necropsy study to clinical, hemodynamic, and ECG variables demonstrating relation of 12- lead QRS amplitude to peak systolic transaortic pressure gradient. *Am Heart J* 1982;103:210–221.

**4.** Ross MR, Roberts WC. Severe atherosclerotic coronary artery disease, healed myocardial infarction and chronic congestive heart failure: analysis of 81 patients studied at necropsy. *Am J Cardiol* 1986;57:44–50.

**5.** Roberts WC, Siegel RJ, McManus BM. Idiopathic dilated cardiomyopathy: analysis of 152 necropsy patients. *Am J Cardiol* 1987;60:1340–1355.

**6.** Roberts CS, Roberts WC. Morphologic features (of hypertrophic cardiomyopathy). Progress in Cardiology 2/2; Zipes DP, Rowlands DJ, eds. Philadelphia: Lea & Febiger, 1989:3–32.

**7.** Arbustini E, Dal Bello B, Morbini P, Grasso M, Diegoli M, Fasani R, Pilotto A, Bellini O, Pellegrini C, Martinelli L, Campana C, Gavazzi A, Specchia G, Vigano M, Roberts WC. Frequency and characteristics of coronary thrombosis in the epicardial coronary arteries after cardiac transplantation. *Am J Cardiol* 1996;78:795–800.

**8.** Arbustini E, Roberts WC. Morphologic observation in the epicardial coronary arteries and their surroundings late after cardiac transplantation (Allograft vascular disease). *Am J Cardiol* 1996;78:814–820.

**9.** Keren A, Billingham ME, Weintraub D, Stinson EB, Popp RL. Mildly dilated congestive cardiomyopathy. *Circulation* 1985;72:302–309.

**10.** Schaper J, Froede R, Hein S, Buck A, Hashizume H, Speiser B, Friedl A, Bleese N. Impairment of the myocardial ultrastructure changes of the cytoskeleton in dilated cardiomyopathy. *Circulation* 1991;83:504–514.

**11.** Becker AE, Heijams CD, Essed CE. Chronic non-ischemic congestive heart disease and endomyocardial biopsies. Worth the extra? *Eur Heart J* 1991;12:218–223.

**12.** Ardehali A, Laks H, Drinkwater DC, Ziv ET, Sorensen TJ, Hamilton MA, Warner-Stevenson L, Moriguchi JB, Kobashigawa JA, edited by Terasaki and Cecka. Cardiac transplantation at UCLA. *Clinical Transpl* 1993:119–127.

**13.** Beltrami CA, Finato N, Rocco M, Feruglio GA, Puricelli C, Cigola E, Sonnenblick EH, Olivetti G, Anversa P. The cellular basis of dilated cardiomyopathy in humans. *J Mol Cell Cardiol* 1995;27:291–305.

**14.** Narula J, Haider N, Virmani R, DiSalvo TG, Kolodgie FD, Hajjar RJ, Schmidt U, Semigran MJ, Dec GW, Khaw B-A. Apoptosis in myocytes in end-stage heart failure. *N Engl J Med* 1996;335:1182–1189.

# Cardiac transplantation 40 years after a stab wound to the heart

WILLIAM C. ROBERTS, MD, SABRINA D. PHILLIPS, MD, JUAN M. ESCOBAR, MD, AND JOHN E. CAPEHART, MD

A 62-year-old man underwent cardiac transplantation in November 2000. In 1959, at the age of 22, he was stabbed in the chest with an 8" butcher knife that was "inserted to the handle." He survived the stabbing and went to the hospital but was discharged within an hour or so without any intervention. He functioned well the next 48 hours. Then, while changing a flat tire on his car, he suddenly began feeling very ill and was taken to a local hospital, where he was found to have a widened cardiac silhouette. He underwent a "7-hour cardiac operation" via a left lateral thoracotomy. His pericardial sac was filled with blood, and a perforating wound in the right ventricular wall was closed. No other details of the cardiac procedure are available. Following recovery from the operation, he felt well again until 1990, when he noted the onset of exertional dyspnea and decreased stamina.

During the next 6 years, the dyspnea slowly but progressively worsened and, in 1996 at age 59, he underwent evaluation by a cardiologist. Cardiac catheterization disclosed angiographically normal epicardial coronary arteries and a left ventricular ejection fraction of approximately 25%. Echocardiogram disclosed left ventricular dimensions of 6.3 cm in end diastole and 5.7 cm in peak systole. A diagnosis of idiopathic dilated cardiomyopathy was made, and appropriate therapy was instituted. A dual-chamber transvenous pacemaker was inserted because of complete heart block, which apparently had been present for decades.

In March 1999, the patient was reevaluated because of further worsening of symptoms of heart failure. At that time, his pulmonary arterial pressure was 55/22 mg Hg; mean pulmonary artery wedge pressure, 15 mm Hg; body mass index, 30 kg/m$^2$; and blood pressure, 135/90 mm Hg. On cardiopulmonary stress test, he was able to exercise for only 2 minutes and 14 seconds on a Naughton protocol, achieving a peak exercise oxygen consumption of 10 cc/kg/min. At baseline, his heart rate was 64, and at peak exercise, it was still only 64 beats a minute. The minute ventilation went from 15 to 46 L per minute (79% of predicted), despite the fact that the heart rate did not change. The room air blood gases disclosed a pH of 7.46; partial pressure of carbon dioxide, 39; partial pressure of oxygen, 58; forced expiratory volume in 1 second, 1.7; and forced vital capacity, 2.71. At this time, the patient was on enalapril, hydrochlorothiazide, allopurinol, spironolactone, digoxin, and aspirin. He had had systemic hypertension for many years before being on any hypertensive therapy. He smoked 20 cigarettes daily for about 40 years.

Because of progressive worsening of the heart failure, cardiac transplantation was performed. The procedure went smoothly. The excised heart weighed 707 g, and a number of adhesions were present on the epicardial surface. Both ventricular cavities were quite dilated *(Figure, next page)*. A small scar was present in the anterior wall of the right ventricle, and a large transmural scar was present in the most basal portion of the ventricular septum in its central portion *(Figure)*. There was no scarring in the left ventricular free wall. The 4 cardiac valves were normal. The epicardial coronary arteries were large and virtually devoid of atherosclerotic plaques.

• • •

The unusual finding in the heart was the large transmural scar in the ventricular septum and a smaller scar in the right ventricular free wall. The stab wound to the heart 40 years earlier led to a 2-day delay of hemopericardium and an emergency cardiac operation. The details of the operation 40 years ago are not available, but no sutures or prosthetic material was present in the ventricular septum, indicating that no procedure was done within the heart. It is likely, however, that the knife penetrated not only the right ventricular free wall but also the ventricular septum, producing a ventricular septal defect in the muscular portion of the ventricular septum. The ventricular septal defect later closed, because the ventricular septum was intact and no precordial murmur had ever been heard. The heart failure was probably a combination of 40 years of complete heart block, causing considerable dilatation of both ventricular cavities with superimposed systemic hypertension for many years. The area of the atrioventricular bundle was extensively scarred.

In summary, we describe a patient who underwent cardiac transplantation because of heart failure and was found to have a large scar in his ventricular septum and fibrosis of his atrioventricular nodal area, suggesting that he had complete heart block for 40 years. The ventricular dilatation likely was the result of both complete heart block and superimposed systemic hypertension.

From the Division of Cardiology, Department of Medicine (Roberts, Phillips, and Escobar), and the Department of Cardiothoracic Surgery (Capehart), Baylor University Medical Center, Dallas, Texas.

**Corresponding author:** William C. Roberts, MD, Baylor Cardiovascular Institute, Baylor University Medical Center, 3500 Gaston Avenue, Dallas, Texas 75246.

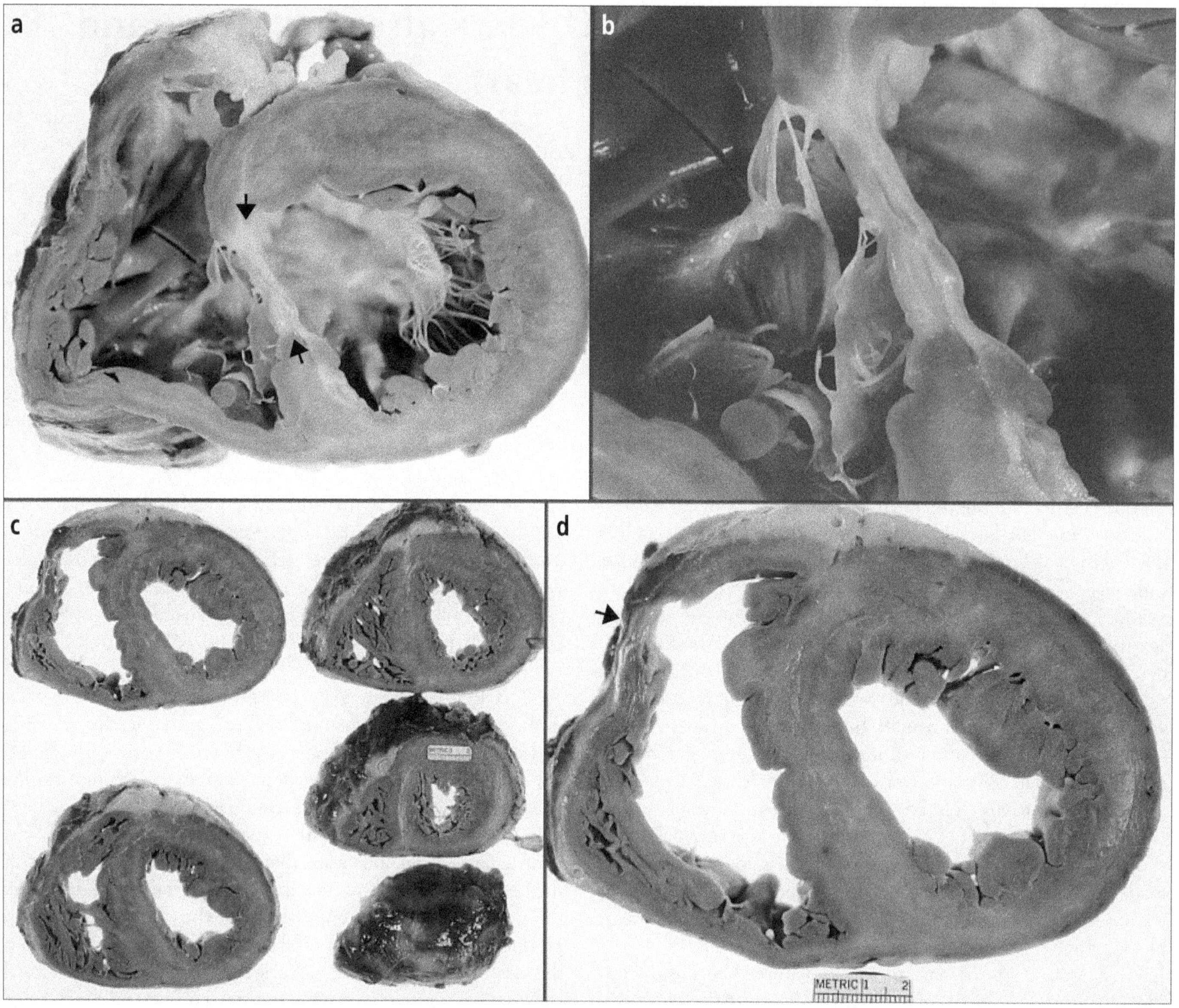


**Figure.** The heart removed for transplant. **(a)** The base of the heart, showing a large transmural scar in the mid portion of the ventricular septum (between the arrows) and dilated right and left ventricular cavities. **(b)** A close-up view of the large scar in the ventricular septum. **(c)** Transverse cuts of the more apical portions of the left ventricular cavity, showing the walls to be thickened and the cavities to be mildly to moderately dilated. **(d)** A magnification of a slice from (a); the arrow points to where the knife entered the anterior wall of the right ventricle.

# Heart Transplantation for Undiagnosed Cardiac Sarcoidosis

Alan S. Donsky, MD, Juan Escobar, MD, John Capehart, MD, and William C. Roberts, MD

Heart transplantation (HT) for cardiac sarcoidosis is rare. Only 6 patients having HT for cardiac sarcoidosis have been previously reported[1–4] (Table 1). In 2 of them, the diagnosis of cardiac sarcoidosis was not known at the time of HT. In this report, we describe a patient who underwent HT for presumed idiopathic dilated cardiomyopathy (IDC), but on examination, the explanted heart was found to have extensive cardiac sarcoidosis.

• • •

A 53-year-old white man was well until age 41 when he developed exertional dyspnea and palpitations. Examination at that time disclosed a blood pressure of 110/70 mm Hg, and a heart rate of 60 beats/min. There was no jugular venous distention or peripheral edema present but an S3 and S4 gallop was heard on auscultation. An electrocardiogram showed normal sinus rhythm with a prolonged PR interval (240 ms) and complete left bundle branch block (QRS duration 160 ms) (Figure 1). Total 12-lead QRS voltage = 110 mm (10 mm = 1 mV). An echocardiogram disclosed dilation of the right and left ventricles (left ventricular end-diastolic diameter = 60 mm, and peak systolic diameter = 38 mm) and global hypokinesia with an ejection fraction of 25%. Exercise thallium stress tests showed no resting or exercise-induced perfusion defects. IDC was diagnosed. Two years later he developed symptomatic sustained ventricular tachycardia requiring electrical cardioversion and implantation of an automatic implantable cardioverter-defibrillator.

Despite optimal medical management, his heart failure progressed. A repeat echocardiogram at age 49 showed that his ejection fraction had fallen to 15%. Right-sided cardiac catheterization showed a cardiac index of 1.5 L/min/m$^2$, a pulmonary artery pressure of 43/24 mm Hg, and a mean pulmonary wedge pressure of 26 mm Hg. At age 53 (September 1999) he underwent orthotopic HT.

Examination of the native (recipient) heart showed extensive focal scarring of the right ventricular wall, the cephalad portion of the ventricular septum, and the lateral, anterior, and posterior left ventricular walls (Figure 2). The heart weighed 510 g. All epicardial coronary arteries were widely patent. Microscopic sections disclosed numerous multinucleated giant cells and lymphocytes, mainly within the scarred areas (Figure 3).

As of May 1, 2002, the patient is asymptomatic. None of his post-transplant biopsy specimens have shown recurrence of sarcoid.

• • •

Sarcoidosis is an idiopathic, systemic, granulomatous disease that can affect any organ system, although the lymph nodes and lungs are most often affected. Cardiac involvement was first described by Bernstein et al[5] in 1929. Not much was known about cardiac sarcoidosis until Gozo et al[6] reviewed 70 autopsy cases of patients who died from primary cardiac sarcoidosis. The average age of death was 40 years. The most common clinical manifestations were conduction disturbances, ventricular arrhythmias, and congestive heart failure. In 1977, Roberts and colleagues[7] reported on 113 necropsy patients with cardiac sarcoidosis. They found that sarcoid granulomas and scars most often involved the left ventricular free wall and the cephalad portion of the ventricular septum. Furthermore, they observed that patients in whom sarcoidosis had caused cardiac dysfunction had little or no clinical evidence of dysfunction in any other organ system. The incidence of cardiac involvement in patients with pulmonary sarcoidosis was studied by Silverman and colleagues[8] in 1978. They reviewed 84 autopsy cases of pulmonary sarcoidosis in the files of The Johns Hopkins Hospital and found grossly visible myocardial sarcoid lesions in only 4 patients (5%), although another 19 (23%) had non-caseating granulomas in microscopic sections of myocardium. Our patient had severe cardiac dysfunction caused by sarcoidosis without extracardiac symptoms.

*Differentiating cardiac sarcoidosis from IDC* can be difficult. Yazaki et al[9] retrospectively compared 15 patients having cardiac sarcoidosis and left ventricular systolic dysfunction (ejection fraction <40% and left ventricular end-diastolic diameter >55 mm) with 30 patients with IDC. The sarcoidosis group had a statistically significant higher frequency of complete heart block (67% vs 0%), right bundle branch block (57% vs 17%), and abnormal left ventricular wall thickness (73% vs 17%). Flemming[10] found that patients with cardiac sarcoidosis who developed complete heart block developed it at a much younger age than those with idiopathic heart block, so that complete heart block in a young patient may be a clue to undiagnosed cardiac sarcoidosis.

*Endomyocardial biopsy* can confirm the diagnosis of cardiac sarcoidosis by the presence of non-caseating epithelioid granulomas.

From the Departments of Internal Medicine (Division of Cardiology) and Cardiothoracic Surgery and Pathology, the Heart and Vascular Institute, Baylor University Medical Center, Dallas, Texas. Dr. Roberts' address is: Baylor Heart and Vascular Institute, Baylor University Medical Center, 3600 Gaston Avenue, Dallas, Texas 75246. Manuscript received January 9, 2002; revised manuscript received and accepted February 25, 2002.

**TABLE 1** Clinical and Morphologic Cardiac Data in Previously Reported Patients Having Cardiac Transplantation for Cardiac Sarcoidosis

| Case | First Author | Publication Year | Age at HT (yrs) | Race | Sex | Pre-HT Dx of Sarcoid | Reason for HT | Died (months Lived after HT) | Occurrence of Sarcoid After HT | Native Heart Weight (g) | Location of Granulomas RA | RV | LA | LV | AS | VS | Dilated RV | LV | BBB | CHB | VT | Prolonged PR Interval |
|---|---|---|---|---|---|---|---|---|---|---|---|---|---|---|---|---|---|---|---|---|---|---|
| 1 | Gokel | 1985 | 37 | - | M | + (Bx) | - | + (8) | - | - | - | - | - | - | - | - | - | - | - | - | - | - |
| 2 | Valantine | 1987 | 46 | W | M | 0 | VT | + (42) | 0 (A) | 630 | - | + | - | + | - | + | 0 | 0 | + (R) | 0 | + | + |
| 3 | Valantine | 1987 | 47 | B | M | + (Bx) | CHF | 0 (16+) | 0 (Bx) | 420 | "Widespread" | | | | | | 0 | + | 0 | 0 | + | + |
| 4 | Valantine | 1987 | 51 | W | F | 0 (Bx) | CHF | 0 (20+) | 0 (Bx) | 400 | - | 0 | - | + | - | + | - | - | + (R) | 0 | 0 | + |
| 5 | Oni | 1992 | 34 | - | M | + (Bx) | CHF | 0 (13+) | + (Bx) | - | - | - | - | - | - | - | + | + | 0 | 0 | + | 0 |
| 6 | Ankersmi | 2001 | 30 | - | M | + (Bx) | CHF | 0 (1+) | - | - | - | - | - | - | - | - | + | + | 0 | 0 | + | 0 |

A = autopsy; AS = atrial septum; B = black; BBB = bundle branch block; Bx = biopsy; CHB = complete heart block; CHF = congestive heart failure; Dx = diagnosis; LA = left atrium; LV = left ventricle; R = right; RA = right atrium; RV = right ventricle; VS = ventricular septum; VT = ventricular tachycardia; W = white; - = no information available.

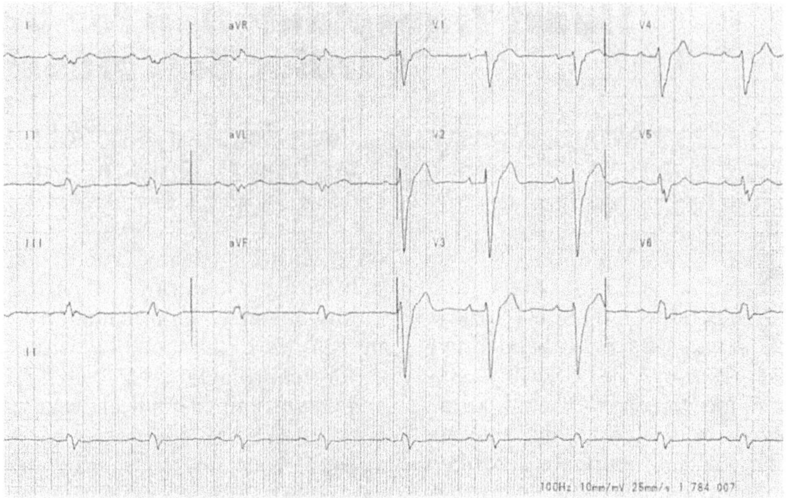


**FIGURE 1. Electrocardiogram in the patient described. The electrocardiogram shows sinus rhythm, prolonged PR interval (0.24 second), and complete left bundle branch block (QRS duration = 0.16 second).**

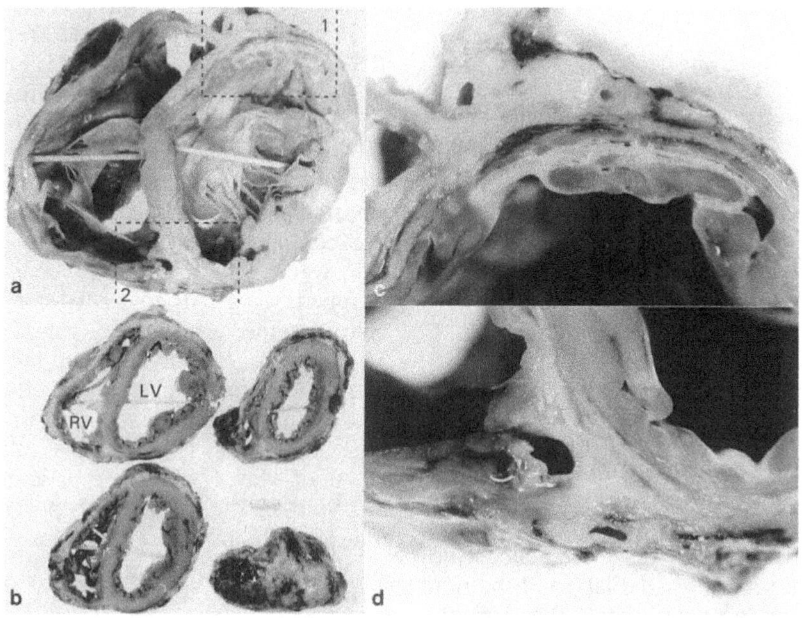


**FIGURE 2. The heart in the patient described. *a*, view of the base of the heart after excision of the more apical portion of the right and left ventricles. Both ventricular cavities are considerably dilated. The area 1 *(shown in box with broken line)* is magnified in *c*. The left ventricular free wall and ventricular septum and a portion of anterior wall of the right ventricle (RV) in its outflow track is severely scarred and the wall is thinned. A close-up of area 2 is shown in *d*. Again the posterior portion of the left ventricular free wall, the right ventricular aspect of the ventricular septum, and a portion of the right ventricular free wall adjacent to the septum are severely scarred. *b*, transverse views of the right and left ventricular cavities and walls in the more apical portions of the heart. The ventricular cavities again are quite dilated. LV = left ventricle.**

Its diagnostic yield is difficult to determine because the gold standard for the diagnosis of cardiac sarcoidosis is autopsy. Several studies, however, have reported on its diagnostic yield in patients with suspected cardiac sarcoidosis. In 1 study of 26 patients in whom cardiac sarcoidosis was "strongly suspected," only 5 (19%) had noncaseating granulomas on biopsy.[11] In another study involving 8 patients, only 2 had noncaseating granulomas.[12] This low yield is likely due to the patchy nature of the granulomas and their predilection for the

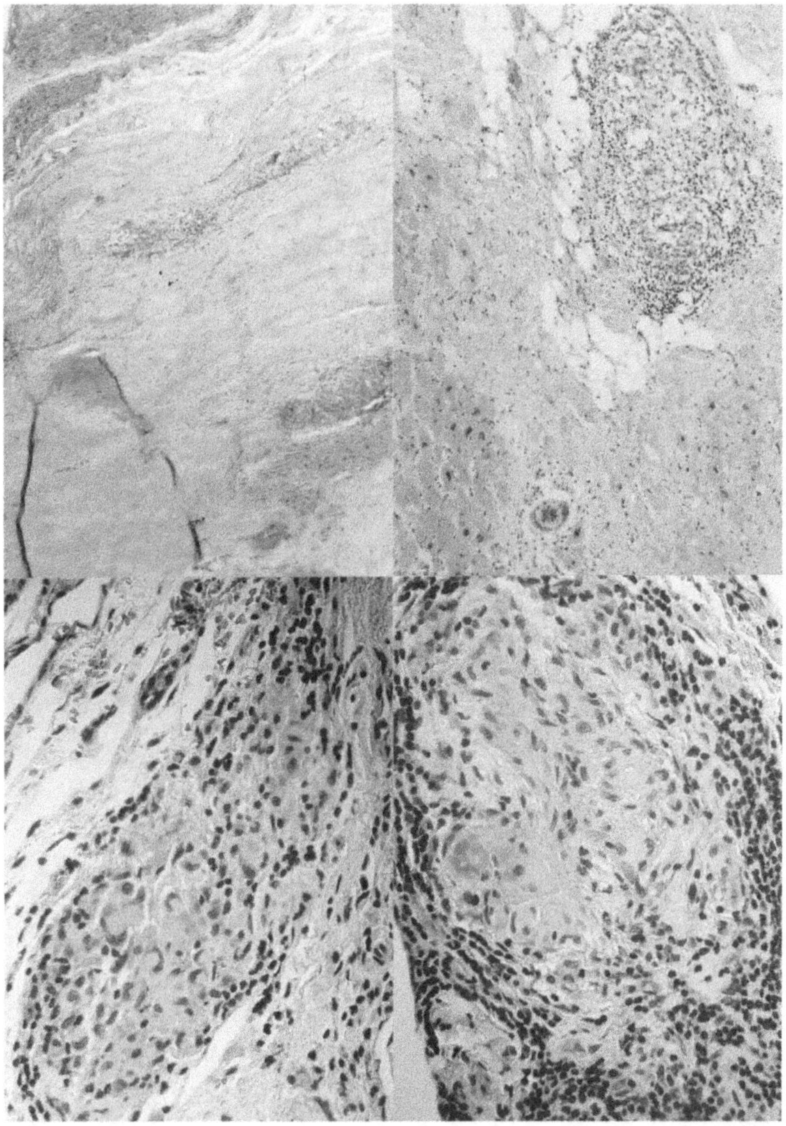

**FIGURE 3. Photomicrographs of various portions of the left ventricular wall in the patient described showing typical sarcoid granulomas. *Upper left,* in an area of severe scarring, 3 "hard" sarcoid granulomas are seen. *Upper right,* 1 large and 1 small giant-celled granuloma is seen in an area adjacent to scarring and myocardial fibers. *Lower left and lower right,* 2 granulomas from the myocardial wall showing typical giant cells and epithelioid cells with associated lymphocytes. Hematoxylin eosin stains, X 40 *(upper left)*, X 100 *(upper right)*, and X 400 *(lower left and lower right)*, reduced by 39%.**

cephalad portion of the ventricular septum, which is less accessible to biopsy.

*Echocardiography* may show abnormal wall thickness, left ventricular systolic dysfunction, or pericardial effusion.[10,13] Only 1 study has actually compared echocardiographic findings in patients with cardiac sarcoidosis to those with IDC.[8] In that study of 15 patients with cardiac sarcoidosis, 11 had either thinning (6 patients), thickening (4 patients), or both (1 patient) of the left ventricular wall, whereas only 5 of the 30 patients with IDC had any abnormality in wall thickness. No other differences were noted between the 2 groups. Despite extensive sarcoid involvement in our patient, abnormal wall thickness was not seen on the echocardiogram.

*Resting myocardial scintigraphy* with thallium-201 may show segmental areas of decreased uptake in up to 30% of patients with sarcoidosis, even those without cardiac symptoms.[14] The unusual feature of these defects is that they tend to disappear after the administration of dipyridamole or on redistribution scanning.[15] Patients with coronary artery disease tend to have fixed perfusion defects or defects seen only after the administration of dipyridamole. Accumulation of gallium-67 is considered an indicator of active inflammation and thus may predict a positive response to steroids.[16] Our patient had repeated nuclear perfusion scans, all of which failed to disclose any resting or exercise-induced defects despite extensive sarcoid involvement of his heart.

*Magnetic resonance imaging* (MRI) has recently been used to diagnose cardiac sarcoidosis as well as to evaluate the response to corticosteroid treatment.[17–21] Several modalities are available including enhancement with gadolinium.[17] In a patient with biopsy-proved cardiac sarcoidosis, MRI showed multiple discrete, high-signal lesions within the anterolateral and posterior left ventricular wall and septum as well as thickening of the cephalad portion of the septum.[21] MRI has not been systematically compared with other imaging modalities, but case reports have shown the ability of MRI to detect cardiac sarcoidosis when other studies have failed to do so.[18,20] Furthermore, its superior reproducibility makes MRI ideal for follow-up studies to monitor response to treatment.

**In summary, this report describes a 53-year-old man who underwent HT for severe heart failure thought to be due to IDC when, in fact, examination of the explanted heart revealed significant sarcoid involvement. Only 2 such cases of HT for undiagnosed cardiac sarcoidosis have been previously reported.**


1. Valantine HA, Tazelaar HD, Macoviak J, Mullin AV, Hunt SA, Fowler MB, Billingham ME, Schroeder JS. Cardiac sarcoidosis: response to steroids and transplantation. *J Heart Transplant* 1987;6:244–250.

2. Gokel JM, Reichart B, Struck E. Human cardiac transplantation—evaluation of morphological changes in serial endomyocardial biopsies. *Path Res Pract* 1985;178:354–364.

3. Ankersmit HJ, Wieselthaler GA, Moser B, Taghavi S, Grimm M, Roth G, Gorlitzer M, Tschernich H, Horvat R, Wolner E. Automated implantable cardiac defibrillator and biventricular Thoratec assist

device as bridge to transplantation in a patient with sarcoidosis. *J Thorac Cardiovasc Surg* 2001;121: 1198–1199.

**4.** Oni AA, Hershberger RE, Norman DJ, Ray J, Hovaguimian H, Cobanoglu AM, Hosenpud JD. Recurrence of sarcoidosis in a cardiac allograft: control with augmented corticosteroids. *J Heart Lung Transplant* 1992;11:367–369.

**5.** Bernstein M, Konzelmann FW, Sidlick DM. Boeck's sarcoid: report of a case with visceral involvement. *Arch Intern Med* 1929;44:721–734.

**6.** Gozo EG, Cosnow I, Cohen HC, Okum L. The heart in sarcoidosis. *Chest* 1971;60:379–388.

**7.** Roberts WC, McAllister HA, Ferrans VJ. Sarcoidosis of the heart. A clinicopathologic study of 35 necropsy patients (group I) and review of 78 previously described necropsy patients (group II). *Am J Med* 1977;63:86–108.

**8.** Silverman KJ, Hutchins GM, Buckley BH. Cardiac sarcoid: a clinicopathologic study of 84 unselected patients with systemic sarcoidosis. *Circulation* 1978;58:1204–1211.

**9.** Yazaki Y, Isobe M, Hiramitsu S, Morimoto S, Hiroe M, Omichi C, Nakano T, Saeki M, Izumi T, Sekiguchi M. Comparison of clinical features and prognosis of cardiac sarcoidosis and idiopathic dilated cardiomyopathy. *Am J Cardiol* 1998;82:537–540.

**10.** Fleming HA. Cardiac sarcoidosis. *Sem Resp Med* 1986;8:65–71.

**11.** Uemura A, Morimoto S, Hiramitsu S, Kato Y, Ito T, Hishida H. Histologic diagnostic rate of cardiac sarcoidosis: evaluation of endomyocardial biopsies. *Am Heart J* 1999;138:299–302.

**12.** Ratner SJ, Fenoglio JJ, Ursell PC. Utility of endomyocardial biopsy in the diagnosis of cardiac sarcoidosis. *Chest* 1986;90:528–533.

**13.** Lewin RF, Mor R, Spitzer S, Arditti A, Hellman C, Agmon J. Echocardiographic evaluation of patients with systemic sarcoidosis. *Am Heart J* 1985; 110:116–122.

**14.** Kinney EI, Jackson GL, Reeves WC, Zelis R. Thallium scan myocardial defects and echocardiographic abnormalities in patients with sarcoidosis without clinical cardiac dysfunction. An analysis of 44 patients. *Am J Med* 1980;96:497–503.

**15.** Tellier P, Paycha F, Antony I, Nitenberg A, Valeyre D, Foult J, Battesti J. Reversibility by dipyridamole of thallium-201 myocardial scan defects in patients with sarcoidosis. *Am J Med* 1988;85:189–193.

**16.** Okayama K, Kurata C, Tawarahara K, Yasushi W, Chida K, Sato A. Diagnosis and prognostic value of myocardial scintigraphy with thallium-201 and gallium-67 in cardiac sarcoidosis. *Chest* 1995;107: 330–334.

**17.** Shimada T, Shimada K, Sakane T, Ochiai K, Tsukihashi H, Fukui M, Inoue S, Katoh H, Murakami Y, Ishibashi Y, Maruyama R. Diagnosis of cardiac sarcoidosis and evaluation of the effects of steroid therapy by gadolinium-DPTA-enhanced magnetic resonance imaging. *Am J Med* 2001;110: 520–527.

**18.** Doherty MJ, Kumar SK, Nicholson AA, McGivern DV. Cardiac sarcoidosis: the value of magnetic resonance imaging in diagnosing and assessment of response to treatment. *Resp Med* 1997;92: 697–699.

**19.** Chandra M, Silverman ME, Oshinski J, Pettigrew R. Diagnosis of cardiac sarcoidosis aided by MRI. *Chest* 1996;110:562–565.

**20.** Smedema JP, Doubell AF. Cardiac sarcoidosis—the value of magnetic resonance imaging. A case report and brief review of the literature. *Cardiovasc J South Afr* 2000;11:218–222.

**21.** Riedy K, Fisher M, Belic N, Koenigsberg DI. MR imaging of myocardial sarcoidosis. *AJR* 1988; 151:915–916.

# Heart failure resulting from chemotherapy for testicular neoplasm: a follow-up on a patient reported 20 years earlier

David Dmitry Boltan, MD, Shelley Anne Hall, MD, and William Clifford Roberts, MD

In 1986 Doll and associates (1) from Phoenix and Nashville reported on 4 patients who developed acute vascular ischemic events after cisplatin-based combination chemotherapy for germ-cell tumor of the testis. Case 1 in their study is the patient described here 20 years later.

• • •

A 47-year-old man, who was born in July 1959, had been well until August 1982, when at age 23 he noted a left-upper-quadrant mass and bilateral testicular enlargement. A computed tomography examination a year later disclosed a retroperitoneal mass. The patient's serum alpha-fetoprotein level was 4058 mg/mL. Bilateral orchiectomy showed yolk sac carcinoma. The patient was treated at 3-week intervals with 4 cycles of cisplatin 20 mg/m$^2$ body surface area intravenously on days 1 through 5; vinblastine, 0.15 mg/kg body weight intravenously on days 1 and 2; and bleomycin, 30 units intravenously weekly for 12 weeks.

A complete remission was obtained, but over the next year the patient developed Raynaud's phenomenon affecting the digits in his fingers. In June 1985, 18 months after completion of chemotherapy, he developed substernal chest pain, and a series of electrocardiograms and cardiac enzyme tests were consistent with anterior wall acute myocardial infarction. In September 1985, 3 months later, coronary angiography showed no abnormalities. Administration of ergonovine maleate precipitated chest discomfort accompanied by diffuse right coronary spasm exceeding 40% diameter reduction. Anginal symptoms and coronary spasm were promptly relieved by nitroglycerin. A left ventriculogram showed anterolateral and apical hypokinesis and a mildly decreased ejection fraction.

In December 1985, the patient was hospitalized for overt heart failure. He continued to work without rehospitalization until 1992 (age 33), when he was advised to stop working because of heart failure. Atrial fibrillation appeared shortly thereafter, and it was paroxysmal. Cardiac catheterization in November 2002 disclosed normal right-sided cardiac pressures, normal pulmonary arterial wedge pressure (11 mm Hg), normal coronary arteries by angiogram, and a slightly decreased cardiac index (2.3 L/min/m$^2$).

In 1995 a stent was placed in an artery in the patient's leg for reasons that are unclear, and shortly thereafter he had 2 transient ischemic attacks. A thrombus was found in the left side of his heart, and warfarin was instituted. His left ventricular ejection fraction at that time was 24%, and the left ventricular cavity had a maximal diameter of 9.3 cm.

In April 1997, his serum total cholesterol was 249; low-density lipoprotein cholesterol, 184; high-density lipoprotein cholesterol, 34; and triglycerides, 156 mg/dL. He was placed on simvastatin 10 mg daily in 2000.

In April 2005 when he was 45, an echocardiogram continued to show the maximal left ventricular cavity diameter to be 9.3 cm, and there was generalized left ventricular hypokinesia with apical akinesia and an ejection fraction of about 10%. The serum total cholesterol now was 170; low-density lipoprotein cholesterol, 122; high-density lipoprotein cholesterol, 34; and triglycerides, 112 mg/dL. Repeat cardiac catheterization in July 2005 disclosed the following pressures in mm Hg: pulmonary artery wedge mean, 29, a 34, v 41; pulmonary artery, 51/26; and right atrial mean 6, a 10, v 9. The cardiac index was 1.9 L/min/m$^2$.

Cardiac transplantation was performed on September 18, 2005. Conversation with the patient on February 20, 2006, disclosed that he was asymptomatic and feeling well. The operatively excised native heart weighed 820 g. The amount of subepicardial adipose tissue was considerably increased such that the basal portion of the heart floated in formaldehyde. Both ventricular cavities but particularly the left one were greatly dilated *(Figure)*. Two transmural scars were present: one in the anterior wall and one in the posterior wall. The scarring extended from the apex to base. About half of the apical wall was scarred. In contrast, only a small portion of the anteroseptal wall was scarred in its most basal portion. The right coronary artery was narrowed about 50% in cross-sectional area at one site. The lumens of the left main, left anterior descending, and left circumflex coronary arteries were widely patent. Histologic sections of the ventricular walls confirmed the scarring. No foci or myofiber necrosis or inflammation were present.

From the Department of Internal Medicine (Boltan, Hall, Roberts) and the Department of Pathology (Roberts), Baylor Heart and Vascular Institute and Baylor University Medical Center, Dallas, Texas.

**Corresponding author:** William C. Roberts, MD, Baylor Heart and Vascular Institute, 621 North Hall Street, Dallas, Texas 75226 (e-mail: wc.roberts@BaylorHealth.edu).

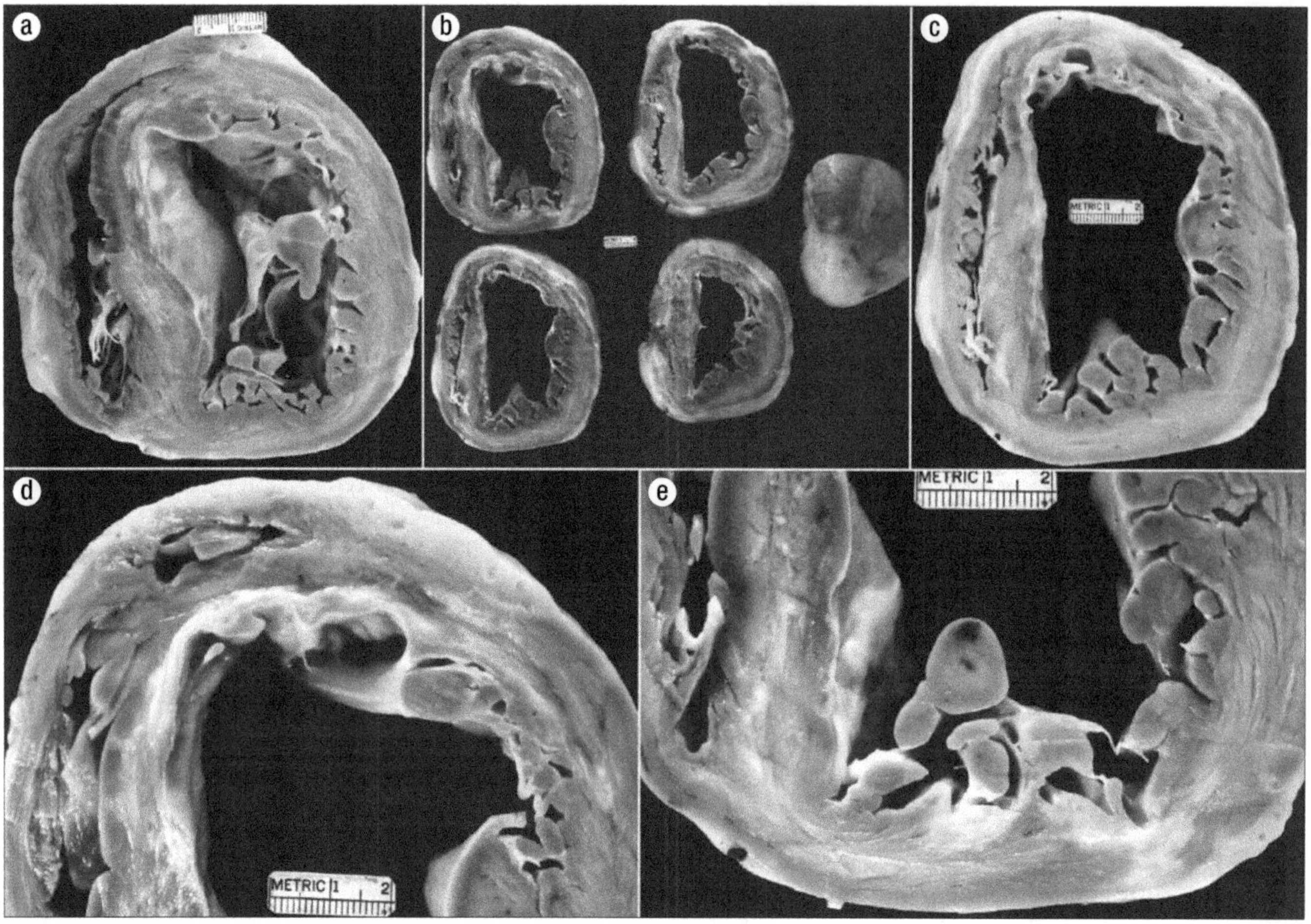


**Figure.** The native heart after cardiac transplantation. **(a)** View of both ventricles showing portions of both tricuspid and mitral valves. The anterior and anteroseptal walls are scarred. **(b)** View of 1-cm thick slices of the ventricles going from base (upper left) to apex (right). **(c)** Close-up view showing the transmural scar on the anterior wall. **(d)** Very close-up view of the anterior wall scar. **(e)** Very close-up view of the posterior wall scar. (Photographs by Jong Mi Ko.)

• • •

The patient described here had chemotherapy for a malignant testicular neoplasm. Although it eliminated the neoplasm, the chemotherapy produced vasospasm as confirmed by Raynaud's phenomenon; the precipitation of chest pain on administration of ergonovine maleate; and narrowing (up to 40% in diameter) of the right coronary artery. Eighteen months after completion of the chemotherapy, the patient, when only 25 years of age, had documented acute myocardial infarction. Three months later, an angiogram confirmed the presence of normal coronary arteries.

Examination of the operatively excised heart after cardiac transplantation disclosed 2 separate left ventricular scars, one anteriorly and one posteriorly, and a hugely dilated left ventricular cavity and essentially normal coronary arteries.

It is fairly well established that individuals who have an acute myocardial infarction and later appear to have normal coronary arteries have a good prognosis and indeed are generally free of clinical evidence of myocardial ischemia or heart failure (2). The patient described herein had 2 separate myocardial infarcts, and the extensiveness of the myocardial damage probably explains the degree of left ventricular dilatation and heart failure.

It is important to realize that the patient did not have coronary angiography *at the time of* the acute infarct but 3 months later. Therefore, we cannot be certain of the status of the coronary arteries at the time of the myocardial infarct. A thrombus or embolus in a coronary artery could have been present at the time of the infarct and could have retracted, organized, and recanalized subsequently such that it was angiographically "normal" later (3). Myocardial infarction as a consequence of coronary spasm has rarely if ever been confirmed.

In conclusion, chemotherapy destroyed the malignant cancer but also damaged the heart; the resulting heart failure would have been fatal had not cardiac transplantation intervened. The chemotherapy killed the cancer but at the same time destroyed the previously normal heart.


1. Doll DC, List AF, Greco FA, Hainsworth JD, Hande KR, Johnson DH. Acute vascular ischemic events after cisplatin-based combination chemotherapy for germ-cell tumors of the testis. *Ann Intern Med* 1986;105(1):48–51.
2. Golzio PG, Orzan F, Ferrero P, Bobbio M, Bergerone S, Di Leo M, Trevi GP. Myocardial infarction with normal coronary arteries: ten-year follow-up. *Ital Heart J* 2004;5(10):732–738.
3. Arnett EN, Roberts WC. Acute myocardial infarction and angiographically normal coronary arteries. An unproven combination. *Circulation* 1976;53(3):395–400.

# Cardiac Transplantation for Cardiac Sarcoidosis With Initial Diagnosis by Examination of the Left Ventricular Apical "Core" Excised for Insertion of a Left Ventricular Assist Device for Severe Chronic Heart Failure

William Clifford Roberts, MD[a,b,d,*], Travis James Vowels[d], Jong Mi Ko, BA[d], John Edward Capehart, MD[c], and Shelley Anne Hall, MD[a,d]

**Three quinquagenarians who underwent insertion of a left ventricular assist device (LVAD) because of severe heart failure and for whom histologic examination of the left ventricular apical "core" (removed to insert the device) showed noncaseating giant cell granulomas typical of sarcoidosis are described. Later, cardiac transplantation showed widespread sarcoid granulomas in the walls of the right and left ventricles and ventricular septum in 2 patients and extensive scarring in the third patient in the absence of coronary narrowing. Previously, 11 patients who underwent cardiac transplantation because of cardiac sarcoidosis had been reported, and in 1 of these patients, diagnosis was also initially made by examination of the left ventricular core excised at the time of insertion of an LVAD. In conclusion, excision of a portion of left ventricular wall to enable insertion of a therapeutic device (LVAD) can also serve as the means of definitive diagnosis of the underlying cardiac condition.**  **(Am J Cardiol 2009;103:110–114)**

Although it may involve virtually any body organ, sarcoidosis infrequently involved the heart, and when it did, it usually did not cause dysfunction of ≥1 noncardiac organ.[1] Cardiac sarcoidosis was usually not diagnosed until percutaneous cardiac biopsy or at necropsy. Earlier, we reported a patient who underwent cardiac transplantation for severe heart failure and diagnosis of cardiac sarcoidosis was not made until morphologic examination of the recipient heart.[2] We found sarcoid granulomas in the left ventricular apical "core" in 3 patients who had a left ventricular assist device (LVAD) inserted because of severe heart failure. Initial diagnosis of cardiac sarcoidosis by this means is most unusual and prompted this report.

## Methods and Results

Pertinent findings in each of the 3 patients are listed in Table 1. All were aged in their 50s and 2 were men. All were mildly overweight (body mass indexes 27.0, 26.5, and 27.0 kg/m$^2$). Chronic heart failure before cardiac transplantation had been present for 3, 4, and 5 years, respectively. Two patients had transient runs of ventricular tachycardia, including 1 with documented ventricular fibrillation. Two had complete branch bundle block and 1 had complete heart block. All had cardioverter defibrillators implanted and 2 had pacemakers implanted. Coronary angiograms showed the epicardial coronary arteries to be either normal (2 patients) or narrowed <50% in diameter (patient 3; Table 1). All 3 had indirect systemic peak systolic blood pressures ≤100 mm Hg. Two were anemic. Only 1 (patient 2) underwent a percutaneous myocardial biopsy, which was negative for sarcoid. Patient 2 also had biopsy-proven sarcoidosis of the lung 16 years earlier (age 36 years) and had been treated with prednisone (10 mg/day) during all 16 years. Spirometry 3 months before cardiac transplantation showed forced vital capacity to be 2.76 L (59% of predicted), forced expiratory volume in 1 second was 1.78 L (49% of predicted), total lung capacity was 76% of predicted value, and diffusing capacity was 57% of predicted value. Times from insertion of the LVAD to cardiac transplantation were 11, 53, and 522 days. Patients 1 and 3 had never been treated with prednisone or other type of corticosteroid, and diagnosis of sarcoid had not been made before the left ventricular apical core had been examined histologically.

Examination of the surgically excised recipient heart showed 2 to have increased cardiac mass. Both ventricular cavities were dilated in all 3 hearts (Figures 1 to 4). (On pretransplantation echocardiograms in patients 1 and 3, right ventricular cavities were 2.6 and 2.3 cm and left ventricular cavities were 9.4 and 5.7 cm, respectively.) All 3 had extensive scarring in the ventricular walls and 2 had numerous noncaseating granulomas.[3] The patient without noncaseating granulomas (patient 1) in the ventricular walls on examination after cardiac transplantation had extensive scarring and foci of lymphocytes in the areas of scarring.

Cardiac transplantation was performed in patient 1 on January 14, 2005; in patient 2, on July 9, 2005; and in

Departments of [a]Internal Medicine, (Division of Cardiology), [b]Pathology, and [c]Cardiothoracic Surgery and the [d]Baylor Heart and Vascular Institute; and Baylor University Medical Center, Dallas, Texas. Manuscript received August 26, 2008; accepted August 27, 2008.

*Corresponding author: Tel: 214-820-7911; Fax: 214-820-7533.
*E-mail address:* wc.roberts@baylorhealth.edu (W.C. Roberts).

Table 1
Clinical and cardiac morphologic findings in 3 patients with cardiac sarcoidosis diagnosed for the first time by histologic examination of the left ventricular apical core excised for insertion of left ventricular assist device for severe heart failure

| Patient No. | Age at Heart Transplantation | Race | Sex | AF | VT | VF | Heart Block | Hct (%) | Pressures (mm Hg) | | | | CI (L/min/m$^2$) | EF (%) | ICD | PM | Heart Weight (g) | Location of Sarcoid | | | Cavity (cm) | |
|---|---|---|---|---|---|---|---|---|---|---|---|---|---|---|---|---|---|---|---|---|---|---|
| | | | | | | | | | LV | RV | PA | PAW mean | | | | | | RV | VS | LV | RV | LV |
| 1 | 50 | W | M | + | + | + | + (LBBB) | 38 | 127/33 | 81/19 | 81/40 | 51 | 1.0 | 10 | + | 0 | 604 | 0* | 0* | +* | 8.0 | 7.0 |
| 2 | 52 | W | M | + | 0 | 0 | + (RBBB) | 26 | N/A | N/A | 51/23 | 24 | 1.6 | 15 | + | + | 480 | + | + | + | 5.2 | 4.2 |
| 3 | 59 | B | F | 0 | + | 0 | + (CHB) | 42 | N/A | 33/11 | 35/16 | 24 | 1.3 | 25 | + | + | 371 | + | + | + | 7.5 | 5.0 |

* Sarcoid granulomas present in the left ventricular apical core removed for insertion of the LVAD. The walls of the left ventricle, ventricular septum, and right ventricle in the excised native heart (at transplantation) had extensive scarring, but no granulomas. Focal collections of lymphocytes were present in the scarred ventricular walls.

AF = atrial fibrillation; B = black; CHB = complete heart block; CI = cardiac index; EF = ejection fraction; Hct = hematocrit; ICD = implantable cardioverter-defibrillator; LBBB = left bundle branch block; LV = left ventricle; PA = pulmonary artery; PAW = pulmonary artery wedge; PM = pacemaker; RBBB = right bundle branch block; RV = right ventricle; VF = ventricular fibrillation; VS = ventricular septum; VT = ventricular tachycardia; W = white.

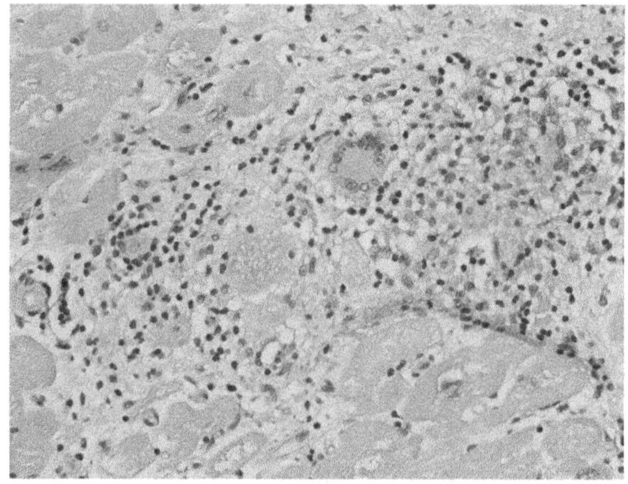

Figure 1. Patient 1. Photomicrograph of sarcoid granuloma in the left ventricular apical core removed 11 days before cardiac transplantation. (Hematoxylin-eosin stain; original magnification ×400.)

patient 3, on July 10, 2006. All 3 patients are alive and active as of August 15, 2008.

The Baylor University Medical Center, Dallas, Texas, Internal Review Board approved the study.

## Discussion

The unique feature of the 3 cases briefly described in this report is the initial diagnosis of cardiac sarcoidosis by histologic examination of the left ventricular apical core excised at the time of insertion of a LVAD for severe heart failure of unclear cause. One other patient with a similar diagnostic scenario was reported previously.[4]

We found 11 previously published case reports of patients who underwent cardiac transplantation for severe heart failure (10 patients) or recurring refractory ventricular arrhythmias (1 patient) secondary to cardiac sarcoidosis (Table 2).[2,4–11] Right-sided intracardiac biopsies after cardiac transplantation were reported later in 7 of these 11 patients, and in 2, noncaseating granulomas were found, indicating recurrence of cardiac sarcoidosis, but this time in the donor heart. The positive biopsies were performed 6 and 19 months after transplantation. Biopsies in 5 other patients were negative for sarcoid 6 to 96 months (mean 29) after transplantation. The other 2 patients died 6 days and 42 months after transplantation. Each of the 3 patients described in this report had right-sided biopsies 15, 24, and 14 months performed after cardiac transplantation and none had noncaseating granulomas in the excised cardiac specimens.

Although not performed for cardiac sarcoidosis, Bartram et al[12] reported findings in a 9-year-old boy who developed systemic sarcoidosis (unclear whether the heart was involved) nearly 9 years after orthotopic heart transplantation for Shone syndrome (supravalvular mitral ring, mitral valve stenosis, valvular and supravalvular aortic stenosis, and aortic coarctation).

Zaidi et al[13] reviewed the United Network for Organ Sharing database to assess survival of patients with sar-

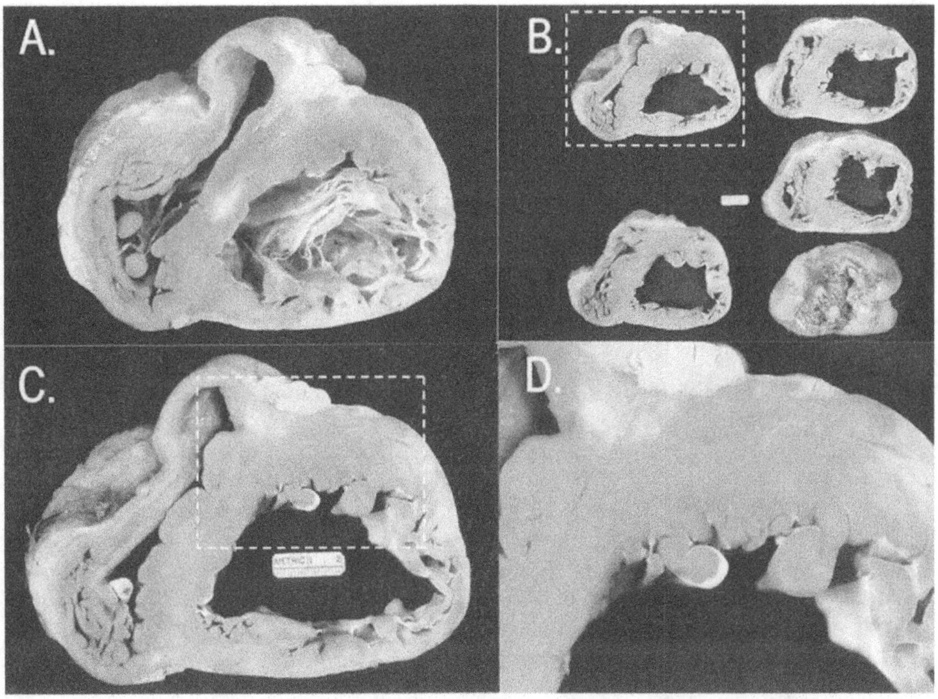


Figure 2. Patient 1. Explanted heart. *(A)* Base shows extensive lateral wall left ventricular scarring and focal ventricular septal scarring by sarcoidosis. Both ventricular cavities are dilated. *(B)* One-centimeter thick slices of the ventricular walls show that scarring extends from base to apex. *(C)* Close-up of 1 ventricular slice shown in *B*. *(D)* Close-up of subepicardial scar in the anterior portion of the ventricular septum shown in *C*.

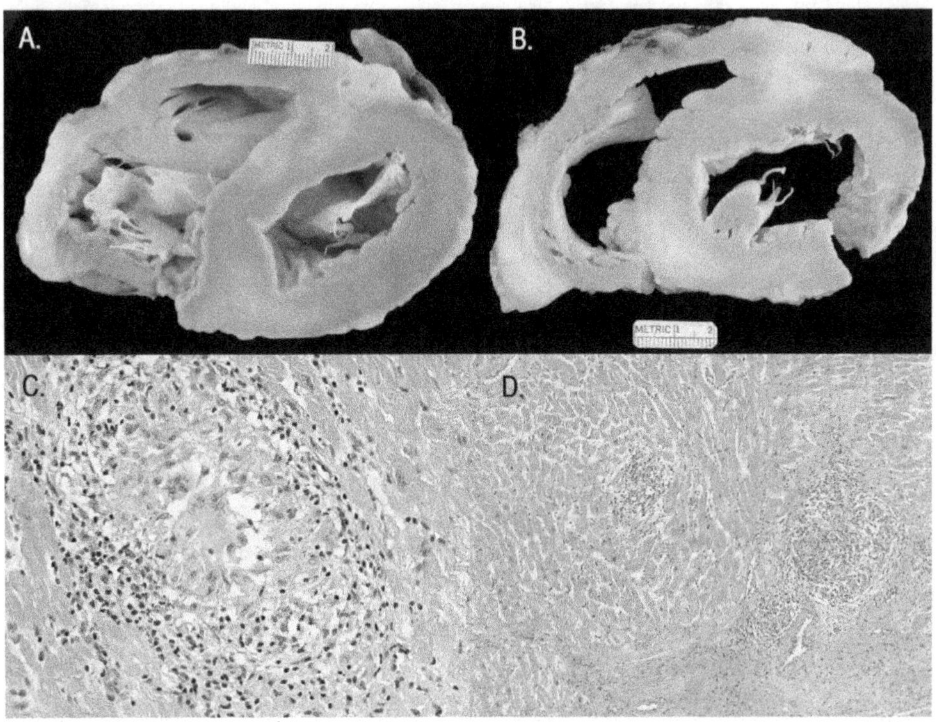


Figure 3. Patient 2. *(A)* Base of heart and *(B)* 1 slice of ventricular walls caudal to the base. Scars are present in the ventricular septum and posterior left ventricular walls. Both cavities are dilated. *(C)* Photomicrograph of a sarcoid granuloma in the left ventricular core removed to insert the LVAD. *(D)* Photomicrograph of portion of explanted heart shows 2 sarcoid granulomas. (Hematoxylin-eosin stain; original magnification *[C]* ×400, *[D]* ×100.)

coidosis treated using heart transplantation. During an 18-year period, 65 patients (40 men, 25 women) with sarcoidosis underwent orthotopic heart transplantation. There were 4 operative deaths and 12 late deaths at a mean follow-up of 40 months. One-year posttransplantation, survival was better for patients with sarcoid undergoing orthotopic transplantation compared with patients undergoing transplantation for nonsarcoid conditions

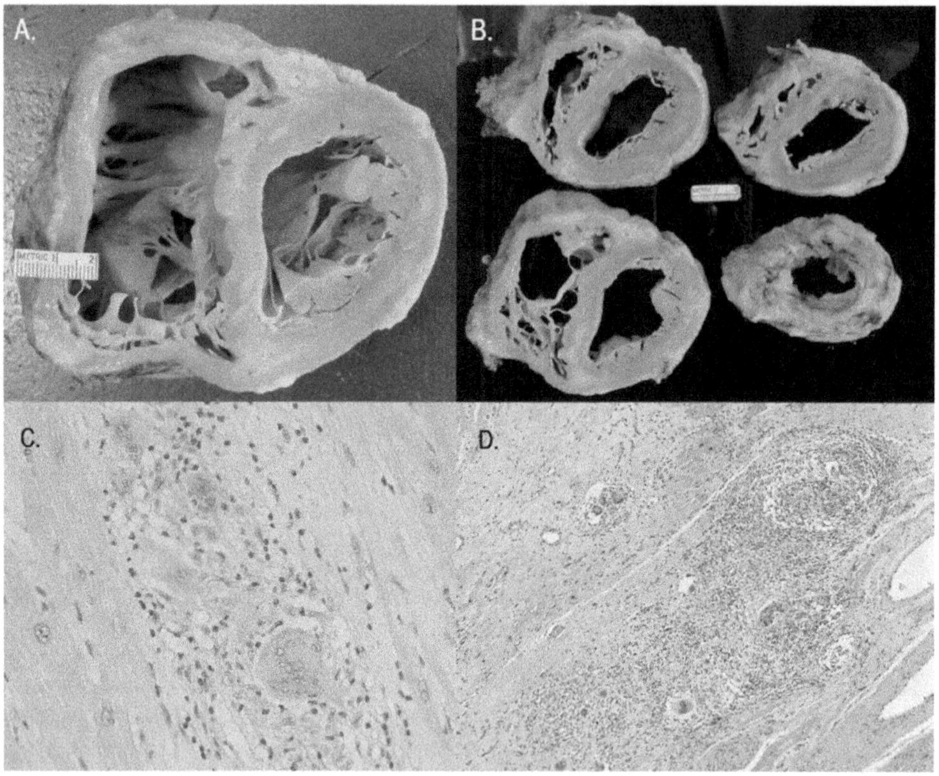


Figure 4. Patient 3. *(A)* Base of heart shows very dilated ventricular cavities and patchy scars in the ventricular septum and left ventricular free wall. *(B)* Slices of ventricular walls caudal to the base again show focal scars. *(C)* Photomicrograph shows sarcoid granuloma in the left ventricular core excised at time of placement of the LVAD. *(D)* Photomicrograph of sarcoid granulomas in the explanted heart. (Hematoxylin-eosin stain; original magnification *[C]* ×400, *[D]* ×100.)

(88% vs 85%; p = 0.03). The investigators concluded that diagnosis of sarcoidosis should not disqualify potential transplantation candidates.

1. Roberts WC, McAllister HA Jr, Ferrans VJ. Sarcoidosis of the heart. A clinicopathologic study of 35 necropsy patients (group I) and review of 78 previously described necropsy patients (group II). *Am J Med* 1977;63:86–108.
2. Donsky AS, Escobar J, Capehart J, Roberts WC. Heart transplantation for undiagnosed cardiac sarcoidosis. *Am J Cardiol* 2002;89:1447–1449.
3. Shirani J, Roberts WC. Subepicardial myocardial lesions. *Am Heart J* 1993;125:1346–1352.
4. Yagar JE, Hernandez AF, Steenbergen C, Persing B, Russell SD, Milano C, Felker GM. Recurrence of cardiac sarcoidosis in a heart transplant recipient. *J Heart Lung Transplant* 2005;24:1988–1990.
5. Gokel JM, Reichart B, Struck E. Human cardiac transplantation—evaluation of morphologic changes in serial endomyocardial biopsies. *Path Res Pract* 1985;79:354–365.
6. Valantine HA, Tazelaar HD, Macoviak J, Mullin AV, Hunt SA, Fowler MB, Billingham ME, Schroeder JS. Cardiac sarcoidosis: response to steroids and transplantation. *J Heart Transplant* 1987;6:244–250.
7. Oni AA, Hershberger RE, Norman DJ, Ray J, Hovaguimian H, Cobanoglu AM, Hosenpud JD. Recurrence of sarcoidosis in a cardiac allograft: control with augmented corticosteroids. *J Heart Lung Transplant* 1992;11:367–369.
8. Ankersmit HJ, Wieselthaler GA, Moser B, Taghavi S, Grimm M, Roth G, Gorlitzer M, Tschernich H, Horvat R, Wolner E. Automated implantable cardiac defibrillator and biventricular thoratec assist device as bridge to transplantation in a patient with sarcoidosis. *J Thorac Cardiovasc Surg* 2001;121:1198–1199.
9. Treaba DO, Benson MD, Assad LW, Dainauskas JR. Sarcoidosis and immunoglobulin lambda II light-chain amyloidosis diagnosed after orthotopic heart transplantation: a case report and review of the literature. *Mod Pathol* 2005;18:451–455.
10. Halushka MK, Yuh DD, Russell SD. Right ventricle-dominant cardiac sarcoidosis with sparing of the left ventricle. *J Heart Lung Transplant* 2006;25:479–482.
11. Greif M, Petrakopoulou P, Weiss M, Reithmann C, Reichart B, Nabauer M, Steinbeck G. Cardiac sarcoidosis concealed by arrhythmogenic right ventricular dysplasia/cardiomyopathy. *Nat Clin Pract Cardiovasc Med* 2008;5:231–236.
12. Bartram U, Thul J, Bauer J, Wössmann W, Schranz D. Systemic sarcoidosis after cardiac transplantation in a 9-year-old child. *J Heart Lung Transplant* 2006;25:1263–1267.
13. Zaidi AR, Zaidi A, Vaitkus PT. Outcome of heart transplantation in patients with sarcoid cardiomyopathy. *J Heart Lung Transplant* 2007;26:714–717.

Table 2
Clinical and morphologic cardiac data in previously reported case reports of patients undergoing cardiac transplantation for cardiac sarcoidosis

| Case | Reference | Year Published | Age at HT (yrs) | Race | Sex | Pre-HT Dx of Sarcoid | Reason for HT | Native Heart Weight (g) | Location of Granulomas | | | Dilated | | BBB | CHB | VT | PR >0.20 s | Died (mo after HT) | Recurrence of Cardiac Sarcoid After HT |
|---|---|---|---|---|---|---|---|---|---|---|---|---|---|---|---|---|---|---|---|
| | | | | | | | | | RV | VS | LV | RV | LV | | | | | | |
| 1 | Gokel et al[5] | 1985 | 37 | N/A | M | + (Bx) | HF | N/A | – | – | – | – | – | – | – | – | – | + (8) | – |
| 2 | Valantine et al[6] | 1987 | 46 | W | M | 0 | VT | 630 | + | + | + | 0 | 0 | + [R] | 0 | + | + | + (42) | 0 (A) |
| 3 | Valantine et al[6] | 1987 | 47 | B | M | + (Bx) | HF | 420 | "Widespread" | | | 0 | + | 0 | 0 | + | + | 0 (16+) | 0 (Bx) |
| 4 | Valantine et al[6] | 1987 | 51 | W | F | 0 | HF | 400 | 0 | + | + | – | – | + [R] | 0 | 0 | + | 0 (20+) | 0 (Bx) |
| 5 | Oni et al[7] | 1992 | 34 | N/A | M | + (Bx) | HF | N/A | – | – | – | + | + | 0 | 0 | + | 0 | 0 (13+) | + (Bx) |
| 6 | Ankersmit et al[8] | 2001 | 30 | N/A | M | + (Bx) | HF | N/A | – | – | – | + | + | 0 | 0 | + | 0 | 0 (1+) | – |
| 7 | Donsky et al[2] | 2002 | 53 | W | M | 0 | HF | 510 | + | + | + | + | + | + [L] | 0 | + | + | 0 (105+) | 0 (Bx) |
| 8 | Yager et al[4] | 2005 | 26 | B | M | + (LVAD) | HF | N/A | – | – | – | – | – | 0 | 0 | 0 | 0 | 0 (24+) | + (Bx) |
| 9 | Treaba et al[9] | 2005 | 53 | B | M | 0 | HF | N/A | + | + | + | – | – | 0 | + | 0 | 0 | + (0.2) | 0 (A) |
| 10 | Halushka et al[10] | 2006 | 53 | W | M | + (Bx) | HF | 380 | + | + | + | + | 0 | 0 | 0 | + | 0 | 0 (6+) | 0 (Bx) |
| 11 | Greif et al[11] | 2008 | 37 | N/A | M | 0 | HF | N/A | + | + | + | + | 0 | + [L] | 0 | + | 0 | 0 (8+) | 0 (Bx) |

A = autopsy; B = black; BBB = bundle branch block; Bx = biopsy of myocardium; CHB = complete heart block; Dx = diagnosis; HF = heart failure; HT = heart transplantation; L = left; LV = left ventricle; R = right; RV = right ventricle; VS = ventricular septum; VT = ventricular tachycardia; W = white.

# Diagnosing cardiac sarcoidosis clinically without tissue confirmation

Poonam S. Sharma, MD, Jordon G. Lubahn, MD, Alan S. Donsky, MD, Anthony Dong H. Yoon, MD, Melissa M. Carry, MD, Paul A. Grayburn, MD, Prescilla Barrientos Wood, MD, Jong Mi Ko, BA, Elizabeth C. Burton, MD, and William Clifford Roberts, MD

A 52-year-old woman is described in whom cardiac sarcoidosis was diagnosed clinically on the basis of high-grade heart block, recurring ventricular tachyarrhythmias, and acute cardiac decompensation. Confirmation of sarcoidosis was not determined until necropsy. When it causes cardiac dysfunction, sarcoidosis rarely causes dysfunction of another body organ, although small sarcoid granulomas may also be present in noncardiac organs or tissues. In the present patient, neurosarcoidosis accompanied the cardiac sarcoidosis, but it was the latter that produced the life-threatening symptoms and was fatal.

Sarcoidosis is characterized by the presence of noncaseating giant-cell granulomas in more than one body organ. Although these granulomas may be present in virtually any organ, most commonly they occur in the lungs and in adjacent lymph nodes (1), but they are rare in the spinal cord. Symptoms usually appear gradually. Diagnosis often is made by chest radiograph showing hilar adenopathy with or without pulmonary parenchymal lesions before appearance of symptoms. Occasionally, sarcoidosis presents with symptoms related to the heart, and in such circumstances the manifestations usually are acute, consisting of a ventricular arrhythmia or a high grade of heart block or symptoms of heart failure (2). When sarcoidosis causes cardiac dysfunction, infrequently is there dysfunction of another body organ (2). To emphasize the fact that patients with cardiac sarcoidosis severe enough to cause cardiac dysfunction rarely have more than minimal involvement of noncardiac body organs, we describe the following case.

## DESCRIPTION OF PATIENT

A 52-year-old nonsmoking, overweight African American female bus driver, who was born in February 1956, had been well until November 2007 when she noted right-sided mid back pain and, in December 2007, impaired vision in the right eye. The right optic disc was swollen and pale. The back pain made it difficult for her to dress herself, it was burning and shooting in nature, and it radiated to her right arm and breast. The impaired vision in the right eye caused blurriness and occasional double vision and was associated with pain with eye movement. Magnetic resonance imaging in January 2008 disclosed multiple small thoracic spine neural foramen tumors and abnormal contrast enhancement in the right retrobulbar fat and along the right optic nerve sheath, and a 15-mm "low-density" lesion in the left lower lobe of the lung was detected by computed tomography. The hilar and mediastinal structures were normal. Treadmill stress echocardiogram disclosed intermittent right bundle branch block throughout exercise and sinus bradycardia at rest, but no ST changes. A four-beat run of atrial tachycardia with aberrant conduction occurred during exercise. No wall-motion abnormalities were seen. Because of the eye problem, she was started on prednisone 80 mg daily and tapered to 10 mg for 7 months. She was off prednisone for the last 5 months of her life. Her vision improved in the right eye from 20/400 to 20/40 as a consequence of treatment.

Repeat chest radiograph in July 2008 disclosed no abnormalities. Echocardiogram disclosed normal-sized ventricular cavities and hyperdynamic left ventricular systolic function. Left ventricular diastolic function, however, was abnormal.

The eye problem cleared and, except for continued periodic right-sided back pain, occasional leg numbness, and some difficulty walking up stairs, she was active and continued working as a bus driver until December 26, 2008, when severe dyspnea appeared. She was found to have complete heart block, and a pacemaker was inserted. The dyspnea, however, persisted and within a week was accompanied by severe substernal chest pain radiating to both arms, dizziness, and worsening dyspnea. She was rehospitalized on January 6, 2009. The erythrocyte sedimentation rate was 76 mm in 1 hour; hematocrit, 31%; troponin, 2.92 ng/mL; and B-type natriuretic peptide, 1183 pg/mL. At cardiac catheterization, the epicardial coronary arteries were normal. The left ventricular ejection fraction was about 55%. Pressures (in mm Hg) were as follows: pulmonary artery, 45/26; pulmonary wedge a wave, 28, v wave, 33, and mean, 26; right atrial a wave, 18, v wave, 23, and mean, 15; left ventricle, 105/14; and aorta, 109/64. A left ventricular angiogram showed a mildly hypokinetic posterobasal wall

From the Department of Internal Medicine (Sharma, Lubahn), Division of Cardiology (Donsky, Yoon, Carry, Grayburn, Roberts), Department of Pathology (Wood, Burton, Roberts), and the Baylor Heart and Vascular Institute (Grayburn, Ko, Roberts), Baylor University Medical Center, Dallas, Texas.

**Corresponding author:** William C. Roberts, MD, Baylor Heart and Vascular Institute, Baylor University Medical Center, 3500 Gaston Avenue, Dallas, Texas 75246 (e-mail: wc.roberts@BaylorHealth.edu).

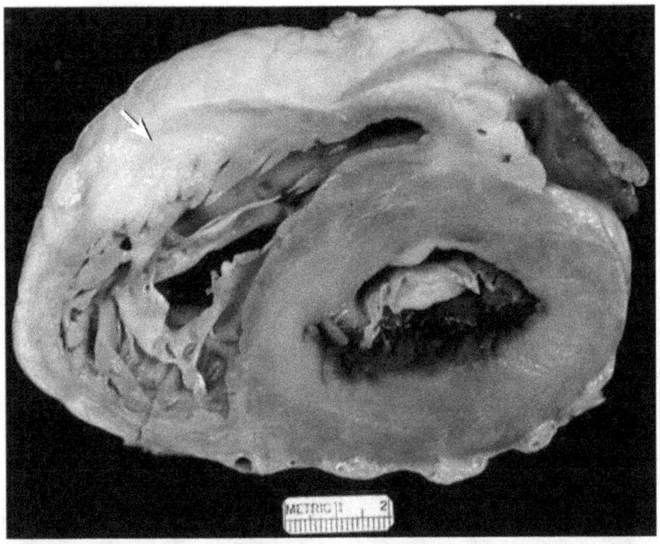


**Figure 1.** The base of the heart, showing a large sarcoid nodule in the right ventricular free wall anteriorly (arrow).

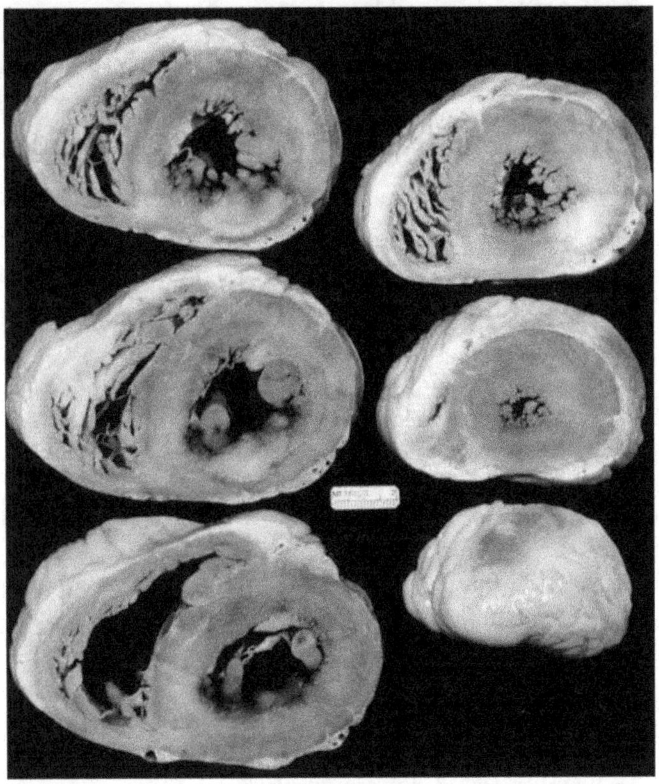

**Figure 2.** Cross-sections of the ventricular walls and cavities showing multiple sarcoid granulomas. One sarcoid focus involves a portion of the posteromedial papillary muscle of the left ventricle, and this deposit may have played a role in causing the mitral regurgitation.

and 2+/4+ mitral regurgitation. Ventricular tachycardia occurred during the procedure. An echocardiogram on January 16 showed depressed right and left ventricular systolic function (ejection fraction 45%), a restrictive left ventricular diastolic filling pattern, and severe mitral regurgitation. The heart failure progressively worsened, the blood pressure dropped, and ventricular tachycardia refractory to cardioversion occurred followed subsequently by fatal ventricular fibrillation on January 22, 2009.

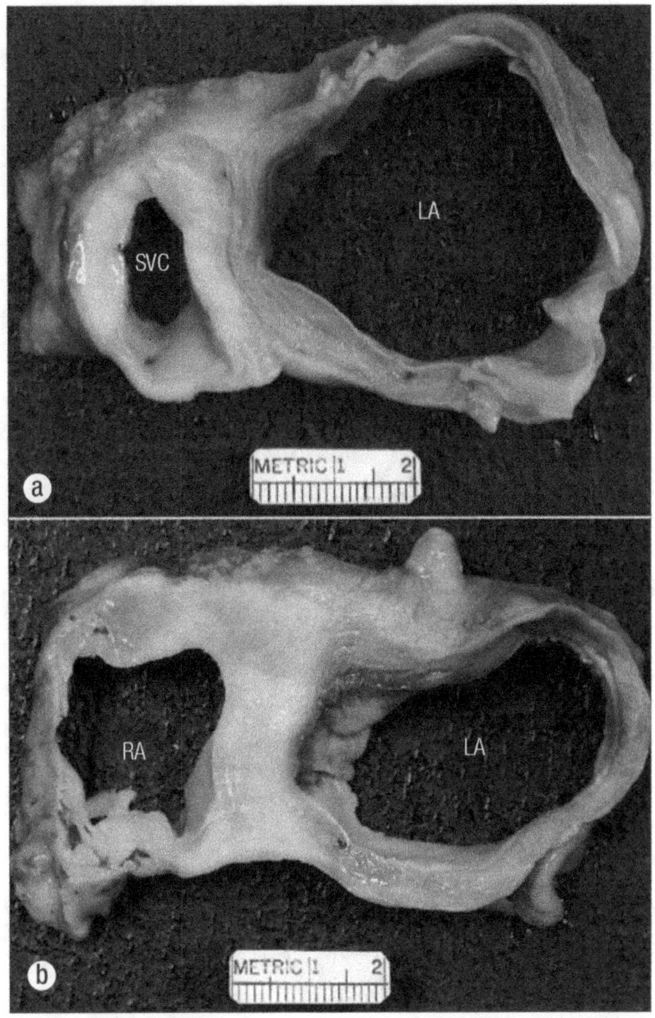


**Figure 3. (a)** The superior vena cava (SVC) entering the right atrium (RA), with the wall of this large vein replaced by sarcoid granulomas. **(b)** The more caudal portion of the RA and left atrium (LA), showing sarcoid granuloma in the right atrial wall posteriorly and in the atrial septum.

At necropsy, the heart weighed 485 g. The epicardial coronary arteries were normal. Multiple lesions were present in the right and left ventricular free walls and in the ventricular septum *(Figures 1 and 2)*. Additionally, the wall of the superior vena cava as it entered the right atrium and portions of the right atrial wall and atrial septum were infiltrated by similar lesions, which histologically were noncaseating giant-cell granulomas *(Figure 3)*. Sarcoid granulomas in the right ventricular wall are shown in *Figure 4* and in the left ventricular wall in *Figure 5*. The four cardiac valves were anatomically normal.

The lung parenchyma was normal grossly except for one lesion in the lower lobe of the left lung, and it too was a sarcoid granuloma *(Figures 6 and 7)*. At least two hilar lymph nodes were infiltrated by similar granulomas: one was normal sized, and one about 4 times larger than normal (Figure 7a).

The spinal cord tumors, seen by magnetic resonance, proved to be sarcoid granulomas *(Figure 8)*. Similar granulomas were present in the single kidney (one had been removed earlier for donation to a family member for renal transplantation).

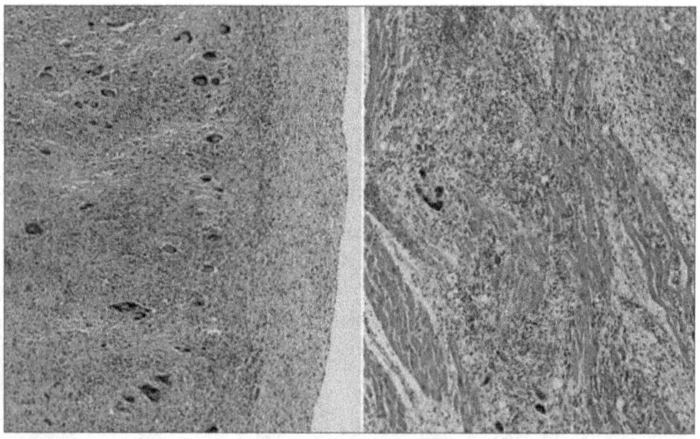

Figure 4. Granulomas in the right ventricular wall. Hematoxylin and eosin stains, each ×100. Stains for fungi and acid-fast organisms were negative.

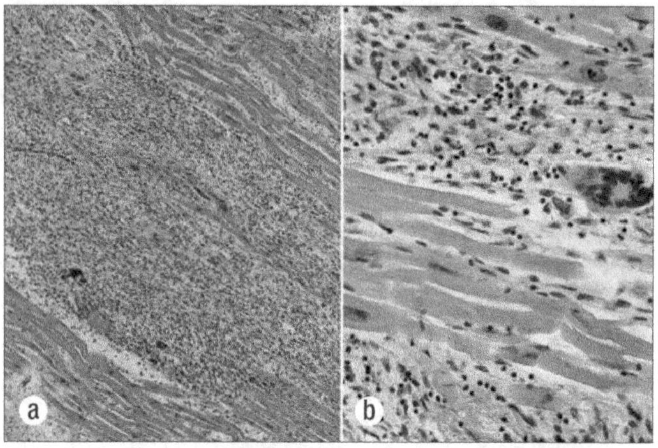


Figure 5. Sarcoid myocarditis in the left ventricular wall. Hematoxylin and eosin stains, (a) ×100, (b) ×400.

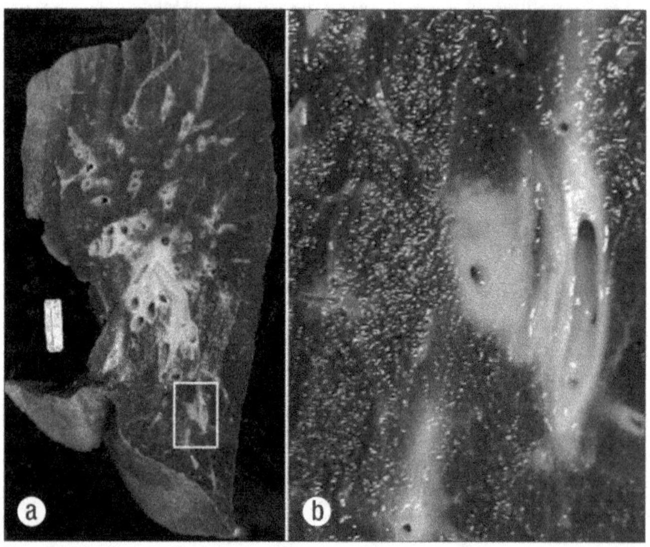


Figure 6. (a) Longitudinal section of the lung showing a single sarcoid granuloma. (b) A close-up of the area in the square.

## DISCUSSION

The patient described had classic features of cardiac sarcoidosis, namely a high degree of heart block (third degree), recurring ventricular arrhythmias, and both systolic and diastolic cardiac dysfunction resulting in severe heart failure. Because of this triad of cardiac manifestations, cardiac sarcoidosis was diagnosed clinically. Necropsy confirmed the diagnosis of sarcoidosis, which involved extensively the heart, thoracic spinal cord, and hilar lymph nodes (only one of which was enlarged), and minimally the lung and kidney. The cause of her back pain was sarcoid granulomas within the spinal cord. Although its cause about a year before death was never definitely determined, the visual disturbance prompted the initiation of prednisone therapy, which eliminated the eye problem and obviously is the treatment of choice for sarcoidosis.

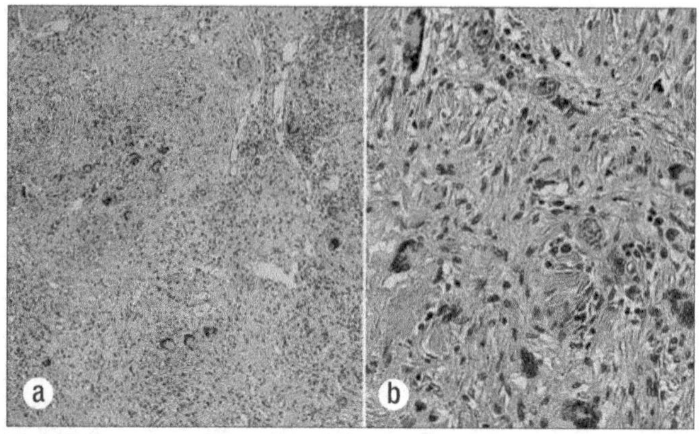


Figure 7. Sarcoid granulomas in the (a) hilar lymph node and (b) lung. Hematoxylin and eosin stains, ×100 (a), ×400 (b).

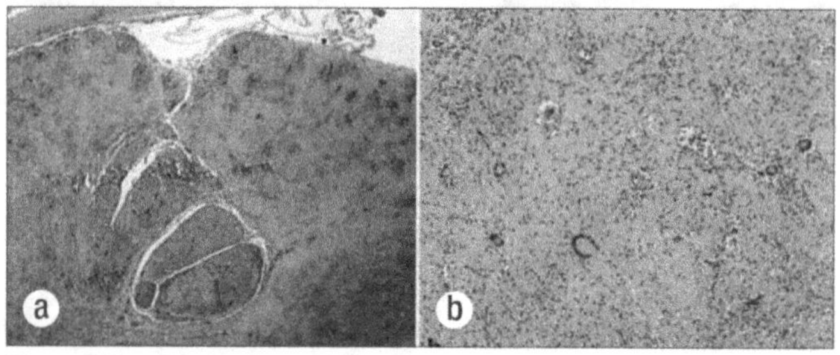


Figure 8. Sarcoid granulomas in the thoracic spinal cord. Hematoxylin and eosin stains, (a) ×2, (b) ×100.

A very unusual feature of the present case is the occurrence of sarcoid granulomas in the spinal cord, which led to some nonlimiting symptoms. Others also have reported neurosarcoid involvement in patients with cardiac sarcoidosis (3, 4). Saleh and colleagues (3) reviewed 172 patients with spinal cord sarcoidosis, and 7 (4%) had cardiac involvement. Perry and Vuitch (4), however, found no cases of neurosarcoidosis among 14 autopsied patients with fatal cardiac sarcoidosis.

1. Crystal RG, Roberts WC, Hunninghake GW, Gadek JE, Fulmer JD, Line BR. Pulmonary sarcoidosis: a disease characterized and perpetuated by activated lung T-lymphocytes. *Ann Intern Med* 1981;94(1):73–94.
2. Roberts WC, McAllister HA Jr, Ferrans VJ. Sarcoidosis of the heart. A clinicopathologic study of 35 necropsy patients (group I) and review of 78 previously described necropsy patients (group II). *Am J Med* 1977;63(1):86–108.
3. Saleh S, Saw C, Marzouk K, Sharma O. Sarcoidosis of the spinal cord: literature review and report of eight cases. *J Natl Med Assoc* 2006;98(6):965–976.
4. Perry A, Vuitch F. Causes of death in patients with sarcoidosis. A morphologic study of 38 autopsies with clinicopathologic correlations. *Arch Pathol Lab Med* 1995;119(2):167–172.

# Some Previously Neglected Examples of Arrhythmogenic Right Ventricular Dysplasia/Cardiomyopathy and Frequency of Its Various Reported Manifestations

William Clifford Roberts, MD[a,b,c,*], Jong Mi Ko, BA[c], Johannes Jacob Kuiper, MD[d], Shelley Anne Hall, MD[d], and Dan Marshall Meyer, MD[d,e]

**Four patients are described with either parchment-like thinning or partial but extensive myocyte depletion with severe fatty or fibrofatty infiltration of the free wall of the right ventricle in its outflow tract, including 2 previously reported patients who also had focal parchment-like thinning of the left ventricular free wall. Three had documented ventricular tachycardia, and the remaining patient had sudden death as his first and only manifestation of heart disease. Three patients had severe heart failure: in 1, it was fatal, and the other 2 underwent cardiac transplantation. Necropsy cases of parchment-heart syndrome before 1980 are reviewed, as well as large series of cases with arrhythmogenic right ventricular dysplasia (ARVD) reported subsequently. It is suggested that ARVD is not an ideal name for this condition, because malignant ventricular arrhythmias are not universal, the left ventricular free wall and/or ventricular septum are sometimes involved, and the name "ARVD" neglects the fact that severe heart failure may be prominent in these patients. The right ventricular wall can be thin or parchment-like, or it may not be thinned but consist mainly of adipose tissue with or without focal fibrous tissue and a few islands of myocytes. Nevertheless, because the name "ARVD" has been commonly used and recognized for >30 years, it is probably best retained for this condition.**  **(Am J Cardiol 2010;106:268–274)**

In 1905, Osler[1] reported a man in his 40s who had died suddenly and unexpectedly while walking up a hill, and necropsy disclosed "parchment-like" thinning of portions of the right and left ventricular free walls in the absence of coronary narrowing or apparent cardiac valve dysfunction. In 1950, Segall[2] described in more detail the patient briefly reported by Osler.[1] The second patient reported (in 1952) to have a parchment-like heart was a 23-year-old woman who had chronic, eventually fatal heart failure and focal thinning of the walls of both ventricles.[3] The third patient, a 7-year-old girl with severe right-sided heart failure and severe thinning of much of the right ventricular free wall, was described by Uhl,[4] also in 1952. Thereafter, through 1980, ≥23 additional patients with parchment-like thinning of the right ventricular wall were reported (Table 1).[5–22] Except for the initial patient reported by Osler[1] and later by Segall[2] and 2 patients reported by Waller et al[23] in 1980, all had myocardial wall thinning limited to the wall of the right ventricle. The 1 patient reported by Osler[1] and later by Segall,[2] the 1 patient reported by Castleman and Sprague,[3] and the 2 patients reported by Waller et al[23] all had congenital hypoplasia of portions of the right and left ventricular free walls in the absence of associated coronary or valvular heart disease. The term "arrhythmogenic right ventricular dysplasia" (ARVD) was first proposed by Fontaine et al[24] in 1977 in a book chapter describing 6 patients with sustained ventricular tachycardia without heart failure and was put on the popular screen by Marcus et al in 1982.[25] Since that time, numerous publications have appeared describing its clinical, radiographic, electrocardiographic, and hemodynamic features. The present report briefly describes again the 2 cases reported by Waller et al[23] in 1980 and describes 2 additional patients, neither diagnosed clinically, with this syndrome treated by cardiac transplantation.

## Patients Studied

Pertinent clinical and morphologic features of the 4 patients are listed in Table 2 and illustrated in Figures 1 to 6. One of the 2 earlier cases (patient 1) had severe, eventually fatal heart failure, and in the other (patient 2), sudden death was the first and only manifestation of his cardiac disease.[23] Patients 3 and 4 had severe intractable heart failure and as a consequence underwent cardiac transplantation. Patient 2's mother and sister had pacemakers. Patient 3 had ventricular tachycardia at 12 years of age treated by an ablation procedure, without recurrence thereafter. Patient 4 also had runs of ventricular tachycardia, and patients 3 and 4 underwent intracardiac defibrillator device insertion.

## Comments

Described and illustrated herein are 4 patients with clinical and morphologic features of ARVD. Three patients had severe heart failure, 1 fatal and 2 severe enough to warrant

[a]Department of Internal Medicine, Division of Cardiology, [b]Department of Pathology, [c]Baylor Heart and Vascular Institute, [d]Baylor Regional Transplant Institute, and the [e]Department of Cardiothoracic Surgery, Baylor University Medical Center, Dallas, Texas. Manuscript received December 2, 2009; revised manuscript received and accepted March 4, 2010.

*Corresponding author: Tel: 214-820-7911; fax: 214-820-7533.

*E-mail address:* wc.roberts@baylorhealth.edu (W.C. Roberts).

Table 1

Clinical and morphologic observations in necropsy patients with parchment hearts reported from 1905 to 1979

| Study | Age at Death | Gender | HF | Symptom Duration (months) | CE (X-Ray) | Abnormal Results on ECG | Mode of Death | HW (g) | Location of Thinned Ventricular Myocardium | | | |
|---|---|---|---|---|---|---|---|---|---|---|---|---|
| | | | | | | | | | RV | | | LV |
| | | | | | | | | | I | A | O | |
| **Patients aged ≤5 years** | | | | | | | | | | | | |
| Haworth et al (1975)[5] | 1 day | M | + | 1/30 | + | + | HF | — | + | + | 0 | — |
| Diaz et al (1973)[6] | 4 mo | M | + | 4 | + | + | HF | — | + | 0 | 0 | 0 |
| Novak et al (1957)[7] | 5 mo | M | + | 5 | + | + | HF | — | + | + | 0 | 0 |
| Arcilla et al (1961)[8] | 6 mo | M | + | 6 | + | + | HF | — | + | + | + | 0 |
| Uhl (1952)[4] | 7 mo | F | + | 4 | + | + | HF | — | + | + | 0 | 0 |
| Cumming et al (1965)[9] | 7 mo | F | + | 4 | + | + | PO | 48 | 0 | + | 0 | 0 |
| Aherne (1973)[10] | 7 mo | F | + | 3 | + | + | HF | — | + | + | + | 0 |
| Perrin and Mehrizi (1965)[11] | 10 mo | M | + | 7 | + | + | HF | — | 0 | + | 0 | 0 |
| Sherman (1963)[12] | 15 mo | F | + | 12 | + | + | HF | — | + | + | + | 0 |
| Kinare et al (1969)[13] | 60 mo | F | + | 60 | + | + | HF | 130 | + | + | + | 0 |
| **Patients aged >15 years** | | | | | | | | | | | | |
| Abe et al (1973)[14] | 17 yrs | F | + | 48 | + | + | PO | 400 | 0 | + | + | 0 |
| Murata et al (1976)[15] | 18 yrs | F | + | 12 | + | + | HF | 400 | 0 | + | + | 0 |
| Froment et al (1968)[16] | 19 yrs | M | + | — | + | — | HF | 350 | 0 | + | 0 | — |
| Vecht et al (1979)[17] | 19 yrs | M | + | 132 | + | + | PO | 435 | + | 0 | 0 | — |
| Castleman and Sprague (1952)[3] | 24 yrs | F | + | 12 | + | + | HF | 300 | + | + | + | 0 |
| Froment et al (1968)[16] | 26 yrs | M | + | — | + | — | HF | 430 | 0 | + | 0 | — |
| Bharati et al (1978)[18] | 29 yrs | F | + | 108 | + | + | HF+CHB | 545 | + | + | + | 0 |
| Osler (1905)[1] (Segall [1950][2]) | 40 s | M | — | — | — | — | SD | 168 | + | + | + | + |
| Reeve and MacDonald (1964)[19] | 47 yrs | F | + | 432 | + | + | CVA | 290 | + | 0 | 0 | 0 |
| Forssman and Bjorkman (1972)[20] | 47 yrs | M | 0 | — | — | + | SD | — | 0 | + | 0 | — |
| Gould et al (1967)[21] | 66 yrs | M | 0 | 0 | 0 | 0 | L | 600 | + | + | 0 | 0 |
| Sugiura et al (1970)[22] | 84 yrs | F | 0 | 0 | 0 | 0 | AP | 220 | 0 | 0 | + | 0 |

Modified with permission from *Am J Cardiol*.[23]

A = ventricular apex; AP = acute pneumonia; CE = cardiac enlargement; CHB = complete heart block; CVA = cerebrovascular accident; ECG = electrocardiography; HF = heart failure; HW = heart weight; I = inflow tract; L = leukemia; LV = left ventricle; O = outflow tract; PO = early postoperatively; RV = right ventricle; SD = sudden death; — = no information available; + = present or positive; 0 = negative or absent.

Table 2

Clinical and morphologic features in the 4 patients described with arrhythmogenic right ventricular dysplasia

| Variable | Patient | | | |
|---|---|---|---|---|
| | 1 | 2 | 3 | 4 |
| Age (years) at death or CT | 61 | 55 | 26 | 44 |
| Gender | Male | Female | Male | Male |
| Age at symptom onset (years) | 61 | 53 | 12 | 42 |
| Heart failure, chronic | 0 | ++++ | ++++ | ++++ |
| Ventricular arrhythmia | — | + | + | + |
| Bundle branch block | — | + | + | + |
| Body mass index (kg/m$^2$) | — | 17 | 24 | 22 |
| Diagnosis of ARVD clinically | 0 | 0 | 0 | 0 |
| Clinical diagnosis | SD | Pericardial disease | IDC | HC |
| Intracardiac defibrillator implanted | 0 | 0 | + | + (2004) |
| Indirect blood pressure (mm Hg) | 130/70 | 115/80* | 100/60 | 90/60 |
| 4-chamber dilatation | 0 | 0 | + | + |
| Pulmonary arterial pressure (mm Hg) (s/d) | — | 28/20* | 50/30 (mean 38) | 19/12 (mean 14) |
| Cardiac index (L/min/m$^2$) | — | — | 0.8 | 1.9 |
| Ejection fraction (%) | — | 65* | 15 | 25 |
| Heart weight (g) | 350 | 320 | 595 | 323 |

* Cardiac catheterization was performed 21 months before death, and heart failure at that time was purely right sided.

CT = cardiac transplantation; HC = hypertrophic cardiomyopathy; IDC = idiopathic dilated cardiomyopathy; s/d = peak systole/end diastole. Other abbreviations as in Table 1.

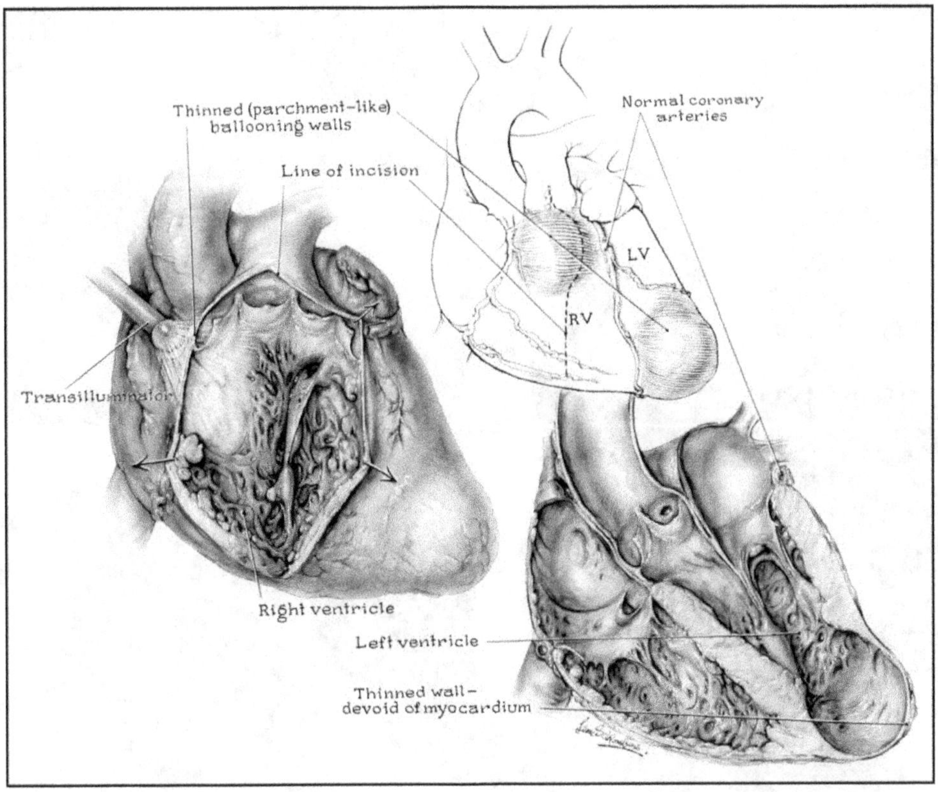


Figure 1. Case 1: drawing of the heart showing the thinned portions of walls of the right ventricle (RV) and left ventricle (LV). Reproduced with permission from *Am J Cardiol*.[23]

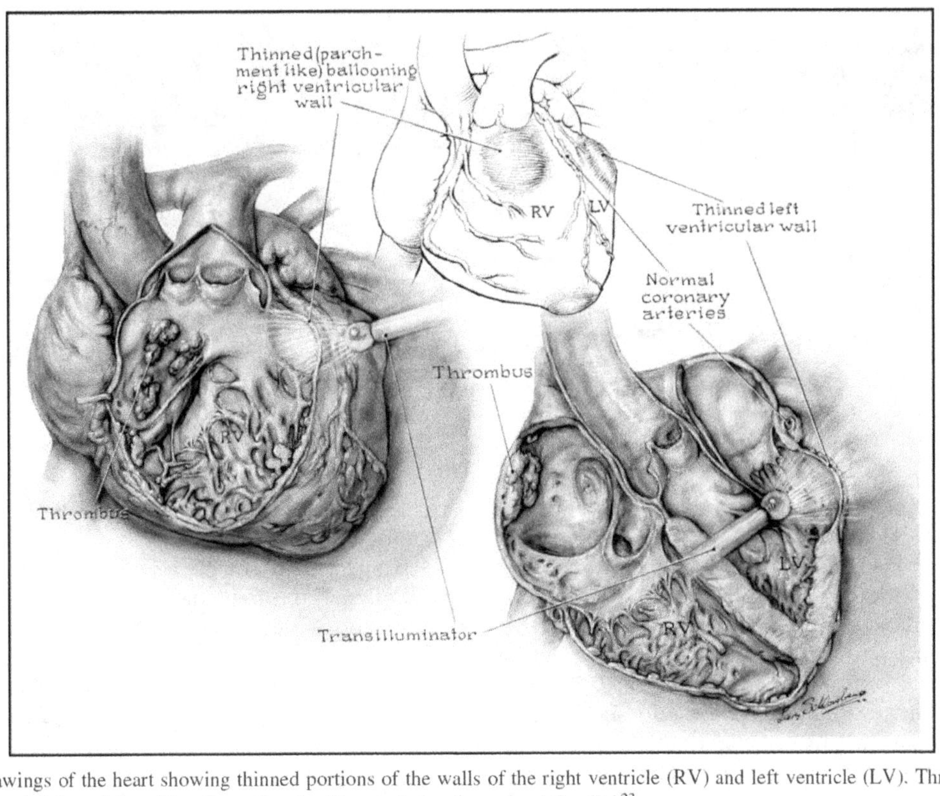


Figure 2. Case 2: drawings of the heart showing thinned portions of the walls of the right ventricle (RV) and left ventricle (LV). Thrombi were present in the right ventricular and right atrial cavities. Reproduced with permission from *Am J Cardiol*.[23]

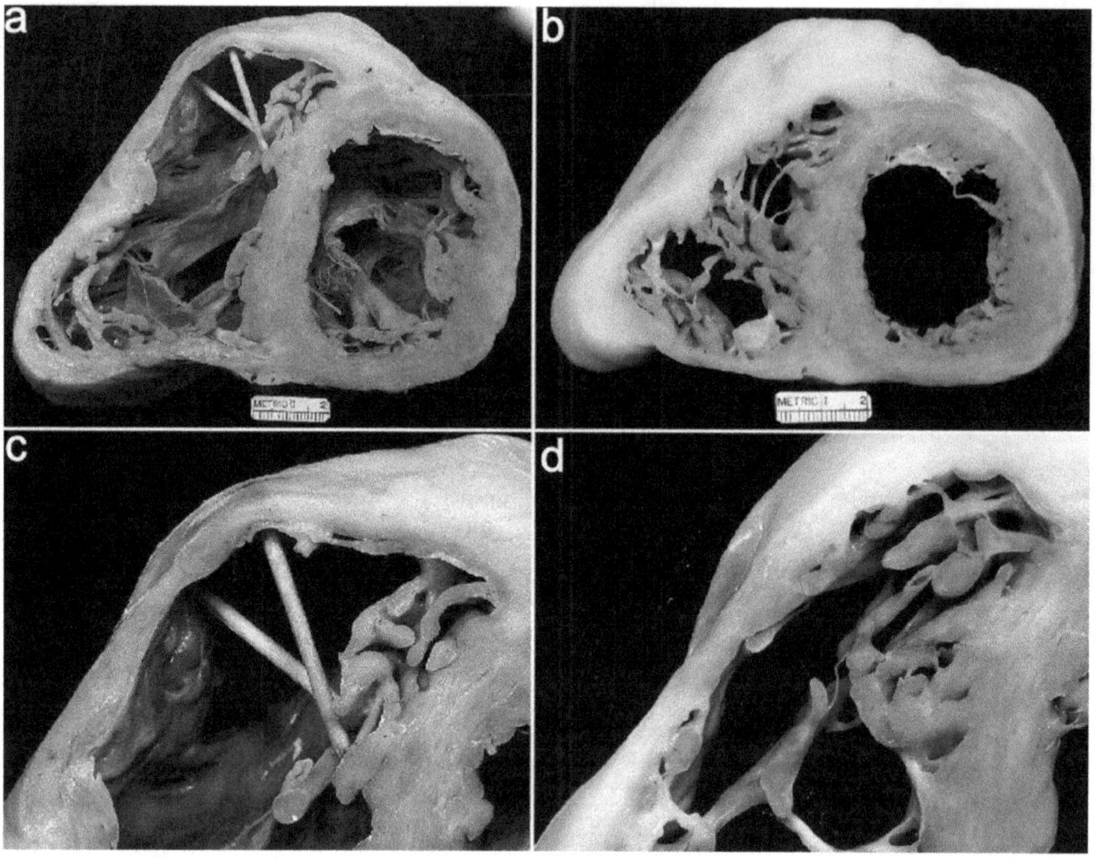

Figure 3. Case 3: cardiac ventricular walls and cavities showing marked dilatation of both cavities *(a,b)* and thinning of the wall in the right ventricular outflow tract *(c,d)*. The amount of subepicardial adipose tissue is excessive.

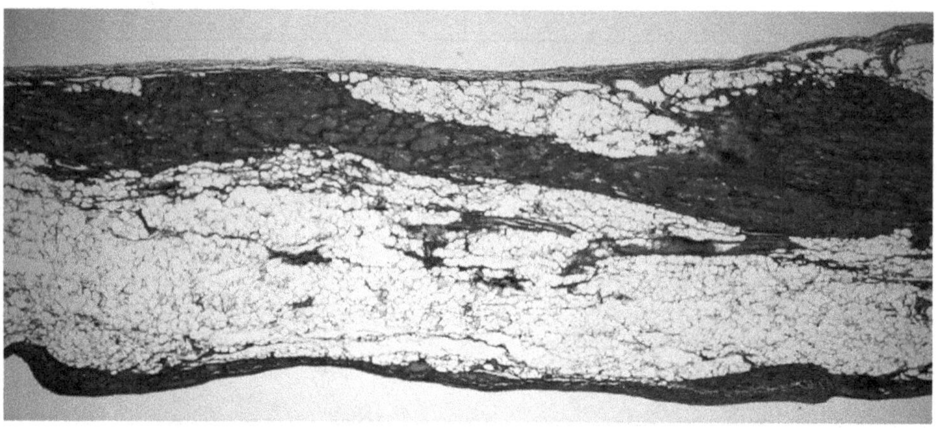

Figure 4. Case 3: photomicrograph (Masson stain, 20×) of the right ventricular wall in its outflow tract. Most of the wall consists of adipose tissue. A thin band of myocardium *(red)* with excessive interstitial fibrous tissue *(blue)* is present.

cardiac transplantation. The other patient died suddenly and unexpectedly, and sudden death was his first manifestation of cardiac disease. Two patients had parchment-like thinning of the right ventricular wall in its outflow portion, and both also had similar thinning in the left ventricular free wall: at its apex in 1 and at its posterobasal portion in the other (Figures 1 and 2). Patients 3 and 4 had fatty infiltrations and partial but severe myocyte depletion in the right ventricular outflow tract. None of the 4 patients had coronary arterial or valvular heart disease. Three had documented ventricular tachycardia, and the 1 who died suddenly while walking presumably also had a "malignant" ventricular arrhythmia.

Table 3 lists selected studies of patients reported with ARVD and the frequency in them of ventricular tachycardia, sudden death, chronic heart failure, left ventricular "dysplasia," and cardiac transplantation.[25–45] Ventricular tachycardia was the most frequent manifestation, but the accuracy of this percentage is unclear. The patients included in the first few studies were referred because of the ventricular arrhythmia, and the necropsy studies had few data on the frequency of these arrhythmias. Sudden, unexpected

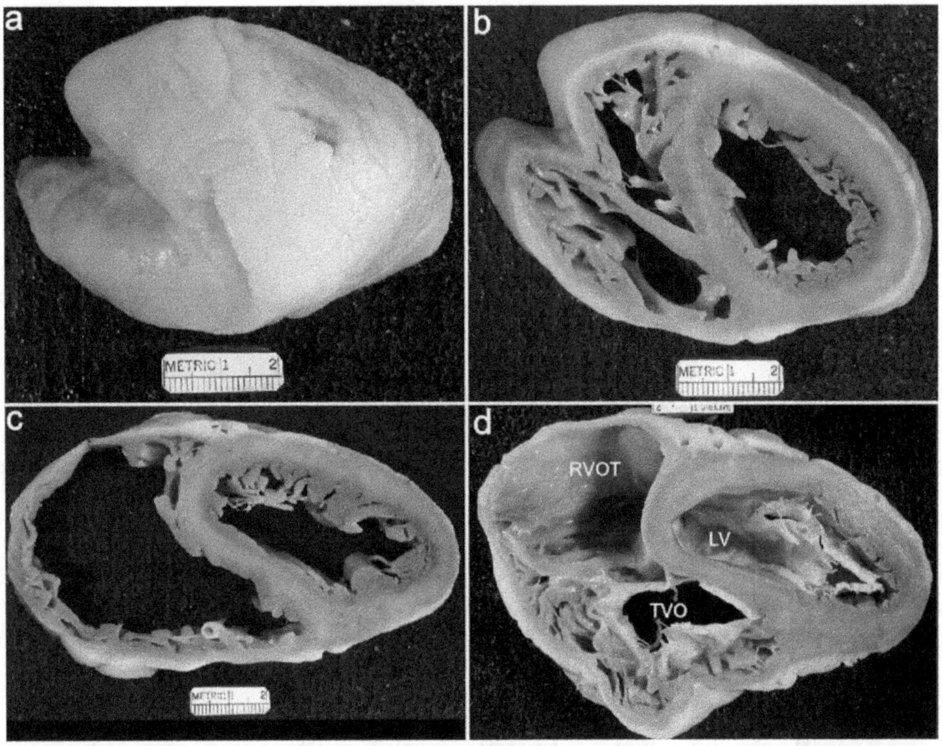


Figure 5. Case 4: heart. *(a)* View from the cardiac apex showing excessive subepicardial adipose tissue and a V-shaped indentation in the right ventricular wall. *(b)* Transverse cut showing the cavities and walls of both cardiac ventricles. The indentation of the right ventricular free wall was caused by the "pull" of a moderator and extending from the right ventricular aspect of the ventricular septum to the right ventricular free wall. *(c)* A more basal view of both ventricles showing the marked dilatation of both cavities, the right greater than the left. *(d)* View showing the very dilated and thin-walled right ventricular outflow tract. LV = left ventricular cavity; RVOT = right ventricular outflow tract; TVO = tricuspid valve orifice.

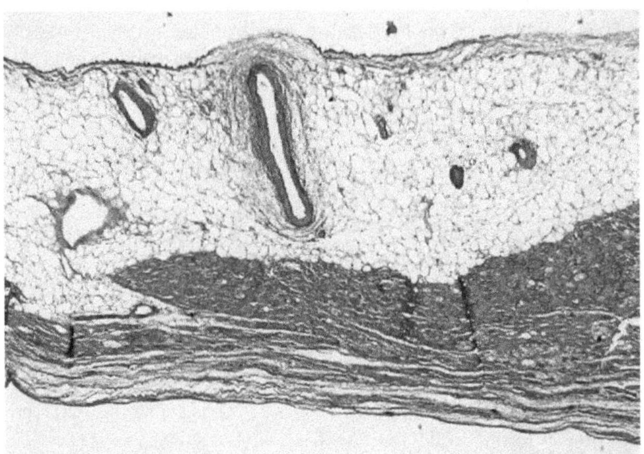

Figure 6. Case 4: photomicrograph (Masson stain, 40×) of the wall of the right ventricle in its outflow portion showing the wall to consist mainly of adipose tissue and scarred *(blue)* myocardium *(red)*.

death was the next most frequent manifestation. Chronic heart failure, as occurred in 3 of our 4 patients, was far less common. Some type of left ventricular dysfunction or wall motion abnormality was mentioned in a number of reports. Relatively few patients underwent cardiac transplantation.

Gerlis et al[46] distinguished between Uhl's anomaly and ARVD but suggested, as we do, that the term "Uhl's anomaly" has frequently been used to describe cases that should be considered examples of ARVD. From a study of 5 patients (2 with Uhl's anomaly and 3 with ARVD) and review of many published cases, these investigators proposed that "Uhl's anomaly" might best be limited to cases in which there is a paper-thin right ventricular free wall, with complete absence of myocardium and "apposition of the endocardial and epicardial layers," and that ARVD be characterized by cases with localized fibrofatty tissue replacement of the right ventricular free wall.

Although most clinicians now call this condition ARVD, that term does not recognize that the only common denominator of this condition is marked focal thinning of the right ventricular free wall or infiltration of that wall by adipose tissue with or without fibrous tissue. Similar focal thinning or fatty or fibrous replacement of the left ventricular free wall may also occur.[23,43,47–53] Although no reports of ARVD have included patients without focal right ventricular free wall thinning or virtual fatty replacement, it is possible that patients with isolated focal left ventricular free wall thinning—diverticuli or left ventricular aneurysm in the absence of coronary arterial narrowing or sarcoidosis—may also be a part of ARVD. Recently, Coats et al[54] described such a case. That heart failure may be its most prominent feature and that it may occur in the absence of a malignant ventricular arrhythmia is not suggested by the term "ARVD." Nevertheless, the phrase is probably here to stay.

1. Osler W. The Principles and Practice of Medicine. 6th ed. New York: Appleton Century Crofts, 1905:820.
2. Segall HN. Parchment heart (Osler). *Am Heart J* 1950;40:948–950.

Table 3
Patients reported with arrhythmic right ventricular dysplasia from 1982 to 2005

| Study | Number of Patients | M | F | Age (years) Range (Mean) | VT | SD | HF | LVD | CT | Follow-up (Years) Range (Mean) | Death |
|---|---|---|---|---|---|---|---|---|---|---|---|
| | | | | **Mainly clinical studies** | | | | | | | |
| Marcus et al (1982)[25] | 24 | 16 | 8 | 17–65 (39) | 22 | 0 | 0 | 1 | 0 | 0.1–12.7 (3) | 2* |
| Reiter et al (1983)[26] | 7 | 4 | 3 | 13–69 (39) | 7 | 1 | 0 | 0 | 0 | — | 0 |
| Manyari et al (1983)[27] | 6 | 4 | 2 | 21–60 (41) | 6 | 0 | 0 | 5† | 0 | — | 0 |
| Blomström-Lundqvist et al (1987)[28] | 15 | 10 | 5 | 7–50 (27) | 14 | 2 | 3 | 3 | 0 | 1.5–28 (9) | 3 |
| Marcus et al‡ (1989)[29] | 6 | 5 | 1 | 26–41 (34) | 4 | 0 | 0 | 0 | 0 | 1–20 | |
| Lemery et al (1989)[30] | 12 | — | — | 21–54 (33) | 12 | 0 | 0 | 2 | 0 | 2.5–15 (8) | 1 |
| Pinamonti et al (1995)[31] | 45 | 27 | 18 | 0.33–59 (32) | 14 | 3 | 6 | 10 | 1 | 1–23 (8.2) | 8 |
| Kullo et al (1995)[32] | 20 | 8 | 12 | 3–60 (30) | 9 | 2 | 5 | 10 | 2 | 2–17 (7) | 4 |
| Hulot et al (2004)[33] | 130 | 100 | 30 | 10–73 (—) | 102 | 7 | 8 | 13 | 0 | 8 ± 8 | 24 |
| Dalal et al (2005)[34] | 100§ | 51 | 49 | 2–70 (—) | 47/69 | 31 | 5 | 0 | 2 | 0–37 (median 6) | 34 |
| Tops et al (2009)[35] | 52 | 22 | 30 | 41 ± 12 | 14 | 0 | 0 | 0 | 0 | — | 0 |
| Marcus et al (2009)[36] | 95 | 35 | 60 | 38 ± 14 | 72 | 0 | 6 | 0 | 0 | 1.3 ± 1.1 | 0 |
| | | | | **Mainly morphologic studies** | | | | | | | |
| Basso et al (1996)[38] | 30‖ | 20 | 10 | 15–65 (28) | 15/19 | 24 | 3 | 14 | 3 | — | 27 |
| Corrado et al (1997)[40] | 42 | 27 | 15 | 9–65 (30) | 17 | 34 | 8 | 32¶ | 4 | — | 38 |
| Burke et al (1998)[41] | 25 | 20 | 5 | 13–72 (31) | 10** | 23 | 2 | 16 | 0 | — | 25 |
| Fornes et al (1998)[42] | 20 | 9 | 11 | 17–80 (41) | — | 20 | 0 | 8 | 0 | — | 20 |
| Lobo et al (1999)[43] | 26†† | 14 | 3 | 16–60 (—) | — | 15 | — | 17/22 | 2 | | 15 |
| D'Amati et al (2001)[44] | 27 | 16 | 11 | 12–66 (—) | 9/22‡‡ | 11/12 | 15 | 15 | 15 | — | 12 |
| Tabib et al (2003)[45] | 200 | 108 | 92 | 1–65 (33) | 4 | 158 | 0 | 8 | 0 | — | 200 |

* Five more patients died as described in Marcus et al's[29] 1989 follow-up study. Seven of the 25 patients subsequently developed chronic HF.

† Left ventricular wall motion abnormalities.

‡ This study provides follow-up in 20 of the 22 patients initially alive when reported by Marcus et al[25] in 1982; it adds 6 new patients studied by Marcus et al and provides follow-up for the 7 patients reported by Reiter et al[26] in 1983.

§ These patients were also included in Jain R, Dalal D, Daly A, Tichnell C, James C, Evenson A, Jain R, Abraham T, Tan BY, Tandri H, Russell SD, Judge D, Calkins H. Electrocardiographic features of arrhythmogenic right ventricular dysplasia. *Circulation* 2009;120:477–487.

‖ These 30 patients include the 12 previously reported by Thiene et al[37] in 1988. Only 4 of these 30 had the diagnosis of arrhythmogenic right ventricular cardiomyopathy made during life. This number was 36 in Corrado D, Basso C, Thiene G. Sudden cardiac death in young people with apparently normal heart. *Cardiovasc Res* 2001;50:399–408.

¶ Observed histologically only in 15 and both grossly and histologically in 17.

** "Arrhythmic or syncope."

†† Gender not given for 9 patients.

‡‡ Included only patients with electrocardiograms.

CT = cardiac transplantation; F = female; HF = heart failure; LVD = left ventricular dysplasia; M = men; SD = sudden death; VT = ventricular tachycardia.


3. Castleman B, Sprague HB. Case records of the Massachusetts General Hospital. Weekly clinicopathological exercises. *N Engl J Med* 1952;246:785–790.
4. Uhl HS. A previously undescribed congenital malformation of the heart: almost total absence of the myocardium of the right ventricle. *Bull Johns Hopkins Hosp* 1952;91:197–209.
5. Haworth SG, Shinebourne EA, Miller GAH. Right to left interatrial shunting with normal right ventricular pressure. *Br Heart J* 1975;37:386–391.
6. Diaz LP, Jimenez MQ, Granados FM, Martinez VP, Batres GM. Congenital absence of myocardium of right ventricle: Uhl's anomaly. *Br Heart J* 1973;35:570–572.
7. Novak G, Szanto PB, Gasul B, Dillon E. Congenital aplasia of the myocardium of the right ventricle. *Proc Inst Med Chic* 1957;21:334–339.
8. Arcilia RA, Gasul BM. Congenital aplasia or marked hypoplasia of the myocardium. *J Pediatr* 1961;58:381–388.
9. Cumming GR, Bowman JM, Whytehead L. Congenital aplasia of the myocardium of the right ventricle (Uhl's anomaly). *Am Heart J* 1965;70:671–676.
10. Aherne WA. Uhl's anomaly [abstract]. *Arch Dis Child* 1973;48:160.
11. Perrin EV, Mehrizi A. Isolated free-wall hypoplasia of the right ventricle. *Am J Dis Child* 1965;109:558–566.
12. Sherman FE. An Atlas of Congenital Heart Disease. Philadelphia: Lea & Febiger, 1963:270, 290–291.
13. Kinare SG, Panday SR, Deshmukh SM. Congenital aplasia of the right ventricular myocardium (Uhl's anomaly). *Chest* 1969;55:429–431.
14. Abe T, Kuribayashi R, Sato M, Nieda S, Abe S. Congenital hypoplasia of the right ventricular myocardium (Uhl's anomaly). A case report and review of literature. *J Cardiovasc Surg* 1973;14:431–438.
15. Murata K, Matsuo H, Yoshitake Y, Ishizawa Y, Shigiya R, Okamato K. Functionally atrialized parchment-like right ventricle with extensive myocardial fibrosis of left ventricle. *Jpn Heart J* 1976;17:428–435.
16. Froment R, Perrin A, Loire R, Dalloz CJ. Ventricule droit papyrace du jeune adultre par dystrophie congenitale. *Arch Mal Coeur* 1968;61:477–503.
17. Vecht RJ, Carmichael JS, Gopal R, Philip G. Uhl's anomaly. *Br Heart J* 1979;41:676–682.
18. Bharati S, Ciraulo DA, Bilitch M, Rosen KM, Lev M. Inexcitable right ventricle and bilateral bundle branch block in Uhl's disease. *Circulation* 1978;57:636–644.
19. Reeve R, MacDonald D. Partial absence of the right ventricular musculature—partial parchment heart. *Am J Cardiol* 1964;14:415–419.
20. Forssman O, Bjorkman G. Absence of the solid part of the right ventricular musculature. *Acta Pathol Microbiol Scand[A]* 1972;80:263–270.

21. Gould K, Guttman AB, Carrasco J, Lyon AF. Partial absence of the right ventricular musculature. A congenital lesion. *Am J Med* 1967; 42:636–641.
22. Sugiura M, Hayashi T, Ueno K. Partial absence of the right ventricular muscle in an aged. *Jpn Heart J* 1970;11:582–585.
23. Waller BF, Smith ER, Blackbourne BD, Arce FP, Sarkar NN, Roberts WC. Congenital hypoplasia of portions of both right and left ventricular myocardial walls. Clinical and necropsy observations in two patients with parchment heart syndrome. *Am J Cardiol* 1980;46:885–891.
24. Fontaine G, Guiraudon G, Frank R, Vedel J, Grosgogeat Y, Cabrol C, Facquet J. Stimulation studies and epicardial mapping in ventricular tachycardia: study of mechanism and selection for surgery. In: Kulbertus H, ed. Reentrant Arrhythmias, Mechanism and Treatment. Lancaster, Pennsylvania: MTP Publishing, 1977:334.
25. Marcus FI, Fontaine GH, Guiraudon G, Frank R, Laurenceau JL, Malergue C, Grosgogeat Y. Right ventricular dysplasia: a report of 24 adult cases. *Circulation* 1982;65:384–398.
26. Reiter MJ, Smith WM, Gallagher JJ. Clinical spectrum morphology. *Am J Cardiol* 1983;51:113–121.
27. Manyari DE, Klein GJ, Gulamhusein S, Boughner D, Guiraudon GM, Wyse G, Mitchell B, Kostuk WJ. Arrhythmogenic right ventricular dysplasia: a generalized cardiomyopathy? *Circulation* 1983;68:251–257.
28. Blomström-Lundqvist C, Sabel KG, Olsson SB. A long term follow-up of 15 patients with Arrhythmogenic right ventricular dysplasia. *Br Heart J* 1987;58:477–488.
29. Marcus FI, Fontaine GH, Frank R, Gallagher JJ, Reiter MJ. Long-term follow-up in patients with arrhythmogenic right ventricular disease. *Eur Heart J* 1989;10(suppl):68–73.
30. Lemery R, Brugada P, Janssen J, Cheriex E, Dugernier T, Wellens HJJ. Nonischemic sustained ventricular tachycardia: clinical outcome in 12 patients with arrhythmogenic right ventricular dysplasia. *J Am Coll Cardiol* 1989;14:96–105.
31. Pinamonti B, Di Lenarda A, Sinagra G, Silvestri F, Bussani R, Camerini F. Long-term evolution of right ventricular dysplasia-cardiomyopathy. *Am Heart J* 1995;129:412–415.
32. Kullo IJ, Edwards WD, Seward JB. Right ventricular dysplasia: the Mayo Clinic experience. *Mayo Clin Proc* 1995;70:541–548.
33. Hulot JS, Jouven X, Empana JP, Frank R, Fontaine G. Natural history and risk stratification of arrhythmogenic right ventricular dysplasia/cardiomyopathy. *Circulation* 2004;110:1879–1884.
34. Dalal D, Nasir K, Bomma C, Prakasa K, Tandri H, Piccini J, Roguin A, Tichnell C, James C, Russell SD, Judge DP, Abraham T, Spevak PJ, Bluemke DA, Calkins H. Arrhythmogenic right ventricular dysplasia. A United States experience. *Circulation* 2005;112:3823–3832.
35. Tops LF, Prakasa K, Tandri H, Dalal D, Jain R, Dimaano VL, Dombroski D, James C, Tichnell C, Daly A, Marcus F, Schalij MJ, Bax JJ, Bluemke D, Calkins H, Abraham TP. Prevalence and pathophysiologic attributes of ventricular dyssynchrony in arrhythmogenic right ventricular dysplasia/cardiomyopathy. *J Am Coll Cardiol* 2009;54:445–451.
36. Marcus GM, Glidden DV, Polonsky B, Zareba W, Smith LM, Cannom D, Estes NAM III, Marcus F, Scheinman MM. Efficacy of antiarrhythmic drugs in arrhythmogenic right ventricular cardiomyopathy. A report from the North American ARVC registry. *J Am Coll Cardiol* 2009;54:609–615.
37. Thiene G, Nava A, Corrado D, Rossi L, Pennelli N. Right ventricular cardiomyopathy and sudden death in young people. *N Engl J Med* 1988;318:129–133.
38. Basso C, Thiene G, Corrado D, Angelini A, Nava A, Valente M. Arrhythmogenic right ventricular cardiomyopathy. *Circulation* 1996; 94:983–991.
39. Basso C, Corrado D, Marcus F. Arrhythmogenic right ventricular cardiomyopathy. *Lancet* 2009;373:1289–1300.
40. Corrado D, Basso C, Thiene G, McKenna WJ, Davies M, Fontaliran F, Nava A, Silvestri F, Blomström-Lundqvist C, Wlodarska EK. Spectrum of clinicopathologic manifestations of arrhythmogenic right ventricular cardiomyopathy/dysplasia: a multicenter study. *J Am Coll Cardiol* 1997;30:1512–1520.
41. Burke AP, Farb A, Tashko G, Virmani R. Arrhythmogenic right ventricular cardiomyopathy and fatty replacement of the right ventricular myocardium. Are they different diseases? *Circulation* 1998;97: 1571–1580.
42. Fornes P, Ratel S, Lecomte D. Pathology of arrhythmogenic right ventricular cardiomyopathy/dysplasia-an autopsy study of 20 forensic cases. *J Forensic Sci* 1998;43:777–783.
43. Lobo FV, Silver MD, Butany J, Heggtveit HA. Left ventricular involvement in right ventricular dysplasia/cardiomyopathy. *Can J Cardiol* 1999;15:1239–1247.
44. D'Amati G, Leone O, Di Gioia CRT, Magelli C, Arpesella G, Grillo P, Marino B, Fiore F, Gallo P. Arrhythmogenic right ventricular cardiomyopathy: clinicopathologic correlation based on a revised definition of pathologic patterns. *Hum Pathol* 2001;32:1078–1086.
45. Tabib A, Loire R, Chalabreysse L, Meyronnet D, Miras A, Malicier D, Thivolet F, Chevalier P, Bouvagnet P. Circumstances of death and gross and microscopic observations in a series of 200 cases of sudden death associated with arrhythmogenic right ventricular cardiomyopathy and/or dysplasia. *Circulation* 2003;108:3000–3005.
46. Gerlis LM, Schmidt-Ott SC, Ho SY, Anderson RH. Dysplastic conditions of the right ventricular myocardium: Uhl's anomaly v arrhythmogenic right ventricular dysplasia. *Br Heart J* 1993;69:142–150.
47. Webb JG, Kerr CR, Huckell VF, Mizgala HF, Ricci DR. Left ventricular abnormalities in arrhythmogenic right ventricular dysplasia. *Am J Cardiol* 58;1986:568–570.
48. Horimoto M, Funayama N, Satoh M, Igarashi T, Sekiguchi M. Histological evidence of left ventricular involvement in arrhythmogenic right ventricular dysplasia. *Jpn Circ J* 1989;53:1530–1534.
49. Nishikawa H, Kasai A, Ono N, Unno M, Kakuta Y, Nishimura S, Nishiyama S, Nakanishi S, Seki A, Nakano T. Two cases of biventricular dysplasia associated with ventricular tachycardia and familial occurrence of sudden death. *J Cardiol* 1991;21:735–747.
50. Shoji T, Kaneko M, Onodera K, Konnno A, Hasegawa T, Ikeda T, Minase T, Uchiyama S, Iwamoto M. Arrhythmogenic right ventricular dysplasia with massive involvement of the left ventricle. *Can J Cardiol* 1991;7:303–307.
51. Pinamonti B, Sinagra G, Salvi A, Di Lenarda A, Morgera T, Silvestri F, Bussani R, Camerini F. Left ventricular involvement in right ventricular dysplasia. *Am Heart J* 1992;123:711–724.
52. Gallo P, D'Amati G, Pelliccia F. Pathologic evidence of extensive left ventricular involvement in arrhythmogenic right ventricular cardiomyopathy. *Hum Pathol* 1992;23:948–952.
53. Sugrue DD, Edwards WD, Olney BA. Histolgic abnormalities of the left ventricle in a patient with arrhythmogenic right ventricular dysplasia. *Heart Vessels* 1958;1:179–181.
54. Coats CJ, Quarta G, Flett AS, Pantazis AA, McKenna WJ, Moon JC. Arrhythmogenic left ventricular cardiomyopathy. *Circulation* 2009; 120:2613–2614.

# Profound Left Ventricular Remodeling Associated With LAMP2 Cardiomyopathy

Barry J. Maron, MD[a,b,*], William C. Roberts, MD[c], Carolyn Y. Ho, MD[d], Carrie Kitner, RN[a,b], Tammy S. Haas, RN[a], Gregory B. Wright, MD[e], Nader Moazami, MD[b], and David S. Feldman, MD[b]

**Lysosome-associated membrane protein (LAMP2) cardiomyopathy is an X-linked and highly progressive myocardial storage disorder associated with diminished survival, which clinically resembles sarcomeric hypertrophic cardiomyopathy. As shown here in a young woman, the natural history of LAMP2 may demonstrate an extreme profile of left ventricular remodeling with regression of hypertrophy (i.e. marked wall thinning), chamber dilatation, and severe systolic dysfunction, all of which are associated with widespread transmural scarring. © 2010 Published by Elsevier Inc. (Am J Cardiol 2010;106:1194–1196)**

Mutations in the X-linked lysosome-associated membrane protein gene (LAMP2) result in a storage disease known as LAMP2 cardiomyopathy, a morphologic phenocopy of sarcomeric hypertrophic cardiomyopathy.[1,2]

[a]Hypertrophic Cardiomyopathy Center, Minneapolis Heart Institute Foundation, Minneapolis, Minnesota; [b]Abbott Northwestern Hospital, Minneapolis, Minnesota; [c]Baylor Cardiovascular Research Institute, Dallas, Texas; [d]Cardiovascular Division, Brigham and Women's Hospital, Harvard Medical School, Boston, Massachusetts; and [e]Children's Heart Clinic, Minneapolis, Minnesota. Manuscript received March 12, 2010; revised manuscript received and accepted April 20, 2010.

This study was supported in part by a grant from the Hearst Foundations, San Francisco, California.

*Corresponding author: Tel: 612-863-3996; fax: 612-863-3875.
*E-mail address:* hcm.maron@mhif.org (B.J. Maron).

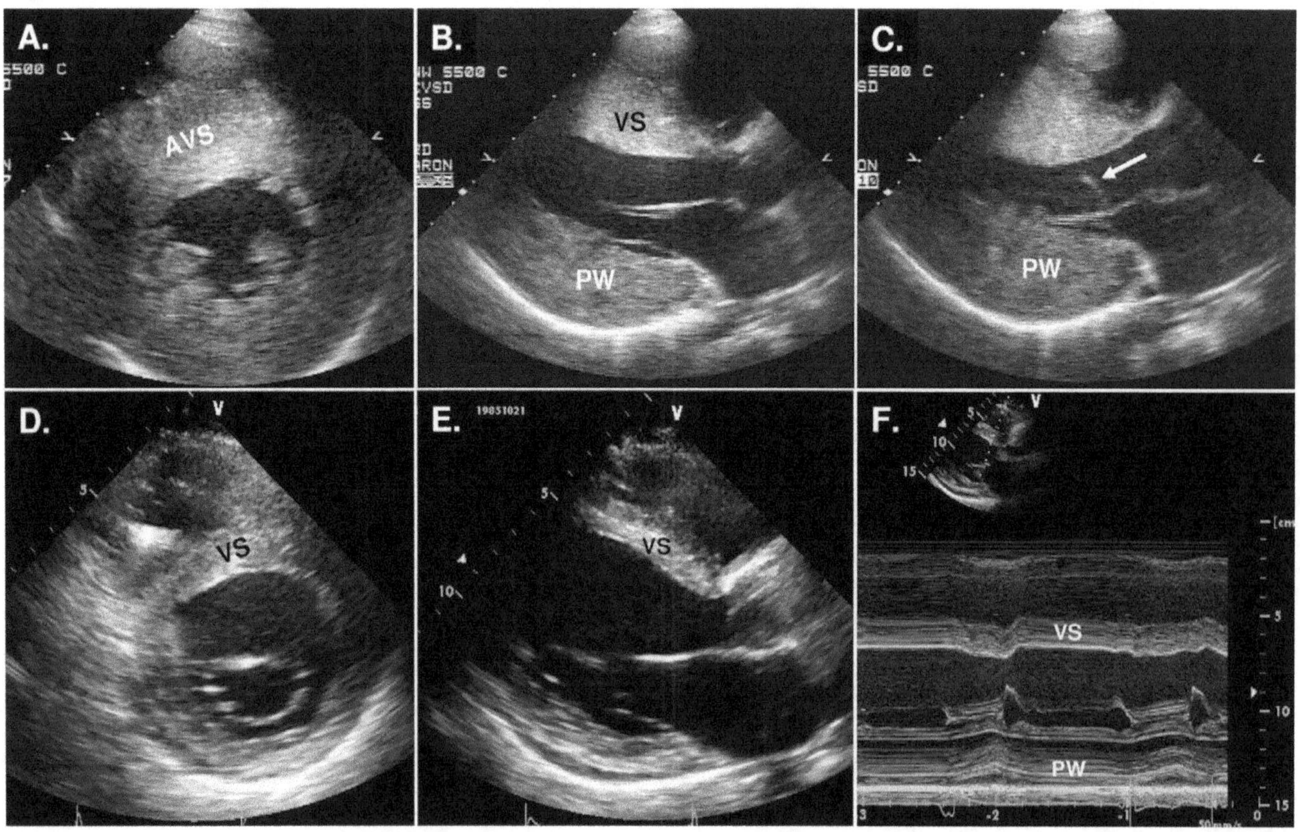


Figure 1. Severe LV remodeling in LAMP2 cardiomyopathy at 13 years of age *(A–C)* and 24 years of age *(D–F)*. *(A)* Parasternal short-axis view at end-diastole; the thickness of the anterior ventricular septum (AVS) is 30 mm, and hypertrophy is distributed diffusely throughout LV free wall. *(B)* End-diastolic parasternal long-axis view shows the ventricular septum (VS) and posterior LV free wall (PW) of equal thickness, each at 30 mm. *(C)* In systole, moderate systolic anterior motion *(arrow)* without septal contact is seen. *(D,E)*. Prior to transplant, VS thickness is only 13 mm, and the LV free wall has also thinned. *(F)* M-mode echocardiogram shows thinned VS and PW.

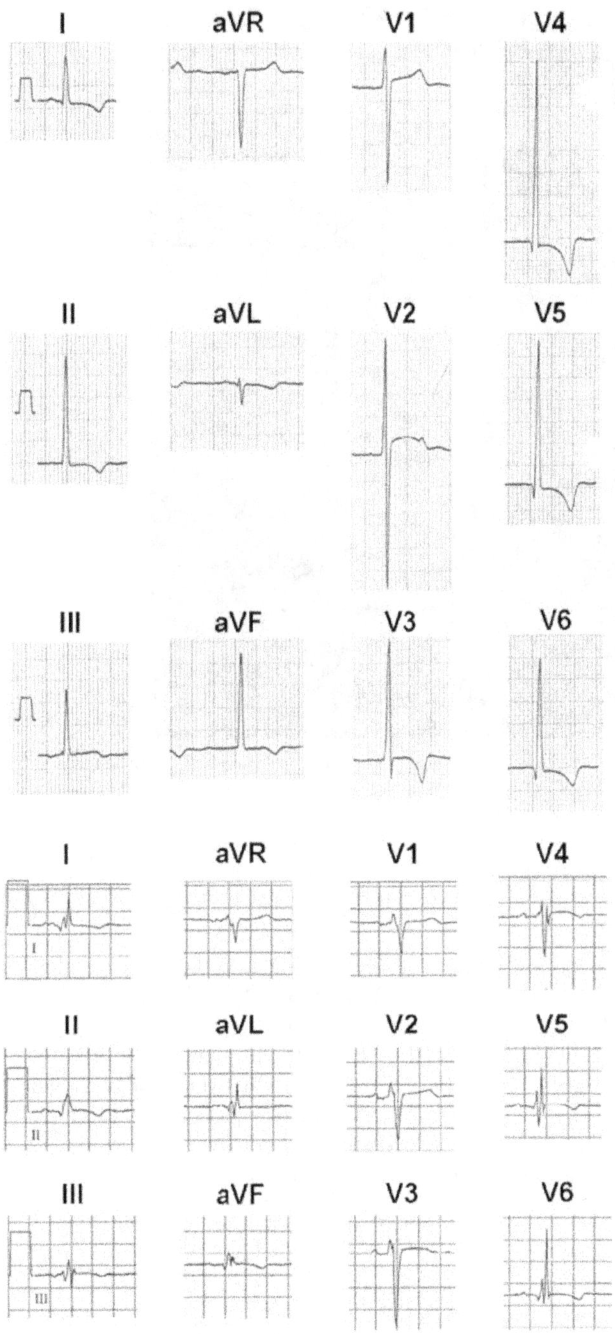


Figure 2. Evolution of the 12-lead electrocardiographic pattern. *(Top)* At 13 years of age, LV hypertrophy with tall R waves (to 80 mm in lead V4) and diffuse T-wave inversion are seen, recorded at 1/2 standard. *(Bottom)* At 24 years of age, low voltage and diffuse T-wave inversions are seen.

LAMP2 mutations are associated with a particularly adverse natural history and a clinical course characterized by progressive (often abrupt) deterioration, with heart failure and malignant ventricular tachyarrhythmias. Of 7 young patients with LAMP2 cardiomyopathy in a recent report,[2] 6 died and/or required heart transplantation before 25 years of age. The unique events documented in the seventh and remaining patient, now 24 years old (and the only female patient), are the subject of this report.

Table 1
Extreme left ventricular remodeling in lysosome-associated membrane protein cardiomyopathy (LAMP2)

| Parameter | Initial Evaluation | Most Recent Evaluation |
|---|---|---|
| Age (years) | 13 | 24 |
| Ventricular septal thickness (mm) | 30* | 13 |
| LV end-diastole (mm) | 38 | 60 |
| Left atrium (mm) | 36 | 34 |
| Ejection fraction (%) | 70 | 17 |
| Cardiac index (ml/min/m$^2$) | — | 1.1 |
| SAM | Moderate† | 0 |
| Electrocardiographic findings | Diffuse T-wave inversion, increased voltages (precordial R wave, 80 mm) | Diffuse T-wave inversion, decreased voltages, intraventricular conduction block (QRS duration 132 ms) |
| NYHA functional class | I | IV |
| Symptoms | Syncope × 2 | Exertional and rest dyspnea, chest pain and fatigue, PND, acute heart failure × 2 |
| Drugs | None | Furosemide, lisinopril, metoprolol |

NYHA = New York Heart Association; PND = paroxysmal nocturnal dyspnea; SAM = systolic anterior motion.

* Posterior LV free wall thickness 30 mm; posterior septum and anterolateral free wall thickness each 20 mm.

† Without mitral-septal contact.

## Case Report

Although the patient experienced an appropriate defibrillator intervention for rapid sustained ventricular tachycardia (222 beats/min) at 18 years of age, she remained asymptomatic until 23 years of age, when she experienced an abrupt deterioration in functional state (requiring several admissions for heart failure) due to profound left ventricular (LV) remodeling.

This process showed a more rapid evolution and began earlier in life than is typical of the end-stage phase of sarcomeric hypertrophic cardiomyopathy,[3] involving a striking decrease in LV wall thickness from 30 to 13 mm (a 57% change). There was also an increase in transverse LV cavity dimension from 38 to 60 mm (a 57% change), loss of mitral valve systolic anterior motion, and a reduction in the ejection fraction from 70% to 17% (a 76% change) (Figure 1 and Table 1). The 12-lead electrocardiographic pattern also changed markedly, with striking reductions in precordial and standard lead voltages (Figure 2).

Detailed analysis of sequential echocardiograms and clinical events showed that LV remodeling began at 21 years of age, at a time when the patient was asymptomatic, constituting a mismatch between cardiac structural changes and clinical state. This remodeling process and clinical progression evolved in the following sequence: (1) a decrease in the ejection fraction while asymptomatic, (2) a regression of LV wall thick-

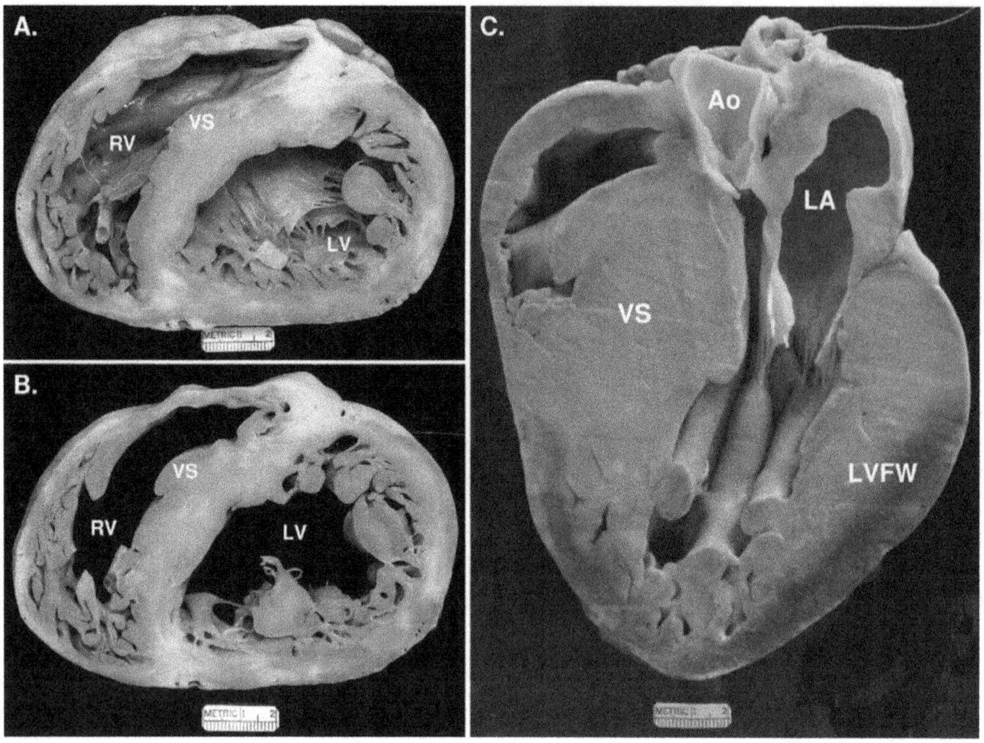


Figure 3. Explanted heart from a 24-year-old woman with LAMP2 cardiomyopathy. *(A)* Proximal cross section at the mitral valve level. *(B)* More distal cross section at the papillary muscle level. In *(A)* and *(B)*, extensive and diffuse transmural and subepicardial scarring of the ventricular septum (VS), LV free wall, and right ventricle (RV), associated with cavity dilatation and marked wall thinning (only 3-, 6-, and 9-mm thickness evident in some areas). The coronary arteries are widely patent. *(C)* For comparison, gross heart at autopsy from an asymptomatic patient with LAMP2 cardiomyopathy who died suddenly at 12 years of age, refractory to cardioverter-defibrillator intervention. In contrast to the patient with LAMP2 cardiomyopathy shown in *(A)* and *(B)*, there is preserved and marked thickness of the VS (65 mm) and LV free wall (LVFW). Ao = aorta; LA = left atrium. Reproduced with permission from *JAMA*.[2]

ness, (3) an enlargement of the LV cavity, and (4) heart failure symptoms rapidly progressive over about 10 months from 23 to 24 years of age. On April 4, 2010, the patient underwent successful heart transplantation. At that time, she was in cardiogenic shock with an ejection fraction of 5% and had intestinal ischemia from poor cardiac output. She was discharged on the eighth postoperative day.

## Comments

LAMP2 cardiomyopathy is an important phenocopy of sarcomeric hypertrophic cardiomyopathy, given its profound natural history with survival uncommon beyond 25 years of age and the need to consider heart transplantation early and prospectively.[2] Although only a small number of cases have been reported, pathways of disease progression appear diverse. For example, the transplanted patient reported here showed a remarkable degree of LV remodeling, characterized by LV wall thinning due to replacement scarring, chamber dilation, marked diastolic dysfunction and an ejection fraction <20%, associated with extreme functional deterioration to New York Heart Association class IV. Notably, this process evolved for 6 years after an aborted sudden-death event in which the implanted defibrillator terminated a life-threatening ventricular tachyarrhythmia.

In contrast, sudden death intervened without remodeling and functional deterioration in another patient with LAMP2 cardiomyopathy, also shown in Figure 3.[2]

1. Arad M, Maron BJ, Gorham JM, Johnson WH, Saul JP, Perez-Atayde AR, Spirito P, Wright GB, Kanter RJ, Seidman CE, Seidman JG. Glycogen storage diseases presenting as hypertrophic cardiomyopathy. *N Engl J Med* 2005;352:362–372.
2. Maron BJ, Roberts WC, Arad M, Haas TS, Spirito P, Wright GB, Almquist AK, Baffa JM, Saul JP, Ho CY, Seidman J, Seidman CE. Clinical outcome and phenotypic expression in LAMP2 cardiomyopathy. *JAMA* 2009;301:1253–1259.
3. Harris KM, Spirito P, Maron MS, Zenovich AG, Formisano F, Lesser JR, Mackey-Bojack S, Manning WJ, Udelson JE, Maron BJ. Prevalence, clinical profile and significance of left ventricular remodeling in the end-stage phase of hypertrophic cardiomyopathy. *Circulation* 2006; 114:216–225.

# Examination of Isolated Ventricular Noncompaction (Hypertrabeculation) as a Distinct Entity in Adults

William Clifford Roberts, MD[a,b,d,*], Sumit Jagdish Karia, MD[a], Jong Mi Ko, BA[d], Paul Arthur Grayburn, MD[a,d], Betsy Ann George, MD[a], Shelley Anne Hall, MD[a], Johannes Jacob Kuiper, MD[a,d], and Dan Marshall Meyer, MD[c,e]

**Three patients (2 women) 36, 45, and 49 years of age underwent cardiac transplantation for what was diagnosed clinically as nonischemic dilated cardiomyopathy. Examination of the transthoracic echocardiogram and explanted heart in each disclosed marked hypertrabeculation involving the free wall of the very dilated left ventricle, a finding consistent with what has been termed "isolated ventricular noncompaction" (IVNC). Although these 3 cases anatomically fulfilled the echocardiographic definition of IVNC, review of previous publications containing gross photographs of the heart suggests that IVNC is overdiagnosed at least morphologically.**  **(Am J Cardiol 2011;108:747–752)**

Although newborns with aortic valve atresia unassociated with mitral valve atresia have true sinusoids from the endocardium that burrow into the myocardium, the endocardium is smooth and devoid of trabeculations.[1] Therefore, it is not proper in our view to consider the left ventricle in aortic valve atresia unassociated with mitral valve atresia an example of ventricular noncompaction as has been done. The first description of what later came to be termed "isolated ventricular noncompaction" (IVNC) in an adult was by Engberding and Bender[2] who described a 33-year-old woman with heart failure, left bundle branch block, marked left ventricular dilatation, and echocardiographically demonstrated large trabeculations (called "sinusoids" by the investigators) within the left ventricular cavity. Subsequently, numerous reports have appeared describing—mainly by echocardiogram—features of IVNC.[3–36] The present report describes morphologic features of hearts in 3 adults who underwent cardiac transplantation and the explanted hearts were characteristic of IVNC. In addition, previous published reports illustrating the heart at necropsy or after cardiac transplantation are reviewed to determine if IVNC is overdiagnosed at least morphologically.

## Methods

Pertinent clinical and morphologic features in each of the 3 patients are presented in Table 1, and transthoracic echocardiographic and morphologic features are illustrated in Figures 1 through 6. All 3 patients had evidence of chronic heart failure for 7, 10, and 12 years before cardiac transplantation at 36, 45, and 49 years of age, respectively. Three had episodes of ventricular tachycardia, and patient 2 had ventricular tachycardia ablation procedures on >1 occasion. All 3 had elevated pulmonary arterial pressures, low systemic arterial pressures, low cardiac indices, and very low left ventricular ejection fractions. All 3 by angiography had normal epicardial coronary arteries. None had a neuromuscular disorder. Examination of explanted hearts from all patients disclosed increased cardiac weight and hugely dilated left ventricular cavities with noncompacted portions of left ventricular free walls ≥2 times as thick as the compacted portions of these walls. Patient 1 had an organizing thrombus in the apex of the left ventricle. Patient 3 had an episode typical of transient ischemic attack. Patients 2 and 3 each had small transmural left ventricular free wall scars. Histologically, myofibers in each were hypertrophied, inflammatory cells were absent, and interstitial fibrous tissue was focally increased in the ventricular walls.

## Comments

Each of the 3 patients described had excessive ventricular trabeculations in very dilated left ventricles, bundle branch block, periodic ventricular tachycardia, severe heart failure, and finally cardiac transplantation.

What is IVNC in adults? Is it really a distinctive entity? Oechslin et al[6] from Zurich described 34 adults with IVNC and stated that ". . . the characteristic discriminating feature . . . [of IVNC is a] . . . two layered myocardial wall structure with both a thin epicardial compacted zone and an extremely thickened endocardial non-compacted zone with deep recesses filled with blood from the ventricular cavity." In 2006 alone, 3 reports described 61, 53, and 57 patients, respectively, >15 years of age with IVNC, each from sep-

Departments of [a]Internal Medicine, [b]Pathology, and [c]Cardiothoracic Surgery, and the [d]Baylor Heart and Vascular Institute, Baylor University Medical Center, Dallas, Texas; [e]Department of Thoracic and Cardiovascular Surgery, University of Texas Southwestern Medical Center, Dallas, Texas. Manuscript received February 22, 2011; revised manuscript received and accepted April 24, 2011.

*Corresponding author: Tel: 214-820-7911; fax: 214-820-7533.

*E-mail address:* wc.roberts@baylorhealth.edu (W.C. Roberts)

Table 1
Features of the three patients described

| Variable | Patient 1 | Patient 2 | Patient 3 |
|---|---|---|---|
| Age (years) at cardiac transplantation | 36 | 45 | 49 |
| Month and year of cardiac transplantation | October 2008 | March 2011 | May 2011 |
| Gender | Woman | Man | Woman |
| Age (years) at onset of signs and symptoms of cardiac dysfunction | 26 | 33 | 42 |
| Chronic heart failure | + | + | + |
| Atrial fibrillation | + | 0 | + |
| Ventricular tachycardia | + | + | + |
| Intracardiac pressures (mm Hg) | | | |
| Mean pulmonary arterial wedge | 29 | 35 | 25* |
| Pulmonary artery (peak systolic pressure/end-diastolic pressure) | 60/30 | 55/27 | 54/22* |
| Right ventricle (peak systolic pressure/end-diastolic pressure) | 60/5 | 55/18 | 54/17* |
| Right atrium (mean) | 14 | 8 | 14* |
| Aorta (peak systolic pressure/end-diastolic pressure) | 90/60† | 90/50† | 100/80* |
| Cardiac index ($L/min/m^2$) | 1.8 | 1.8 | 2.0* |
| Left ventricular ejection fraction (%) | 10 | 15 | 5 |
| Automatic implantable cardioverter–defibrillator cardiac resynchronizing therapy | + | + | + |
| Left bundle branch block | + | + | 0 |
| Total cholesterol (mg/dl) | 110 | 160 | 147 |
| Body mass index ($kg/m^2$) | 19.6 | 26.6 | 22.1 |
| Heart weight (g) | 420 | 530 | 360 |
| Maximal left ventricular cavity (cm) | 7.0 | 7.0 | 8.0 |
| Scar, left ventricular wall | 0 | + | + |

* Recorded 14 months before heart transplantation.
† Indirect pressure.

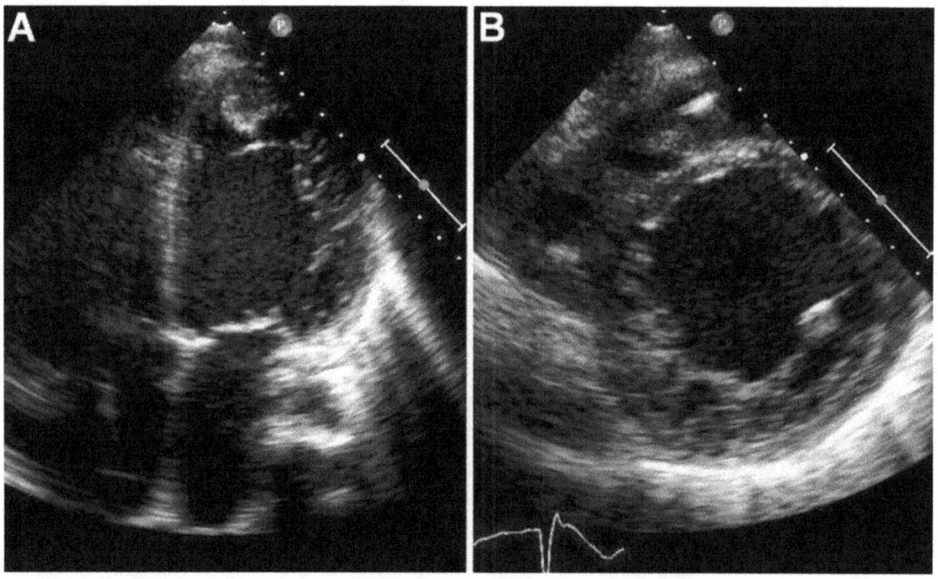


Figure 1. Patient 1. Echocardiogram. *(A)* Four-chamber view shows a dilated left ventricular cavity with excessive trabeculations and a thrombus in the apex. *(B)* Short-axis view demonstrates trabeculations better than in the 4-chamber view.

arate single medical centers.[13,21,22] In 2007 another 65 adults were reported,[23] in 2008 another 60 adults were reported,[33] and in 2010, 140 more adults were reported, each study from single medical centers.[22] In addition, many other case studies and small series of patients have been described.

In the many publications on IVNC, most from Europe, we found 18 gross photographs of the heart in adults in peer-reviewed journals.[3–20] Of these, in the view of 1 of the authors (W.C.R.), only 7 of the 18 cases represent clear examples of IVNC (hypertrabeculation).[3,4,7,8,11,13] Burke et al[11] were the only investigators to report and illustrate morphologically 2 adults with IVNC. One was an 18-year-old man who underwent cardiac transplantation for chronic heart failure. The second was a 30-year-old man who died suddenly and had a nondilated left ventricular cavity. (A beautiful example of IVNC was a heart prepared by Dr. William D. Edwards and published in an *Up-to-Date* piece in 2011 authored by Dr. H.M. Connolly and Dr. C.H.A. Jost.) The photograph shown of

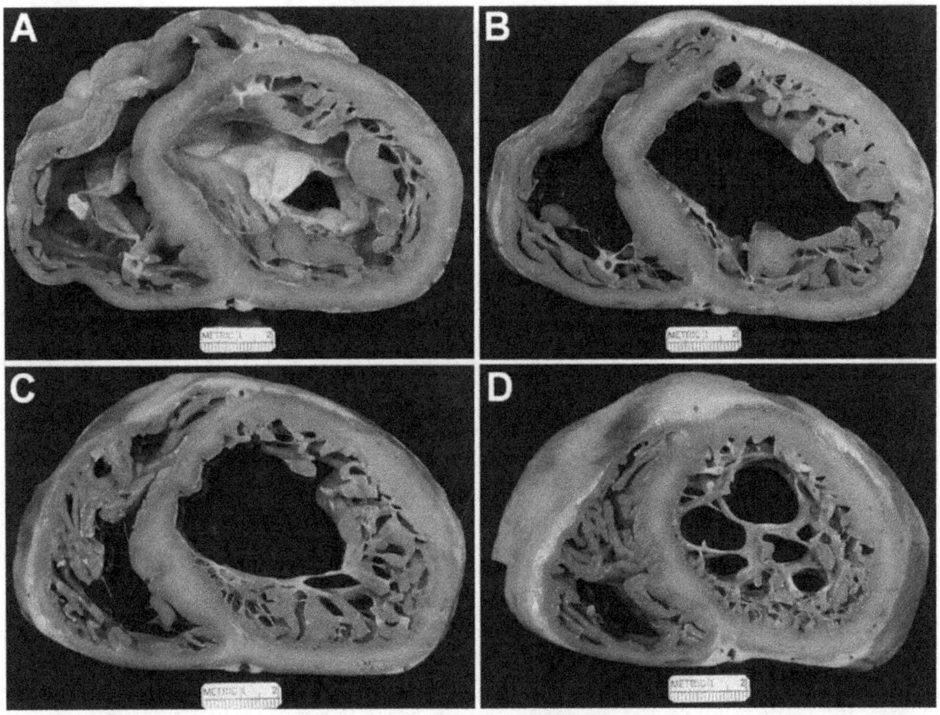


Figure 2. Patient 1. Explanted heart. Views of the right and left ventricles at 4 different levels: *(A)* near the base exposing the tricuspid and mitral valves, *(B, C)* intermediate levels, and *(D)* near the apex. The noncompacted portion of the free wall of the left ventricle is thicker than the compacted portion of the wall.

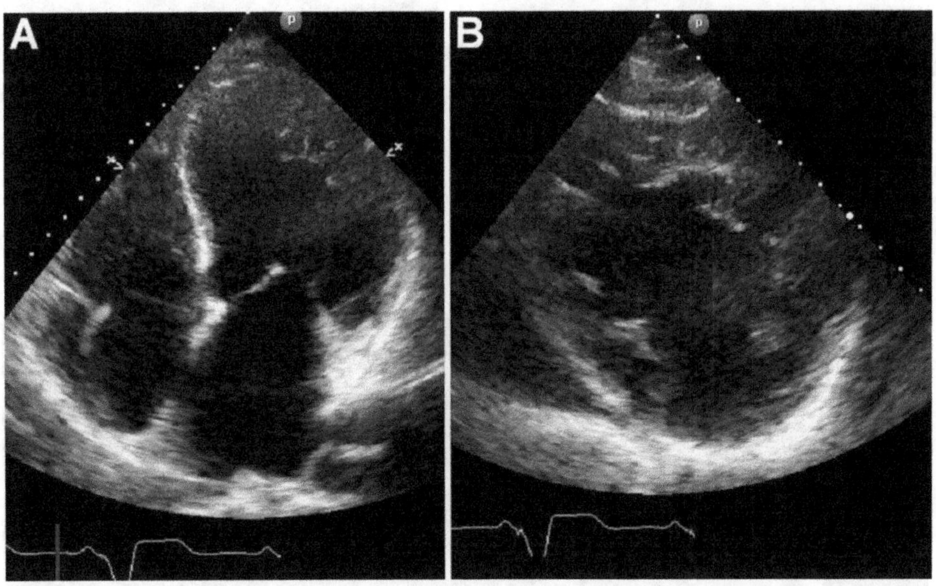


Figure 3. Patient 2. Echocardiogram. *(A)* Four-chamber view shows a dilated left ventricular cavity with excessive trabeculations. *(B)* Short-axis view demonstrates trabeculations better than in the 4-chamber view.

the heart in 1 report appears to be a classic example of cor pulmonale.[6] Most published illustrated hearts were opened when fresh by cuts according to the flow of blood. These cuts result in flattened cardiac chambers and then comparison of the thickness of the compacted to that of the noncompacted portions of the cardiac ventricles is more difficult to discern. Cuts of the ventricles made parallel to the posterior atrioventricular sulcus after fixation appears to provide the best opportunity of demonstrating ventricular hypertrabeculation if present.

In Table 2 we attempt to show various characteristics of patients with 4 different types of cardiomyopathies. The various clinical features of IVNC and idiopathic dilated cardiomyopathy are virtually identical. Clearly, hypertrophic cardiomyopathy is the most distinctive. Whether IVNC deserves a special characterization is debatable.

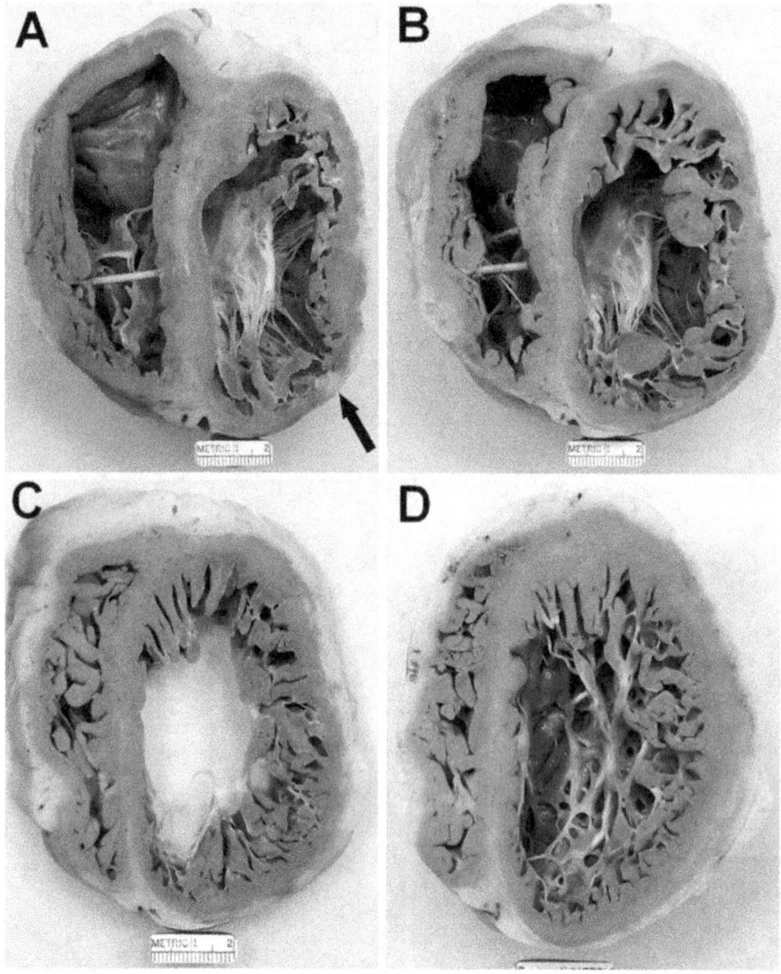


Figure 4. Patient 2. Views of the right and left ventricles at 4 different levels: *(A)* near the base exposing the tricuspid and mitral valves, *(B, C)* intermediate levels, and *(D)* near the apex. A small scar *(arrow)* is present in the left ventricular wall. The noncompacted portion of the left ventricular free wall is thicker than the compacted portion, which is especially thin in the basilar portion *(A, B)*.

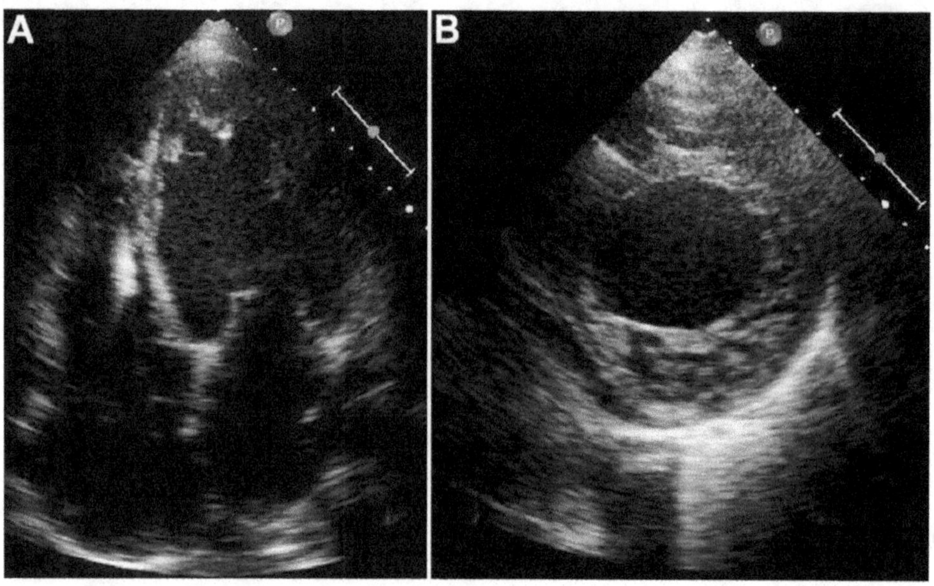


Figure 5. Patient 3. Echocardiogram. *(A)* Four-chamber view shows a dilated left ventricular cavity with excessive trabeculations. *(B)* Short-axis view demonstrates excessive trabeculations in the left ventricular cavity.

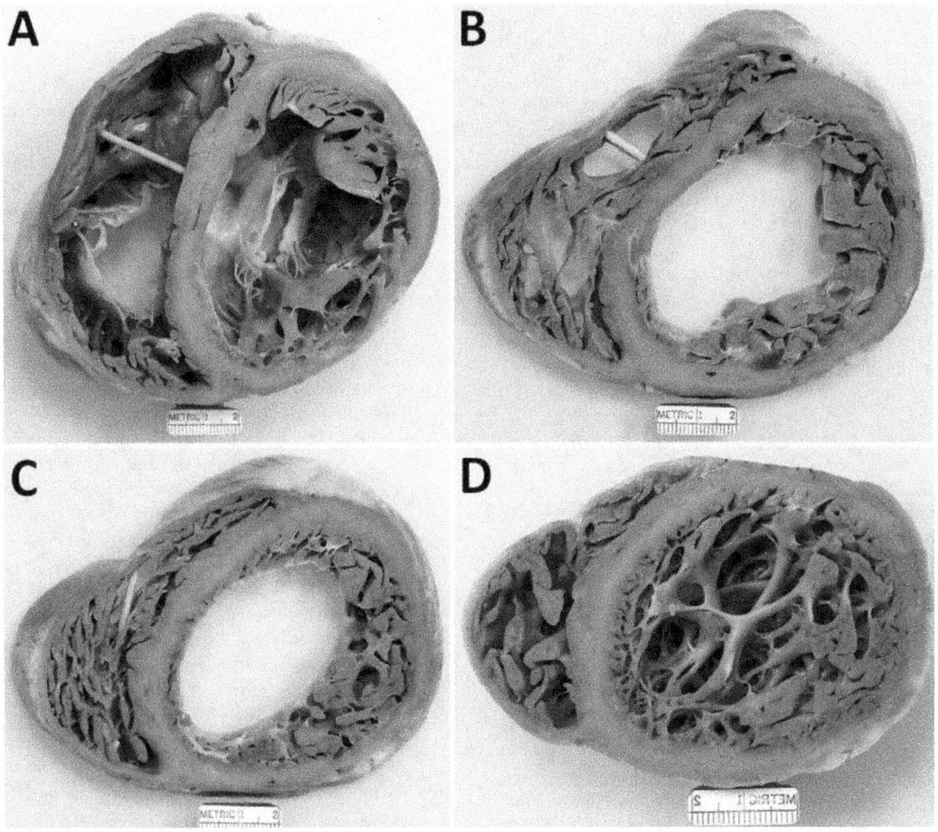


Figure 6. Patient 3. Views of the right and left ventricles at 4 different levels: *(A)* near the base exposing the tricuspid and mitral valves, *(B, C)* intermediate levels, and *(D)* near the apex. *C* corresponds almost precisely with the echocardiogram shown in Figure 5B. The noncompacted portion of the left ventricular free wall is thicker than the compacted portion, which is particularly thin in the basilar portion *(A)*.

Table 2
Clinical features of four major cardiomyopathies

| Variable | IVNC | IDC | ARVD | HC |
|---|---|---|---|---|
| Ages | All | All | All | All |
| Men | +++ | +++ | +++ | +++ |
| Women | + | + | + | + |
| Heart failure | +++ | +++ | ++ | ++ |
| Atrial arrhythmias | ++ | +++ | +++ | + |
| Ventricular arrhythmias | +++ | +++ | +++ | +++ |
| Bundle branch block | +++ | ++ | +++ | + |
| Heart block | + | + | +++ | + |
| Epsilon waves | 0 | 0 | + | 0 |
| Right + left ventricular dilatation | +++ | +++ | +++ | 0 |
| Atrial dilatation | ++ | ++ | ++ | +++ |
| Sudden death | + | + | ++ | +++ |
| Heart failure death | +++ | +++ | ++ | + |
| Left ventricular scars | + | + | + | ++ |
| Tricuspid and/or mitral regurgitation | ++ | ++ | ++ | +++ |
| Familial | + | + | +++ | +++ |
| Heart weight | ↑↑ | ↑↑ | ↑↑ | ↑↑↑ |
| Ejection fraction | ↓↓↓ | ↓↓↓ | ↓↓ | ↑ |

ARVD = arrhythmogenic right ventricular dysplasia; HC = hypertrophic cardiomyopathy; IDC = idiopathic dilated cardiomyopathy; IVNC = isolated ventricular noncompaction; + = positive or present; ↑ = increased; ↓ = decreased.

1. Roberts WC, Perry LW, Chandra RS, Myers GE, Shapiro SR, Scott LP. Aortic valve atresia: a new classification based on necropsy study of 73 cases. *Am J Cardiol* 1976;37:753–756.
2. Engberding R, Bender F. Identification of a rare congenital anomaly of the myocardium by two-dimensional echocardiography: persistence of isolated myocardial sinusoids. *Am J Cardiol* 1984;53:1733–1734.
3. Jenni R, Goebel N, Tartini R, Schneider J, Arbenz U, Oelz O. Persisting myocardial sinusoids of both ventricles as an isolated anomaly: echocardiographic, angiographic, and pathologic anatomical findings. *Cardiovasc Interv Radiol* 1986;9:127–131.
4. Steiner I, Hrubecký J, Pleskot J, Kokštejn Z. Persistence of spongy myocardium with embryonic blood supply in an adult. *Cardiovasc Pathol* 1996;5:47–53.
5. Ritter M, Oechslin E, Sütsch G, Attenhofer C, Schneider J, Jenni R. Isolated noncompaction of the myocardium in adults. *Mayo Clin Proc* 1997;72:26–31.
6. Oechslin EN, Jost CH, Rojas JR, Kaufmann PA, Jenni R. Long-term follow-up of 34 adults with isolated left ventricular noncompaction: a distinct cardiomyopathy with poor prognosis. *J Am Coll Cardiol* 2000; 36:493–500.
7. Jenni R, Oechslin E, Schneider J, Attenhofer Jost C, Kaufmann PA. Echocardiographic and pathoanatomical characteristics of isolated left ventricular non-compaction: a step towards classification as a distinct cardiomyopathy. *Heart* 2001;86:666–671.
8. Zambrano E, Marshalko SJ, Jaffe CC, Hui P. Isolated noncompaction of the ventricular myocardium: clinical and molecular aspects of a rare cardiomyopathy. *Lab Invest* 2002;82:117–122.
9. Finsterer J, Stöllberger C, Feichtinger H. Histological appearance of left ventricular hypertrabeculation/noncompaction. *Cardiology* 2002; 98:162–164.
10. Hughes SE, McKenna WJ. New insights into the pathology of inherited cardiomyopathy. *Heart* 2005;91:257–264.
11. Burke A, Mont E, Kutys R, Virmani R. Left ventricular noncompaction: a pathological study of 14 cases. *Hum Pathol* 2005;36:403–411.
12. Pujadas S, Bordes R, Bayes-Genis A. Ventricular non-compaction cardiomyopathy: CMR and pathology findings. *Heart* 2005;91:582.

13. Biagini E, Ragni L, Ferlito M, Pasquale F, Lofiego C, Leone O, Rocchi G, Perugini E, Zagnoni S, Branzi A, Picchio FM, Rapezzi C. Different types of cardiomyopathy associated with isolated ventricular noncompaction. *Am J Cardiol* 2006;98:821–824.
14. Engberding R, Yelbuz TM, Breithardt G. Isolated noncompaction of the left ventricular myocardium—a review of the literature two decades after the initial case description. *Clin Res Cardiol* 2007;96:481–488.
15. Finsterer J, Stöllberger C, Feichtinger H. Noncompaction in Duchenne muscular dystrophy: frustrated attempt to create a compensatory left ventricle? *Cardiology* 2006;105:223–225.
16. Finsterer J, Stöllberger C, Feichtinger H. Noncompaction and endocarditis in suspected mitochondrial disorder. *Int J Cardiol* 2008; 123(suppl):e45–e47.
17. Karner J, Keller H, Stöllberger C, Feichtinger H, Finsterer J. Deficiency of mannose-binding lectin, myopathy, calcified endomyocardial fibrosis, and left ventricular noncompaction. *Heart Lung* 2008;37: 476–478.
18. Finsterer J, Stöllberger C, Bonner E. Left ventricular hypertrabeculation/noncompaction associated with coronary heart disease and myopathy. *Int J Cardiol* 2011;148:e53–e55.
19. Stöllberger C, Ormin V, Finsterer J. Fatal outcome of aortic-valve endocarditis in noncompaction/hypertrabeculation. *Int J Cardiol* 2009 [Epub ahead of print].
20. Stöllberger C, Finsterer J, Sodeck GH, Grassberger M, Zimpfer D. Stroke from noncompaction overlooked by echocardiography. *Int J Cardiol* 2011;148:357–358.
21. Espinola-Zavaleta N, Soto ME, Castellanos LM, Játiva-Chávez S, Keirns C. Non-compacted cardiomyopathy: clinical–echocardiographic study. *Cardiovasc Ultrasound* 2006;4:35.
22. Aras D, Tufekcioglu O, Ergun K, Ozeke O, Yildiz A, Topaloglu S, Deveci B, Sahin O, Kisacik HL, Korkmaz S. Clinical features of isolated ventricular noncompaction in adults long-term clinical course, echocardiographic properties, and predictors of left ventricular failure. *J Card Fail* 2006;12:726–733.
23. Lofiego C, Biagini E, Pasquale F, Ferlito M, Rocchi G, Perugini E, Bacchi-Reggiani L, Boriani G, Leone O, Caliskan K, ten Cate FJ, Picchio FM, Branzi A, Rapezzi C. Wide spectrum of presentation and variable outcomes of isolated left ventricular non-compaction. *Heart* 2007;93:65–71.
24. Stöllberger C, Blazek G, Wegner C, Winkler-Dworak M, Finsterer J. Neuromuscular and cardiac comorbidity determines survival in 140 patients with left ventricular hypertrabeculation/noncompaction. *Int J Cardiol* 2010 [Epub ahead of print].
25. Conces DJ Jr, Ryan T, Tarver RD. Noncompaction of ventricular myocardium: CT appearance. *AJR Am J Roentgenol* 1991;156:717–718.
26. Agmon Y, Connolly HM, Olson LJ, Khandheria BK, Seward JB. Noncompaction of the ventricular myocardium. *J Am Soc Echocardiogr* 1999;12:859–863.
27. Hamamichi Y, Ichida F, Hashimoto I, Uese KH, Miyawaki T, Tsukano S, Ono Y, Echigo S, Kamiya T. Isolated noncompaction of the ventricular myocardium: ultrafast computer tomography and magnetic resonance imaging. *Int J Cardiovasc Imaging* 2001;17:305–314.
28. Koo BK, Choi D, Ha JW, Kang SM, Chung N, Cho SY. Isolated noncompaction of the ventricular myocardium: contrast echocardiographic findings and review of the literature. *Echocardiography* 2002; 19:153–156.
29. Daimon Y, Watanabe S, Takeda S, Hijikata Y, Komuro I. Two-layered appearance of noncompaction of the ventricular myocardium on magnetic resonance imaging. *Circ J* 2002;66:619–621.
30. Stöllberger C, Finsterer J, Blazek G. Left ventricular hypertrabeculation/noncompaction and association with additional cardiac abnormalities and neuromuscular disorders. *Am J Cardiol* 2002;90:899–902.
31. de Groot-de Laat LE, Krenning BJ, ten Cate FJ, Roelandt JR. Usefulness of contrast echocardiography for diagnosis of left ventricular noncompaction. *Am J Cardiol* 2005;95:1131–1134.
32. Murphy RT, Thaman R, Blanes JG, Ward D, Sevdalis E, Papra E, Kiotsekoglou A, Tome MT, Pellerin D, McKenna WJ, Elliott PM. Natural history and familial characteristics of isolated left ventricular non-compaction. *Eur Heart J* 2005;26:187–192.
33. Belanger AR, Miller MA, Donthireddi UR, Najovits AJ, Goldman ME. New classification scheme of left ventricular noncompaction and correlation with ventricular performance. *Am J Cardiol* 2008; 102:92–96.
34. Ichida F, Tsubata S, Bowles KR, Haneda N, Uese K, Miyawaki T, Dreyer WJ, Messina J, Li H, Bowles NE, Towbin JA. Novel gene mutations in patients with left ventricular noncompaction or Barth syndrome. *Circulation* 2001;103:1256–1263.
35. Jenni R, Wyss CA, Oechslin EN, Kaufmann PA. Isolated ventricular noncompaction is associated with coronary microcirculatory dysfunction. *J Am Coll Cardiol* 2002;39:450–454.
36. Bozić I, Fabijanić D, Carević V, Polić S. Echocardiography in the diagnosis and management of isolated left ventricular noncompaction: case reports and review of the literature. *J Clin Ultrasound* 2006;34: 416–421.

# Cardiac Transplantation in Adults With Aortic Valve Disease With Focus on the Bicuspid Aortic Valve

William Clifford Roberts, MD[a,b,d,*], Carey Camille Roberts[d,e], Jong Mi Ko, BA[d], Shelley Anne Hall, MD[a,d], and John Edward Capehart, MD[c]

The frequency of congenitally bicuspid aortic valves in patients having cardiac transplantation (CT) is unknown. We reviewed 243 explanted hearts in patients having CT at Baylor University Medical Center, Dallas from June 1997 through November 2011 to determine the frequency of a bicuspid aortic valve in this population. Of the 243 explanted hearts, 7 (2.9%) were found to have a congenitally bicuspid aortic valve: 3 had severe aortic valve stenosis and before CT had had the aortic valve replaced; the other 4 had normally functioning bicuspid valves and underwent CT for cardiomyopathy (ischemic in 1, idiopathic in 2, and hypertrophic in 1). Review of previously published reports of CT and aortic valve disease disclosed that 4 patients had had aortic valve replacement (AVR) from 2 to 8 years before CT, 3 had AVR or aortic valve repair of the donor heart at the time of CT, and 4 had AVR or transcatheter aortic valve implantation from 1 to 14 years after CT. Some of these aortic valve replacements, before, at the time of, or after CT were in patients with congenitally bicuspid aortic valves. In conclusion, congenitally bicuspid aortic valves were found in 7 of 243 explanted hearts in patients having CT at a single medical center in a 14-year period: 4 had functioned normally and 3 were severely stenotic. Previous reports of patients having AVR or repair before, during, and after CT were reviewed.  (Am J Cardiol 2012;109:1212–1214)

Cardiac transplantation (CT) is performed mainly in patients with ischemic or idiopathic dilated cardiomyopathy and infrequently in patients with valvular heart disease. This report describes the frequency of finding a bicuspid aortic valve in patients undergoing CT at a single medical center in a 14-year period and reviews previously published reports of patients having aortic valve replacement (AVR) or repair before, at the time of, and after CT.

## Methods

From June 1997 through November 2011, CT was performed at Baylor University Medical Center, Dallas in 243 patients and in each the recipient heart was submitted to the cardiovascular division of the surgical pathology department. Each heart was examined and described by 1 of the authors (W.C.R.) and photographed. Among the 243 hearts studied, 9 had structural (primary) cardiac valve disease: 1 had had mitral valve replacement 2 times, originally for rheumatic mitral stenosis; 1 had replacement of both mitral and aortic valves for pure regurgitation secondary to radiation therapy for Hodgkin's disease many years previously; and the remaining 7 patients had congenitally bicuspid aortic valves, 3 stenotic valves had been replaced and the other 4 were functionally normal (Table 1).

This study was approved by the institutional review board at Baylor University Medical Center and informed consent was waived.

## Results

Pertinent data in each of the 7 patients—all men—are presented in Table 1. Four of the 7 patients (cases 1 to 4) had normally functioning congenitally bicuspid aortic valves discovered during examination of the recipient heart: 2 of these patients had idiopathic dilated cardiomyopathy,[1] 1 had hypertrophic cardiomyopathy, and 1 had ischemic cardiomyopathy.

The remaining 3 patients (cases 5 to 7) had had AVR for aortic valve stenosis and all 3 had congenitally bicuspid aortic valves (Figure 1). Case 7 also had coronary artery bypass grafting at the time of AVR. The interval from AVR to CT in these 3 patients was 8, 4.7, and 5.2 years, respectively. During the interval from AVR to CT, heart failure persisted and eventually progressed in each to New York Heart Association class IV without evidence of significant dysfunction of the mechanical prosthesis or the bioprosthesis in the aortic valve position. Case 6 had a left ventricular assist device inserted 5 months before CT. All 3 patients had left ventricular ejection fractions during the months before CT of ≤20%. All 3 patients are alive as of October 28, 2011. The hearts in each of the 3 patients who had CT after AVR had very dilated left ventricular cavities (maximum internal diameter 5.5, 6.0, and 7.5 cm, respectively), hearts of increased weight (650, 730, and 615 g, respectively, not including the portion of the atrial walls to which the donor heart was connected), and 2 had transmural left ventricular

Departments of [a]Internal Medicine (Division of Cardiology), [b]Pathology, [c]Cardiothoracic Surgery, and [d]Baylor Heart and Vascular Institute, Baylor University Medical Center, Dallas, Texas; [e]Junior, The University of Georgia, Athens, Georgia. Manuscript received November 29, 2011; revised manuscript received and accepted December 1, 2011.

The study was funded by the Baylor Health Care System Foundation, Dallas, Texas.

*Corresponding author: Tel: 214-820-7911; fax: 214-820-7533.

*E-mail address:* wc.roberts@baylorhealth.edu (W.C. Roberts).

Table 1
Pertinent data in seven men having cardiac transplantation and congenitally bicuspid aortic valves with or without aortic valve replacement

| Patient Number | Age at CT (years) | Diagnosis | AVR | Year of AVR | Interval (years) AVR → CT | LVAD | BMI (kg/m$^2$) | LVEF (%) | Date of CT | HW (g) | LV Diameter (cm) | RV Diameter (cm) | CABG | CABG Date | LV Scar |
|---|---|---|---|---|---|---|---|---|---|---|---|---|---|---|---|
| 1 | 35 | HC | 0 | — | — | + | 28.2 | 5 | 10/13/2011 | 435 | 6.0 | 1.0 | 0 | — | 0 |
| 2 | 46 | IDC | 0 | — | — | + | 29.9 | 15 | 12/23/2001 | 565 | 5.0 | 2.5 | 0 | — | 0 |
| 3 | 47* | IDC | 0 | — | — | + | 30.3 | 10 | 4/25/2001 | 705 | 5.0 | 3.0 | 0 | — | 0 |
| 4 | 60 | IC | 0 | — | — | 0 | 27.5 | 7 | 7/1/2011 | 635 | 8.0 | 5.0 | + | 2005 | + |
| 5 | 30 | AS | + (SJM) | 1991 | 8 | 0 | 25.0 | 10 | 10/14/1999 | 650 | 5.5 | 2.8 | 0 | — | + |
| 6 | 56 | AS | + (Bio) | 2002 | 4.7 | + | 28.3 | 5 | 7/1/2007 | 730 | 6.0 | 4.0 | 0 | — | 0 |
| 7 | 65 | AS | + (SJM) | 1997 | 5.2 | 0 | 18.4 | 20 | 1/16/2003 | 615 | 7.5 | 3.0 | + | 1997 | + |

— = not applicable; AS = aortic stenosis; AVR = aortic valve replacement; Bio = bioprosthesis; BMI = body mass index; CABG = coronary artery bypass grafting; CT = cardiac transplantation; HC = hypertrophic cardiomyopathy; HW = heart weight; IC = ischemic cardiomyopathy; IDC = idiopathic dilated cardiomyopathy; LV = left ventricular; LVAD = left ventricular assist device; LVEF = left ventricular ejection fraction; RV = right ventricular; SJM = St. Jude Medical mechanical prosthesis.

* Died March 22, 2011, or 10 years after cardiac transplantation.

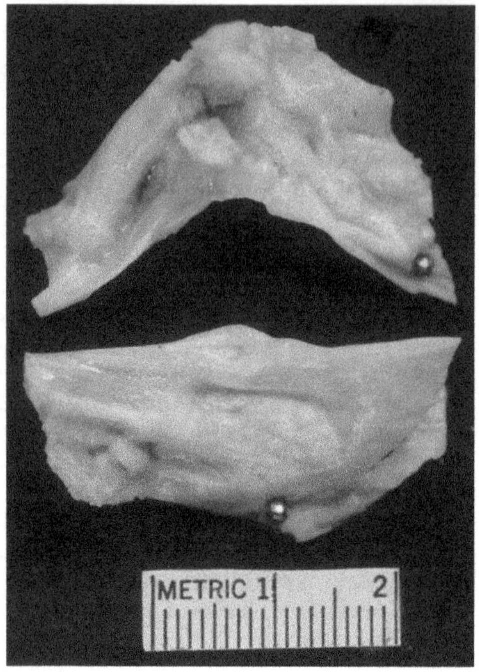


Figure 1. Case 6 (Table 1). Operatively excised severely stenotic congenitally bicuspid aortic valve.

scars, only 1 (case 7) of whom had narrowed coronary arteries. Case 6 had focally thickened left ventricular mural endocardium (possibly the consequence of the left ventricular assist device inserted 5 months previously).

## Discussion

A common denominator in each of the heretofore described men was the presence of a congenitally malformed bicuspid aortic valve. In 4, the malformed valve functioned normally and was unrecognized during life. CT was performed in 2 of them because of idiopathic dilated cardiomyopathy, in 1 for ischemic cardiomyopathy, and in 1 for hypertrophic cardiomyopathy.

The remaining 3 patients had AVR for aortic stenosis superimposed on their malformed valve and of them 1 had concomitant coronary bypass grafting. The decision to do CT in these 3 patients rather than repeat AVR was based on the presence of progressively worsening heart failure without evidence of dysfunction of the mechanical prosthesis or bioprosthesis in the aortic valve position, extremely dilated left ventricular cavities ($\geq$5 cm) in ventricular systole, and extremely low left ventricular ejection fractions ($\leq$20%). These 3 patients may have had underlying dilated cardiomyopathy in addition to aortic stenosis.

The frequency of congenitally malformed aortic valves is unclear but probably is about 1% of the population, an involvement of about 3 million Americans.[2] In the present study, 7 congenitally malformed valves were found in 243 patients undergoing CT.

The present report is not the first to describe aortic valve disease and CT (Figure 2). Park et al[3] described a 33-year-old man who underwent orthotopic CT after 2 previous valve replacements for active infective endocarditis involving the native mitral and aortic valves followed by infection

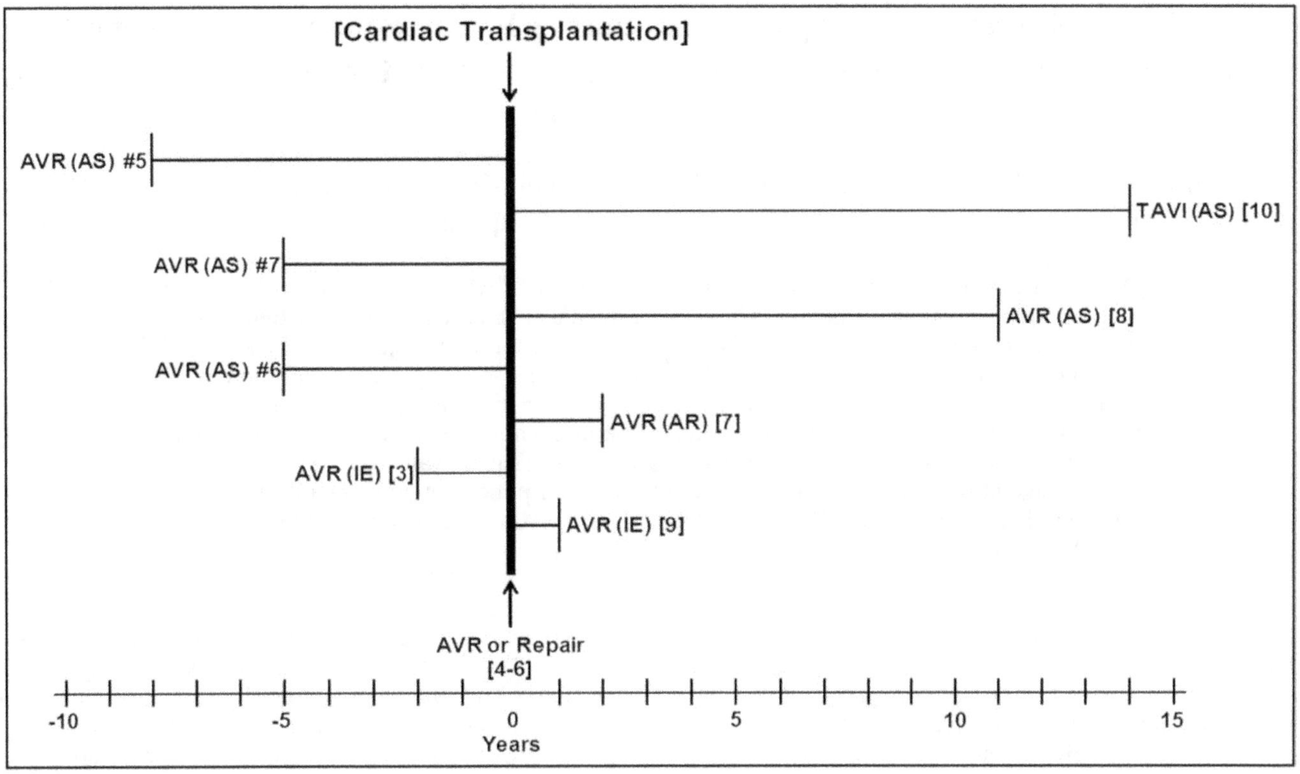


Figure 2. This diagram shows the present cases (5 to 7) and the previously reported patients *(reference in brackets)* having cardiac transplantation and aortic valve replacement or repair, before, at the time of, or after cardiac transplantation. Time in years *(horizontal axis)* is presented before (minus), at the time of, and after cardiac transplantation for aortic stenosis (AS) and/or regurgitation (AR). Several patients clearly had malfunctioning congenitally bicuspid aortic valves. IE = infective endocarditis; TAVI = transcatheter aortic valve implantation (without replacement).

involving the prosthetic aortic valve. Navia et al[4] repaired a purely regurgitant aortic valve in the donor heart before using it for CT. Rao et al[5] and Larobina et al[6] found a donor's heart to have a very stenotic aortic valve and replaced it before CT. Goenen et al[7] found a donor heart to have a mildly regurgitant congenitally bicuspid aortic valve, used the heart for CT, but 2 years after CT did AVR in the donor heart because of development of severe aortic regurgitation. Joyce et al[8] described severe aortic stenosis involving a congenitally bicuspid aortic valve in a donor heart 11 years after CT with successful AVR. Sayeed et al[9] performed AVR for infective endocarditis in a donor heart a year after CT. And finally, Seiffert et al[10] performed successfully transcatheter aortic valve implantation (without replacement) in a 67-year-old heart transplant recipient for severe symptomatic aortic stenosis 14 years after CT.

1. Roberts WC, Siegel RJ, McManus BM. Idiopathic dilated cardiomyopathy: analysis of 152 necropsy patients. *Am J Cardiol* 1987;60:1340–1355.
2. Roberts WC. The congenitally bicuspid aortic valve. A study of 85 autopsy cases. *Am J Cardiol* 1970;26:72–83.
3. Park SJ, Sullivan HJ, Lonchyna V, Hinkamp TJ, Pifarre R. Heart transplantation for complicated and recurrent early prosthetic valve endocarditis. *J Heart Lung Transplant* 1993;12:802–803.
4. Navia JL, Atik FA, Marullo A, Starling RC, Garcia M, Vega PR, Smedira NG, McCarthy PM. Bench repair of donor aortic valve with minimal access orthotopic heart transplantation. *Ann Thorac Surg* 2005;80:313–315.
5. Rao JN, Prendergast B, Dark JH. Orthotopic heart transplantation with concurrent aortic valve replacement and coronary artery bypass grafting. *J Heart Lung Transplant* 2000;19:897–899.
6. Larobina ME, Mariani JA, Rowland MA. Aortic valve replacement for aortic stenosis during orthotopic cardiac transplant. *Ann Thorac Surg* 2008;86:1979–1982.
7. Goenen MJ, Jacquet L, De Kock M, Van Dyck M, Schoevardts JC, Chalant CH. Aortic valve replacement thirty-one months after orthotopic heart transplantation. *J Heart Lung Transplant* 1991;10:604–607.
8. Joyce DL, Russell SD, Conte JV, Cattaneo SM. Aortic valve replacement in a diseased bicuspid valve eleven years after transplantation. *Interact Cardiovasc Thorac Surg* 2009;8:594–595.
9. Sayeed R, Drain AJ, Sivasothy PS, Large SR, Wallwork J. Aortic valve replacement for late infective endocarditis after heart-lung transplantation. *Trans Proc* 2005;37:4537–4539.
10. Seiffert M, Meyer S, Franzen O, Conradi L, Baldus S, Schirmer J, Deuse T, Costard-Jaeckle A, Reichenspurner H, Treede H. Transcatheter aortic valve implantation in a heart transplant recipient: a case report. *Trans Proc* 2010;42:4661–4663.

# Dramatically Different Phenotypic Expressions of Hypertrophic Cardiomyopathy in Male Cousins Undergoing Cardiac Transplantation With Identical Disease-Causing Gene Mutation

William C. Roberts, MD[a,b,d,*], Carey Camille Roberts[d], Jong Mi Ko, BA[d], Paul A. Grayburn, MD[b,d], Anumeha Tandon, MD[b], Johannes J. Kuiper, MD[b], John E. Capehart, MD[c], and Shelley A. Hall, MD[b]

**Described herein are certain findings in 2 male cousins who underwent cardiac transplantation for severe heart failure (HF), one of the diastolic type (ejection fraction ≈65%), and one of the systolic type (ejection fraction ≈20%), both the consequence of hypertrophic cardiomyopathy (HC), and each had identical disease-causing gene mutations. The implanted heart in one had normal-sized ventricular cavities and no grossly visible ventricular wall lesions (except in one papillary muscle) and the other patient had severely dilated ventricular cavities and multiple extensive ventricular wall scars. The heart mass and the age of onset of symptoms was similar in each patient. A number of other family members had evidence of HC.**  **(Am J Cardiol 2013;111:1818–1822)**

Hypertrophic cardiomyopathy (HC) is a genetically transmitted cardiac disease with a diverse variety of clinical and morphologic manifestations. Its frequency of 1 in 500 persons is similar to that of familial hypercholesterolemia.[1] Some patients with HC remain asymptomatic or nearly so throughout a long life; others die suddenly, usually prematurely; many have symptoms related to left ventricular outflow obstruction and once the obstruction is relieved the symptoms vanish or at least decrease in frequency, and some patients develop end-stage HF that can be relieved only by cardiac transplantation (CT).[2–4] Recently, we encountered 2 male cousins with HC, both of whom underwent CT, and examination of the recipient heart disclosed nearly opposite morphologic features of the disease although both had identical disease-causing gene mutations. A description of certain findings in them is the purpose of this report.

## Patient Descriptions

Pertinent clinical and morphologic findings in the 2 patients are tabulated in Table 1. The pedigrees of the family are illustrated in Figure 1. Both were African American men, one had CT at age 45 and the other, at age 48 years. One became symptomatic from HF about 6 years before CT, the other 7 years, before CT. Both had class IV HF. Each also had one or more episodes of syncope, atrial fibrillation, and runs of ventricular tachycardia. Neither had a precordial murmur. Neither had obstruction to outflow from either the right or left ventricle. Both had normal epicardial coronary arteries. The left ventricular ejection fractions were strikingly different. In case #1 it was ≈65%, and in case #2, ≈20%. Both patients had elevated pulmonary arterial pressures. Both had cardiac defibrillators implanted several years before CT. Patient #2 had a left ventricular assist device. Echocardiograms before CT are shown in Figures 2–4.

Table 1
Certain clinical and morphologic findings in the 2 African American male cousins who underwent cardiac transplantation for end-stage heart failure secondary to hypertrophic cardiomyopathy

| Variable | Case #1 | Case #2 |
|---|---|---|
| Age (yrs) at cardiac transplantation | 45 | 48 |
| Age (yrs) onset symptoms | 39 | 41 |
| Heart failure class IV | + | + |
| Chest pain | 0 | + |
| Syncope | + | + |
| Precordial murmur | 0 | 0 |
| Atrial fibrillation | + | + |
| Ventricular tachycardia | + | + |
| Body mass index (Kg/m$^2$) | 26.5 | 30.6 |
| Left ventricular ejection fraction | 65% | 20% |
| Cardiac index (l/min/m$^2$) | 1.3 | 1.8 |
| Pulmonary artery peak systolic pressure (mm Hg) | 82 | 56 |
| Coronary narrowing by angiogram | 0 | 0 |
| Left ventricular assist device inserted | 0 | + |
| Heart weight (g) | 410 | 410 |
| Scars (0-4+), left ventricular wall and ventricular septum | 0* | +(4+) |
| Dilated right ventricle | 0 | + |
| Dilated left ventricle | 0 | + |
| Mitral valve | normal | normal |
| Mural endocardial thickening in the left ventricular outflow tract in apposition to anterior mitral leaflet | 0 | 0 |
| Mitral annular calcium | 3+/4+ | 0 |
| Abnormal intramural coronary arteries | 0 | + |

* Scarring in one left ventricular papillary muscles.

[a]Department of Pathology, [b]Department of Internal Medicine, Division of Cardiology, [c]Department of Cardiothoracic Surgery, and [d]Baylor Heart and Vascular Institute, Baylor University Medical Center, Dallas, Texas. Manuscript received September 19, 2012; revised manuscript received and accepted February 6, 2013.

See page 1822 for disclosure information.

*Corresponding author: Tel: 214-820-7911; fax: 214-820-7533.

*E-mail address:* wc.roberts@baylorhealth.edu (W.C. Roberts).

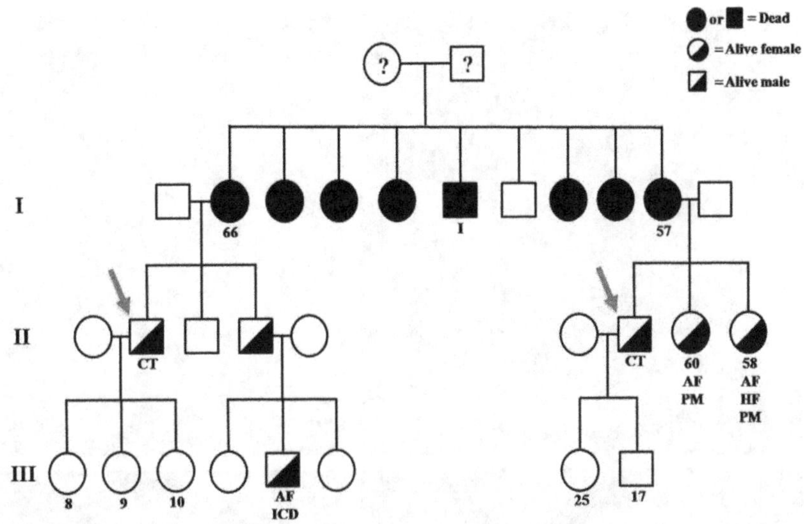


Figure 1. Pedigree of the family of case #1 *(left)* and case #2 *(right)*. Whether or not the grand parents had heart disease is unclear but 8 of their 9 children died of heart disease, several of them suddenly and prematurely, and others from heart failure of varying durations. The *arrows* designate the 2 patients described herein. The numbers represent the ages at death or presently (2012). AF = atrial fibrillation; CT = cardiac transplantation; HF = heart failure; I = stillbirth; ICD = intracardiac defibrillator; PM = pacemaker.

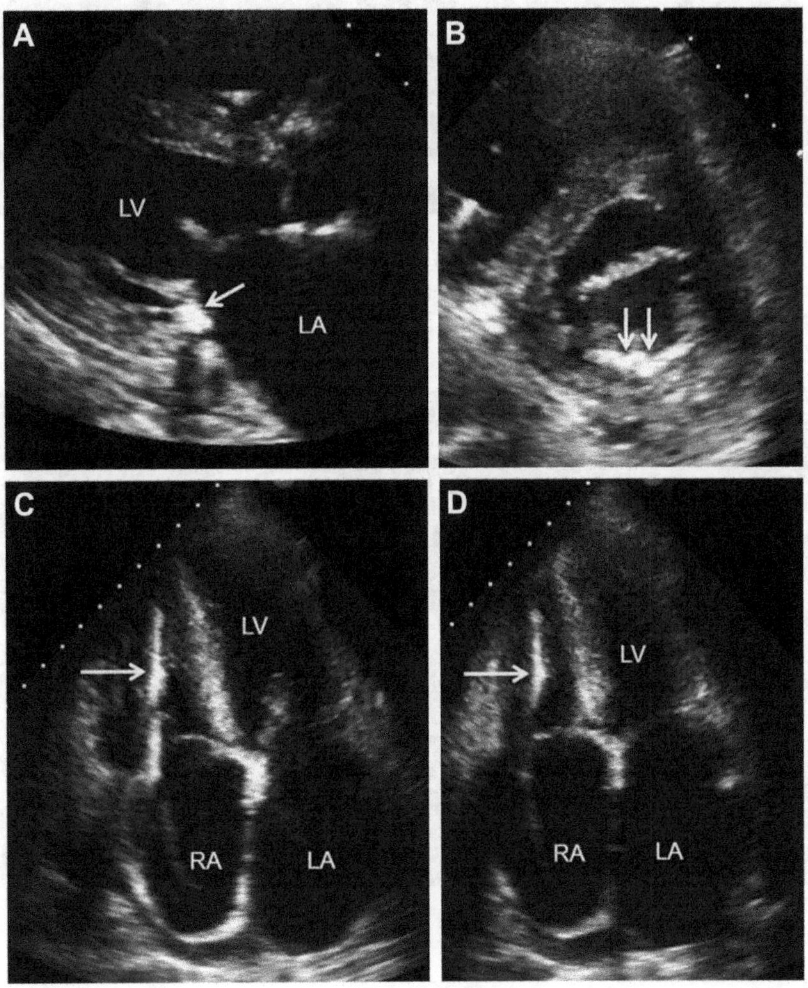


Figure 2. Echocardiogram in patient #1. *(A)* Parasternal long-axis view showing a very dilated left atrium (LA) and a non-dilated left ventricle (LV). The *arrow* points to calcium in the mitral annular area. *(B)* Parasternal short-axis view of the ventricles. The *arrows* again point to calcium deposits in the mitral valve area. *(C)* Four-chamber view during ventricular diastole. The *arrow* points to the intracardiac defibrillator catheter. *(D)* Four-chamber view in ventricular systole. Cavity size is much smaller than in diastole, consistent with a left ventricular ejection fraction of ≈65%.

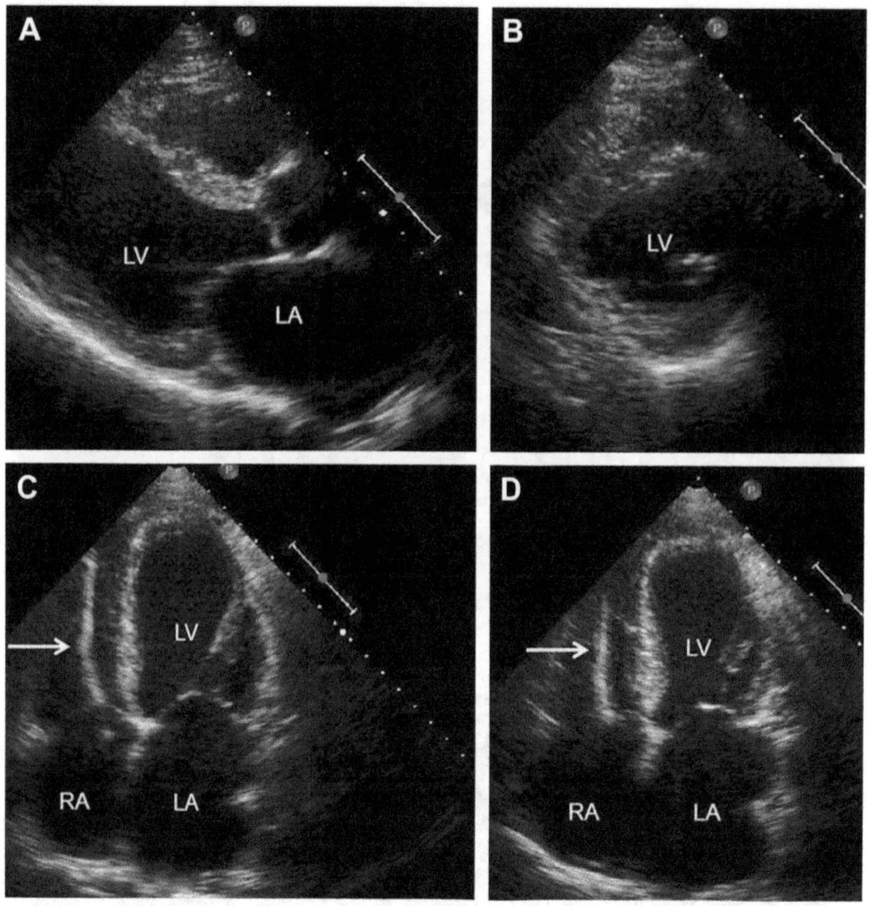


Figure 3. Echocardiogram is patient #2. *(A)* Parasternal long-axis view showing very dilated left ventricle (LV) and left atrium (LA). *(B)* Parasternal short-axis view of the left ventricle. *(C)* Four-chamber view showing the very dilated left ventricles in ventricular diastole with its thin walls. The *arrow* points to the implanted intracardiac defibrillator catheter. RA = right atrium. *(D)* Same view in ventricular systole, with minimal change in ventricular size and wall thickness indicative of markedly depressed systolic function.

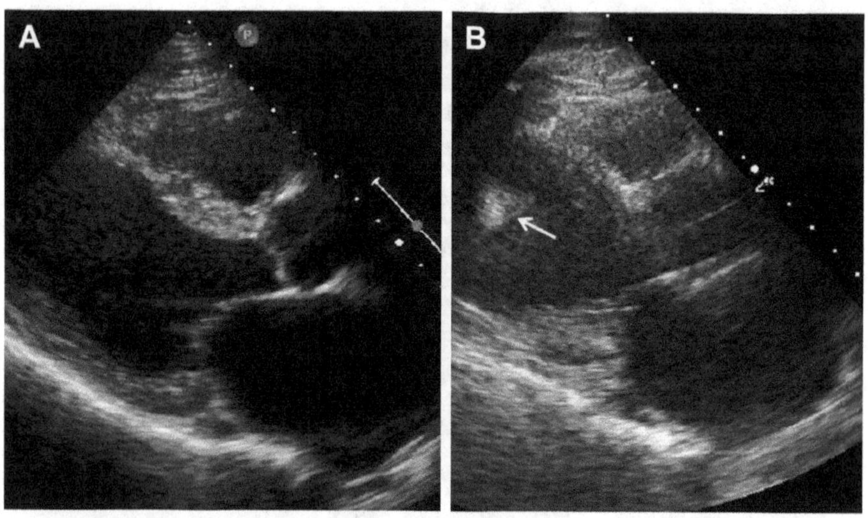


Figure 4. Echocardiogram in patient #2 before *(A)* and after *(B)* insertion of a left ventricular assist device *(arrow)*. The size of the left ventricular cavity is larger before than after insertion of the device.

The explanted heart in each patient weighed 410 g (portions of the atrial walls are not included in the weight) (Figures 5 and 6). Both hearts contained excessive subepicardial adipose tissue. In case #1, neither cardiac ventricles was dilated. Except for one left ventricular papillary muscle, no grossly visible myocardial scars were

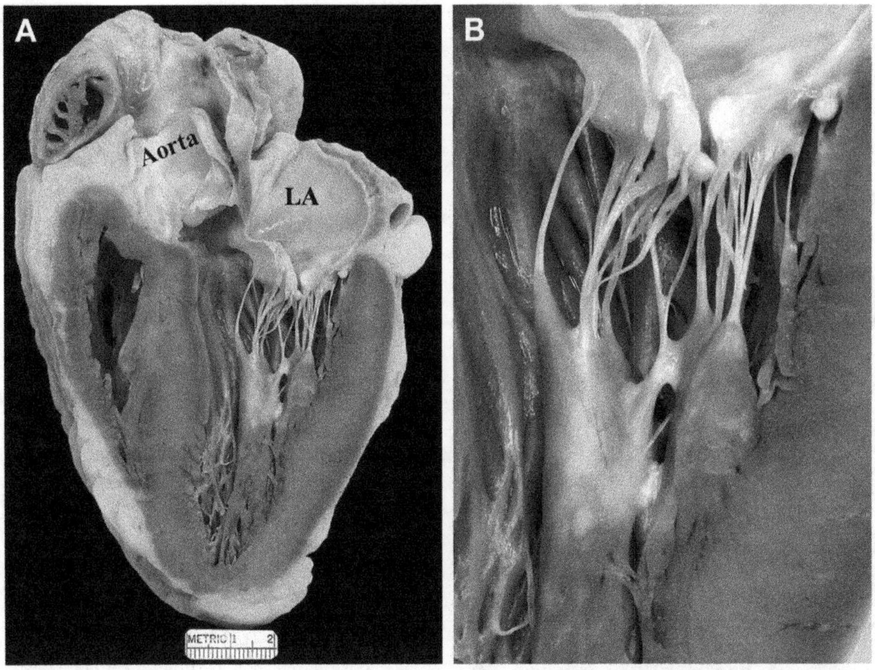


Figure 5. Case #1. *(A)* Longitudinal view of the left ventricle, right ventricular outflow tract, aortic valve, mitral valve, and left atrium. The thickness of the ventricular septum is a bit greater than that of the left ventricular free wall. The apical portion of the posteromedial papillary muscle is scarred. Calcium is present in the mitral annular region. *(B)* Close-up of the scarred papillary muscle.

present. In case #2, in contrast, there was extensive, usually transmural, scarring of the left ventricular free wall and ventricular septum with some scarring also in the right ventricular free wall. The ventricular cavities were dilated in case #2 but not as dilated as would have occurred had not a left ventricular assist device been inserted 29 months earlier. Neither patient had mural endocardial thickening in the ventricular septum in apposition to the anterior mitral leaflet, the anatomic feature of systolic anterior motion of the anterior mitral leaflet with septal contact. Patient #1, but not patient #2, had calcium in the mitral annular region.[5] Histologic study demonstrated considerable enlargement of the myocardial fibers in both patients. The intramural coronary arteries in patient #2 were increased in number and size and the lumens in many were narrowed. The quantity of interstitial fibrous tissue between myofibers was increased in both patients.

Several months after CT, both patients had blood samples (in EDTA) sent to Gene Dx (207 Perry Parkway, Gaithersburg, Maryland 20877) for "hypertrophic cardiomyopathy panel" analysis. Both patients had the p.Arg 186Gln (CGG>GAG)(R186Q) mutation in exon 8 of the troponin I (TNN13) gene (NM_000363.4), confirming that both patients had the identical disease-causing gene mutation despite strikingly different phenotypic expressions.

## Discussion

Although HC is a genetically transmitted disease with an autosomal dominant trait, the penetrance into the family of the 2 cousins described herein is particularly striking. Some family members died suddenly, usually prematurely, others developed severe heart failure, and others developed various arrhythmias and conduction disturbances with intracardiac pacemakers and implantable intracardiac defibrillators implanted.

Cardiac transplantation for patients with HC is relatively infrequent, and most patients with HC having CT have severe systolic heart failure and no obstruction to either left or right ventricular outflow. Warren and colleagues[6] in 1988 appear to have been the first to describe CT for HC. Both of their patients had severe diastolic heart failure with normal sized ventricular cavities, apparently similar to our patient #1. Shirani and colleagues[7] in 1993 described 10 patients with HC who had CT and all of them had severe systolic heart failure with severe left ventricular and ventricular septal scarring, similar to that in our patient #2. Hecht and associates[8] in the same year described 2 patients with end-stage systolic heart failure who underwent CT. Contu and colleagues[9] in 2004 described 14 patients with HC who underwent CT, 13 of whom underwent CT for severe heart failure, presumably systolic in type, and 1 for malignant ventricular arrhythmias. Biagini and associates[10] in 2008 described 18 patients with HC who underwent CT, 17 of whom had severe systolic heart failure and severely dilated ventricular cavities and 1 of whom had severe diastolic heart failure with normal sized ventricular cavities. Maron and colleagues[11] in 2010 acquired data from the United Network of Organ-Sharing Registry and found among 26, 706 patients $\geq$18 years of age having CT that 303 (1%) had CT for HC. Among those 303 patients it is unclear how many had systolic or diastolic HF. They found that survival after CT was at least similar to that in non-HC patients having CT and maybe better. And finally, Kato and colleagues[12] in 2012 described 41 patients with HC who underwent CT, 39 (95%) for "refractory heart failure" and 2

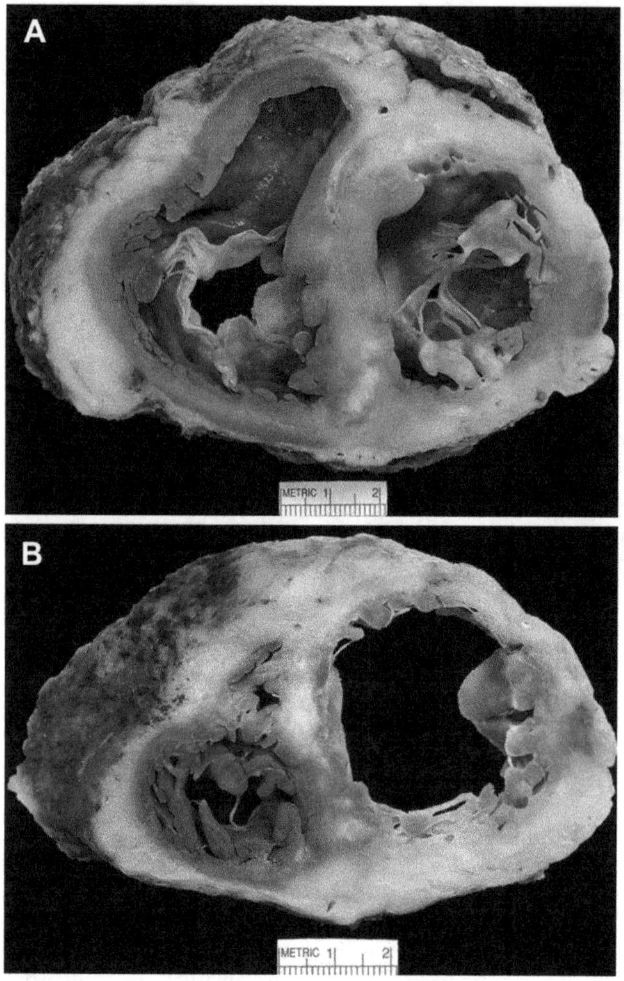


Figure 6. Case #2. Basal portion of the heart *(A)* and more caudal portion *(B)* showing extensive scarring in the left ventricular free wall and ventricular septum and scarring in the moderator band of the right ventricle. Both ventricular cavities dilated.

from "recurrent ventricular arrhythmias." Prior to CT only 14 (34%) of the 41 patients had a dilated left ventricular cavity (left ventricular end-diastolic dimension >55 mm) and 27 patients (66%) had smaller left ventricular cavities. Survival of their 41 HC patients after CT was better than that for their 771 non-HC patients. Thus, CT is a useful procedure for the relatively small percentage of patients with HC who develop end-stage HF or refractory ventricular arrhythmias unassociated with left or right ventricular outflow obstruction.

**Acknowledgment:** We thank Ms. Carolyn Q. Alexander, RN, BSN, for arranging the acquisition of the genetic tests in each of the 2 patients.

## Disclosures

The authors have no conflicts of interest to disclose.


1. Maron BJ, Gardin JM, Flack JM, Gidding SS, Kurosaki TT, Bild DE. Prevalence of hypertrophic cardiomyopathy in a general population of young adults: echocardiographic analysis of 4111 subjects in the CARDIA study. *Circulation* 1995;92:785–789.
2. Maron BJ. Hypertrophic cardiomyopathy. *Lancet* 1997;350:127–133.
3. Spirito P, Seidman CE, McKenna WJ, Maron BJ. The management of hypertrophic cardiomyopathy. *New Eng J Med* 1997;366:775–785.
4. Maron BJ, Maron MS, Wigle ED, Bruanwald E. The 50-year history, controversy, and clinical implication of left ventricular outflow tract obstruction in hypertrophic cardiomyopathy. From idiopathic cardiomyopathy subaortic stenosis to hypertrophic cardiomyopathy. *J Am Coll Cardiol* 2009;54:191–200.
5. Motamed HE, Roberts WC. Frequency and significance of mitral anular calcium in hypertrophic cardiomyopathy: analysis of 200 necropsy patients. *Am J Cardiol* 1987;60:877–884.
6. Warren SE, Cohn LH, Schoen FJ, Mudge GH Jr, Lorell BH. Advanced diastolic heart failure in familial hypertrophic cardiomyopathy managed with cardiac transplantation. *J Appl Cardiol* 1988;3:415–422.
7. Shirani J, Maron BJ, Cannon RO III, Shahin S, Roberts WC. Clinicopathologic features of hypertrophic cardiomyopathy managed by cardiac transplantation. *Am J Cardiol* 1993;72:434–440.
8. Hecht GM, Heinrich GK, Roberts WC, Maron BJ. Coexistence of sudden cardiac death and end-stage heart failure in familial hypertrophic cardiomyopathy. *J Am Coll Cardiol* 1993;22:489–497.
9. Coutu M, Parrault LP, White M, Pelletier GB, Racine N, Poirier NC, Carrier M. Cardiac transplantation for hypertrophic cardiomyopathy: a valid therapeutic option. *J Heart Lung Transplant* 2004;43:413–417.
10. Biagini E, Spirito P, Leone O, Piccio FM, Coccolo F, Ragni L, Lofiego C, Grigioni F, Potena L, Rocchi G, Bacchi-Reggiani L, Boriani G, Prandstraller D, Arbustini E, Branzi A, Rapezzi C. Heart transplantation in hypertrophic cardiomyopathy. *Am J Cardiol* 2008;101:387–392.
11. Maron MS, Kalsmith BM, Udelson JE, Li W, DeNofrio D. Survival after cardiac transplantation in patients with hypertrophic cardiomyopathy. *Circ Heart Fail* 2010;3:574–579.
12. Kato TS, Takayama H, Yoshizawa S, Morboe C, Schulze PS, Farr M, Naka Y, Mancini D, Maurer MS. Cardiac transplantation in patients with hypertrophic cardiomyopathy. *Am J Cardiol* 2012;110:568–574.

# Comparison of Total 12-Lead QRS Voltage in a Variety of Cardiac Conditions and Its Usefulness in Predicting Increased Cardiac Mass

William C. Roberts, MD[a,b,*], Giovanni Filardo, PhD[c,d,e,f], Jong Mi Ko, BA[b], Robert J. Siegel, MD[g], Allen L. Dollar, MD[g], Elizabeth M. Ross, MD[g], and Jamshid Shirani, MD[g]

**Echocardiography provides a more accurate method to determine increased cardiac mass than does electrocardiography. Nevertheless, most offices of physicians do not possess echocardiographic machines, but many possess electrocardiographic machines. Many electrocardiographic criteria have been used to determine increased cardiac mass, but few of the criteria have been measured against cardiac weight determined at necropsy or after cardiac transplantation. Such was the purpose of the present study. Cardiac weight at necropsy or after transplantation was determined in 359 patients with 11 different cardiac conditions, and total 12-lead electrocardiographic QRS voltage (from the peak of the R wave to the nadir of either the Q or the S wave, whichever was deeper) was measured in each patient. Even in hearts with massively increased cardiac mass (>1,000 g), the total 12-lead QRS voltage was clearly increased (>175 mm) in only 94%, but this criterion was superior to that of previously described electrocardiographic criteria for "left ventricular hypertrophy." Hearts with excessive adipose tissue infrequently had increased total 12-lead QRS voltage despite increased cardiac weight. Likewise, patients with fatal cardiac amyloidosis had hearts of increased weight but quite low total 12-lead QRS voltage. In conclusion, 12-lead QRS voltage is useful in predicting increased cardiac mass, but that predictability is dependent in part on the cause of the increased cardiac mass.**  **(Am J Cardiol 2013;112:904–909)**

Various electrocardiographic criteria have been used to predict left ventricular hypertrophy (LVH), but few have been compared with the actual weight of the heart at necropsy or after cardiac transplantation. Exceptions are the studies by Griep[1] in 1959, and by Allenstein and Hiroyoshi[2] in 1960. The most common criterion used in the past 60 years is that recommended in 1949 by Sokolow and Lyon,[3] who studied 12-lead electrocardiograms in patients who were believed to have LVH on the basis of "a cardiac disorder capable of producing increased strain on the left ventricle (such as hypertension, aortic valve lesions, coarctation of the aorta, patent ductus arteriosus)." These investigators produced a variety of electrocardiographic criteria for LVH, including among others R in lead $V_5$ + $S_1$ in lead $V_1$ $\geq$35 mm. A number of other criteria have been suggested subsequently (Table 1).[4–11] Siegel and Roberts[12] in 1982 proposed that measuring the total amplitude (from the peak of the R wave to the nadir of either the Q or the S wave, whichever was deeper) of the QRS complex in all 12 electrocardiographic leads was a better determinant of cardiac mass than the previously reported criteria (Figure 1). Subsequently, several investigators from the same laboratory measured total 12-lead QRS voltage in a variety of cardiac conditions and in each compared it with the heart weight determined by the same investigators.[13–22] Here, we review their findings in 11 different cardiac conditions.

## Methods

To be included in this study, a heart had to be studied in the Pathology Branch of the National Heart, Lung, and Blood Institute of the National Institutes of Health (Bethesda, Maryland). An accurate heart weight and a 12-lead electrocardiogram had to be available in all cases to be included in this study. The patients were divided into 11 groups (Table 2). The electrocardiographic QRS voltage was measured in each of the 12 leads, as demonstrated in Figure 1. In patients with >1 twelve-lead electrocardiogram available, the one measured was the one recorded closest to the patient's death or closest to cardiac transplantation. The medical records were reviewed in all cases to provide pertinent clinical information. All hearts were examined and classified morphologically by one investigator (WCR). The QRS measurements were

[a]Departments of Internal Medicine and Pathology; [b]Baylor Heart and Vascular Institute, Dallas, Texas; [c]Institute for Health Care Research and Improvement, Baylor Health Care System; [d]Cardiovascular Epidemiology, Baylor University Medical Center, Dallas, Texas; [e]Cardiovascular Epidemiology, The Heart Hospital Baylor, Plano, Texas; [f]Southern Methodist University, Dallas, Texas; and [g]Pathology Branch, National Heart, Lung, and Blood Institute, National Institutes of Health, Bethesda, Maryland. Manuscript received April 3, 2013; revised manuscript received and accepted April 23, 2013.

Present address (RJS): Cedars-Sinai Medical Center, Division of Cardiology, 8700 Beverly Boulevard, Suite 5623, Los Angeles, CA 90048.

Present address (ALD): Emory University School of Medicine (Cardiology), 49 Jesse Hill Drive, Atlanta, GA 30303.

Present address (EMR): 2021 K Street, NW, Suite 315, Washington, DC 20006.

Present address (JS): St. Luke's University Health Network Cardiology, 801 Ostrum Street, Bethlehem, PA 18015.

This work was supported by grants from Baylor Health Care System Foundation.

See page 909 for disclosure information.

*Corresponding author: Tel: (214) 820-7911; fax: (214) 820-7533.

*E-mail address:* wc.roberts@baylorhealth.edu (W.C. Roberts).

Table 1
Recommended or modified electrocardiographic criteria for determining left ventricular hypertrophy as to 17 patients with hearts at necropsy weighing >1,000 grams*

| No. | QRS Complex Measured | Value Considered Upper Limit of Normal (mm) | No. (%) of 17 Patients Above Normal Limit |
|---|---|---|---|
| 1a | $SV_1 + RV_5$ or $V_6$ (larger) | 35 | 12 (71%) |
| 1b | $SV_1 + RV_5$ or $V_6$ (larger) | 40 | 11 (65%) |
| 2a | $SV_1$ or $V_2$ (larger) + $RV_5$ or $V_6$ (larger) | 35 | 15 (88%) |
| 2b | $SV_1$ or $V_2$ (larger) + $RV_5$ or $V_6$ (larger) | 40 | 14 (82%) |
| 3a | $SV_1$ or $V_2$ (larger) + $RV_6$ | 35 | 15 (88%) |
| 3b | $SV_1$ or $V_2$ (larger) + $RV_6$ | 40 | 13 (76%) |
| 4a | $SV_2 + RV_5$ | 35 | 14 (82%) |
| 4b | $SV_2 + RV_5$ | 40 | 14 (82%) |
| 5a | Deepest $SV_1 - V_3$ + tallest $RV_4 - V_6$ | 35 | 14 (82%) |
| 5b | Deepest $SV_1 - V_3$ + tallest $RV_4 - V_6$ | 40 | 13 (76%) |
| 5c | Deepest $SV_1 - V_3$ + tallest $RV_4 - V_6$ | 45 | 13 (76%) |
| 5d | Deepest $SV_1 - V_3$ + tallest $RV_4 - V_6$ | 50 | 13 (76%) |
| 6a | Tallest R + deepest S in any V lead | 35 | 14 (82%) |
| 6b | Tallest R + deepest S in any V lead | 40 | 14 (82%) |
| 7a | Deepest $SV_1 - V_3$ | 25 | 14 (82%) |
| 7b | Deepest $SV_1 - V_3$ | 30 | 12 (71%) |
| 8a | Tallest $RV_4 - V_6$ | 25 | 9 (53%) |
| 8b | Tallest $RV_4 - V_6$ | 30 | 8 (27%) |
| 9a | Deepest $SV_1 - V_2$ | 25 | 14 (82%) |
| 9b | Deepest $SV_1 - V_2$ | 30 | 12 (71%) |
| 10a | Tallest $RV_5$ or $V_6$ | 25 | 9 (53%) |
| 10b | Tallest $RV_5$ or $V_6$ | 30 | 8 (27%) |
| 11 | $RV_6 > RV_5$ | $\leq 1$ | 13 (76%) |
| 12a | Tallest limb-lead R + deepest limb-lead S | 15 | 15 (88%) |
| 12b | Tallest limb-lead R + deepest limb-lead S | 20 | 12 (71%) |
| 13a | $R_1 + S_3$ | 15 | 12 (71%) |
| 13b | $R_1 + S_3$ | 20 | 10 (59%) |
| 14a | Tallest limb-lead R | 10 | 14 (82%) |
| 14b | Tallest limb-lead R | 15 | 6 (35%) |
| 15a | Deepest limb-lead S | 10 | 10 (59%) |
| 15b | Deepest limb-lead S | 15 | 6 (35%) |
| 16 | $R_1$ | 10 | 11 (65%) |
| 17 | $S_3$ | 10 | 7 (41%) |
| 18a | Total 12-lead QRS voltage | 175 | 16 (94%) |
| 18b | Total 12-lead QRS voltage | 200 | 15 (88%) |
| 18c | Total 12-lead QRS voltage | 225 | 13 (76%) |
| 18d | Total 12-lead QRS voltage | 250 | 13 (76%) |

* From Roberts and Podolak.[13]

performed by the first author of each study and "spot checked" by WCR when not the first author.

Means, SDs, and percentages were calculated to describe the study cohort (n = 359). A multivariate linear regression model was used to assess the adjusted association between patients' heart weight (grams) and 12-lead QRS voltage (millimeters).[23] Covariates included gender, age, and cardiac condition. Restricted cubic splines were used for all continuous variables.[24] Adjusted p values and plots of the association between patient's heart weight and 12-lead QRS voltage were also estimated.

## Results

A total of 359 patients, 208 men (58%) and 151 women (42%), were included and divided into 11 groups (Table 2). Their ages ranged from 14 to 85 years; of the 359 patients, 8 (2%) were aged ≤20 years, including 1 aged 20 years, 5 aged 19 years, 1 aged 16 years, and 1 aged 14 years. The heart weights in the 359 patients ranged from 150 to 1,360 g, and the mean heart weights were of increased mass (heart weight >350 g in women and >400 g in men) in 8 of the 11 groups in men and in 10 of the 11 groups in women. Total 12-lead QRS voltage (measured with normal [10 mm] standardization [10 mm = 1 mV]) ranged from 58 to 601 mm. In 8 of the 11 groups, the mean total 12-lead QRS voltage was lower in male than in female patients; in contrast, the mean heart weight was higher in male than in female patients in 9 of the 11 groups. Additionally, the ratio of total 12-lead QRS voltage (millimeters) to heart weight (grams) was lower in male than in female patients in all 11 groups. Figure 2 depicts the adjusted (by age and gender) association between heart weight and total 12-lead QRS voltage in the 10 patient groups and in the normal group. (Individual patient-level data in the aortic stenosis patient group were not available.) The electrocardiograms obtained in the patients who underwent

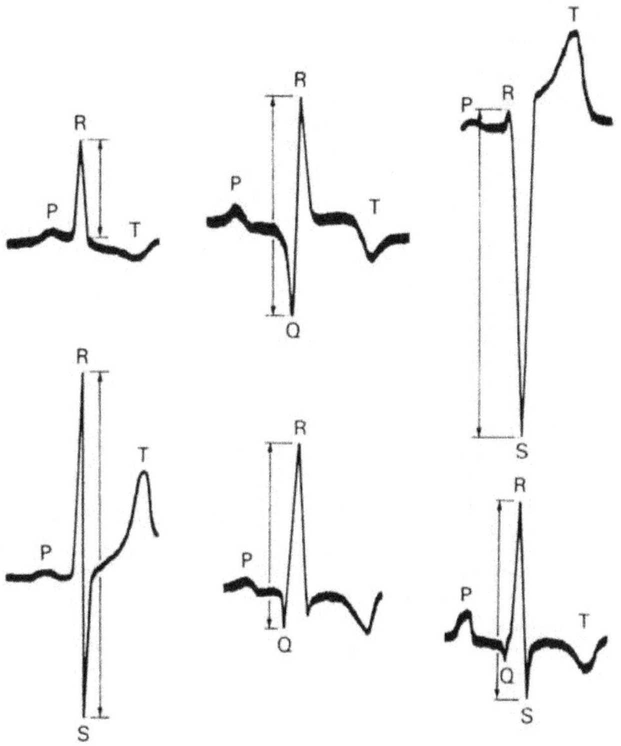


Figure 1. Various QRS complexes showing how each was measured. Reproduced from Siegel and Roberts[12] with permission of the publisher.

cardiac operations were the ones recorded immediately preoperatively.

**Hearts weighing >1,000 g[13]:** Of these 17 patients, 16 (94%) were men aged 29 to 64 years (mean 42). The one woman's heart weighed 1,250 g (3.6 times the upper limit of normal), and her total 12-lead QRS voltage, 601 mm, was the largest of any of the 359 patients. The cause of the massive cardiomegaly in these 17 patients was isolated pure aortic regurgitation (5 patients), combined pure aortic regurgitation and pure mitral regurgitation (4 patients), pure aortic regurgitation plus ventricular septal defect (2 patients), aortic stenosis and regurgitation (2 patients), aortic regurgitation plus mitral stenosis with regurgitation (1 patient), hypertrophic cardiomyopathy (2 patients), and ventricular septal defect with mitral stenosis (1 patient). The total 12-lead QRS voltage was highest in this group than in any of the others.

**Aortic valve stenosis[12]:** These 50 patients, aged 16 to 65 years (mean 48), had peak systolic transvalvular pressure gradients ranging from 52 to 180 mm Hg (mean 98) and peak left ventricular systolic pressures ranging from 149 to 270 mm Hg (average 210). All had anatomically normal mitral valves. Aortic valve replacement had been done in 38 patients (76%), and all died <6 weeks after the operation; 2 others died during anesthesia induction. The aortic valve was unicuspid unicommissural in 5 patients (12%), congenitally bicuspid in 29 patients (58%), and tricuspid in 15 patients (30%). Because the total 12-lead QRS amplitude (millimeters) roughly equaled the peak left ventricular systolic pressure (millimeters of mercury), Siegel and Roberts[13] suggested that the total 12-lead QRS voltage (millimeters) minus the systemic arterial systolic pressure (millimeters of mercury) roughly equaled the peak systolic pressure gradient (millimeters of mercury) between the left ventricle and the systemic artery.

**Aortic regurgitation[14]:** These 30 patients, aged 19 to 65 years (mean 45), all had chronic pure (no element of aortic stenosis) severe aortic regurgitation secondary to infective endocarditis that had healed (8 patients), syphilis (6 patients), ankylosing spondylitis (5 patients), Marfan syndrome (5 patients), and uncertain or other causes (6 patients). Nineteen patients (63%) had undergone aortic valve replacement, and all died <60 days after the operation. Only 2 of these 30 hearts weighed >1,000 g (1,010 and 1,100 g).

**Mitral regurgitation[15]:** These 24 patients, aged 21 to 84 years (mean 42), all had chronic isolated severe pure (no element of stenosis) mitral regurgitation. The cause of the regurgitation was attributed to rheumatic disease (14 patients), mitral valve prolapse (7 patients), and infective endocarditis that had healed (3 patients). Nine patients (30%) had undergone mitral valve replacement.

**Hypertrophic cardiomyopathy (studied at necropsy)[16]:** These 57 patients ranged in age from 14 to 87 years (mean 49). Cardiac catheterization data within 2 years of death were available in 42 patients: left ventricular to systemic arterial peak pressure gradient at rest >10 mm Hg was present in 32 patients (77%) and with provocation in 35 patients (85%). The resting peak systolic gradients ranged from 12 to 162 mm Hg (mean 79) and the provoked gradients, from 40 to 190 mm Hg (mean 104). There were no differences between patients with and without outflow pressure gradients with regard to heart weight, ventricular septal thickness, total 12-lead QRS amplitude, and Romhilt-Estes score.[6] The mean Sokolow-Lyon index was insignificantly different: 37 in the obstructive group and 28 in the nonobstructive group.

**Hypertrophic cardiomyopathy (studied after cardiac transplantation)[17]:** These 10 patients, aged 19 to 46 years (mean 35), all had severe chronic heart failure, and only 1 had left ventricular outflow obstruction. Nine had dilated left ventricular cavities, and 8 had extensive left ventricular wall scarring without narrowing of the epicardial coronary arteries. Six of the 9 had left ventricular ejection fractions <50%.

**Idiopathic dilated cardiomyopathy[18]:** These 49 patients, aged 19 to 75 years (mean 45), had typical clinical and morphologic cardiac features of this condition.

**Lipomatous hypertrophy of the atrial septum[19]:** The thickness of the atrial septum cephalad to the fossa ovalis is these 28 patients ranged from 2.0 to 5.0 cm (mean 2.8). The 12 men ranged in age from 48 to 84 years (mean 67) and the 16 women, from 59 to 83 years (mean 74). The total 12-lead QRS voltage in the men ranged from 93 to 241 mm (mean 140) and in the women from 59 to 266 mm (mean 124). The heart weights in the men averaged 576 g and in the women, 502 g.

**Carcinoid syndrome[20]:** Of these 36 patients, 21 (57%) had carcinoid heart disease and 15 (43%) did not. The 2 groups were similar in mean age (54 vs 55 years), duration of clinical illness (4.7 vs 6.3 years), body weight (50 vs 52 kg), and systemic blood pressure (117/77 vs 128/77 mm Hg). The 2 groups were different in the frequency of the presence

Table 2
Total 12-lead QRS voltage, heart weight, and age of groups of 331 patients with various cardiac conditions

| Condition | Gender | Number of Cases | Ages (yrs), Range (Mean) | Total 12-Lead QRS Voltage (mm), Mean | Patients With 12-Lead QRS Voltage >175 mm | Heart Weight (g), Range (Mean) | Total 12-Lead QRS Voltage (mm)/Heart Weight (g) | Year of Publication | Authors (Reference Number) |
|---|---|---|---|---|---|---|---|---|---|
| Hearts weighing >1,000 g | M | 16 | 29–64 (42) | 140–414 (306) | 16 | 1,005–1,360 (1,102) | 0.28 | 1985 | Roberts and Podolak[13] |
| | F | 1 | 20 | 601 | (94%) | 1,250 | 0.48 | | |
| Aortic valve stenosis | M | 36 | 16–64 (48) | 144–417 (249) | 47 | 440–880 (639) | 0.39 | 1982 | Siegel and Roberts[12] |
| | F | 14 | 16–65 (47) | 193–376 (277) | (94%) | 380–700 (521) | 0.53 | | |
| Aortic regurgitation | M | 22 | 19–59 (44) | 109–428 (271) | 27 | 430–1,100 (717) | 0.38 | 1985 | Roberts and Day[14] |
| | F | 8 | 35–56 (48) | 169–384 (275) | (90%) | 375–950 (638) | 0.43 | | |
| Mitral regurgitation | M | 11 | 24–84 (47) | 111–364 (245) | 17 | 400–775 (629) | 0.39 | 1992 | Glick and Roberts[15] |
| | F | 13 | 21–64 (37) | 114–290 (199) | (71%) | 350–675 (472) | 0.42 | | |
| Hypertrophic cardiomyopathy without cardiac transplantation | M | 21 | 14–68 (46) | 107–339 (190) | 30 | 325–1,070 (671) | 0.28 | 1989 | Dollar and Roberts[16] |
| | F | 36 | 19–87 (51) | 68–327 (201) | (53%) | 290–1,230 (547) | 0.38 | | |
| Hypertrophic cardiomyopathy with cardiac transplantation | M | 6 | 19–46 (35) | 109–201 (142) | 4 | 310–480 (393) | 0.36 | 1993 | Shirani et al[17] |
| | F | 4 | 24–45 (35) | 172–378 (241) | (40%) | 290–650 (408) | 0.59 | | |
| Idiopathic dilated cardiomyopathy | M | 35 | 19–73 (46) | 74–281 (147) | 20 | 400–940 (620) | 0.24 | 1987 | Roberts et al[18] |
| | F | 14 | 22–75 (54) | 75–243 (167) | (41%) | 400–860 (602) | 0.28 | | |
| Lipomatous hypertrophy of the atrial septum | M | 12 | 48–84 (67) | 93–24 (140) | 3 | 410–795 (576) | 0.24 | 1993 | Shirani and Roberts[19] |
| | F | 16 | 59–83 (74) | 59–266 (124) | (11%) | 330–680 (502) | 0.25 | | |
| Carcinoid syndrome | | | | | | | | | |
| With carcinoid heart disease | M | 11 | 39–72 (56) | 58–227 (120) | 2 | 220–480 (350) | 0.34 | 1985 | Ross and Roberts[20] |
| | F | 8 | 28–64 (54) | 58–128 (84) | (11%) | 200–290 (245) | 0.34 | | |
| Without carcinoid heart disease | M | 10 | 42–75 (55) | 89–129 (137) | 2 | 240–570 (350) | 0.39 | | |
| | F | 5 | 28–67 (50) | 102–135 (121) | (13%) | 150–270 (230) | 0.53 | | |
| Cardiac amyloidosis | M | 15 | 32–69 (52) | 60–197 (99) | 2 | 410–850 (570) | 0.17 | 1983 | Roberts and Waller[21] |
| | F | 15 | 21–93 (69) | 58–199 (109) | (7%) | 370–900 (494) | 0.22 | | |
| Cardiac adiposity | M | 13 | 51–73 (64) | 73–159 (114) | 1 | 320–795 (485) | 0.24 | 1995 | Shirani et al[22] |
| | F | 17 | 40–85 (70) | 77–210 (124) | (3%) | 250–575 (395) | 0.31 | | |

of precordial murmurs consistent with tricuspid regurgitation and/or pulmonary stenosis (95% vs 13%), cardiomegaly by chest x-ray (38% vs 0%), low voltage on electrocardiography (47% vs 0%), and location of the primary carcinoid neoplasm. Total 12-lead QRS voltage was similar in each group (105 vs 132 mm; 10 mm = 1 mV). Of those with carcinoid heart disease, 43% died of cardiac causes, whereas in those without carcinoid heart disease, none died of a cardiac cause.

**Cardiac amyloidosis[21]:** All 30 patients, aged 32 to 92 years (mean 59), died from amyloidosis that involved the heart extensively and also multiple other organs. The peak systemic arterial systolic pressure in the 9 patients with hemodynamic studies was ≤110 mm Hg.

**Cardiac adiposity (cor adiposum)[22]:** These 30 patients died from noncardiac causes. The heart weights ranged from 250 to 795 g (mean 435) and were increased (>350 g in women, >400 g in men) in 17 (57%). Adipose tissue constituted 4% to 52% (mean 22%) of the total heart weight (mean weight of adipose tissue = 105 g). No heart had grossly visible evidence of myocardial fibrosis or necrosis. Total 12-lead QRS voltage decreased significantly as the quantity of cardiac adipose tissue increased. As the ratio of adipose tissue to heart weight × 100 increased from 12 ± 3 to 20 ± 4 to 32 ± 9 mm/100 g, the ratio of total 12-lead QRS voltage to heart weight × 100 decreased significantly from 36 ± 9 to 34 ± 9 to 21 ± 6 mm/100 g. The amount of subepicardial fat increased with increasing body weight. Simple visual assessment of the extent of cardiac adiposity and the degree of buoyancy of the heart when placed in a container of water estimated well the amounts of subepicardial fat. If the amount of subepicardial fat was considered normal by visual

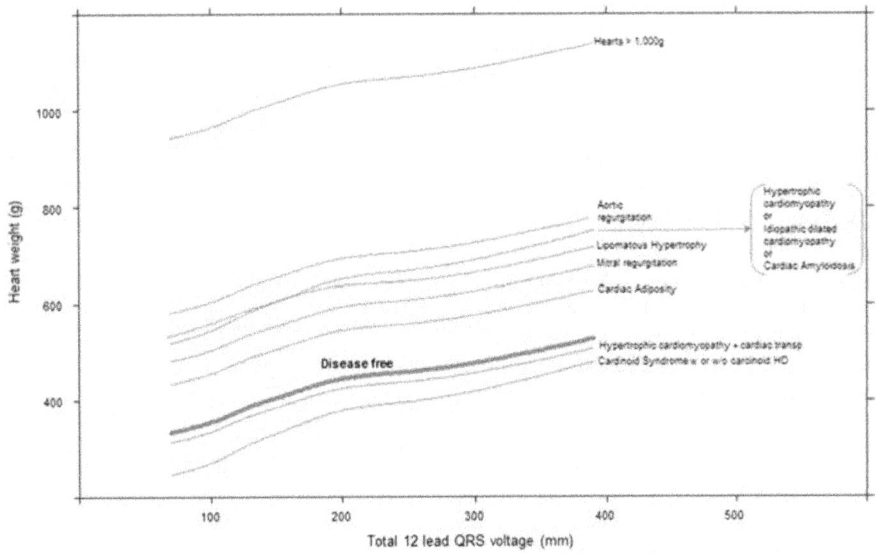


Figure 2. Adjusted (by gender and age) association between patient's heart weight and 12-lead QRS voltage by cardiac condition. HD = heart disease; transp = transplantation.

inspection, then the adipose tissue constituted a mean of 12% (range 4% to 14%) of the heart weight; if the subepicardial tissue was increased but the heart did not float in water, then fat constituted a mean of 20% (range 15% to 28%) of the heart weight; in the 12 hearts that floated in water, a mean of 32% (range 21% to 52%) of the heart weight was composed of adipose tissue.

## Discussion

This study summarizes 11 previously published studies on total 12-lead QRS voltage in 11 different cardiac conditions and compares that voltage with heart weight. The best cut-off point for total 12-lead QRS voltage separating hearts with increased weight compared with those of normal weight has not been fully established. Odom et al[25] determined heart weight in 30 men free of cardiopulmonary disease and found that total 12-lead QRS voltage ranged from 80 to 185 mm (mean 127; 10 mm = 1 mV). These authors considered 175 mm as the best upper range of normal 12-lead QRS voltage. Rodríguez Padial[26] studied M-mode and 2-dimensional echocardiograms and 12-lead electrocardiograms in 74 consecutive patients with systemic hypertension and calculated left ventricular mass. This author found a total 12-lead QRS voltage >120 mm to be a good electrocardiographic criterion and "better than those most frequently used."[27] Yang et al[28] studied total 12-lead QRS voltage in 120 adults free of cardiopulmonary disease and 114 patients with LVH by echocardiography. They found >190 mm to be a good criterion for LVH, with sensitivity of 77%, specificity of 96%, and accuracy of 87%, and suggested that total 12-lead QRS voltage had a relatively high reliability for diagnosing LVH. Pelliccia et al[29] studied total 12-lead QRS voltage in 67 patients with idiopathic dilated cardiomyopathy and found that total 12-lead QRS voltage (also the sum of T/R wave ratios) was the only independent predictor of left ventricular mass determined by either angiography or echocardiography.

In the present study of patients with clear increased cardiac mass at autopsy (>350 g in women, >400 g in men) total 12-lead QRS voltage in 118 men averaged 239 mm (range 107 to 428). These 118 men included 16 with hearts weighing >1,000 g, 36 with aortic stenosis, 22 with pure aortic regurgitation, 11 with pure mitral regurgitation, and 21 with hypertrophic cardiomyopathy (without cardiac transplantation). The upper limit for total 12-lead QRS voltage in women without cardiopulmonary disease has not been established. As listed in Table 2, 12-lead QRS voltage generally was slightly higher in women than men with the same cardiac condition, although heart weight on average was lower in the women than in the men. Clearly, total 12-lead QRS voltage is not perfect in diagnosing increased cardiac mass, but as listed in Table 1, it is more reliable in predicting increased cardiac mass than are previously recommended electrocardiographic criteria for LVH.

There is some variation in the relation of total 12-lead QRS voltage to heart weight depending on the underlying cardiac condition. As listed in Table 2, all 49 patients with idiopathic dilated cardiomyopathy had hearts weighing ≥400 g, and yet the mean total 12-lead QRS voltage in men and women was relatively low (147 and 167 mm, respectively). Wilensky et al[30] showed that QRS voltage in patients with this condition diminishes with time, and therefore, electrocardiograms recorded shortly before death show lower QRS voltages than those recorded at earlier times. Additionally, all 30 patients with fatal cardiac amyloidosis had hearts of increased mass, but mean total 12-lead QRS voltage in them averaged only 104 mm. Possibly as much as half or more of their cardiac mass, however, was contributed by the amyloid deposits in the heart and not by cardiac myocardium. The patients with excessive cardiac adiposity, with or without lipomatous hypertrophy of the atrial septum, also usually had hearts of increased mass with relatively low total 12-lead QRS voltages.

Lanti et al[31] studied electrocardiograms in 154 men without clinical evidence of heart disease and compared electrocardiographic findings in 67 who died suddenly to the 87 who had nonsudden death. They found that 12-lead QRS voltage had a significant and independent relation to sudden death and helped identify subjects at increased risk for sudden coronary death. These investigators also found that the Sokolow-Lyon index was inversely related to nonsudden death.

The strong features of the present study are the following: (1) the 12-lead QRS voltage was determined in a variety of cardiac conditions, and (2) heart weights in all patients studied were available and accurately determined. Relatively few previous studies on electrocardiographic determination of LVH actually compared the electrocardiographic criteria with actual heart weight, and those that did acquired those data from autopsy protocols produced by a variety of prosecutors with varying expertise in cardiovascular disease.

### Disclosures

The authors have no conflicts of interest to disclose.


1. Griep AH. Pitfalls in the electrocardiographic diagnosis of left ventricular hypertrophy: a correlative study of 200 autopsied patients. *Circulation* 1959;20:30–34.
2. Allenstein BJ, Hiroyoshi M. Evaluation of electrocardiographic diagnosis of ventricular hypertrophy based on autopsy comparison. *Circulation* 1960;21:401–412.
3. Sokolow M, Lyon TP. The ventricular complex in left ventricular hypertrophy as obtained by unipolar precordial and limb leads. *Am Heart J* 1949;37:161–186.
4. Holt DH, Spodick DH. The $Rv_6$:$Rv_5$ voltage ratio in left ventricular hypertrophy. *Am Heart J* 1962;63:65–66.
5. Carter WA, Estes EH Jr. Electrocardiographic manifestations of ventricular hypertrophy; a computer study of ECG-anatomic correlations in 319 cases. *Am Heart J* 1964;68:173–182.
6. Romhilt DW, Estes WH Jr. A point-score system for the ECG diagnosis of left ventricular hypertrophy. *Am Heart J* 1968;75: 752–758.
7. Romhilt DW, Bove KE, Norris RJ, Conyers E, Conradi S, Rowlands DT, Scott RC. A critical appraisal of the electrocardiographic criteria for the diagnosis of left ventricular hypertrophy. *Circulation* 1969;40: 185–195.
8. Bennett DH, Evans DW. Correlation of left ventricular mass determined by echocardiography with vectorcardiographic and electrocardiographic voltage measurements. *Br Heart J* 1974;36:981–987.
9. Casale PN, Devereux RB, Alonso DR, Camp E, Kligfield P. Improved sex-specific criteria of left ventricular hypertrophy for clinical and computer interpretation of electrocardiograms: validation with autopsy findings. *Circulation* 1987;3:565–572.
10. Koito H, Spokick DH. Accuracy of the $RV_6$:$RV_5$ voltage ratio for increased left ventricular mass. *Am J Cardiol* 1988;62:985–987.
11. Velury S, Spodick DH. Increased left ventricular mass in patients with lateral low voltage electrocardiograms. *Am J Cardiol* 1992;69: 707–708.
12. Siegel RJ, Roberts WC. Electrocardiographic observations in severe aortic valve stenosis: correlative necropsy study to clinical, hemodynamic, and ECG variables demonstrating relation of 12-lead QRS amplitude to peak systolic transaortic pressure gradient. *Am Heart J* 1982;103:210–221.
13. Roberts WC, Podolak MJ. The king of hearts: analysis of 23 patients with hearts weighing 1000 grams or more. *Am J Cardiol* 1985;55: 485–494.
14. Roberts WC, Day PJ. Electrocardiographic observations in clinically isolated, pure, chronic, severe aortic regurgitation: analysis of 30 necropsy patients aged 19 to 65 years. *Am J Cardiol* 1985;55:431–438.
15. Glick BN, Roberts WC. Usefulness of total 12-lead QRS voltage in diagnosing left ventricular hypertrophy in clinically isolated, pure, chronic, severe mitral regurgitation. *Am J Cardiol* 1992;70:1088–1092.
16. Dollar AL, Roberts WC. Usefulness of total 12-lead QRS voltage compared with other criteria for determining left ventricular hypertrophy in hypertrophic cardiomyopathy: analysis of 57 patients studied at necropsy. *Am J Med* 1989;87:377–381.
17. Shirani J, Maron BJ, Cannon RO III, Shahin S, Roberts WC. Clinicopathologic features of hypertrophic cardiomyopathy managed by cardiac transplantation. *Am J Cardiol* 1993;72:434–440.
18. Roberts WC, Siegel RJ, McManus BM. Idiopathic dilated cardiomyopathy: analysis of 152 necropsy patients. *Am J Cardiol* 1987;60:1340–1355.
19. Shirani J, Roberts WC. Clinical, electrocardiographic and morphologic features of massive fatty deposits ("lipomatous hypertrophy") in the atrial septum. *J Am Coll Cardiol* 1993;22:226–238.
20. Ross EM, Roberts WC. The carcinoid syndrome: comparison of 21 necropsy subjects with carcinoid heart disease to 15 necropsy subjects without carcinoid heart disease. *Am J Heart* 1985;79:339–354.
21. Roberts WC, Waller BF. Cardiac amyloidosis causing cardiac dysfunction: analysis of 54 necropsy patients. *Am J Cardiol* 1983;52:137–146.
22. Shirani J, Berezowski K, Roberts WC. Quantitative measurement of normal and excessive (cor adiposum) subepicardial adipose tissue, its clinical significance, and its effect on electrocardographic QRS voltage. *Am J Cardiol* 1995;76:414–418.
23. Harrell FE Jr. Regression Modeling Strategies: With Application to Linear Models, Logistic Regression, and Survival Analysis. New York: Springer-Verlag, 2001.
24. Filardo G, Hamilton C, Hamman B, Ng HK, Grayburn P. Categorizing BMI may lead to biased results in studies investigating in-hospital mortality after isolated CABG. *J Clin Epidemiol* 2007;60:1132–1139.
25. Odom H II, Davis JL, Dinh H, Baker BJ, Roberts WC, Murphy ML. QRS voltage measurements in autopsied men free of cardiopulmonary disease: a basis for evaluating total QRS voltage as a index of left ventricular hypertrophy. *Am J Cardiol* 1986;58:801–804.
26. Rodríguez Padial L. Usefulness of total 12-lead QRS voltage for determining the presence of left ventricular hypertrophy in systemic hypertension. *Am J Cardiol* 1991;68:261–262.
27. Rodríguez Padial L, Navarro A, Sánchez J. RVG: $RV_5$ voltage ratio in systemic hypertension. *Am J Cardiol* 1990;66:869–871.
28. Yang TH, Deng SY, Cai YC. The normal values of total 12-lead QRS voltage and its significance in diagnosing left ventricular hypertrophy. *Chinese J Cardiol* 1988;16:353–355.
29. Pelliccia F, Critelli G, Cianfrocca C, Nigri A, Reale A. Electrocardiographic correlates with left ventricular morphology in idiopathic dilated cardiomyopathy. *Am J Cardiol* 1991;68:642–647.
30. Wilensky RL, Yudelman P, Cohen A, Fletcher RD, Atkinson J, Virmani R, Roberts WC. Serial electrocardiographic changes in idiopathic dilated cardiomyopathy confirmed at necropsy. *Am J Cardiol* 1988;62:276–283.
31. Lanti M, Puddu PE, Menotti A. Voltage criteria of left ventricular hypertrophy in sudden and nonsudden coronary artery disease mortality: the Italian section of the seven countries study. *Am J Cardiol* 1990;66:1181–1185.

# Morphologic Features of Cardiac Sarcoidosis in Native Hearts of Patients Having Cardiac Transplantation

William C. Roberts, MD[a,b,c,*], Monica S. Chung, MS[a], Jong Mi Ko, BA[a], John E. Capehart, MD[d], and Shelley A. Hall, MD[c]

**Described herein are 10 patients who underwent cardiac transplantation (CT) for severe chronic systolic heart failure resulting from cardiac sarcoidosis. None had the diagnosis of sarcoidosis established before CT except for the 3 patients who earlier had had a portion of left ventricular wall excised for insertion of a left ventricular assist device and non-caseating granulomas were present in the removed myocardium. Although none of the 10 patients had significant narrowing of any of the epicardial coronary arteries, all had focal scarring of the walls of the left and right ventricles and ventricular septum and all had dilated ventricular cavities. The patients with the most ventricular wall scarring tended to have the fewest sarcoid granulomas in the ventricular walls. Two patients had no sarcoid granulomas in the excised heart although one did have typical sarcoid granulomas in the portion of left ventricular wall excised to insert a left ventricular assist device. Patients with cardiac sarcoidosis severe enough to warrant CT had characteristic cardiac ventricular morphologic findings, and no dysfunction of other non-cardiac organs, making clinical diagnosis of cardiac sarcoidosis rather difficult.**  **(Am J Cardiol 2014;113:706–712)**

Although sarcoidosis of the heart has been recognized for over 70 years, most reports have appeared in the last 30 years. The condition continues to fascinate physicians because of its multiple modes of presentation—ventricular arrhythmias with or without cardiac arrest, various forms of heart block, heart failure, mitral regurgitation, left ventricular aneurysm—and its difficulty in diagnosis.[1–4] Single case reports on the topic continue to appear as well as frequent reviews.[5–12] In the last 2 decades a number of patients with cardiac sarcoidosis have undergone cardiac transplantation (CT) and few of them have had the condition diagnosed before CT or at least before cardiac biopsy (including the histologic examination of a portion of the left ventricular wall excised for insertion of a left ventricular assist device) (Table 1).[13–19] Since 1993, we have studied the hearts of 10 patients who underwent CT for severe chronic heart failure found to be the result of cardiac sarcoidosis. Our purpose was to subjectively quantify the relative density of the cardiac non-caseating granulomas in the myocardium and the extent and characteristics of the resulting scarring in the walls of the cardiac ventricles.

[a]Baylor Heart and Vascular Institute, [b]Department of Pathology, [c]Division of Cardiology, Department of Internal Medicine, and [d]Department of Cardiothoracic Surgery, Baylor University Medical Center, Dallas, Texas. Manuscript received October 15, 2013; revised manuscript received and accepted November 9, 2013.

Monica S. Chung is a second-year medical student at Texas Tech University Health Science Center, Paul L. Foster School of Medicine, El Paso, Texas.

See page 712 for disclosure information.

*Corresponding author: Tel: (214) 820-7911; fax: (214) 820-7533.

*E-mail address:* wc.roberts@baylorhealth.edu (W.C. Roberts).

## Methods

The explanted hearts were sent to the surgical pathology division of the Baylor University Medical Center department of pathology. All hearts were examined and described by WCR and, after "cleaning" and fixation in formalin, weighed, and opened by him. At least 5 sections from the walls of the cardiac ventricles (endocardium through to epicardium) were processed, stained, and examined. From each paraffin block, 2 sections were cut: one was stained by both hematoxylin/eosin and the other by Masson, and each was examined by WCR. The medical records were then examined by MSC, JMK, and WCR.

The quantity of scarring in the left ventricular free wall, ventricular septum, and right ventricular free wall was graded subjectively by WCR on a scale of zero to 4+. Likewise, the density of sarcoid granulomas in the ventricular myocardium was graded zero (none seen) to 4+ (granulomas present in virtually all microscopic fields magnified ×40).

## Results

From January 1993 through June 2013, a total of 346 isolated CTs were performed at Baylor University Medical Center. Of them, examination of the explanted hearts disclosed that 10 (3%) had cardiac sarcoidosis. Pertinent clinical and cardiac morphologic findings in them are summarized in Table 2. Their ages at the time of CT ranged from 38 to 55 years (mean 48); 6 were women and 4 were men; 4 of 6 women were black and all 4 men were white. Symptoms of cardiac dysfunction in the 10 patients were present from 1 to 15 years (mean 7). Of the 10 patients, electrocardiograms before CT were available to examine in 9; of the 5 without a pacemaker, total 12-lead QRS voltage varied from 74 to 168 mm (1 mm = 1 millivolt) (mean 132)[20] (Table 2). Body mass index (10 patients) ranged from 19.0 to 32.0 kg/m$^2$

Table 1
Reported frequency of cardiac sarcoidosis among patients having cardiac transplantation (CT)

| First Author (Reference) | Year of Publication | Total CT (Years of CT) | No. (%) With Sarcoidosis | Ages of S Patients (Years) | F/M | W/B | Dx S Before CT | Extra Cardiac Sarcoid | Died | Cardiac Sarcoid Recurrence |
|---|---|---|---|---|---|---|---|---|---|---|
| Zaidi[13] | 2007 | 38,230 (1987–2005) | 65 (0.2%) | 4–71 (m 45) | 25/40 | 44/19 | — | — | 16 | — |
| Miliman[14] | 2008 | 250 (1990–2006) | 4 (2%) | 25–57 | 3/1 | 4/0 | 1 | 0 | 2 | 0 |
| Luk[15] | 2009 | 296 (1987–2006) | 6 (2%) | — | — | — | 1 | — | — | — |
| Chang[16] | 2012 | 411 (2003–2011) | 5 (1%) | 31–40 | 1/4 | — | 1 | 0 | 0 | 0 |
| Akashi[17] | 2012 | 825 (1997–2010) | 14 (2%) | 42–67 | 7/7 | 5/7 | 6 | 7* | 6 | 2 |
| Totals | | 40,012 | 94 (2.3%) | 4–67 | 36/52 | 53/26 | 9/1,782 | 7 | 24/88 (27%) | 2/23 (9%) |

B = black; Dx = diagnosis; F = female; M = male; S = sarcoidosis; W = white; — = no information.
* Lungs in all 7.

(mean 25.3). The lowest left ventricular ejection fractions ranged from 10% to 20% (mean 16). Three patients at the time of CT had a left ventricular assist device (Nos 6, 7, and 8, Table 2).

The weights in the hearts in the 4 men ranged from 440 to 605 g (mean 506) and in the 6 women, from 370 to 600 g (mean 476). The maximal internal dimension of the left ventricular cavity ranged from 5.0 to 9.0 cm (mean 6.3); the maximal internal diameter of the right ventricular cavity (right ventricular free wall to ventricular septum at posterior wall at the base) ranged from 2.0 to 9.0 cm (mean 4.5).

Grossly visible scars were present in the left and right ventricular free walls and in the ventricular septum in all 10 patients (Figures 1 to 4) and none of the 10 patients had narrowing of any significant degrees in any of the epicardial coronary arteries. The left ventricular scars were most often transmural but often were also or only subepicardial (outer one-half of the myocardial wall). Scars in the right ventricular free wall were transmural (full thickness scarring). Scars in the ventricular septum also varied in extent: some were transmural and when not were often centrally located in the septum or in the right ventricular half rather than the left ventricular half of the septum. No grossly visible scars or other lesions were observed in the walls of either the right atrium or left atrium, but much of these walls were retained in the recipient to connect to the donor heart. No patient had sarcoid lesions in the cardiac valves, coronary arteries or subepicardial adipose tissue.

The numbers of or density of the sarcoid granulomas in the ventricular walls varied considerably. Some patients had granulomas in virtually every microscopic field magnified ×40 (graded 4+). On the other extreme, 2 patients (#5 and #7, Table 2) had no granulomas in multiple sections of the explanted heart although one of them had typical sarcoid granulomas in the portion of left ventricular free wall excised for insertion of a left ventricular assist device. The patient (#5) in whom granulomas were never observed in the heart had ventricular wall scarring similar to that in the other patients with cardiac granulomas.

An attempt was made to correlate the amount of ventricular wall scarring to the density of giant-cell granulomas in the myocardium. In the 2 patients (#5 and #7, Table 2) without granulomas in the explanted heart each had severe and extensive ventricular wall scarring (grade 4+). Two others (#2 and #10, Table 2) had nearly as extensive ventricular wall scarring (grade 3+) and few (grade 1+) sarcoid granulomas in the heart. Patient #4 (Table 2, Figure 6) had 4+ ventricular wall scarring and 3+ density of sarcoid granulomas in the ventricular walls. The correlation between ventricular wall scarring and the density of cardiac granulomas was less clear in the other 6 patients.

No meaningful correlation was found between the duration of symptoms of heart failure and the extent of left ventricular scarring.

## Discussion

All 10 patients included in this study underwent CT for chronic systolic heart failure. In none was the diagnosis of cardiac sarcoidosis made clinically although all 3 patients who underwent insertion of a left ventricular assist device had non-caseating granulomas in the portion of left ventricular wall excised to insert the device. The amount of ventricular wall scarring was considerable in all 10 patients but the number of granulomas in the ventricular myocardium varied considerably in them. Two of the 10 patients had no granulomas in the operatively excised native heart although one of them did have classic sarcoid granulomas in the left ventricular wall removed to insert the left ventricular assist device. One might reasonably question how the other patient without cardiac granulomas was included in the study. The answer is that the quantity of and distribution of the ventricular fibrous tissue in this patient (#5, Table 2) was similar to that in the other 9 patients, none of whom had significant coronary narrowing. The scarring often preferentially involved the subepicardial portions of left ventricular free wall, and also the ventricular septum. Portions of right ventricular free wall were usually involved. We know of no other condition which produces such a distinctive type and distribution of ventricular scarring.

Would diagnosis of cardiac sarcoidosis before CT in these patients with severe systolic heart failure been beneficial to the patient? The answer has not been determined because this diagnosis has been so infrequent before CT.[13–17] Some patients with cardiac sarcoidosis have been benefited by corticosteroid therapy and pre-CT diagnosis would allow a trial of this therapy. Is corticosteroid therapy beneficial after CT for cardiac sarcoidosis? The answer has not been determined. Recurrence of sarcoid in the donor heart has occurred and therefore the answer may be "yes."[21,22]

One feature of cardiac sarcoidosis is clear. Although patients with cardiac sarcoidosis may have non-caseating

Table 2
Pertinent data in the 10 patients having cardiac transplantation (CT) for sarcoidosis

| Patient | Age at CT (Years) | Race | Age at Onset of Symptoms (Years) | Duration of Symptoms (Years) | Total 12-lead QRS Voltage (ECG) | ECG Date | BMI (kg/m²) | Pressures (mm Hg) | | | | | CI (L/min/m²) | Lowest LVEF (%) | LV AD | Date of CT | HW (g) | Largest Diameter (cm) | | Grossly Visible Scar (0–4+) | | | Density Of LV Sarcoid Granulomas (0–4+) | Figure Number |
|---|---|---|---|---|---|---|---|---|---|---|---|---|---|---|---|---|---|---|---|---|---|---|---|---|
| | | | | | | | | PA (s/d) | RV (s/d) | RA (Mean) | LV (s/d) | Aorta (s/d) | | | | | | LV | RV | LV | VS | RV | | |
| **WOMEN** | | | | | | | | | | | | | | | | | | | | | | | | |
| 1 | 50 | B | 38 | 12 | 113* | 10/05/2008 | 27.0 | — | 43/—† | 10† | — | — | — | 20 | 0 | 1/28/2012 | 440 | 7.5 | 4.0 | 3+ | 2+ | 1+ | 4+ | 1 |
| 2 | 52 | B | 48 | 4 | — | — | 28.7 | 59/28 | 59/15 | 9 | 115/34 | 115/79 | 1.7 | 20 | 0 | 9/4/2010 | 440 | 5.5 | 2.0 | 3+ | 2+ | 1+ | 1+ | 2 |
| 3 | 56 | W | 55 | 1 | — | — | 25.7 | — | — | — | 109/33 | 104/79 | — | 15 | 0 | 10/30/2009 | 445 | 5.5 | 3.5 | 4+ | 4+ | 4+ | 4+ | |
| 4 | 58 | W | 54 | 4 | 74 | 3/10/2012 | 26.4 | 20/11 | — | 8 | — | — | 2.2 | 20 | 0 | 3/10/2012 | 560 | 5.0 | 2.5 | 4+ | 4+ | 2+ | 3+ | 3,6 |
| 5 | 62 | B | 49 | 13 | 168 | 2/18/2013 | 19.0 | 36/14 | 62/—† | 20† | — | — | 2.6 | 10 | 0 | 3/16/2013 | 600 | 7.5 | 6.0 | 4+ | 0 | 2+ | 0 | 4 |
| 6 | 59† | B | 55 | 4 | — | — | 20.8 | 44/21 | — | — | — | — | 1.8 | 20 | + | 7/9/2006 | 370 | 5.0 | 7.5 | 2+ | 2+ | 0 | 4+ | 6 |
| **MEN** | | | | | | | | | | | | | | | | | | | | | | | | |
| 7 | 50‡,§ | W | 47 | 3 | 147 | 1/02/2005 | 24.7 | 97/45 | 92/15 | 11 | — | — | 1.7 | 10 | + | 1/14/2005 | 605 | 7.0 | 2.5 | 4+ | 1+ | 0 | 0‖ | |
| 8 | 52‡,§ | W | 48 | 4 | 158* | 11/22/2002 | 21.6 | 51/23 | 49/6 | 6 | — | — | 1.6 | 20 | + | 7/8/2005 | 440 | 5.0 | 3.5 | 2+ | 2+ | 0 | 4+ | |
| 9 | 54¶ | W | 41 | 13 | — | — | 27.5 | 32/14 | 32/12 | 8 | — | — | 2.1 | 10 | 0 | 9/5/1999 | 510 | 9.0 | 9.0 | 1+ | 1+ | 1+ | 4+ | |
| 10 | 63 | W | 48 | 15 | — | — | 32 | 23/8 | 24/7 | −1 | — | — | 1.6 | 15 | 0 | 1/6/2013 | 470 | 6.0 | 4.0 | 3+ | 1+ | 4+ | 1+ | 5 |

B = black; BMI = body mass index; CI = cardiac index; ECG = electrocardiogram; HW = heart weight; IC = ischemic cardiomyopathy; LV = left ventricular; LVAD = left ventricular assist device; LVEF = left ventricular ejection fraction; PA = pulmonary artery; RA = right atrial; RV = right ventricular; S = sarcoidosis; VS = ventricular septum; W = white.

* Electrocardiogram recorded 3 or 4 years before CT.

† Values from echocardiogram.

‡ These 3 patients were included in a previous report (*Am J Cardiol* 2009;103:110–114)[19].

§ Diagnosis of cardiac sarcoid made from histologic study of "left ventricular core" excised for insertion of a left ventricular device.

‖ Sarcoid granulomas present in the left ventricular "core" but not in the excised native heart.

¶ Case previously published (*Am J Cardiol* 2002;89:1447–1450)[18].

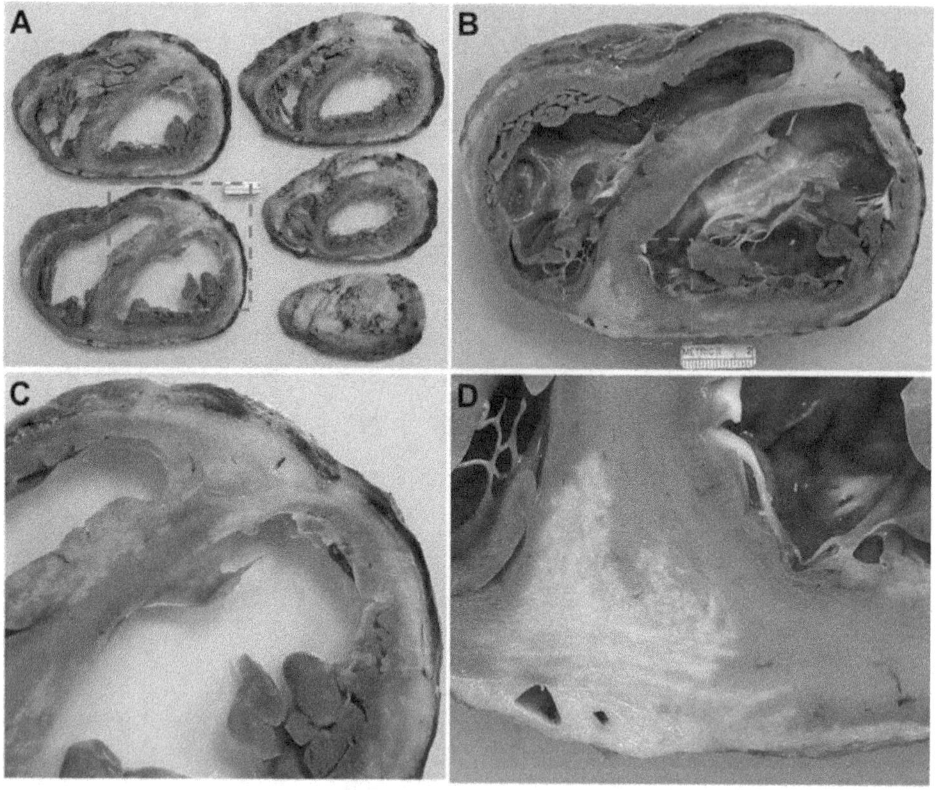

Figure 1. Patient 1, Table 1. Heart in a 50-year-old man who had had symptoms of heart failure for approximately 12 years. *(A)* Sections of the ventricles approximately 1 cm in thickness showing lesions in the right ventricular wall and pectinate muscles, ventricular septum and left ventricular free wall. Some of the scarring, as in the lower left figure of the left ventricular free wall, is subepicardial only. *(B)* Section of the base of the heart exposing the tricuspid and mitral valves, again showing the extensive scarring in the ventricular septum and left ventricular free wall. The anterior descending coronary artery is wide open. *(C)* Close-up view of the anterior wall of left ventricle, right ventricle, and ventricular septum. *(D)* Close-up of the posterior left ventricular free wall showing a large sarcoid granulomatous lesion in the ventricular septum posteriorly.

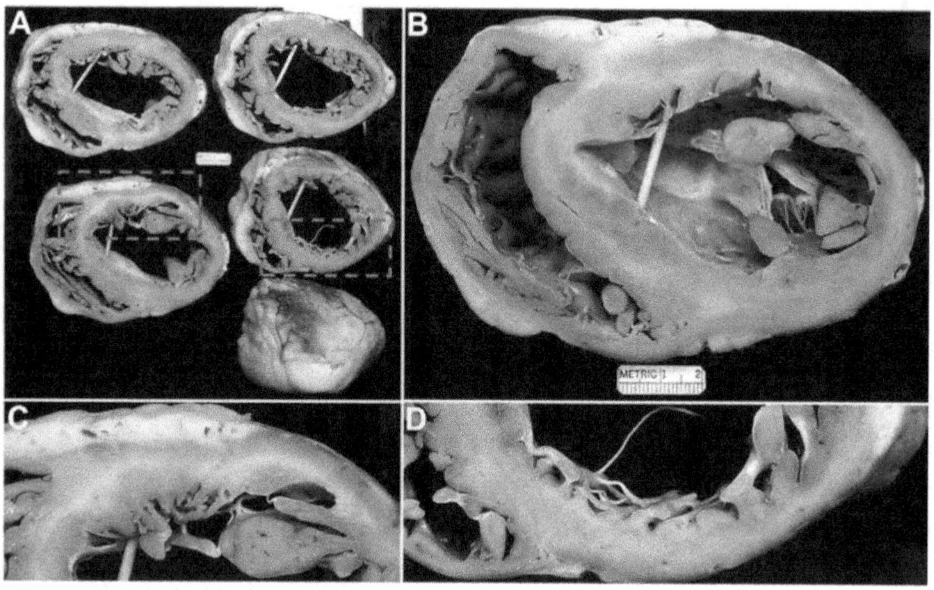

Figure 2. Patient 2, Table 1. *(A)* Views of the various ventricular slices, each about a cm in thickness. Extensive scarring is seen in the left ventricular free wall and ventricular septum anteriorly. *(B)* Close-up of the basal portion showing the mitral valve and the scarring in the ventricular septum and left ventricular free wall. *(C)* Close-up of the anterior left ventricular free wall. The coronary arteries are wide open. *(D)* Close-up view of the posterior wall of left ventricle shown in the brackets in *(A)*. The scarring is mainly subepicardial with relative sparing of the subendocardial portion.

granulomas in other body organs (always in lymph nodes[1]), dysfunction of the involved non-cardiac organ is uncommon. Thus, patients with severe pulmonary sarcoidosis or ocular sarcoid, infrequently have cardiac dysfunction, although an occasional granuloma may be present in myocardium. In other words, patients with sarcoidosis either

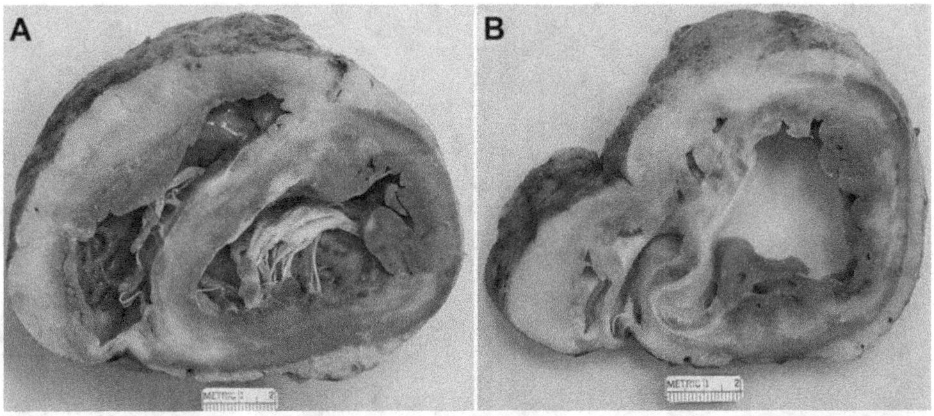


Figure 3. Patient 4, Table 1. *(A)* View of the base of the heart showing extensive scarring in the ventricular septum and also in the left ventricular and right ventricular free walls. Both tricuspid and mitral leaflets are visible. The quantity of subadipose tissue is such that the heart floated in a container of formaldehyde. *(B)* Close-up of a transverse section in the more apical portion, showing an internal aneurysm at the posterior portion of the ventricular septum and left ventricular free wall. The left ventricular free wall scarring is more subepicardial than subendocardial. The scarring in the ventricular septum is transmural.

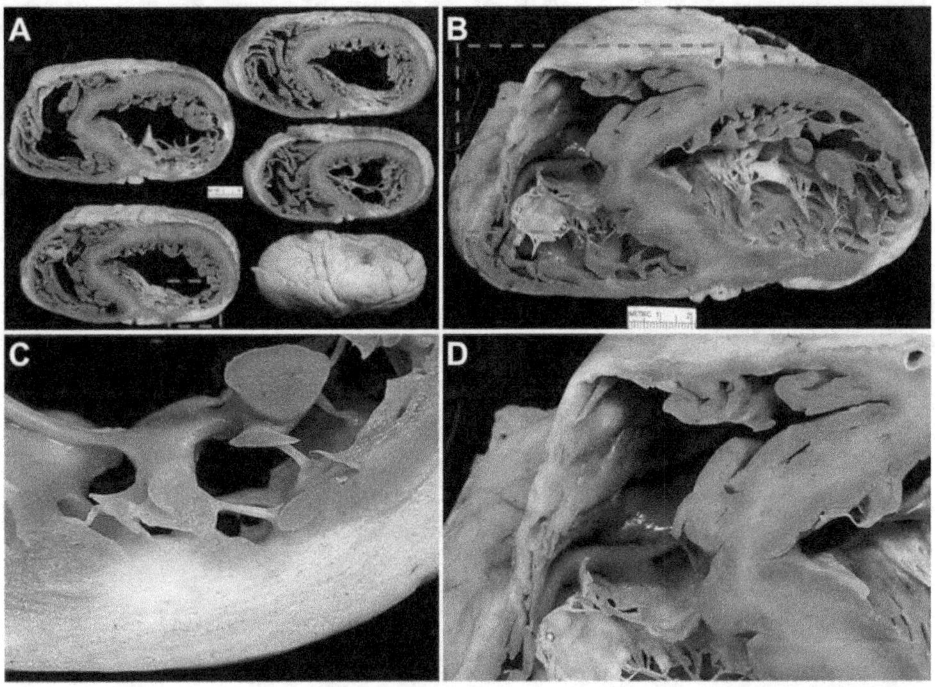


Figure 4. Patient 5, Table 1. *(A)* Transverse sections of the cardiac ventricles showing scarring in the right ventricular anterior wall and left ventricle posterior wall. *(B)* Close-up view of the base showing the tricuspid and mitral valves. The right ventricular free wall is made quite thin by the scarring as is the scarring in the lateral wall of left ventricle. *(C)* Close-up view of the left ventricular free wall showing the scarring to be much greater in the subepicardial region than in the subendocardial region. *(D)* Close-up of the right ventricular free wall showing marked thinning in its anterior lateral portion.

travel the clinical cardiac road or the clinical non-cardiac road, with little to no crossing of the two.

Why is diagnosis of cardiac sarcoidosis so difficult clinically? First, there is nothing specific about the electrocardiogram, echocardiogram, or cardiac catheterization findings. Magnetic resonance imaging and positron emission tomography may be suggestive but biopsy is the only definitive procedure.[23–25] Electrophysiological mapping may be helpful in those patients with ventricular tachycardia.[26] Biopsy of the ventricular septum via the right side of the heart may be negative because the granulomas are focal and can be missed by the biocap. The condition can mimic arrhythmogenic right ventricular dysplasia as demonstrated in our patient #10 (Figure 5) and as reported by others.[27–30]

The positive feature of the present study is the detailed morphologic description and illustrations of the scarring observed in the ventricular walls of these patients with cardiac sarcoidosis. A deficiency is the subjective characterization of the density of sarcoid granulomas and the degree of scarring in the ventricular walls.

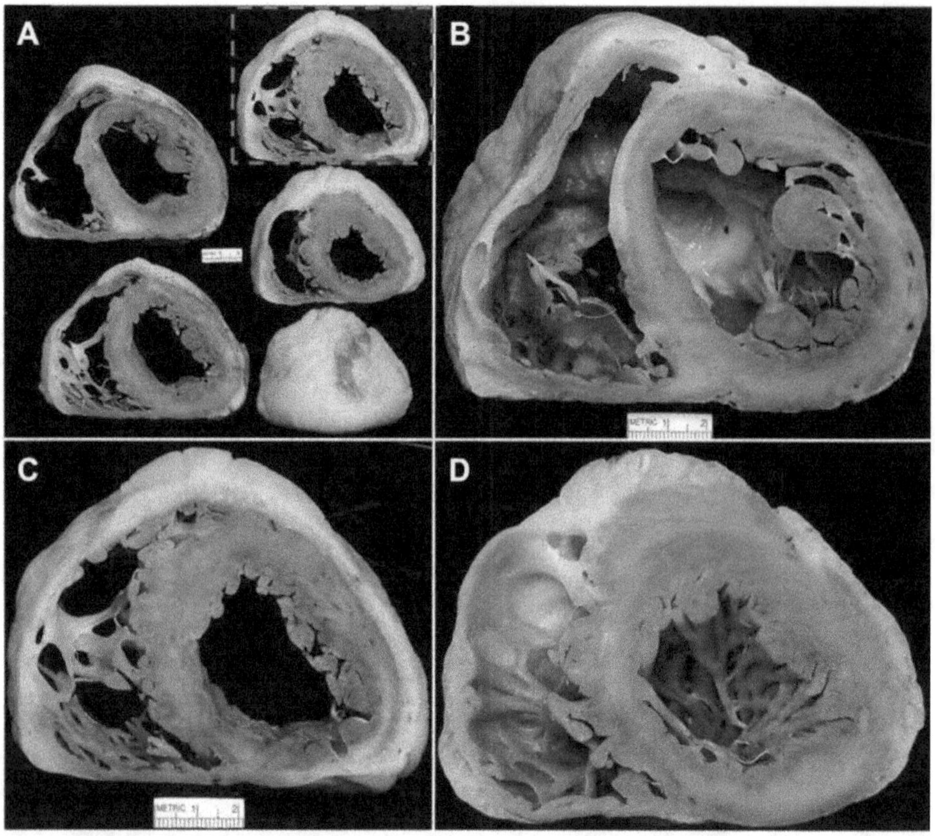

Figure 5. Patient 10, Table 1. *(A)* Close-up views of the various slices of the cardiac ventricles showing extensive scarring in the right ventricular free wall and ventricular septum, and less in the left ventricular free wall. *(B)* Close-up of the cardiac base showing severe scarring of the right ventricular free wall and portions of the ventricular septum and left ventricular free wall. *(C)* Close-up view showing the scarring in the left ventricular free wall to be mainly subepicardial. The scarring in the right ventricular free wall and papillary muscle is transmural. *(D)* View showing the severe thinning of the right ventricular free wall anteriorly such that it would assimilate arrhythmogenic right ventricular cardiomyopathy.

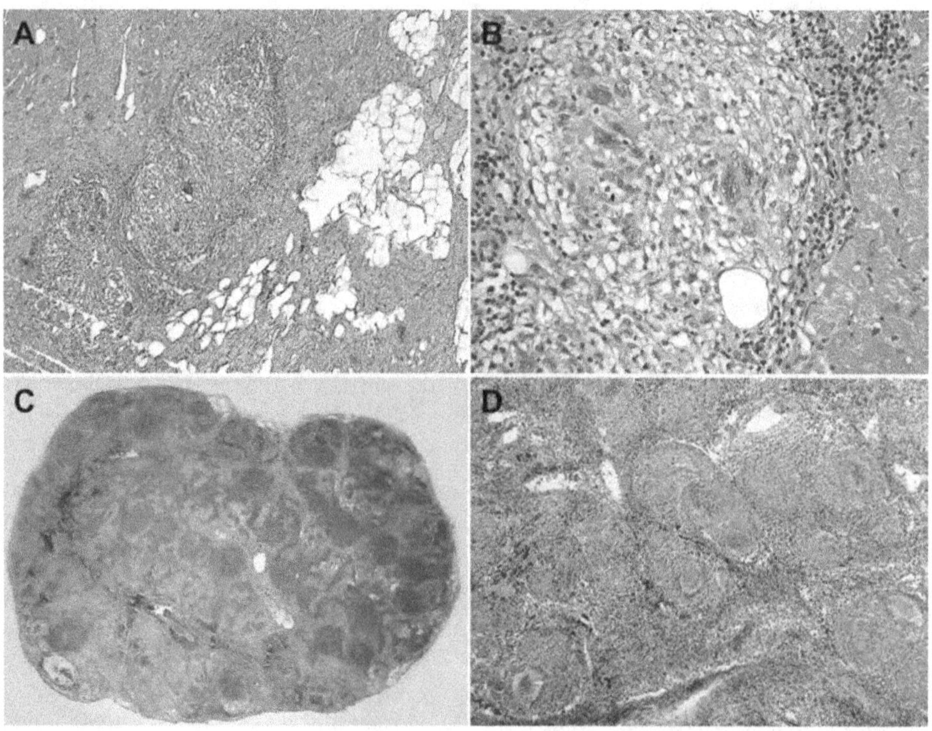

Figure 6. Photomicrographs of cardiac sarcoid granulomas *(A* and *B)* in patient #4 (Table 2) and of lymph node *(C* and *D)* in patient #6 (Table 2). Hematoxylin-eosin stains: *(A)* ×100; *(B)* ×400; *(C)* ×20, and *(D)* ×100. Patient #6 had a mediastinal lymph node excised at the time of CT, the only patient of the 10 to have a lymph node to examine. Giant-cell granulomas typical of sarcoidosis are present in the node.

## Disclosures

The authors have no conflicts of interest to disclose.


1. Roberts WC, McAllister HA Jr, Ferrans VJ. Sarcoidosis of the heart: a clinicopathologic study of 35 necropsy patients (group I) and review of 78 previously described necropsy patients (group II). *Am J Med* 1977;63:86–108.
2. Virmani R, Bures JC, Roberts WC. Cardiac sarcoidosis: a major cause of sudden death in young individuals. *Chest* 1980;77:423–428.
3. Sharma PS, Lubahn JG, Donsky AS, Yoon AD, Carry MM, Grayburn PA, Wood PB, Ko JM, Burton EC, Roberts WC. Diagnosing cardiac sarcoidosis clinically without tissue confirmation. *Proc (Bayl Univ Med Cent)* 2009;22:236–238.
4. Tavora F, Cresswell N, Li L, Ripple M, Solomon C, Burke A. Comparison of necropsy findings in patients with sarcoidosis dying suddenly from cardiac sarcoidosis versus dying suddenly from other causes. *Am J Cardiol* 2009;104:571–577.
5. Kim JS, Judson MA, Donnino R, Gold M, Cooper LT Jr, Prystowsky EN, Prystowsky S. Cardiac sarcoidosis. *Am Heart J* 2009;157:9–21.
6. Lagana SM, Parwani AV, Nichols LC. Cardiac sarcoidosis: a pathology-focused review. *Arch Pathol Lab Med* 2010;134:1039–1046.
7. Dubrey SW, Falk RH. Diagnosis and management of cardiac sarcoidosis. *Prog Cardiovasc Dis* 2010;52:336–346.
8. Yeboah J, Lee C, Sharma OP. Cardiac sarcoidosis: a review 2011. *Curr Opin Pulm Med* 2011:17:308–315.
9. Mantini N, Williams B Jr, Stewart J, Rubinsztain L, Kacharava A. Cardiac sarcoid: a clinician's review on how to approach the patient with cardiac sarcoid. *Clin Cardiol* 2012:35:410–415.
10. Saidha S, Sotirchos ES, Eckstein C. Etiology of sarcoidosis: does infection play a role? *Yale J Biol Med* 2012;85:133–141.
11. Hamzeh NY, Wamboldt FS, Weinberger HD. Management of cardiac sarcoidosis in the United States: a Delphi study. *Chest* 2012:141:154–162.
12. Mitropoulos FA, Floudas CS, Kanakis MA, Vaiopoulos GA. Cardiac sarcoidosis. *Thorac Cardiovasc Surg* 2009;57:187–190.
13. Zaidi AR, Zaidi A, Vaitkus PT. Outcome of heart transplantation in patients with sarcoid cardiomyopathy. *J Heart Lung Transplant* 2007;26:714–717.
14. Milman N, Andersen CB, Mortensen SA, Sander K. Cardiac sarcoidosis and heart transplantation: a report of four consecutive patients. *Sarcoidosis Vasc Diffuse Lung Dis* 2008;25:51–59.
15. Luk A, Metawee M, Ahn E, Gustafsson F, Ross H, Butany J. Do clinical diagnoses correlate with pathological diagnoses in cardiac transplant patients? The importance of endomyocardial biopsy. *Can J Cardiol* 2009:25:e48–e54.
16. Chang TI, Chi NH, Chou NK, Tsao CI, Yu HY, Chen YS, Wang SS. Isolated cardiac sarcoidosis in heart transplantation. *Transplant Proc* 2012;44:903–906.
17. Akashi H, Kato TS, Takayama H, Naka Y, Farr M, Mancini D, Schulze PC. Outcome of patients with cardiac sarcoidosis undergoing cardiac transplantation—single-center retrospective analysis. *J Cardiol* 2012;60:407–410.
18. Donsky AS, Escobar J, Capehart J, Roberts WC. Heart transplantation for undiagnosed cardiac sarcoidosis. *Am J Cardiol* 2002;89: 1447–1450.
19. Roberts WC, Vowels TJ, Ko JM, Capehart JE, Hall SA. Cardiac transplantation for cardiac sarcoidosis with initial diagnosis by examination of the left ventricular apical "core" excised for insertion of a left ventricular assist device for severe chronic heart failure. *Am J Cardiol* 2009;103:110–114.
20. Roberts WC, Filardo G, Ko JM, Siegel RJ, Dollar AL, Ross EM, Shirani J. Comparison of total 12-lead QRS voltage in a variety of cardiac conditions and its usefulness in predicting increased cardiac mass. *Am J Cardiol* 2013;112:904–909.
21. Yager JE, Hernandez AF, Steenbergen C, Persing B, Russell SD, Milano C, Felker GM. Recurrence of cardiac sarcoidosis in a heart transplant recipient. *J Heart Lung Transplant* 2005;24:1988–1990.
22. Luk A, Lee A, Ahn E, Soor GS, Ross HJ, Butany J. Cardiac sarcoidosis: recurrent disease in a heart transplant patient following pulmonary tuberculosis infection. *Can J Cardiol* 2010;26:e273–e275.
23. Ichinose A, Otani H, Oikawa M, Takase K, Saito H, Shimokawa H, Takahashi S. MRI of cardiac sarcoidosis: basal and subepicardial localization of myocardial lesions and their effect on left ventricular function. *Am J Roentgenol* 2008;191:862–869.
24. Greulich S, Deluigi CC, Gloekler S, Wahl A, Zürn C, Kramer U, Nothnagel D, Bültel H, Schumm J, Grün S, Ong P, Wagner A, Schneider S, Nassenstein K, Gawaz M, Sechtem U, Bruder O, Mahrholdt H. CMR imaging predicts death and other adverse events in suspected cardiac sarcoidosis. *JACC Cardiovasc Imaging* 2013;6:501–511.
25. Khan R, Tweedie EJ, Pflugfelder PW, White JA. Cardiac sarcoid in a heart transplant recipient: detection with cardiac magnetic resonance imaging. *Transplant Proc* 2010;42:1976–1978.
26. Koplan BA, Soejima K, Baughman K, Epstein LM, Stevenson WG. Refractory ventricular tachycardia secondary to cardiac sarcoid: electrophysiologic characteristics, mapping, and ablation. *Heart Rhythm* 2006;3:924–929.
27. Vasaiwala SC, Finn C, Delpriore J, Leya F, Gagermeier J, Akar JG, Santucci P, Dajani K, Bova D, Picken MM, Basso C, Marcus F, Wilber DJ. Prospective study of cardiac sarcoid mimicking arrhythmogenic right ventricular dysplasia. *J Cardiovasc Electrophysiol* 2009;20:473–476.
28. Corrado D, Thiene G. Cardiac sarcoidosis mimicking arrhythmogenic right ventricular cardiomyopathy/dysplasia: the renaissance of endomyocardial biopsy? *J Cardiovasc Electrophysiol* 2009;20:477–479.
29. Chia PL, Subbiah RN, Kuchar D, Walker B. Cardiac sarcoidosis masquerading as arrhythmogenic right ventricular cardiomyopathy. *Heart Lung Circ* 2012;21:42–45.
30. Barbou F, Lahutte M, Gontier E. Cardiac sarcoidosis presenting as an arrhythmogenic right ventricular cardiomyopathy. *Heart* 2012;98: 1753–1754.

# Morphologic Features of the Recipient Heart in Patients Having Cardiac Transplantation and Analysis of the Congruence or Incongruence Between the Clinical and Morphologic Diagnoses

*William C. Roberts, MD, Carey Camille Roberts, BS, Jong Mi Ko, BA, Giovanni Filardo, PhD, John Edward Capehart, MD, and Shelley Anne Hall, MD*

**Abstract:** Cardiac transplantation (CT) has been one of the great medical advances of the last nearly 50 years. We studied the explanted hearts of 314 patients having CT at Baylor University Medical Center Dallas from 1993 to 2012, and compared the morphologic diagnoses to the clinical diagnoses before CT. Among the 314 patients the morphologic and clinical diagnoses were congruent in 272 (87%) and incongruent in 42 (13%). Most of the incongruity occurred among the 166 patients with non-ischemic cardiomyopathy (non-IC) (36/166 [22%]), and of that group the major incongruity occurred among the patients with hypertrophic cardiomyopathy (7/17 [41%]), non-compaction left ventricular cardiomyopathy (NCLVC) (3/3 [100%]), mononuclear myocarditis (3/3 [100%]), arrhythmogenic right ventricular cardiomyopathy (ARVC) (4/4 [100%]), and cardiac sarcoidosis (8/8 [100%]). The phrase "non-IC" is a general term that includes several subsets of cardiac diseases and simply means "insignificant narrowing of 1 or more of the epicardial coronary arteries," but it does not specify the specific cause of the heart failure leading to CT. A number of cardiac illustrations are provided to demonstrate the morphologic variability occurring among the patients with IC and non-IC.

(*Medicine* 2014;93: 211–235)

**Abbreviations:** ARVC = arrhythmogenic right ventricular cardiomyopathy, CT = cardiac transplantation, HC = hypertrophic cardiomyopathy, IC = ischemic cardiomyopathy, IDC = idiopathic dilated cardiomyopathy, NCLVC = non-compaction left ventricular cardiomyopathy.

## INTRODUCTION

The first cardiac transplantation (CT) procedure was done in Capetown, South Africa, by Christiaan Barnard in 1967.[3] From that time through 2012, more than 90,000 CT procedures were performed worldwide, approximately 3500 a year with about 2200 of that number being performed in the United States.[30] The immediate pre-op care, the operation, and the first 6-month post-operative care cost about $1,000,000. Although most have been performed in patients with idiopathic dilated cardiomyopathy (IDC) or ischemic cardiomyopathy (IC), CT is also performed, albeit less frequently, for a variety of other cardiac conditions. In 1998 Waller and colleagues reported clinical and morphologic findings in 92 patients who had had CT for IDC, IC, or hypertrophic cardiomyopathy (HC).[71] Of them, 57 had CT at Baylor University Medical Center (BUMC) Dallas from March 1993 through June 1997. (The remaining 35 patients had CT at other institutions and are not included in the present analysis.) Surprisingly, that clinico-pathologic study appears to have been the first to report morphologic findings in a systematic fashion in the recipient hearts in those 3 conditions. The present report was prompted by finding incongruity between the clinical and morphologic diagnoses in some patients having CT, and that incongruity led to a thorough analysis of that frequency in 314 patients who had had CT at BUMC in the past 20 years.

## METHODS

The recipient hearts in each of the 314 patients were submitted to the surgical pathology division of the department of pathology of BUMC Dallas. The patients included had undergone CT at BUMC from March 1993 through June 2012. All hearts during this period were described and classified by 1 of the authors (WCR). Figure 1 displays the number of CTs done at BUMC during each of those 20 years and the 3 major reasons for CT among the 314 patients. Each heart after formalin fixation and "cleaning" was weighed carefully by WCR, opened by him, and photographed (most by JMK). Although some were opened by parasagittal cuts, especially in those patients with HC, the cardiac ventricles in most were incised by transverse cuts parallel to the posterior atrioventricular sulcus. The resulting "bread-loaf" slices were approximately 1 cm in thickness except for the most apical portion, which was about 3 cm thick. The heart was weighed after these cuts and after all extraneous tissues were removed. The left ventricular cavity was measured both from anterior to posterior and from right to left dimensions, and the largest of these cavity numbers were used as the maximal cavity dimension. The right ventricular cavity dimension was the length from the right ventricular aspect of the ventricular septum to the endocardial lining of the right ventricular free wall along the posterior wall of this chamber.

From the Departments of Internal Medicine (Division of Cardiology) (WCR, SAH), Pathology (WCR), and Cardiothoracic Surgery (JEC), and the Baylor Heart and Vascular Institute (WCR, CCR, JMK), Baylor University Medical Center, Dallas, Texas. Carey Camille Roberts is currently a freshman at Georgetown University School of Medicine, Washington, DC.

Correspondence: Dr. William C. Roberts, Baylor Heart and Vascular Institute, Baylor University Medical Center, 3500 Gaston Avenue, Dallas, TX (e-mail: wc.roberts@baylorhealth.edu).

Financial support and conflicts of interest: Support for this investigation was provided by the Baylor Health Care System Foundation. The authors have no conflicts of interest to disclose.



ISSN: 0025-7974

DOI: 10.1097/MD.0000000000000038

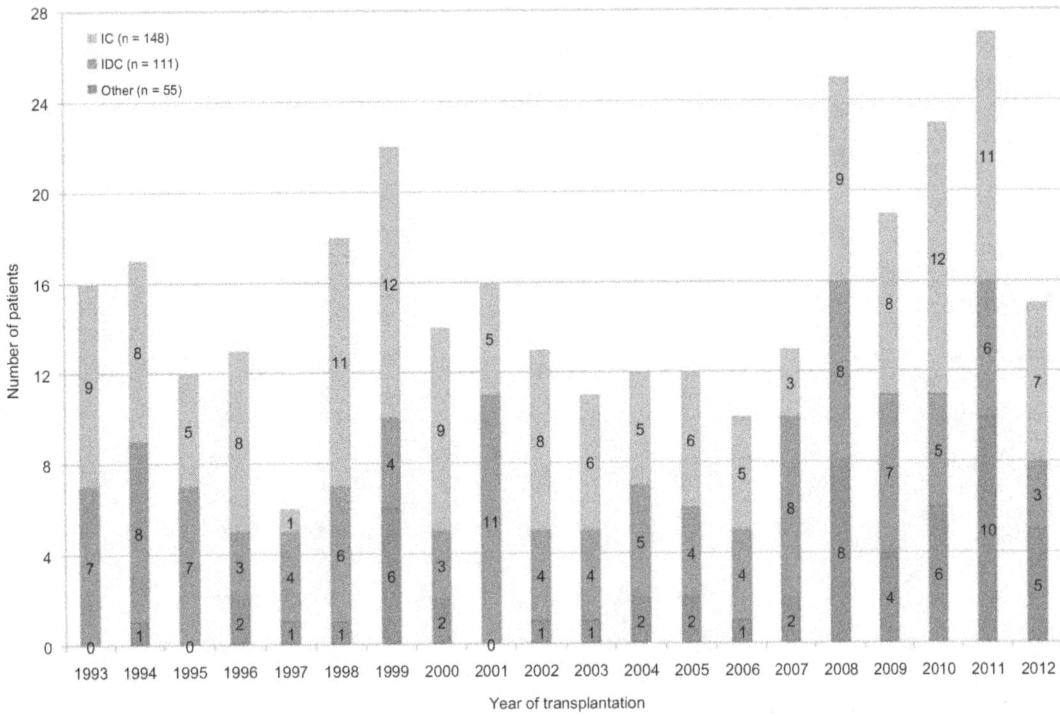


**FIGURE 1.** Bar graph showing the number of cardiac transplantation procedures done each year at Baylor University Medical Center 1993–2012 (through June 2012), and the 3 major reasons for the transplant (IC = ischemic cardiomyopathy [green]; IDC = idiopathic dilated cardiomyopathy [red], and other [blue]).

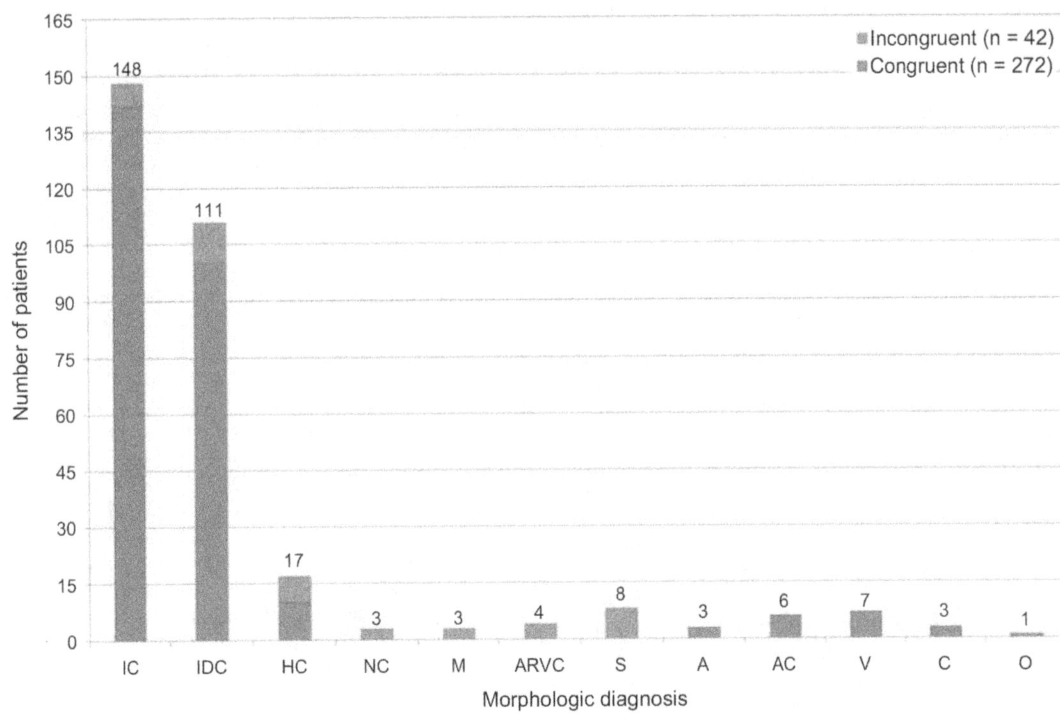


**FIGURE 2.** Bar graph showing frequency of congruence and incongruence among the various conditions cardiac transplantation among the 314 patients. IC = ischemic cardiomyopathy; IDC = idiopathic dilated cardiomyopathy; HC = hypertrophic cardiomyopathy; NC = non-compaction left ventricular cardiomyopathy; M = mononuclear myocarditis; ARVC = arrhythmogenic right ventricular cardiomyopathy; S = sarcoidosis; A = amyloidosis; V = valvular heart disease; C = congenital heart disease; O = other.

**TABLE 1.** Clinical and Morphologic Diagnoses of the 2 Basic Conditions Leading to Cardiac Transplantation: Ischemic Cardiomyopathy and Non-Ischemic Cardiomyopathy, and Incongruence Found Between the Diagnoses (Number of Patients in Each Category With the Clinical and Morphologic Diagnoses)

| Condition | Clinical Diagnosis | Morphologic Diagnosis | Incongruence Between Clinical and Morphologic Diagnosis |
|---|---|---|---|
| Ischemic cardiomyopathy | 142 (96%) | 148 | 6 (4%)* |
| Non-ischemic cardiomyopathy | 130 (78%) | 166 | 36 (22%) |
| Idiopathic dilated | 100 | 111 | 11† |
| Hypertrophic | 10 | 17 | 7‡ |
| Non-compaction left ventricular | 0 | 3 | 3‡ |
| Mononuclear myocarditis | 0 | 3 | 3‡ |
| Arrhythmogenic right ventricular | 0 | 4 | 4‡ |
| Cardiac sarcoidosis | 0 | 8 | 8‡ |
| Cardiac amyloidosis | 3 | 3 | 0 |
| Adriamycin cardiomyopathy | 6 | 6 | 0 |
| Valvular heart disease | 7 | 7 | 0 |
| Cyanotic congenital heart disease | 3 | 3 | 0 |
| Other | 1 | 1 | 0 |
| Total | 272 (87%) | 314 | 42 (13%) |

*All 6 morphologically had normal or near normal coronary arteries.
†All 11 had severe narrowing of 1 or more epicardial coronary arteries by atherosclerotic plaques.
‡All 25 were diagnosed clinically as "non-ischemic cardiomyopathy."

The orifices of the right and left main coronary arteries in the aorta were carefully examined for proper location and degrees of narrowing, if any. Random cuts were made in the 4 major (right, left main, left anterior descending, and left circumflex) coronary arteries, and the arteries were probed (1.5 mm diameter probe) both anterograde and retrograde. The 2 coronary orifices in the aorta were probed to determine any resistance to movement of the probe. Additionally, all incisions into the major coronary arteries were carefully explored for atherosclerotic plaques and luminal narrowing.

Each of the 4 cardiac valves was examined for abnormality.

At least 6 sections of each heart were submitted for preparation of histology slides. They included at least 2 sections of the left ventricular free wall, 1 of ventricular septum, 1 of right ventricular free wall, and 1 each of the walls of left and right atria. If coronary artery bypass grafts were present, sections of them were also prepared. Both hematoxylin-eosin and Masson stains were prepared on all myocardial sections and Movat stains were prepared on all sections of coronary bypass conduits and/or native coronary arteries. If heavy calcific deposits were palpated in the epicardial coronary arteries or in other areas of the heart, usually a radiograph was made of the recipient heart.

The clinical, echocardiographic, hemodynamic, and operative records were sought from the patients' medical records and/or the BUMC Apollo cardiovascular database. Information regarding death of any patient was obtained from the medical records in deaths during hospitalization at the time of CT and from the Social Security Death Index for post-hospitalization deaths. Survival was assessed as March 31, 2013.

Means, standard deviations (SDs), and percentages were calculated to describe the study cohort. The Kaplan-Meier method was used to construct the survival curve for the whole population. The log-rank test statistic was computed to compare unadjusted survival curves between men and women.

The study was approved by the institutional review board at BUMC.

## RESULTS

The main findings in the 314 patients are summarized in Tables 1 and 2. All patients at the time of CT were aged >18 years of age: 230 (73%) were men, and 84 (27%) were women. The patients included had CT only; there were no patients having heart/lung, heart/liver, or heart/bone marrow transplantation. Clinically, the patients were divided into 2 major groups: 1) *ischemic cardiomyopathy* (IC), 148 patients (47%); and 2) *non-ischemic cardiomyopathy* (N-IC), 166 patients (53%). The N-IC patients were subdivided into 11 groups, the 2 largest being IDC, 111 patients (66%), and HC, 17 patients (10%). The remaining 9 groups under N-IC consisted of 38 patients (23% of 166).

The frequency of congruity between the clinical and morphologic diagnoses is summarized in Table 1 and in Figure 2. Both the clinical and morphologic diagnoses were congruous in 272 (87%) of the 314 patients: in 142 (96%) of the 148 patients with IC and in 130 (78%) of the 166 patients with N-IC. Incongruity between the clinical and morphologic diagnoses was most glaring among the patients with HC (10 of 17 [59%]), non-compaction left ventricular cardiomyopathy (0 of 3); arrhythmogenic right ventricular cardiomyopathy (0 of 4), and cardiac sarcoidosis (0 of 8). Details of individual patients in the non-IC subgroups (excluding IDC) are tabulated in Tables 3–10.

### Ischemic Cardiomyopathy

The 148 IC patients had hearts with dilated left ventricular cavities (>3.5 cm: range, 3.5–8.5 cm [mean 5.9]);

**TABLE 2.** Morphologic Findings in Patients Having Cardiac Transplantation, by Cardiac Condition (n=314)

| Variable | IC (n=148) | IDC (n=111) | HC (n=17) | NCLVC (n=3) | M (n=3) | ARVC (n=4) | S (n=8) | A (n=3) | AC (n=6) | V (n=7) | C (n=3) | O (n=1*) |
|---|---|---|---|---|---|---|---|---|---|---|---|---|
| Age (mean), yr | | | | | | | | | | | | |
| Men | 38–70 (58) | 24–69 (51) | 19–68 (51) | 45 | 24, 56 | 21–44 (30) | 50–54 (52) | 57–61 (58) | 30, 55 | 30–65 (50) | 40 | 62 |
| Women | 30–66 (55) | 26–67 (51) | 35–56 (46) | 36, 49 | 46 | NA | 50–59 (55) | NA | 49–69 (62) | 43–64 (56) | 28,38 | NA |
| Sex | | | | | | | | | | | | |
| Male | 129 (87%) | 66 (59%) | 13 (76%) | 1 (33%) | 2 (67%) | 4 (100%) | 3 (38%) | 3 (100%) | 2 (30%) | 5 (71%) | 1 (33%) | 1 (100%) |
| Female | 19 (13%) | 45 (41%) | 4 (24%) | 2 (67%) | 1 (33%) | 0 | 5 (62%) | 0 | 4 (60%) | 2 (29%) | 2 (67%) | 0 |
| Heart weight (mean), g | | | | | | | | | | | | |
| Men | 324–839 (531) | 285–940 (544) | 355–780 (547) | 438 | 443, 545 | 314–686 (521) | 440–604 (518) | 420–550 (494) | 366, 526 | 605–732 (651) | 653 | 707 |
| Women | 255–726 (451) | 232–660 (444) | 220–424 (358) | 380, 422 | 356 | NA | 371–562 (453) | NA | 326–558 (446) | 258–635 (388) | 460,573 | NA |
| Number of major coronary arteries narrowed >50% in cross-sectioned area | | | | | | | | | | | | |
| 0 | 0 | 100 | 13 | 3 | 2 | 4 | 7 | 1 | 5 | 5 | 3 | 1 |
| 1 | 25 | 5 | 3 | 0 | 1 | 0 | 0 | 2 | 1 | 0 | 0 | 0 |
| 2 | 30 | 6 | 0 | 0 | 0 | 0 | 1 | 0 | 0 | 1 | 0 | 0 |
| 3 | 51 | 0 | 1 | 0 | 0 | 0 | 0 | 0 | 0 | 0 | 0 | 0 |
| 4 | 42 | 0 | 0 | 0 | 0 | 0 | 0 | 0 | 0 | 1 | 0 | 0 |
| LV cavity size (mean), cm | 3.5–8.5 (5.9) | 3–10 (6.3) | 3.0–7.5 (5.5) | 7.5–8 (7.5) | 7–9 (8) | 4.5–11 (6.6) | 5–9 (6.3) | 3.0–4.5 (3.8) | 6–8 (6.7) | 3.4–7.5 (5.4) | 5.5–7 (6.1) | 6 |
| RV cavity size (mean), cm | 1.0–5.0 (2.8) | 0.7–9 (3.1) | 1.0–4.5 (2.6) | 2.5–4 (3.2) | 2–2.5 (2.3) | 3–6 (4.6) | 2–9 (4.4) | 3.0–4.0 (3.5) | 2–3 (2.5) | 2–5 (3.3) | 3 | 5.5 |
| Grossly visible LV scarring | 147 | 5 | 13 | 1 | 3 | 1 | 8 | 0 | 0 | 5 | 2 | 1 |
| Grossly visible foci of necrosis | 2 | 0 | 0 | 0 | 0 | 0 | 0 | 0 | 0 | 1 | 0 | 0 |
| Died postoperatively | | | | | | | | | | | | |
| ≤60 d | 6 | 1 | 0 | 0 | 0 | 0 | 0 | 0 | 1 | 1 | 0 | 0 |
| >60 d | 25 | 20 | 3 | 0 | 1 | 0 | 1 | 1 | 0 | 0 | 0 | 1 |
| Previous major cardiac operation | | | | | | | | | | | | |
| Coronary artery bypass grafting | 52 | 2 | 2 | 0 | 0 | 0 | 0 | 0 | 0 | 1 | 0 | 0 |

| | | | | | | | | | | | | |
|---|---|---|---|---|---|---|---|---|---|---|---|---|
| LVAD insertion | 22 | 10 | 6 | 0 | 0 | 0 | 3 | 0 | 0 | 1 | 1 | 0 |
| Valve operation | 2† | 1 | 0 | 0 | 0 | 0 | 0 | 0 | 0 | 7 | 3 | 0 |
| Body mass index ($kg/m^2$) | n = 118 | n = 86 | n = 15 | n = 3 | n = 3 | n = 4 | n = 8 | n = 3 | n = 6 | n = 6 | n = 3 | n = 1 |
| <25.0 | 33 (28%) | 33 (38%) | 6 (40%) | 2 (67%) | 3 (100%) | 2 (50%) | 3 (38%) | 1 (33%) | 2 (33%) | 2 (33%) | 2 (66%) | 0 |
| ≥25.0–30.0 | 62 (53%) | 39 (45%) | 7 (47%) | 1 (33%) | 0 | 2 (50%) | 5 (62%) | 0 | 2 (33%) | 3 (50%) | 1 (33%) | 1 (100%) |
| >30.0–35.0 | 21 (18%) | 12 (14%) | 2 (13%) | 0 | 0 | 0 | 0 | 2 (66%) | 2 (33%) | 1 (17%) | 0 | 0 |
| >35.0–40.0 | 2 (1%) | 2 (2%) | 0 | 0 | 0 | 0 | 0 | 0 | 0 | 0 | 0 | 0 |
| >40.0 | 0 | 0 | 0 | 0 | 0 | 0 | 0 | 0 | 0 | 0 | 0 | 0 |

Abbreviations: A = cardiac amyloidosis, AC = Adriamycin cardiomyopathy, C = congenital heart disease, LV = left ventricular, LVAD = left ventricular assist device, M = myocarditis, NA = not applicable, O = other, RV = right ventricular, S = cardiac sarcoidosis, V = valvular heart disease.
*Previously reported.[48]
†Mitral valve repairs.

1 or more major epicardial coronary arteries narrowed >75% in cross-sectional area by atherosclerotic plaque; 1 or more grossly visible transmural (>50% of wall thickness) scars in the left ventricular free wall with or without similar scars in the ventricular septum and right ventricular free wall; normal or nearly normal cardiac valves; and absent inflammatory, giant, neoplastic cell or non-fibrous infiltrates (such as amyloid).[56] Additionally, the intramural coronary arteries were normal. Of the total 314 patients, 148 (47%) morphologically fulfilled these criteria. Of these 148 patients, 52 (35%) had had a coronary artery bypass grafting procedure previously and 22 (15%) had a left ventricular assist device. Of these 148 patients, 142 (96%) before CT were diagnosed as IC; the remaining 6 patients were diagnosed clinically as IDC because coronary angiograms, some performed several years earlier, had indicated no significant luminal narrowing, although all 6 had transmural left ventricular scars and severe (>75% cross-sectional area) narrowing of 1 or more major coronary arteries. Examples of IC are shown in Figures 3–13.

## Idiopathic Dilated Cardiomyopathy

The 111 IDC patients had dilated left ventricular cavities (4.0–10.0 cm [mean 6.3]); normal or nearly normal cardiac valves; normal epicardium; no inflammatory, giant, neoplastic cells or non-fibrous interstitial infiltrates (such as amyloid) in the cardiac walls; and usually normal epicardial coronary arteries (Figures 14–17).[20,51,54,71] A few patients had some atherosclerotic plaques but the plaques had narrowed the lumen ≤50% in cross-sectional area in 1 or more of the 4 major epicardial coronary arteries. Eleven patients had narrowing of 1 or more major epicardial coronary arteries >75% in cross-sectional area by plaques, but none of them had grossly visible left ventricular or ventricular septal scars. These 11 patients do not fulfill our definition of IDC because of the coronary narrowing, but none of the 11 had 1 or more grossly visible left ventricular scars. In these patients the coronary angiogram appeared to simply underestimate the degree of coronary narrowing. Their lack of myocardial scarring prevents them from being placed in the IC group. It is likely that these 11 patients actually had IDC, but because they lived in a high-cholesterol environment (United States), their coronary arteries developed significant plaque.[55] Five patients with normal epicardial coronary arteries had grossly visible left ventricular free wall and/or ventricular septal scars. The 5 patients were diagnosed morphologically and clinically as IDC.[23]

## Hypertrophic Cardiomyopathy

The 17 HC patients (Table 3) had either normal sized (<4 cm) (5 patients) or dilated (>4 cm) (12 patients) left ventricular cavities and past clinical evidence of non-dilated left ventricular cavities (Figures 18–21).[5,13,21,24,33,36,37,42,49,61] Transmural scarring involved the ventricular septum and left ventricular free walls in 13 patients (76%) with or without grossly visible scarring of portions of the right ventricular free wall. The ventricular septum at sometime in the past or presently was thicker than the left ventricular free wall; typical myofiber disorganization was present in the ventricular septum, and the intramural coronary arteries on histologic study were abnormal in all 13 patients with ventricular wall scarring.[35] None of the 17 HC patients had clinical or hemodynamic evidence of left

TABLE 3. Pertinent Data in 17 Patients Having Cardiac Transplantation for Hypertrophic Cardiomyopathy

| Patient | Age at CT (yr) | Sex | Clinical Diagnosis | BMI (kg/m$^2$) | Lowest LVEF (%) | Year of CT | HW (g) | LV Diameter (cm) | Narrowed Coronary Arteries | Grossly Visible LV Scar* | LVAD |
|---|---|---|---|---|---|---|---|---|---|---|---|
| 1 | 35 | F | Non-IC | 26.9 | 15 | 2010 | 367 | 5.0 | 0 | + | + |
| 2 | 43 | F | HC | – | 60 | 1994 | 220 | 3.7 | 0 | + | 0 |
| 3 | 50 | F | HC | 21.7 | – | 1999 | 422 | 3.7 | 0 | + | 0 |
| 4 | 56 | F | Non-IC | 18.4 | 10 | 2012 | 424 | 7.0 | 0 | + | 0 |
| 5 | 19 | M | HC | 16.8 | 58 | 1999 | 451 | 3.5 | 0 | 0 | 0 |
| 6 | 35 | M | HC | 35.5 | 5 | 2011 | 705 | 6.0 | 0 | + | + |
| 7 | 41 | M | HC | 27.6 | 27 | 2009 | 566 | 6.5 | 0 | + | 0 |
| 8 | 45 | M | Non-IC | 25.7 | 65 | 2010 | 411 | 3.0 | 0 | 0 | 0 |
| 9 | 48 | M | Non-IC | 30.6 | 25 | 2012 | 442 | 4.5 | + | + | + |
| 10 | 50 | M | HC | – | 10 | 1999 | 674 | 7.5 | 0 | 0 | 0 |
| 11 | 54 | M | Non-IC | 28.7 | 20 | 1997 | 637 | 5.5 | 0 | + | 0 |
| 12 | 55 | M | IC[†] | 27.3 | 25 | 1998 | 506 | 4.5 | + | + | + |
| 13 | 58 | M | HC | – | 15 | 1996 | 355 | 6.9 | + | + | 0 |
| 14 | 58 | M | HC & IC[†] | 29.4 | 35 | 1999 | 374 | 7.0 | + | + | + |
| 15 | 63 | M | HC | 21.7 | – | 2011 | 625 | 7.4 | 0 | 0 | 0 |
| 16 | 68 | M | Non-IC | 32.4 | 10 | 2009 | 780 | 7.5 | 0 | + | + |
| 17 | 68 | M | HC | 25.4 | 35 | 2010 | 580 | 3.5 | 0 | + | 0 |

Abbreviations: See previous tables. BMI = body mass index, CT = cardiac transplantation, HW = heart weight, LVEF = left ventricular ejection fraction.

*Excludes papillary muscles.

[†]Each also had coronary artery bypass grafting.

TABLE 4. Pertinent Data in 3 Patients Having Cardiac Transplantation for Non-Compaction Left Ventricular Cardiomyopathy*

| Patient | Age at CT (yr) | Sex | Clinical Diagnosis | BMI (kg/m$^2$) | Lowest LVEF (%) | Year of CT | HW (g) | Diameter (cm) | | LV Scar |
|---|---|---|---|---|---|---|---|---|---|---|
| | | | | | | | | LV | RV | |
| 1 | 36 | F | Non-IC | 22.6 | 15 | 2008 | 422 | 7.0 | 4.0 | 0 |
| 2 | 49 | F | Non-IC | 22.5 | 5 | 2011 | 380 | 7.5 | 3.0 | 0 |
| 3 | 45 | M | Non-IC | 26.1 | 10 | 2011 | 438 | 8.0 | 2.5 | + |

*None had narrowed coronary arteries or coronary artery bypass grafting or a left ventricular assist device.

TABLE 5. Pertinent Data in 3 Patients Having Cardiac Transplantation for Active or Healed Mononuclear Myocarditis*

| Patient | Age at CT (yr) | Sex | Clinical Diagnosis | BMI (kg/m$^2$) | Lowest LVEF (%) | Year of CT | HW (g) | Diameter (cm) | | Narrowed Coronary Arteries | LV Scar |
|---|---|---|---|---|---|---|---|---|---|---|---|
| | | | | | | | | LV | RV | | |
| 1 | 46 | F | Non-IC | 24.6 | 20 | 2008 | 356 | 7.0 | 2.5 | 0 | + |
| 2 | 24 | M | Non-IC | 19.8 | 5 | 2011 | 545 | 9.0 | 2.0 | 0 | + |
| 3 | 56 | M | IC | 18.4 | 10 | 2008 | 443 | 8.0 | 2.5 | + | + |

Abbreviations: See previous tables.

*None had coronary artery bypass grafting or a left ventricular assist device.

**TABLE 6.** Pertinent Data in 4 Men Having Cardiac Transplantation for Arrhythmogenic Right Ventricular Cardiomyopathy*

| Patient | Age at CT (yr) | Clinical Diagnosis | BMI (kg/m²) | Lowest LVEF (%) | Year of CT | HW (g) | Diameter (cm) LV | Diameter (cm) RV | LV Scar | RV Scar |
|---|---|---|---|---|---|---|---|---|---|---|
| 1 | 21 | Non-IC | 26.5 | 10 | 2012 | 489 | 4.5 | 6 | 0 | + |
| 2 | 26 | Non-IC | 24.8 | 10 | 2009 | 594 | 6.0 | 5.5 | 0 | + |
| 3 | 30 | Non-IC | 27.6 | 10 | 2008 | 686 | 11.0 | 3.0 | + | + |
| 4 | 44 | Non-IC | 22.5 | 25 | 2008 | 314 | 5.0 | 4.0 | 0 | + |

Abbreviations: See previous tables.
*None had narrowed coronary arteries or coronary artery bypass grafting or a left ventricular assist device.

**TABLE 7.** Pertinent Data in 8 Patients Having Cardiac Transplantation for Cardiac Sarcoidosis*

| Patient | Age at CT (yr) | Sex | Clinical Diagnosis | BMI (kg/m²) | Lowest LVEF (%) | Year of CT | HW (g) | Diameter (cm) LV | Diameter (cm) RV | Narrowed Coronary Arteries | LV Scar | LVAD |
|---|---|---|---|---|---|---|---|---|---|---|---|---|
| 1 | 50 | F | Non-IC | 27.0 | 20 | 2012 | 442 | 7.5 | 4.0 | 0 | + | 0 |
| 2 | 52 | F | Non-IC | 28.7 | 20 | 2010 | 441 | 5.5 | 2.0 | 0 | + | 0 |
| 3 | 56 | F | Non-IC | 25.7 | 15 | 2009 | 447 | 5.5 | 3.5 | 0 | + | 0 |
| 4 | 58 | F | Non-IC | 26.4 | 20 | 2012 | 562 | 5.0 | 2.5 | 0 | + | 0 |
| 5 | 59 | F | Non-IC | 20.8 | 20 | 2006 | 371 | 5.0 | 7.5 | + | + | + |
| 6 | 50 | M | Non-IC† | 24.7 | 10 | 2005 | 604 | 7.0 | 2.5 | 0 | + | + |
| 7 | 52 | M | Non-IC† | 21.6 | 20 | 2005 | 440 | — | – | 0 | + | + |
| 8 | 54 | M | Non-IC† | 27.5 | 10 | 1999 | 511 | 9.0 | 9.0 | 0 | + | 0 |

Abbreviations: See previous tables.
*None had coronary artery bypass grafting.
†Diagnosis of cardiac sarcoid made from histologic study of "left ventricular core" excised for insertion of a left ventricular assist device.

**TABLE 8.** Pertinent Data in 3 Men Having Cardiac Transplantation for Cardiac Amyloidosis*

| Patient | Age at CT (yr) | Clinical Diagnosis | BMI (kg/m²) | Lowest LVEF (%) | Year of CT | HW (g) | Diameter (cm) LV | Diameter (cm) RV | Narrowed Coronary Arteries | LV Scar |
|---|---|---|---|---|---|---|---|---|---|---|
| 1 | 57 | Amyloidosis | 20.2 | 30 | 2004 | 550 | 4.0 | 3.5 | 0 | 0 |
| 2 | 57 | Amyloidosis | 32.0 | 20 | 2010 | 420 | 4.5 | 3.0 | +† | 0 |
| 3 | 61 | Amyloidosis | 30.6 | 46 | 2008 | 513 | 3.0 | 4.0 | + | 0 |

Abbreviations: See previous tables.
*None had coronary artery bypass grafting or a left ventricular assist device.
†Stent to the right coronary artery in October 2009.

**TABLE 9.** Pertinent Data in 6 Patients Having Cardiac Transplantation for Adriamycin Cardiomyopathy*

| Patient | Age at CT (yr) | Sex | Clinical Diagnosis | BMI (kg/m²) | Lowest LVEF (%) | Year of CT | HW (g) | Diameter (cm) LV | Diameter (cm) RV | Narrowed Coronary Arteries | LV Scar |
|---|---|---|---|---|---|---|---|---|---|---|---|
| 1 | 49 | F | AC | – | – | 2007 | 404 | 8.0 | 2.5 | 0 | 0 |
| 2 | 64 | F | AC | 24.6 | 10 | 2004 | 326 | 6.5 | 3.0 | + | 0 |
| 3 | 65 | F | AC | 25.7 | – | 2011 | 558 | 6.5 | 2.5 | 0 | 0 |
| 4 | 69 | F | AC | 34.3 | 25 | 2011 | 497 | 6.0 | 3.0 | 0 | 0 |
| 5 | 30 | M | AC | 25.9 | 35 | 2008 | 366 | 7.0 | 2.0 | 0 | 0 |
| 6 | 55 | M | AC | 31.6 | 15 | 2011 | 526 | 6.0 | 2.2 | 0 | 0 |

Abbreviations: See previous tables. AC = Adriamycin cardiomyopathy.
*None had coronary artery bypass grafting or a left ventricular assist device.

TABLE 10. Pertinent Data in 6 Patients Having Cardiac Transplantation for Valvular Disease

| Patient | Age at CT (yr) | Sex | Clinical Valve Dysfunction | Valve Replaced | Interval (yr) AVR → CT | BMI (kg/m$^2$) | Lowest LVEF (%) | Year of CT | HW (g) | Diameter (cm) LV | Diameter (cm) RV | Narrowed Coronary Arteries | LV Scar | CABG | LVAD |
|---|---|---|---|---|---|---|---|---|---|---|---|---|---|---|---|
| 1 | 30 | M | AS (BAV) | Aortic | 8 | 25 | 10 | 1999 | 650 | 5.5 | 2.8 | 0 | + | 0 | 0 |
| 2 | 47 | M | AS (BAV) | Aortic* | – | – | – | 1996 | 605 | – | – | 0 | + | 0 | 0 |
| 3 | 56 | M | AS (BAV) | Aortic | 4.7 | 28.3 | 5 | 2007 | 732 | 6.0 | 4.0 | 0 | 0 | 0 | + |
| 4 | 65 | M | AS (BAV) | Aortic | 5.2 | 18.4 | 20 | 2003 | 616 | 7.5 | 3.0 | + | + | +† | 0 |
| 5 | 43 | F | AR‡, MR‡ | Aortic, mitral | – | – | 30 | 2002 | 258 | 3.4 | 2.0 | 0 | 0 | 0 | 0 |
| 6 | 64 | F | MS, MR | Mitral (x2) | – | 31.8 | 25 | 2010 | 635 | 5.5 | 5.0 | 0 | + | 0 | 0 |
| 7 | 60 | F | MR‡ | 0§ | – | 27.1 | 35 | 2011 | 271 | 4.5 | 3.0 | + | + | 0 | 0 |

Abbreviations: See previous tables. AR = aortic regurgitation, AS = aortic stenosis, AVR = aortic valve replacement, BAV = bicuspid aortic valve, CABG = coronary artery bypass grafting, MR = mitral regurgitation, MS = mitral stenosis.

*Procedure at another hospital (non-BUMC).

†CABG done 6 yr before AVR.

‡Radiation therapy for Hodgkin disease.

§Mitral valve repair twice.

TABLE 11. Pertinent Data in 3 Patients Having Cardiac Transplantation for Congenital Heart Disease*

| Patient | Age at CT (yr) | Sex | Clinical Diagnosis | BMI (kg/m$^2$) | Lowest LVEF (%) | Year of CT | HW (g) | LV Diameter (cm) | LV Scar | LVAD |
|---|---|---|---|---|---|---|---|---|---|---|
| 1 | 28 | F | TGA | 19.4 | 10 | 2008 | 460 | 7.0 | + | 0 |
| 2 | 38 | F | RV hypoplasia | 19.6 | 10 | 2011 | 573 | 5.9 | 0 | + |
| 3 | 40 | M | T of F | 27.3 | 10 | 2010 | 653 | 5.5 | + | 0 |

Abbreviations: See previous tables. TGA = transposition of great arteries, T of F = tetralogy of Fallot.

*None had narrowed coronary arteries or coronary artery bypass grafting.

**TABLE 12.** Previously Reported Data on Congruity vs Incongruity Among 296 Patients Having Cardiac Transplantation (From Luk et al[29])

| Cardiac Condition | Clinical Diagnosis (No.) | Morphologic Diagnosis (No.) |
|---|---|---|
| Ischemic cardiomyopathy | 140 | 144 |
| Idiopathic dilated cardiomyopathy | 96 | 54 |
| Hypertrophic cardiomyopathy | 15 | 17 |
| Myocarditis | 8* | 25† |
| Valvular "cardiomyopathy" | 6 | 5 |
| Infiltrative | 5‡ | 4‡ |
| Congenital | 18 | 18 |
| Doxorubicin | 6 | 6 |
| Becker's muscular dystrophy | 1 | 1 |
| Fabry's | 1 | 2 |
| Arrhythmogenic RV cardiomyopathy | 0 | 12 |
| Cardiac sarcoid | 0 | 6 |
| Mitochondrial myopathy | 0 | 1 |
| Iron cardiomyopathy | 0 | 1 |
| TOTAL | 296 | 296 |

Modified and reprinted with permission from Elsevier.[29]
*"Viral myocarditis" in 6, hypersensitive/eosinophilic in 2.
†"Viral myocarditis" in 20, hypersensitive/eosinophilic in 4, and giant cell in 1.
‡Amyloid in 3.

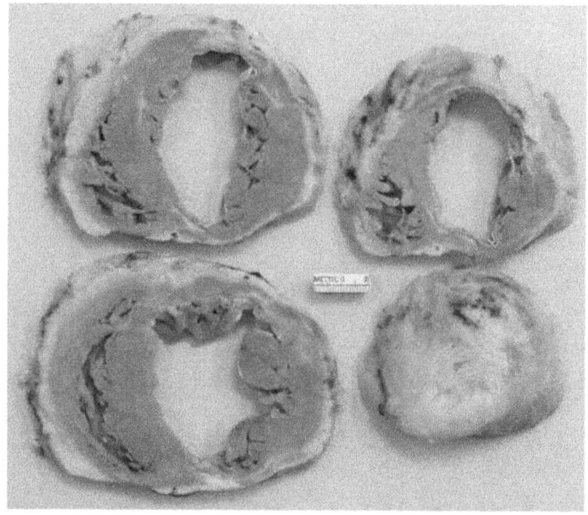

**FIGURE 4.** Ischemic cardiomyopathy. Photographs of sections of the cardiac ventricles caudal to the mitral valve in a 54-year-old woman who had an acute myocardial infarction when she was 33 years of age and underwent percutaneous coronary intervention at that time. At age 39 years, she had another acute myocardial infarct and underwent coronary artery bypass grafting. Cardiac catheterization 2 years later disclosed that all bypass conduits were closed. At age 42 years, she had another percutaneous coronary intervention. The left ventricular ejection fraction shortly before cardiac transplantation was 10%. These views show a healed myocardial infarct in the anterior wall of left ventricle and another in the posterior wall opposite one another. The quantity of subepicardial adipose tissue is clearly increased. The left ventricular cavity is quite dilated.

ventricular outflow obstruction just prior to CT. Four (24%) of the 17 patients also had severe narrowing of 1 or more epicardial coronary arteries, and all 4 had grossly visible left ventricular and ventricular septal scars. Nine other HC patients had left ventricular or ventricular septal scar without narrowing of the epicardial coronary arteries. The clinical diagnosis in 6 of the 17 patients was "non-IC," in 1 patient IC, and in 1 patient both HC and IC. Each of the latter 2 patients had coronary bypass grafting in the remote past before CT. Thus, the clinical and morphologic diagnosis were incongruous in 7 (41%) of these 17 patients.

## Non-Compaction Left Ventricular Cardiomyopathy

Three patients had NCLVC (Table 4, Figures 22 and 23). Each had very dilated ventricular cavities with the non-compacted portion of left ventricular free wall in 1 or

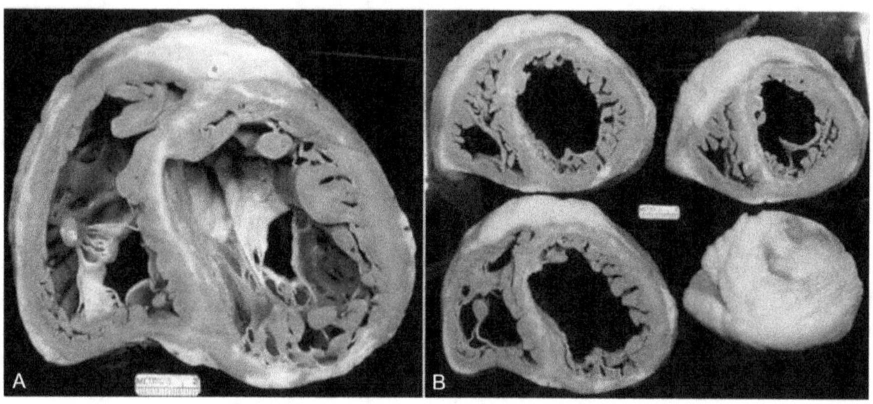



**FIGURE 3.** Ischemic cardiomyopathy. The heart in a 48-year-old man who had had at least 2 acute myocardial infarcts in the past. One is located posteriorly and the other anteriorly. The left ventricular ejection fraction was about 5%. (a) View of the heart showing both tricuspid and mitral valves. Both ventricles are greatly dilated. The 2 healed myocardial infarcts are clearly seen, and they are opposite one another. The left ventricular cavity measures up to 8 cm. (b) Views of the cardiac ventricles caudal to the picture shown on the left. These views show both the anterior and posterior scars are present from apex to base.

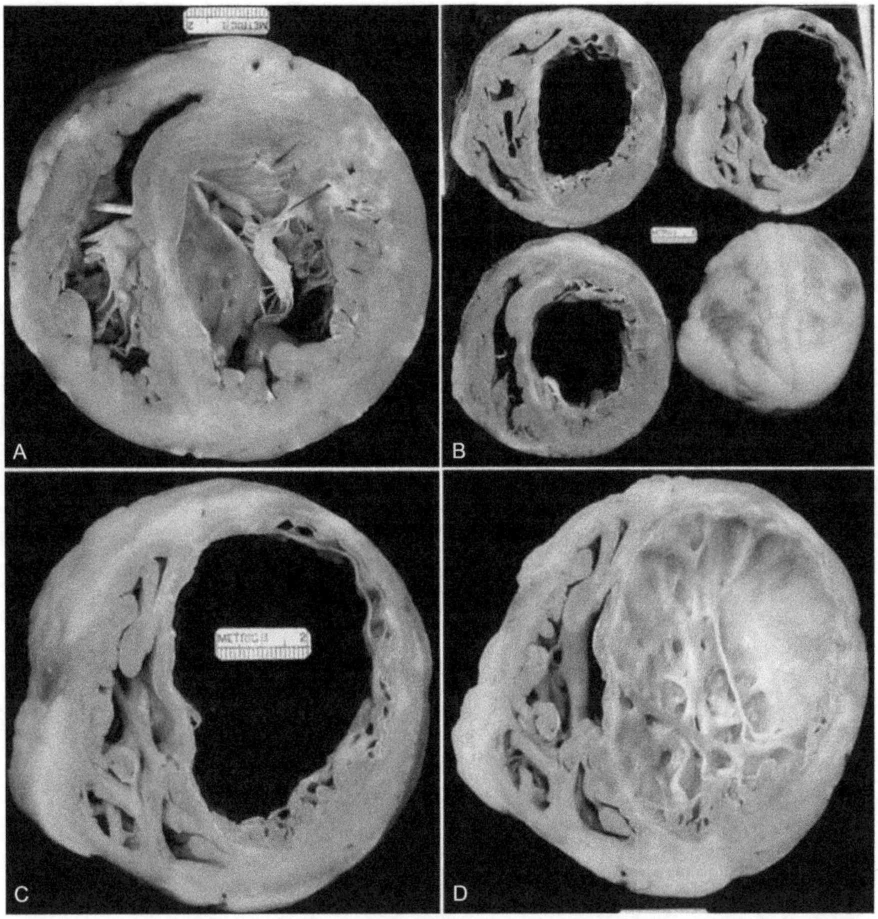


**FIGURE 5.** Ischemic cardiomyopathy. Heart in a 56-year-old man who had a large anterior wall acute myocardial infarct at age 46 years. Subsequently, a stent was inserted into the left anterior descending and left circumflex coronary arteries. His left ventricular ejection fraction shortly before cardiac transplantation was 10%. (a) View of the ventricular cavities at the base showing both tricuspid and mitral valves. A scar is present in the central portion of the ventricular septum and in the anterior left ventricular free wall. (b) Views of the cardiac ventricles caudal to the base showing a huge amount of scaring in the anterior wall of left ventricle with scaring of the entire ventricular septum. Less than half of the left ventricular free wall is devoid of scars. (c) A close-up view of a portion of ventricular walls showing full thickness scarring of the ventricular septum and anterior lateral left ventricular free wall. (d) View of the interior of the left ventricular apex showing the extensive septal and free wall left ventricular scaring.

more areas being >2 times the thickness of the underlying compacted portion of the wall and unassociated with narrowing of the epicardial coronary arteries.[11,45,68] Clinically, each of the 3 patients were diagnosed as "non-IC." One of the 3 patients had a small grossly visible left ventricular scar.

## Mononuclear Myocarditis

Three patients had active or healed mononuclear myocarditis (Table 5, Figures 24 and 25). The key identifying mark of this condition was focal subepicardial left ventricular wall lesions.[19,25,58,60,62,65] Each had mononuclear -cell infiltrates–mainly lymphocytes–in the left ventricular free wall or subepicardial scars with or without mononuclear-cell infiltrates and without granulomas. The hearts were of increased weight (>350 g in women; >400 g in men), and the ventricular cavities were very dilated. One of the 3 patients had significant narrowing by atherosclerotic plaque of 1 or more epicardial coronary arteries. This patient clinically was diagnosed as IC, the other 2 as "non-IC."

## Arrhythmogenic Right Ventricular Cardiomyopathy

Four patients had ARVC; pertinent findings for them are summarized in Table 6 and illustrated in Figure 26.[2,4,8,12,14,28,31,32,46,64,66,70,72,73] All 4 during life were diagnosed as "non-IC." All 4 had thinning of the right ventricular free wall with replacement of the myocardial wall focally by adipose tissue and/or scar tissue without focal thinning (except in 1 patient) of the left ventricular free wall. All 4 had very dilated ventricular chambers. Before CT all 4 had documented runs of ventricular tachycardia. Three had other family members with a similar cardiac disease.

## Cardiac Sarcoidosis

Pertinent findings in the 8 cardiac sarcoidosis patients are summarized in Table 7 and illustrated in Figure 27.[9,15,43,47,52,62,67] All 8 were diagnosed clinically as "non-IC." Six had focal but extensive scars in the free walls of both right and left ventricles and in the ventricular septum

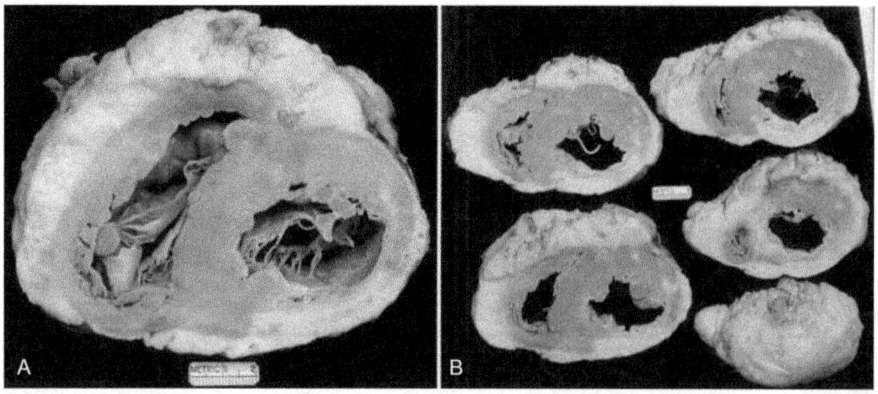

FIGURE 6. Ischemic cardiomyopathy. Heart in a 56-year-old man who at age 49 years had an acute myocardial infarction, and percutaneous coronary intervention with multiple stents was performed. Six months later he underwent coronary artery bypass grafting. Heart failure gradually progressed thereafter such that the left ventricular ejection fraction fell to 25%. (a) View of the basal portion of the heart exposing both tricuspid and mitral valves. The posterior wall of left ventricular is transmurally scarred resulting in the ventricular septum's being thicker than the left ventricular free wall. The quantity of subepicardial adipose tissue is enormous, such that the heart floated in a container of formaldehyde. (b) Views of the ventricles more caudally showing that the posterior wall infarct extends from apex to base.

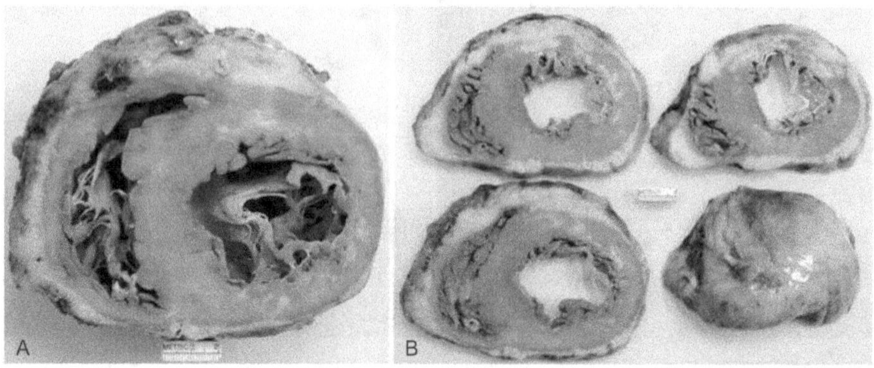

FIGURE 7. Ischemic cardiomyopathy. Views of the heart showing a transmural left ventricular scar from apex to base and a lateral and posterior walls scar which is probably not transmural in a 57-year-old man who had an acute myocardial infarct at age 48 years followed later by a coronary bypass grafting. Heart failure gradually progressed through the years, and his lowest left ventricular ejection fraction was 30%. (a) View of the base of the heart exposing both tricuspid and mitral valves. There is scarring in the anterior wall and in the posterior lateral wall. The lateral wall is much thinner than the ventricular septum. (b) Views of the ventricles more caudally showing extensive transmural anterior wall scarring. The quantity of subepicardial adipose tissue is increased.

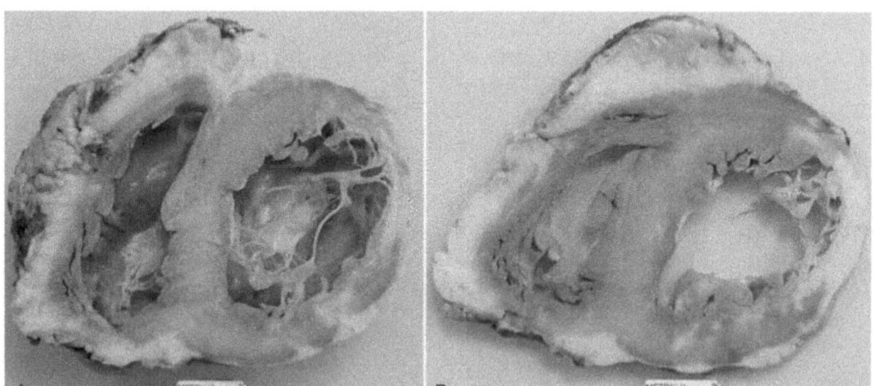

FIGURE 8. Ischemic cardiomyopathy. Heart in a 58-year-old man who had an acute myocardial infarct at age 29 years. A sibling and a parent had had myocardial infarcts at age 42 years. He clearly had heterozygous familial hypercholesterolemia. At age 30 years, he had coronary bypass grafting. His lowest left ventricular ejection fraction was 20%. (a) View of the basal portion of the heart exposing both tricuspid and mitral valves. The anterolateral wall is transmurally scarred such that the ventricular septum is thicker than the left ventricular free wall. (b) A more caudal view of the left ventricular wall showing the severe degree of scarring in the lateral wall with lesser degrees of scarring in the anterior and posterior walls. The quantity of subepicardial adipose tissue is increased.

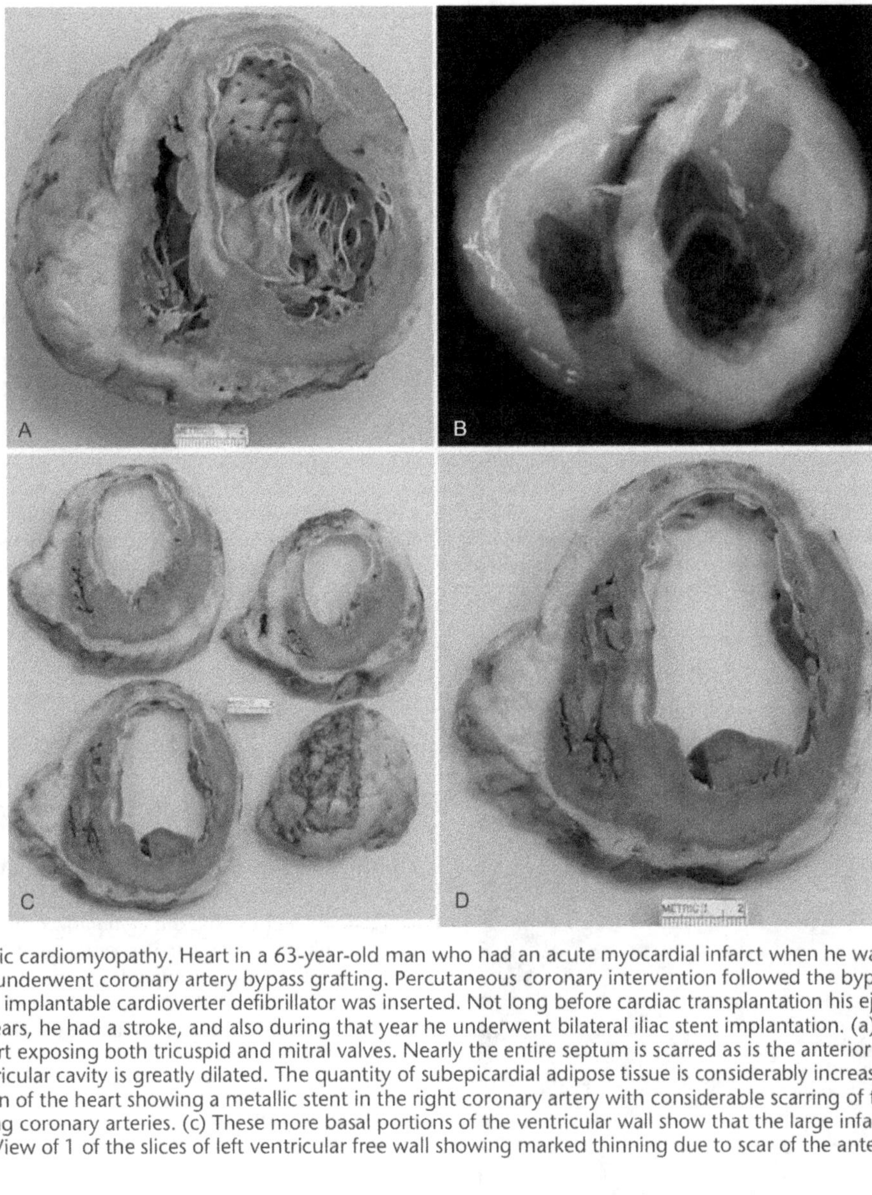


**FIGURE 9.** Ischemic cardiomyopathy. Heart in a 63-year-old man who had an acute myocardial infarct when he was 51 years of age. Subsequently, he underwent coronary artery bypass grafting. Percutaneous coronary intervention followed the bypass operation, and at age 58 years an implantable cardioverter defibrillator was inserted. Not long before cardiac transplantation his ejection fraction was 15%. At age 61 years, he had a stroke, and also during that year he underwent bilateral iliac stent implantation. (a) View of the basal portion of the heart exposing both tricuspid and mitral valves. Nearly the entire septum is scarred as is the anterior left ventricular free wall. The left ventricular cavity is greatly dilated. The quantity of subepicardial adipose tissue is considerably increased. (b) Radiograph of the basal portion of the heart showing a metallic stent in the right coronary artery with considerable scarring of the right and left anterior descending coronary arteries. (c) These more basal portions of the ventricular wall show that the large infarct extends to the cardiac apex. (d) View of 1 of the slices of left ventricular free wall showing marked thinning due to scar of the anterior wall.

without associated narrowing of the epicardial coronary arteries (except for 1 patient), and the scarring tended to be subepicardial. The ventricular chambers were very dilated in all 8 patients. Non-caseating giant cell granulomas were present in the ventricular walls in 7 of the 8 patients. In 1 patient the typical "hard" granulomas were present in the portion of left ventricular free wall excised to insert a left ventricular assist device but not in the recipient heart sometime later. Another patient had right and left ventricular free wall and ventricular septal scarring typical of cardiac sarcoidosis but no granulomas were found in the histologic sections of left ventricular free wall. This case we believe is an example of "burnt out" sarcoidosis.[43]

## Cardiac Amyloidosis

Pertinent findings in the 3 cardiac amyloidosis patients are summarized in Table 8, and the hearts are illustrated in Figure 28.[7,10,16–18,40,53,69] The clinical and morphologic diagnoses were congruous in all 3 patients. The ventricular cavities were either not dilated or dilated to a small degree. The patients had firm—actually rubbery—myocardium, no grossly visible focal myocardial lesions but focal endocardial lesions in either the right atrium or left atrium or both and in the tricuspid valve leaflets. The presence of amyloid was confirmed by Congo-red stains of sections of the heart. Two of the 3 patients had narrowing >75% in cross-sectional area by atherosclerotic plaque, but none had grossly visible ventricular wall scars.

## Adriamycin Cardiomyopathy

Pertinent findings in the 6 patients with Adriamycin cardiomyopathy are summarized in Table 9 and illustrated in Figure 29.[22,26,27,41,44] The clinical and morphologic diagnoses were congruous in each. All 6 had severely dilated ventricular chambers. All had received Adriamycin for cancer treatment.

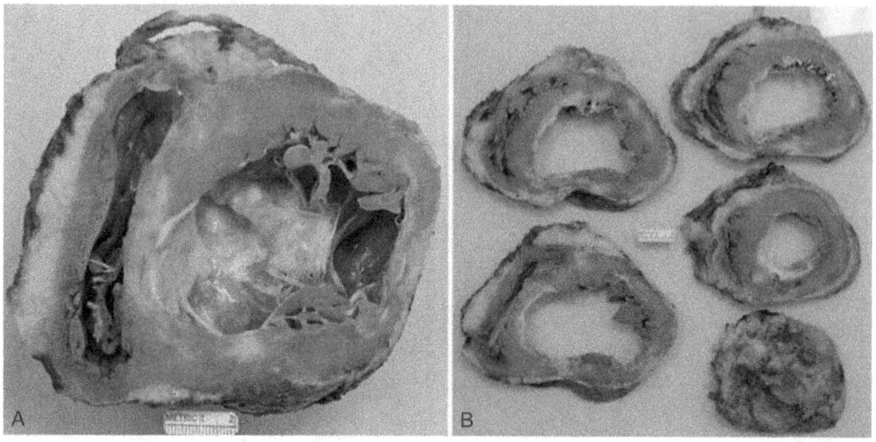



**FIGURE 10.** Ischemic cardiomyopathy. Heart in a 61-year-old man who had a acute myocardial infarct at age 53 years followed by a coronary artery bypass grafting. By age 59 years, his left ventricular ejection fraction was as low as 15%. An intracardiac defibrillator had been inserted also at age 54 years. (a) View of the basal portion of the heart showing a portion of tricuspid valve and a good bit of the anterior mitral leaflet. A large transmural scar is present in the lateral wall between the 2 left ventricular papillary muscles and in the ventricular septum in apposition to the lateral wall infarct. The left ventricular cavity is greatly dilated. (b) View of the more caudal portions of the ventricular wall again showing the 2 infarcts extending almost to the apex of the heart.

## Valvular Heart Disease

Pertinent findings in the 7 patients with valvular heart disease are summarized in Table 10.[39,50,57] Four had aortic valve stenosis initially and repeated valve replacements; 1 had mitral valve replacements for mitral stenosis in 1 and for pure mitral regurgitation in the other. The latter patient also had severe tricuspid valve regurgitation, which had not been approached at a previous operation. The clinical and morphologic diagnoses were congruous in all 7 patients.

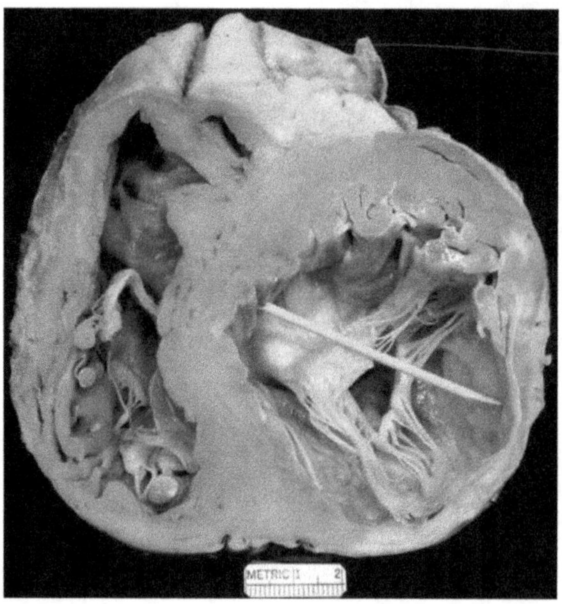

**FIGURE 11.** Ischemic cardiomyopathy. Heart in a 67-year-old man who had a large acute myocardial infarction at age 53 followed by coronary artery bypass grafting. At age 60, he had another bypass grafting operation. Heart failure progressed and was accompanied by several mitral regurgitation. His ejection fraction not long before cardiac transplantation was 10%. The view of the heart shows its basal portion exposing both mitral and tricuspid valves. The posterior and lateral walls of the heart are extremely thin from the extensive scarring. The posteromedial papillary muscle is flattened from the scarring and the anterolateral 1 is atrophied. The ventricular septum as a consequence is much thicker than the left ventricular free wall.

## Cyanotic Congenital Heart Disease

Pertinent findings in the 3 patients with cyanotic congenital heart disease are summarized in Table 11.[38,63] One had complex complete transposition of the great arteries, 1 severe right ventricular hypoplasia, and 1 tetralogy of Fallot. All 3 had had more than 1 previous cardiac operation. The clinical and morphologic diagnosis were congruous in all 3.

## Other

One patient had CT for ventricular septal defect resulting from a stab wound to the heart many years earlier. Details of this patient are described elsewhere.[48]

## Outcomes

The survival probabilities for all 257 patients are shown in Figure 30. Of the 257 (of 314) patients in whom survival data are available, 66 (26%) have died: 8 (12%) within 60 days of CT and 58 (88%) at later periods. The log-rank test show no significant survival differences between men and women (log-rank = 0.479, p value = 0.4926) (Figure 30).

# DISCUSSION

The present study serves 2 major functions: 1) it illustrates by gross photographs of the hearts the variability that occurs morphologically in each of the etiologic categories, and 2) it determines the frequency among the 314 patients of discrepancies between the clinical and morphologic diagnoses. Just like clinical presentations and courses are quite variable among patients with various types of cardiac diseases, the morphologic features in each type of cardiac

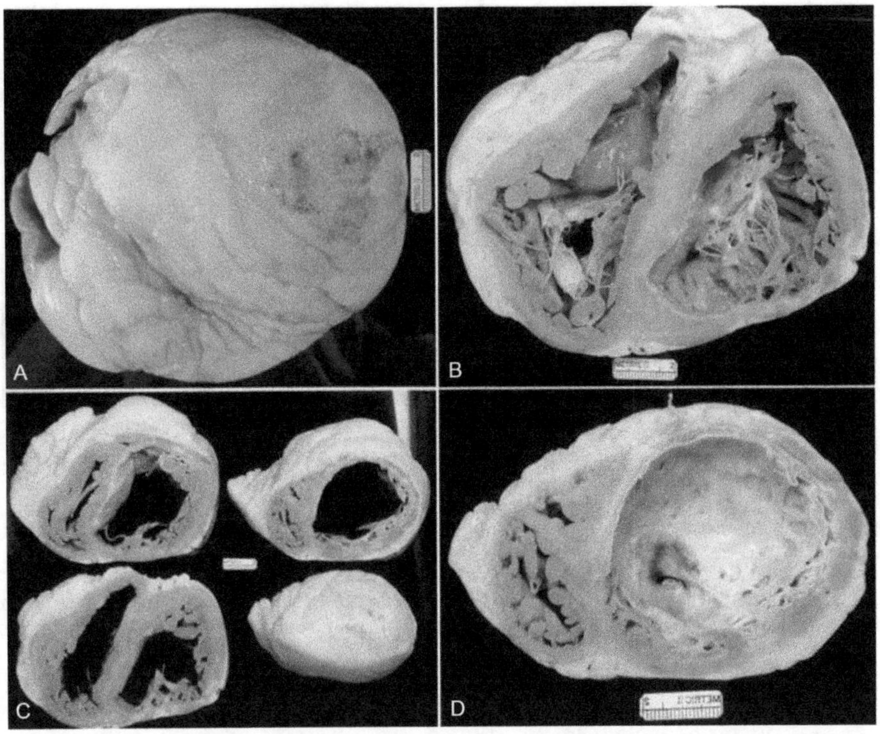

**FIGURE 12.** Ischemic cardiomyopathy. Heart in a 67-year-old man who had a large anterior wall infarct and another posterior wall infarct in the distant past. The exact dates of the infarcts are unclear, but radiograph of the excised heart showed calcium in the wall of the apex of the left ventricle indicating that the infarct was probably at least 10 years earlier. Heart failure had been a problem for many years. The left ventricular ejection fraction not long before cardiac transplantation was as low as 5%. (a) View of the exterior of the heart showing that most of the myocardial walls are covered by adipose tissue. (b) View of the base of the heart exposing both tricuspid and mitral valves. The posterior left ventricular free wall is thinned by scar tissue. (c) Views of the ventricles more caudally now showing both anterior and posterior wall infarcts. (d) View of the apex showing scarring in probably 300° of the 360° left ventricular wall. The heart contained so much adipose tissue that it floated in formaldehyde.

disease are also quite variable. To properly illustrate that variability a number of photographs of recipient hearts are presented.

As part of the second purpose of this report, we determined the frequency of congruity or incongruity between the clinical and morphologic diagnoses among the 314 patients. As shown in Table 1, most (96%) of the patients with IC at morphologic study had been diagnosed with that condition clinically. The discrepancy occurred when 6 patients with IC anatomically had insignificant coronary narrowing by angiography before CT, but nevertheless severe narrowing of 1 or more major epicardial coronary arteries morphologically and extensive left ventricular wall scarring. We defined IC as the presence of severe

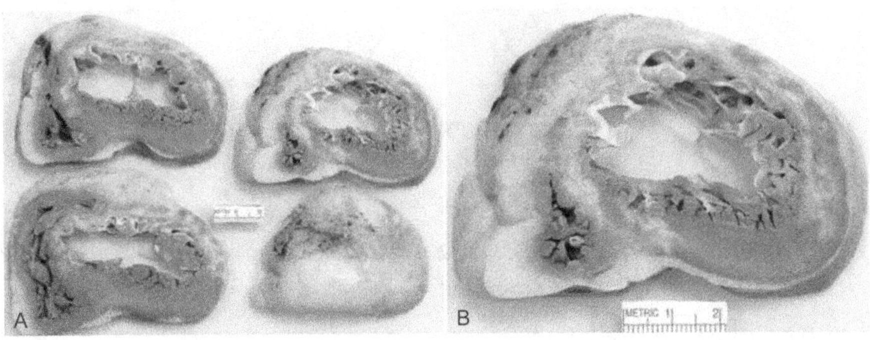

**FIGURE 13.** Ischemic cardiomyopathy. Heart in a 69-year-old man who had a large myocardial infarct, involving the anterior, septal, and lateral walls of the left ventricle only 4 months earlier with severe heart failure thereafter. (a) Sections of the ventricular walls caudal to the atrioventricular valves show a healed septal, anterior, and lateral wall infarct from apex to base. (b) A close-up of 1 of the slices showing the extensive scarring.

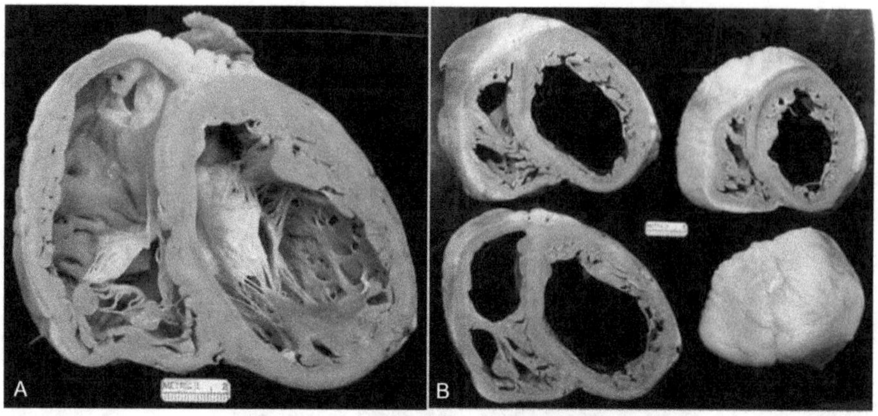

FIGURE 14. Idiopathic dilated cardiomyopathy. Heart of a 68-year-old man who had had evidence of heart failure since age 54 years. He was known to have severe hypothyroidism and was treated appropriately. He had never had chest pain. He did however have evidence of chronic obstructive lung disease and at 1 time was a habitual alcoholic. He also was known to have a fatty liver. The lowest left ventricular ejection fraction before transplantation was 5%. (a) View of the cardiac ventricles at the base exposing the tricuspid, mitral, and pulmonic valves. Both ventricular cavities are enormously dilated, and the walls of the left ventricle, ventricular septum, and right ventricle are free of foci of fibrosis and necrosis. (b) Views of the ventricles caudal to the atrioventricular valves. The moderator band is prominent in the right ventricle. The right coronary artery wall was quite calcified, and the lumen was quite narrowed. Nevertheless, the patient was classified as having idiopathic dilated cardiomyopathy because there were no lesions in the myocardial walls. It appears that this happened to be a patient who had both a narrowed coronary artery and idiopathic dilated cardiomyopathy.

(>75% in cross-sectional area) coronary narrowing accompanied by 1 or more transmural left ventricular wall scars. The reverse occurred in the case of IDC. Of the 111 patients with IDC anatomically (no left ventricular wall lesion grossly), 11 had severe narrowing of 1 or more major epicardial coronary arteries such that these patients in actuality did not fulfill our definitions for either IC or IDC. We suspect, however, that these 11 patients actually had IDC but resided in a high-cholesterol environment (United States), where coronary atherosclerosis is so prevalent.

Most of the incongruity between clinical and morphologic diagnoses occurred in the non-IC subgroups other than IDC. Thus, among the 56 patients with non-IC, excluding the patients with IDC, only 31 (55%) had congruity between the clinical and morphologic diagnoses. Specifically, among the 17 patients with HC, the 3 with NCLVC, the 3 with

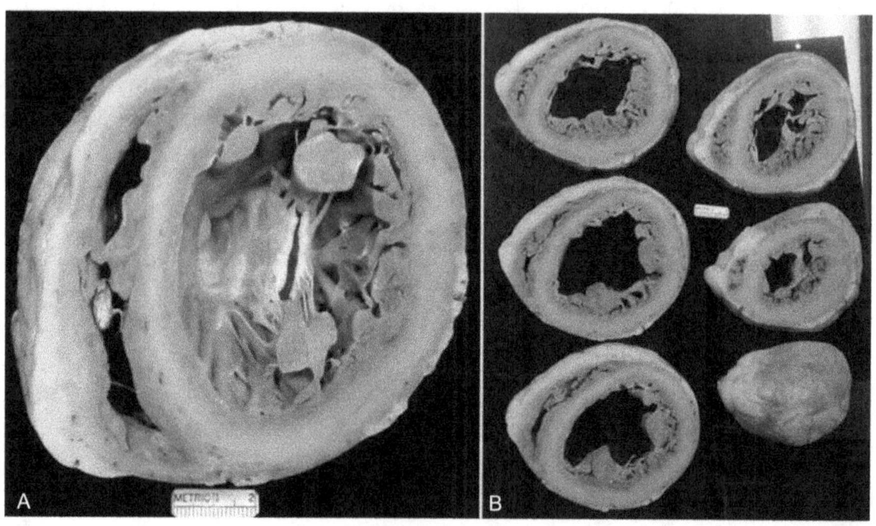

FIGURE 15. Idiopathic dilated cardiomyopathy. Views of the heart in a 61-year-old woman who had had evidence of chronic heart failure since age 51 years. She did reasonably well on medical therapy until age 59 years, when the heart failure worsened considerably and an implantable cardiac defibrillator was inserted. During the 2 years before transplant, the heart failure progressively worsened, and the left ventricular ejection fraction fell to a low of approximately 10%. She never had chest pain. Earlier in life she had had several children. (a) Basal portion of heart exposing well the mitral valve. The left ventricle is greatly enlarged measuring up to 7.5 cm. No foci of fibrosis or necrosis are seen in the ventricular walls. (b) Views of the ventricles caudal to the mitral valve, again showing considerable left ventricular cavity dilatation.

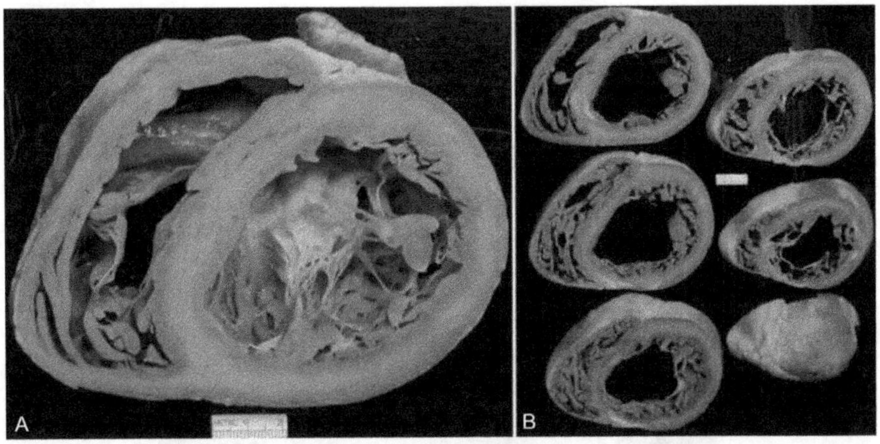

**FIGURE 16.** Idiopathic dilated cardiomyopathy. Heart in a 62-year-old woman who developed evidence of heart failure at age 55 years, which progressed thereafter. During the 7 months before cardiac transplant, the heart failure worsened considerably. Coronary angiography showed the major epicardial coronary arteries to be wide open. (a) Basal portion of heart exposing both tricuspid and mitral valves. Both ventricular cavities are considerably dilated. No foci of fibrosis or necrosis were noted in this portion of the ventricular walls. (b) Views of the ventricles caudal to the atrioventricular valves. In this view the posterior wall is thinned by scar tissue as is the most posterior portion of ventricular septum. The right coronary artery, as well as the others, was wide open. The focal scar may have been due to a coronary embolus many years earlier.

mononuclear myocarditis, the 4 with ARVC, and the 8 with cardiac sarcoidosis, a total of 35 patients, only 11 (31%) had the specific diagnosis made clinically. One could argue that including the single case without cardiac granulomas in the sarcoid group is improper. The type and distribution of the myocardial scarring, however, is absolutely typical of the other cases of cardiac sarcoidosis, a type of scarring not seen by us in any other condition.[43] Additionally, documented sarcoid granulomas in the lungs have been shown to disappear as the scarring increases.[59] Obviously, it is not sufficient to stop clinically with the diagnosis of non-IC cardiomyopathy. Ideally, of course, the specific subgroup needs to be sought even though therapy and outcome might not be altered by that knowledge.

The present study is not the first to compare the frequencies of discrepancies between the clinical and morphologic diagnoses in patients having CT. Bortman and colleagues[6] in 1994 examined the congruity-incongruity issue in 112 patients who underwent their first orthotopic CT at the authors' institution (University of Texas Southwestern

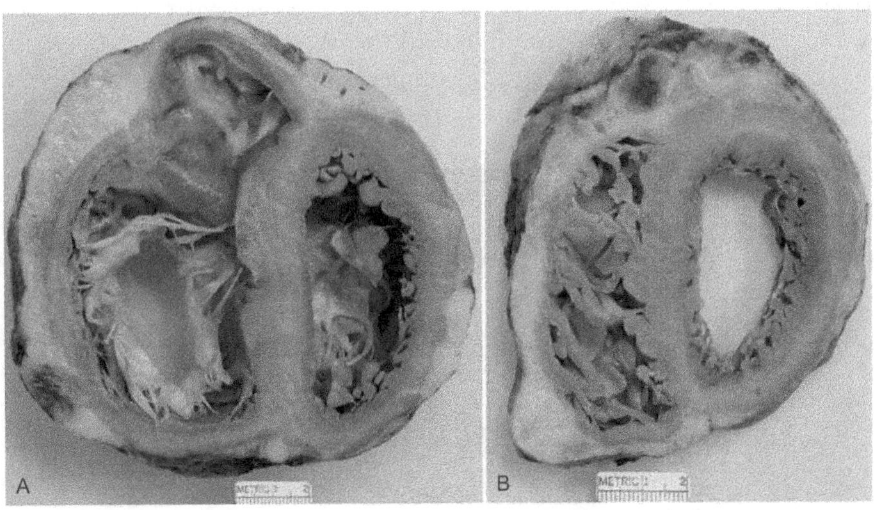

**FIGURE 17.** Idiopathic dilated cardiomyopathy. Heart of a 68-year-old man who was found to have heart failure at age 50 years, and, at the time, also to have severe mitral regurgitation. Coronary angiogram showed the coronary arteries to be wide open. At age 50 years, the patient underwent repair of the mitral valve including the insertion of an annular ring. The mitral regurgitation was reduced from severe to mild, but the heart failure continued and progressed. A left ventricular assist device was inserted before the cardiac transplantation. (a) View of the basal portion of the heart showing dilatation of both right and left ventricular cavities. The tricuspid annulus is quite dilated. No lesions are noted in the ventricular walls although the ventricular septum is thicker than the left ventricular free wall. (b) View more caudal showing impressive pectinate muscles within the right ventricular cavity. Again, no myocardial lesions are noted. The quantity of subepicardial adipose tissue is considerably increased.

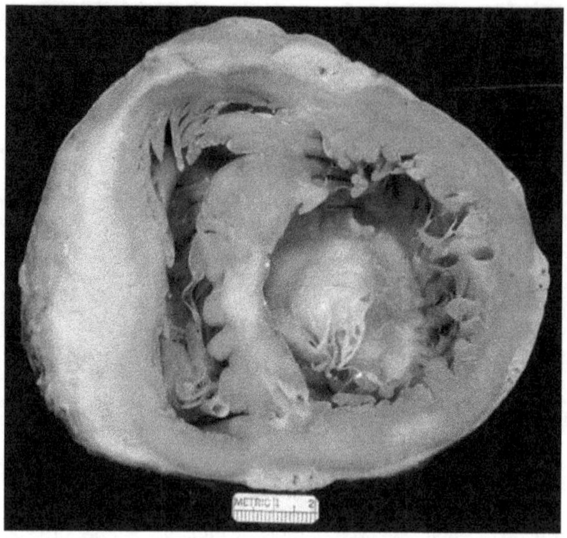

FIGURE 18. Hypertrophic cardiomyopathy. Heart in a 41-year-old man in whom hypertrophic cardiomyopathy was diagnosed when he was 6 years of age. At age 26 years, atrial fibrillation appeared and during the next 15 years he was cardioverted 98 times. He eventually developed complete heart block, and a pacemaker was inserted. At age 30 years, an intracardiac defibrillator was implanted, and at the same time an alcohol septal ablation procedure was performed. Nevertheless, evidence of heart failure persisted and a heart transplant was performed. View of the basal portion exposing both tricuspid and mitral valves. The left ventricular cavity is quite dilated. The focal scar in the ventricular septum may be the result of the alcohol septal ablation. Another small scar is present in the posterior wall of left ventricle. The thickness of the ventricular septum is greater than that of the left ventricular free wall.

Medical Center at Dallas). Among their 64 patients diagnosed with IC clinically, all had severe coronary narrowing morphologically; of their 48 patients with IDC clinically, 12 (25%) morphologically had severe coronary disease, and 3 had acute myocarditis. Thus, of their 112 patients a discrepancy between pre- and post-transplant diagnosis occurred in 15 (13%). Neither gross photographs nor definitions of the entities were provided.

In 1999, Angelini and colleagues[1] from Padua, Italy, studied the agreement or lack thereof between pre- and post-CT diagnoses in 257 patients having CT, and found a discrepancy between clinical and pathologic diagnoses in 20 patients (8%). Among their 87 patients with a clinical diagnoses of IC, 3 had IDC and 1 granulomatous myocarditis; among their 126 patients whose clinical diagnosis was non-IC, 7 morphologically had IC, 5 myocarditis, 1 ARVC, and 1 with NCLVC; among their 10 patients with a clinical diagnosis of HC, 1 had ARVC, and 1 had a cardiac fibroma.[1] No gross photographs of the heart or definitions of the conditions were provided.

In 2009, Luk and colleagues[29] from Toronto, Canada, studied the problem in 296 patients who had had CT from

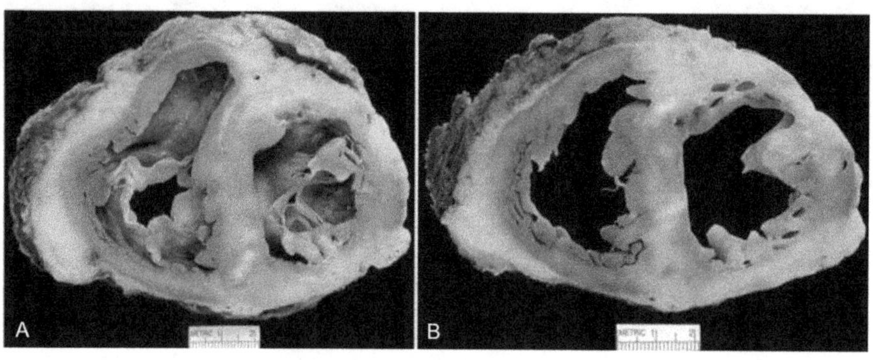


FIGURE 19. Hypertrophic cardiomyopathy. The heart in a 48-year-old man who developed heart failure at age 41 years and had an intracardiac defibrillator inserted shortly thereafter. A left ventricular assist device was inserted 2.3 years before cardiac transplantation. At age 45 years, he developed atrial fibrillation and had several cardioversion procedures performed. A parent and several cousins had heart disease of unclear type and were either asymptomatic or had died from it. (a) View of the base of the heart exposing both tricuspid and mitral valves. There is considerable scarring in the left ventricular and ventricular septal walls and in both papillary muscles. Both cavities are quite dilated. The thickness of the ventricular septum is greater than that of the left ventricular free wall. (b) Another view more caudal showing extensive scarring. The left anterior descending coronary artery is narrowed on this slice, probably the result of extensive scaring surrounding it. (Figure 19a is reprinted with permission from Elsevier.[49])

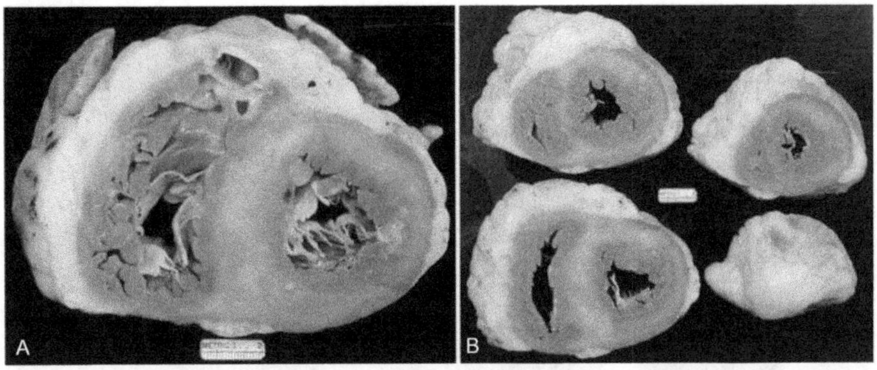

**FIGURE 20.** Hypertrophic cardiomyopathy. This 68-year-old man was diagnosed with hypertrophic cardiomyopathy many years earlier. His major problem was recurrent episodes of ventricular tachycardia, and he underwent an ablation procedure for that. He also had atrial fibrillation and other atrial arrhythmias. An implantable cardiac defibrillator was inserted. He also was obese, had obstructive sleep apnea, and chronic renal disease, stage 3. (a) View of the cardiac base exposing tricuspid, pulmonic, and mitral valves. The thickness of the ventricular septum is greater than that of the left ventricular free wall. The 2 ventricular cavities are only mildly dilated. Calcium was present in the mitral annular area. (b) Views of the ventricles caudal to the views shown on the left.

1987 to 2006 (Table 12). The frequency of the diagnosis made clinically and after examination of the recipient heart is shown in Table 12. It is apparent that the incongruity between the clinical and morphologic diagnoses was relatively frequent. Three gross photographs of the heart were presented. Definitions of the various conditions were not provided.

It is apparent from the present and previous studies that the largest incongruity between clinical and morphologic diagnosis in patients having CT is among the non-IC subtypes, particularly the dilated (end-stage) form of HC, mononuclear myocarditis, cardiac sarcoidosis, ARVC, and NCLVC. Would the use of additional diagnostic "instruments of precision" have allowed more precise pre-CT diagnosis among the non-IC group? Possibly so, particularly more use of magnetic resonance imaging among the patients with HC and sarcoidosis.[35] Would a more

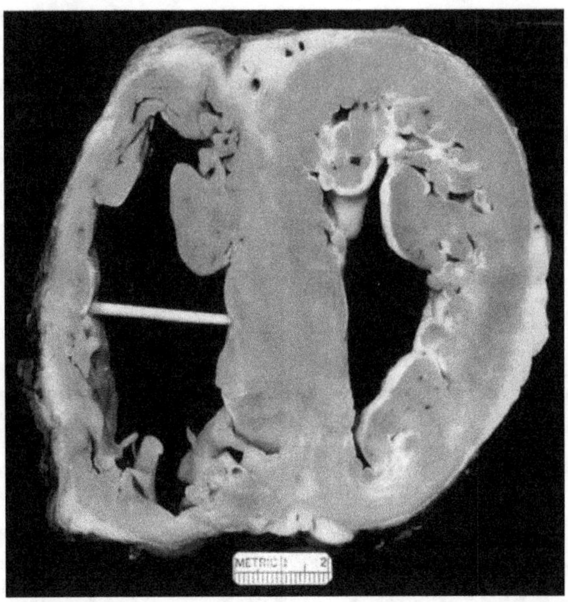

**FIGURE 21.** Hypertrophic cardiomyopathy. View of the heart in a 68-year-old man who was known to have some form of heart disease since age 38 years. The problem during the 30 years was various degrees of heart failure which began progressing about age 55 years. In the 2 years before cardiac transplantation he had multiple hospitalizations for decompensated heart failure. He had an intracardiac defibrillator in place for several years. Because of the severity of the heart failure, a left ventricular assist device was inserted 7 months before cardiac transplantation. The heart failure severity, however, continued, and before heart transplantation the left ventricular ejection fraction was approximately 10%. Both cardiac ventricles are dilated, the right more than the left. The ventricular septum is thicker than the left ventricular free wall. The mural endocardium of the left ventricle is thickened by white fibrous tissue. A scar is present in the posterior portion of the left ventricular free wall and also in the posterior portion of the ventricular septum.

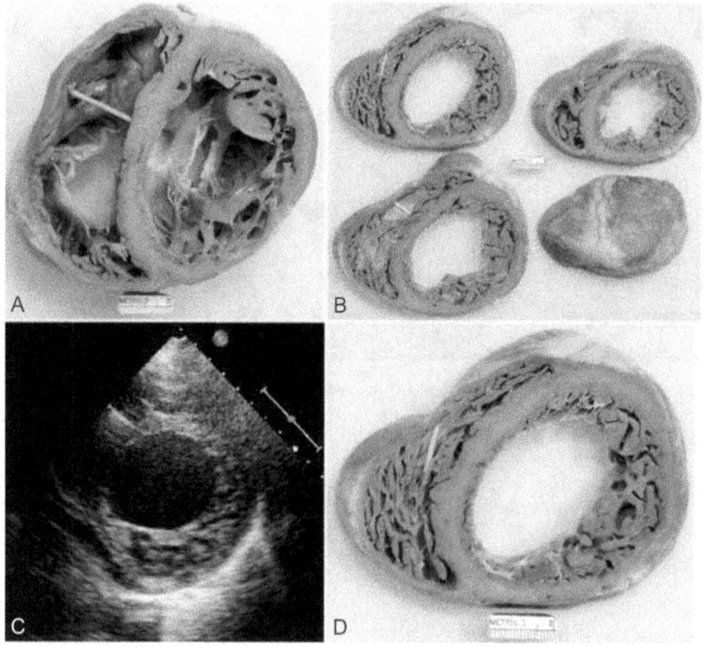

**FIGURE 22.** Left ventricular non-compaction cardiomyopathy. Heart in a 49-year-old man who had been well until age 33 years when symptoms of heart failure appeared. At the time, echocardiogram showed both ventricles to be dilated and the left ventricular systolic function to be severely depressed. A defibrillator was inserted at age 39 years, and cardiac resynchronization therapy at age 43 years. He underwent ablation therapy for multiple episodes of ventricular tachycardia. His left ventricular ejection fraction just before cardiac transplantation was 15%. (a) View of both ventricles just caudal to the tricuspid and mitral valves. The thickness of the ventricular septum is much greater than that of the left ventricular free wall. The compacted portion of left ventricular free wall is much thinner than the non-compacted portion. Both ventricular cavities are greatly dilated. The left ventricular free wall posteriorly is focally scarred. (a) View of the basal portion of the heart exposing the tricuspid and mitral valves. Both ventricles are greatly dilated. The posterolateral wall is focally scarred. The compacted portion of left ventricular free wall is much thinner than the trabeculated portion. (b) Views of sections of the ventricular walls caudal to the view shown in the upper left. (c) Echocardiogram showing hypertrabeculation of the left ventricular free wall. (d) Section of the left ventricular free wall corresponding to the echocardiogram. (Reprinted with permission from Elsevier.[45]).

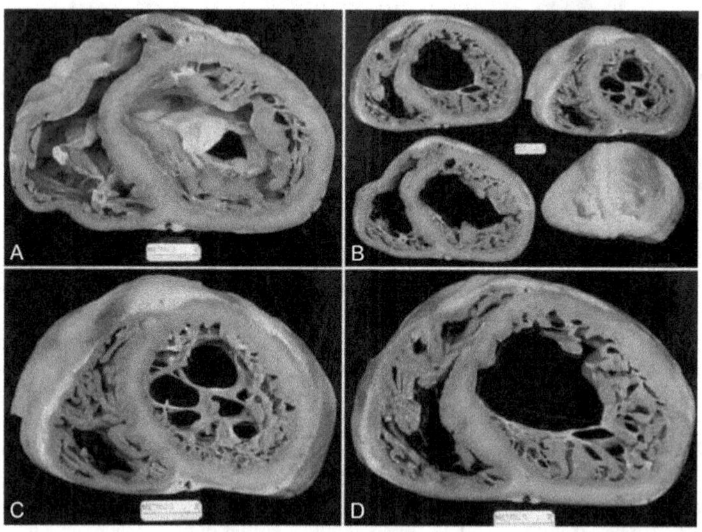

**FIGURE 23.** Left ventricular non-compaction cardiomyopathy. Heart of a 36-year-old woman who was well until approximately age 35 years when she developed evidence of heart failure, which slowly but gradually progressed thereafter such that when she was aged 34 years her left ventricular ejection fraction had fallen to 20% and she was in chronic atrial fibrillation. She also developed runs of ventricular tachycardia for which a defibrillator was inserted. (a) View of the heart showing both tricuspid and mitral valves. Both ventricular cavities are enormously dilated, and the ventricular walls are free of foci of fibrosis and necrosis. (b) Views of the ventricles caudal to the view shown in upper left. (c) Close-up view of 1 of the slices in upper right. (d) View showing the hypertrabeculated or non-compacted portion of the left ventricular wall to be much thicker than the compacted portion. (Reprinted with permission from Elsevier.[45]).

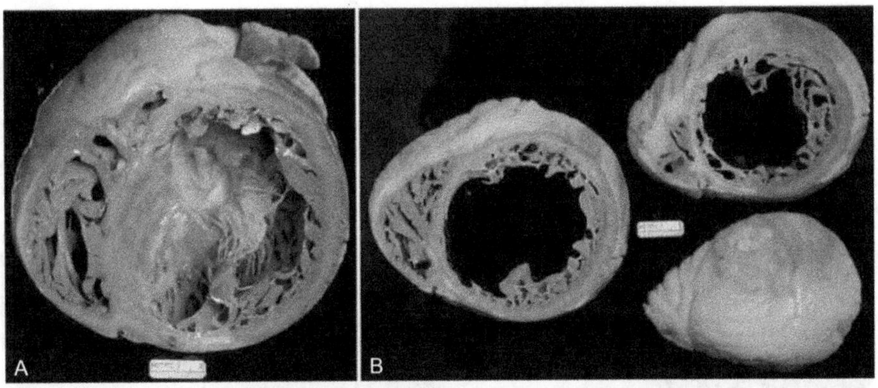


FIGURE 24. Mononuclear myocarditis. The heart in a 56-year-old man who had been well until age 48 years, when he had a cardiac event that resulted in the appearance of heart failure, which progressed thereafter. He also smoked heavily and had evidence of chronic obstructive lung disease. A defibrillator was inserted when he was 53 years old. (a) Basal portion of the heart showing severe dilatation of the left ventricular cavity with transmural scarring in the posterior and anterior left ventricular free wall and in the anterior portion of the ventricular septum. (b) Sections of the ventricular cavities caudal to the view shown on the left. The ventricular septum in 2 of the slices is completely scarred. Histologic section showed focal collections of mononuclear cells in the walls of left ventricle and ventricular septum. The coronary arteries at necropsy were wide open.

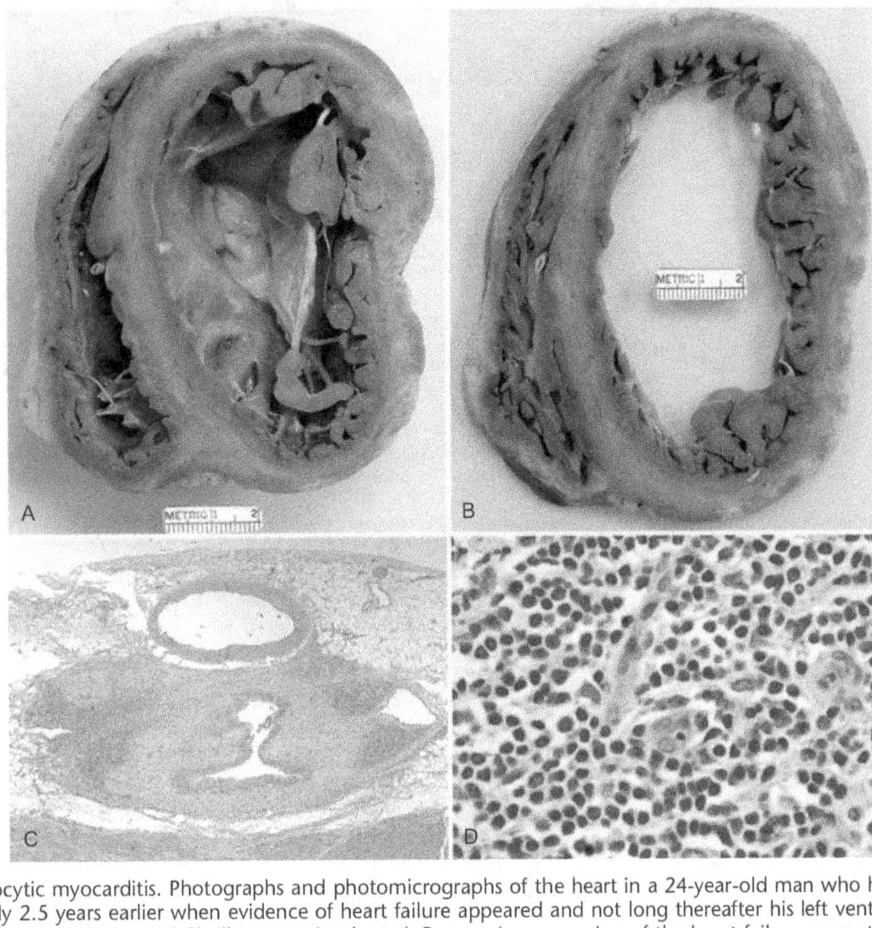


FIGURE 25. Monocytic myocarditis. Photographs and photomicrographs of the heart in a 24-year-old man who had been well until approximately 2.5 years earlier when evidence of heart failure appeared and not long thereafter his left ventricular ejection fraction was approximately 15%. A defibrillator was implanted. Progressive worsening of the heart failure prompted the CT. The echocardiogram 15 months before cardiac transplantation showed his left ventricular ejection fraction to be as low as 5%. (a) View of the cardiac base exposing the mitral valve. (b) Slice of the ventricles more caudal. The scarring and inflammatory cell infiltrates are mainly subepicardial in location. (c) Inflammatory cell collection in the subepicardial adipose tissue (Movat stain ×20). (d) Close-up of the lymphocytes (hematoxylin/eosin stain, ×100).

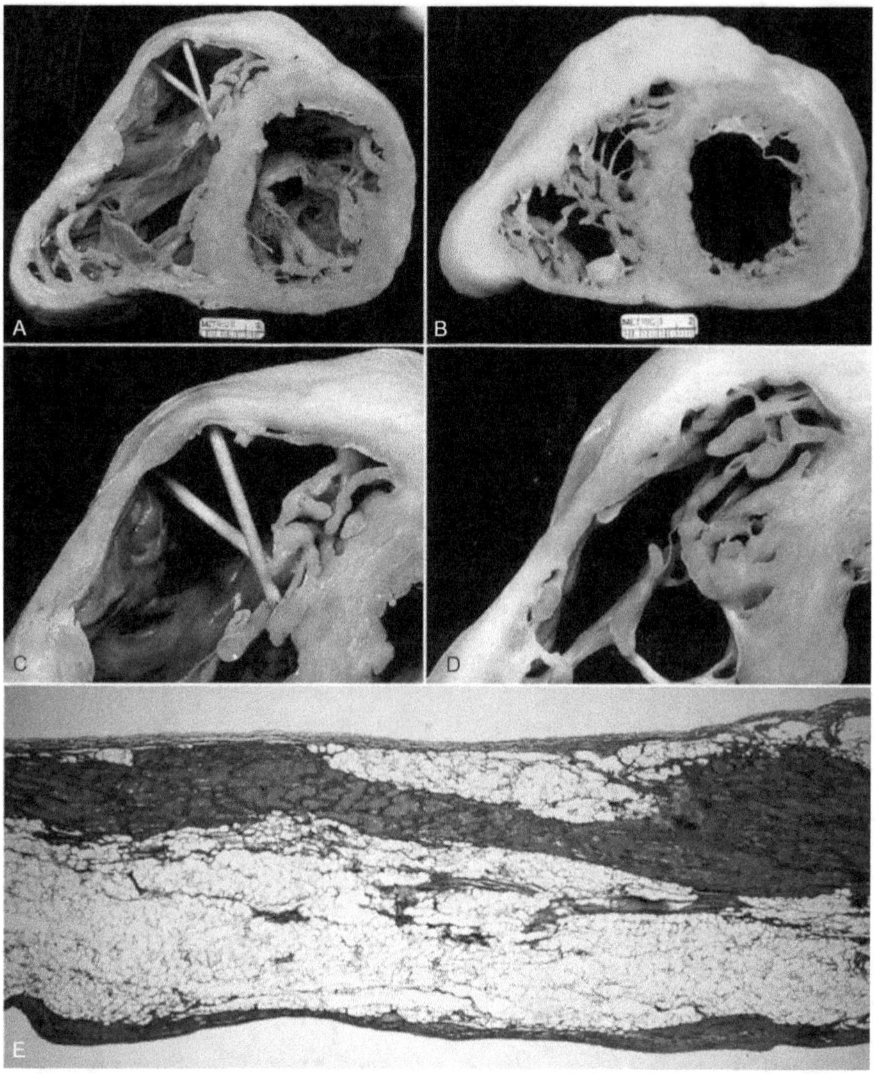


**FIGURE 26.** Arrhythmogenic right ventricular cardiomyopathy. The heart in a 26-year-old man who developed symptoms of heart failure at age 12 years, followed later by ventricular arrhythmias and bundle branch block. His left ventricular ejection fraction fell to 15%. (a) View of the base of the heart showing marked dilatation of both ventricles. The right ventricular wall in its outflow tract is thin (b, c, d). (e) Photomicrograph of the right ventricular wall in the right ventricular outflow tract, which consists of adipose tissue, fibrous tissue, and a few myocardial cells (Masson stain, ×20). (Reprinted with permission from Elsevier.[46]).

accurate pre-CT diagnosis among the non-IC group have led to a re-evaluation of the need for CT in the first place? Or, if clinicians had actually known the specific non-IC diagnosis, would treatment have been different and might CT have been avoided? Among the 314 patients included in this study, the morphologic and clinical diagnoses were incongruent in 42 (13%), including 7 of 17 patients with HC, 3 of 3 with NCLVC, 3 of 3 with mononuclear myocarditis, 4 of 4 with ARVC, and 8 of 8 with cardiac sarcoidosis. This incongruity certainly leaves open the possibility that, if immunosuppressive or immunomodulatory treatment had been used in certain cases, such as specific antiarrhythmic agents for ARVC or intracardiac defibrillator for non-obstructive HC with normal or near-normal left ventricular ejection fraction, this therapy might have made a difference with respect to treatment, outcome, and even potentially the need for CT.

The positive features of the present study include the fact that all hearts were examined and described and all morphologic diagnoses were provided by the same person (WCR), who has been studying cardiovascular diseases for several decades. Had many of the non-IC cases been "grossed" by a first or second year trainee, which is the modus of operation in the surgical pathology laboratory at BUMC—except for the cardiovascular cases—it is unlikely that the cases of burnt-out or end-stage HC, or ARVC, or NCLVC would have been recognized grossly, and histologic examination in these cases would unlikely have provided the proper morphologic diagnoses.

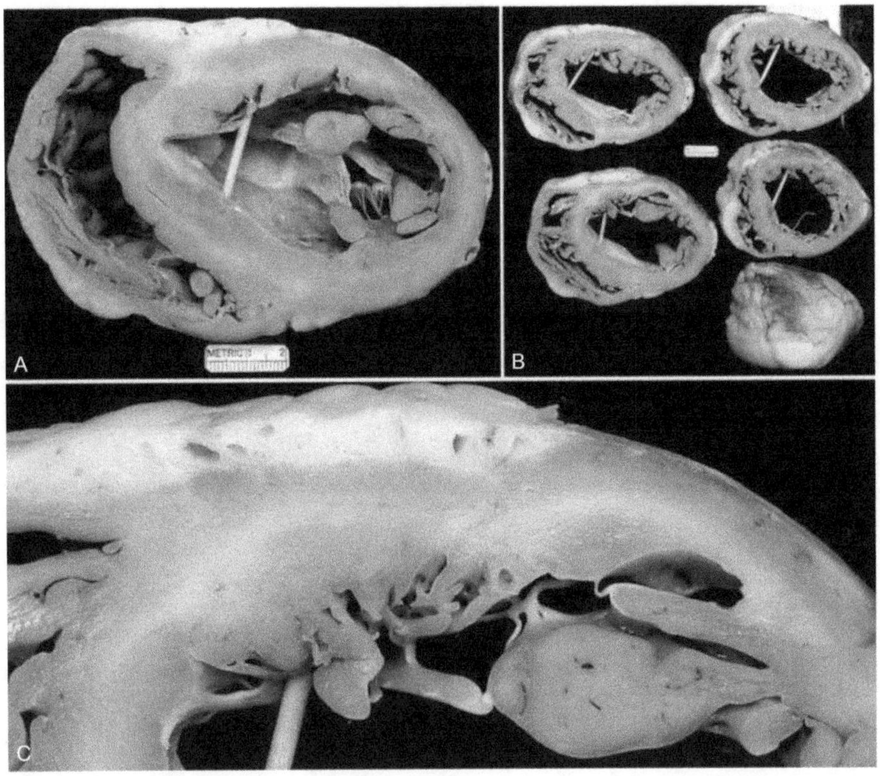

**FIGURE 27.** Cardiac sarcoidosis. Heart in a 52-year-old black woman who had developed evidence of heart failure beginning at age 48 years. It progressed, and an implantable cardiac defibrillator/pacemaker was placed. Runs of ventricular tachycardia occasionally were seen. Cardiac catheterization 8 months before cardiac transplantation disclosed normal coronary arteries, severe global left ventricular hypokinesis, and an estimated ejection fraction of 10%. The pressures in mm Hg were as follows: left ventricle, 115/34; right ventricle, 59/15; pulmonary artery wedge a wave 20, v wave 20, mean 18; right atrium a wave 12, v wave 10, mean 9. The cardiac index was 1.7 L/min per m2. A diagnosis of cardiac sarcoidosis was never entertained clinically. (a) Heart at the base showing the greatly dilated ventricular cavities and scarring in the ventricular septum and left ventricular free wall anteriorly. (b) Cross-section of the ventricles showing the extent of the scarring. (c) Close-up of the left ventricular free wall and ventricular septum showing the scarring. (Reprinted with permission from Elsevier.[43]).

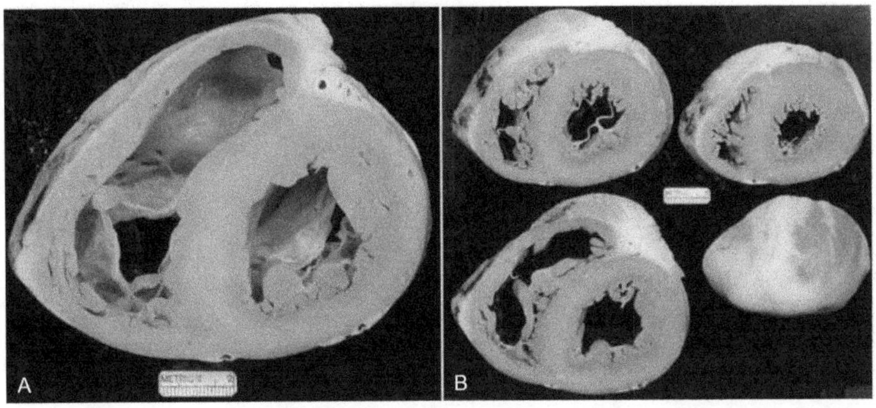

**FIGURE 28.** Cardiac amyloidosis. Heart in a 57-year-old man who had been well until 1 year before cardiac transplantation, when evidence of heart failure appeared. On examination 2 months later he was noted to have periorbital ecchymoses and a biopsy of an abdominal fat pad disclosed amyloidosis. During the year before CT, he lost 40 pounds, and the dyspnea and exercise intolerance progressively worsened. Echocardiogram 5 months before CT disclosed an ejection fraction of 55%, a restrictive diastolic filling pattern, and an "ineffective atrial kick." The heart weighed 420 g and amyloid deposits were extensively present in the walls of all 4 cardiac chambers. The right ventricular cavity was larger than the left ventricular cavity. The epicardial coronary arteries were wide open. Amyloid deposits were extensive in the walls of all 4 cardiac chambers. (a) View of the cardiac base. (b) Views of the more caudal portions of the heart.

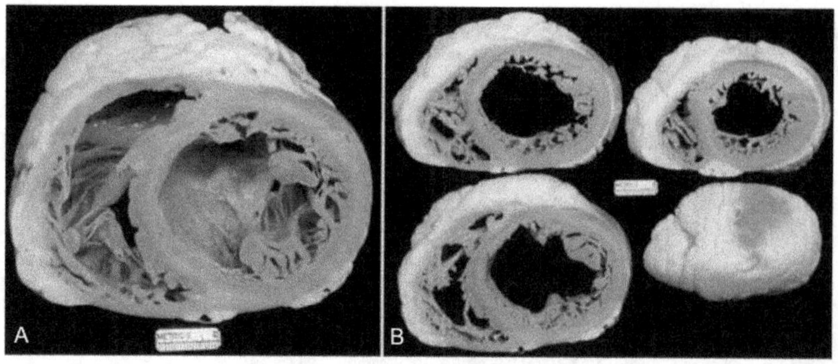


**FIGURE 29.** Adriamycin-induced cardiomyopathy. Heart in a 50-year-old woman who had received Adriamycin at age 38 years (12 years earlier) for cancer of the right breast with total mastectomy. She had evidence of heart failure only a couple of months before CT with rapid progression thereafter such that 1 month before CT her left ventricular ejection fraction was only 10%. The pressures in mm Hg were left ventricle 85/23; aorta 85/50. The cardiac output was 1.2 L/min, the ventricular cavities were severely dilated, and the epicardial coronary arteries were wide open. The heart weighed 405 g and the ventricles were dilated. Histologically, no specific cardiac lesions are present. (a) View of the cardiac base. (b) View of the more caudal cardiac slices.

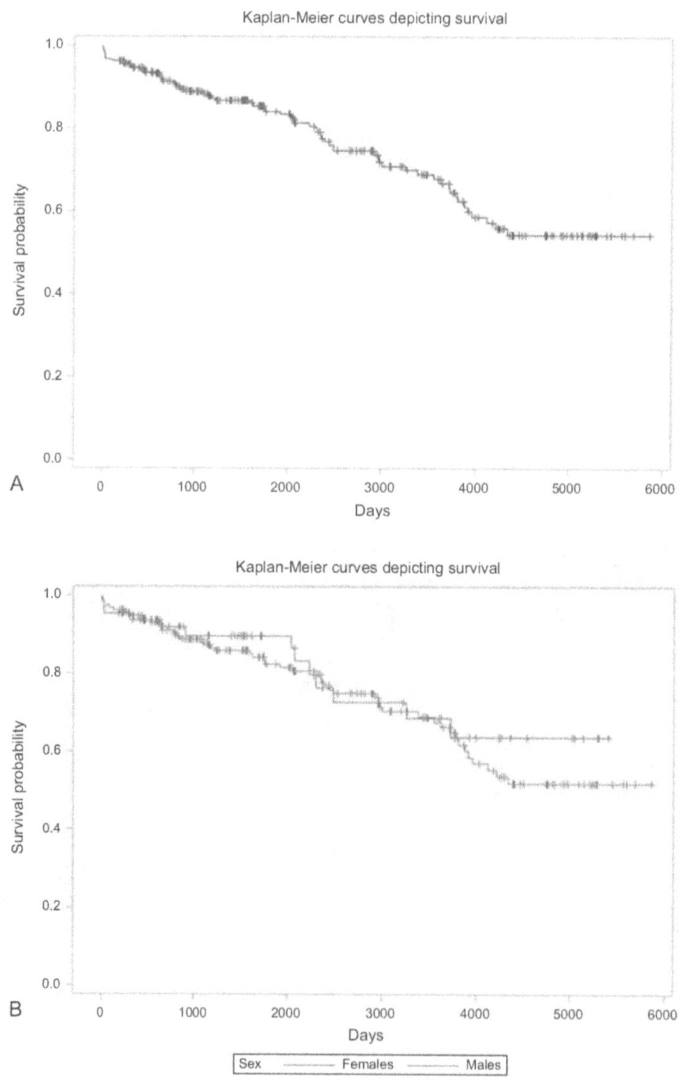


**FIGURE 30.** Kaplan-Meier survival curves for 257 patients whose survival data were available. (a) The unadjusted survival curve. (b) The unadjusted survival curves by sex.

## REFERENCES


1. Angelini A, Boffa GM, Livi U, et al. Discordance between pre and post cardiac transplant diagnosis: implications for pre- and postoperative decision making. *Cardiovasc Pathol*. 1999; 8:17–23.
2. Avella A, d'Amati G, Zachara E, et al. Comparison between electro-anatomic and pathologic findings in a patient with arrhythmogenic right ventricular cardiomyopathy/dysplasia treated with orthotopic cardiac transplant. *Heart Rhythm*. 2010; 7:828–831.
3. Barnard CN. The Operation. A human heart transplant: an interim report of a successful operation performed at Groote Schuur Hospital, Cape Town. *S AFr Med J*. 1967; 41:1271–1274.
4. Basso C, Corrado D, Marcus FI, et al. Arrhythmogenic right ventricular cardiomyopathy. *Lancet*. 2009; 373:1289–1300.
5. Biagini E, Spirito P, Leone O, et al. Heart transplantation in hypertrophic cardiomyopathy. *Am J Cardiol*. 2008; 101:387–392.
6. Bortman G, Sellanes M, Odell DS, et al. Discrepancy between pre- and post-transplant diagnosis of end-stage dilated cardiomyopathy. *Am J Cardiol*. 1994; 74:921–924.
7. Bradshaw SH, Veinot JP. Cardiac amyloidosis: what are the indications for transplant?. *Curr Opin Cardiol*. 2012; 27:143–147.
8. Burke AP, Farb A, Tashko G, et al. Arrhythmogenic right ventricular cardiomyopathy and fatty replacement of the right ventricular myocardium: are they different diseases?. *Circulation*. 1998; 97:1571–1580.
9. Chang TI, Chi NH, Chou NK, et al. Isolated cardiac sarcoidosis in heart transplantation. *Transplant Proc*. 2012; 44:903–906.
10. Conner R, Hosenpud JD, Norman DJ, et al. Heart transplantation for cardiac amyloidosis: successful one-year outcome despite recurrence of the disease. *J Heart Transplant*. 1988; 7:165–167.
11. Conraads V, Paelinck B, Vorlat A, et al. Isolated non- compaction of the left ventricle: A rare indication for transplantation. *J Heart Lung Transplant*. 2001; 20:904–907.
12. Corrado D, Basso C, Thiene G, et al. Spectrum of clinicopathologic manifestations of arrhythmogenic right ventricular cardiomyopathy/dysplasia: a multicenter study. *J Am Coll Cardiol*. 1997; 30: 1512–1520.
13. Coutu M, Perrault LP, White M, et al. Cardiac transplantation for hypertrophic cardiomyopathy: a valid therapeutic option. *J Heart Lung Transplant*. 2004; 23:413–417.
14. Dalal D, Nasir K, Bomma C, et al. Arrhythmogenic right ventricular dysplasia: a United States experience. *Circulation*. 2005; 112:3823–3832.
15. Donsky AS, Escobar J, Capehart J, et al. Heart Transplantation for undiagnosed cardiac sarcoidosis. *Am J Cardiol*. 2002; 89:1447–1450.
16. Dubrey SW, Burke MM, Hawkins PN, et al. Cardiac transplantation for amyloid heart disease: the United Kingdom experience. *J Heart Lung Transplant*. 2004; 23:1142–1153.
17. Dubrey SW, Burke MM, Khaghani A, et al. Long term results of heart transplantation in patients with amyloid heart disease. *Heart*. 2001; 85:202–207.
18. Falk RH. Cardiac amyloidosis: a treatable disease, often overlooked. *Circulation*. 2011; 124:1079–1085.
19. Garner WL, Starling C, Kuiper JJ, et al. Lymphocytic myocarditis as a cause of fulminant fatal heart failure. *Proc (Bayl Univ Med Cent)*. 2006; 19:122–123.
20. Gungor H, Oguz E, Ayik MF, et al. Comparison of heart transplantation patients with ischemic and idiopathic dilated cardiomyopathy. *Transplant Proc*. 2011; 43:3847–3850.
21. Hamada T, Kubo T, Kitaoka H, et al. Clinical features of the dilated phase of hypertrophic cardiomyopathy in comparison with those of dilated cardiomyopathy. *Clin Cardiol*. 2010; 33:E24–E28.
22. Isner JM, Ferrans VJ, Cohen SR, et al. Clinical and morphologic cardiac findings after anthracycline chemotherapy. Analysis of 64 patients studied at necropsy. *Am J Cardiol*. 1983; 51:1167–1174.
23. Isner JM, Virmani R, Itscoitz SB, et al. Left and right ventricular myocardial infarction in idiopathic dilated cardiomyopathy. *Am Heart J*. 1980; 9:235–242.
24. Kato TS, Takayama H, Yoshizawa S, et al. Cardiac transplantation in patients with hypertrophic cardiomyopathy. *Am J Cardiol*. 2012; 110:568–574.
25. Kindermann I, Barth C, Mahfoud F, et al. Update on myocarditis. *J Am Coll Cardiol*. 2012; 59:779–792.
26. Kumar S, Marfatia R, Tannenbaum S, et al. Doxorubicin-induced cardiomyopathy 17 years after chemotherapy. *Tex Heart Inst J*. 2012; 39:424–427.
27. Lennenman AJ, Wang L, Wigger M, et al. Heart transplant survival outcomes for adriamycin-dilated cardiomyopathy. *Am J Cardiol*. 2013; 111:609–612.
28. Lobo FV, Silver MD, Butany J, et al. Left ventricular involvement in right ventricular dysplasia/cardiomyopathy. *Can J Cardiol*. 1999; 15:1239–1247.
29. Luk A, Metawee M, Ahn E, et al. Do clinical diagnoses correlate with pathological diagnoses in cardiac transplant patients? The importance of endomyocardial biopsy. *Can J Cardiol*. 2009; 25:e48–e54.
30. Mancini D, Lietz K. Selection of cardiac transplantation candidates in 2010. *Circulation*. 2010; 122:173–183.
31. Marcus FI, Zareba W, Calkins H, et al. Arrhythmogenic right ventricular cardiomyopathy/dysplasia clinical presentation and diagnostic evaluation: results from the North American Multidisciplinary Study. *Heart Rhythm*. 2009; 6:984–992.
32. Marcus GM, Glidden DV, Polonsky B, et al. Multidisciplinary Study of Right Ventricular Dysplasia Investigators. Efficacy of antiarrhythmic drugs in arrhythmogenic right ventricular cardiomyopathy: a report from the North American ARVC Registry. *J Am Coll Cardiol*. 2009; 54:609–615.
33. Maron BJ, Maron MS, Wigle ED, et al. The 50-year history, controversy, and clinical implications of left ventricular outflow tract obstruction in hypertrophic cardiomyopathy. *J Am Coll Cardiol*. 2009; 54:191–200.
34. Maron BJ, Maron MS. Hypertrophic cardiomyopathy. *Lancet*. 2013; 381:242–255.
35. Maron BJ, Wolfson JK, Epstein SE, et al. Intramural ("small vessel") coronary artery disease in hypertrophic cardiomyopathy. *J Am Coll Cardiol*. 1986; 8:545–557.
36. Maron BJ. Hypertrophic cardiomyopathy. *Lancet*. 1997; 350:127–133.
37. Maron MS, Kalsmith BM, Udelson JE, et al. Survival after cardiac transplantation in patients with hypertrophic cardiomyopathy. *Circ Heart Fail*. 2010; 3:574–579.
38. Parisi F. Heart transplantation in congenital heart disease. *Curr Cardiol Rev*. 2011; 7:50.
39. Pavie A. Heart transplantation for end-stage valvular disease: indications and results. *Curr Opin Cardiol*. 2006; 21:100–105.
40. Pelosi F, Capehart JE, Roberts WC. Effectiveness of cardiac transplantation for primary (AL) cardiac amyloidosis. *Am J Cardiol*. 1997; 79:532–535.
41. Ried M, Rupprecht L, Hirt S, et al. Sequential therapy of primary cardiac lymphoma with cardiectomy, total artificial heart support, and cardiac transplantation. *J Heart Lung Transplant*. 2010; 29: 707–709.
42. Roberts CS, Roberts WC. Morphologic features (of hypertrophic cardiomyopathy). *Progress in Cardiology 2/2*. In: Zipes DP, Rowlands DJ, editor Philadelphia: Lea & Febiger, 1989; pp. 3–32.

43. Roberts WC, Chung MS, Ko JM, et al. Morphologic features of cardiac sarcoidosis in native hearts of patients having cardiac transplantation. *Am J Cardiol.* 2014; 113:706–712.

44. Roberts WC, Glancy DL, DeVita VT. Heart in malignant lymphoma (Hodgkin's disease, lymphosarcoma, reticulum cell sarcoma and mycosis fungoides). A study of 196 autopsy cases. *Am J Cardiol.* 1968; 22:85–107.

45. Roberts WC, Karia SJ, Ko JM, et al. Examination of isolated ventricular non-compaction (hypertrabeculation) as a distinct entity in adults. *Am J Cardiol.* 2011; 108:747–752.

46. Roberts WC, Ko JM, Kuiper JJ, et al. Some previously neglected examples of arrhythmogenic right ventricular dysplasia /cardiomyopathy and frequency of its various reported manifestations. *Am J Cardiol.* 2010; 106:268–274.

47. Roberts WC, McAllister HA, Ferrans VJ. Sarcoidosis of the Heart. A clinicopathologic study of 35 necropsy patients (Group I) and review of 78 previously described necropsy patients (Group II). *Am J Med.* 1977; 63:86–108.

48. Roberts WC, Phillips SD, Escobar JM, et al. Cardiac transplantation 40 years after a stab wound to the heart. *Proc (Bayl Univ Med Cent).* 2001; 14:241–242.

49. Roberts WC, Roberts CC, Ko JM, et al. Dramatically different phenotypic expressions of hypertrophic cardiomyopathy in male cousins undergoing cardiac transplantation with identical disease-causing gene mutation. *Am J Cardiol.* 2013; 111:1818–1822.

50. Roberts WC, Roberts CC, Ko JM, et al. Cardiac transplantation in adults with aortic valve disease with focus on the bicuspid aortic valve. *Am J Cardiol.* 2012; 109:1212–1214.

51. Roberts WC, Siegel RJ, McManus BM. Idiopathic dilated cardiomyopathy: Analysis of 152 necropsy patients. *Am J Cardiol.* 1987; 60:1340–1355.

52. Roberts WC, Vowels TJ, Ko JM, et al. Cardiac transplantation for cardiac sarcoidosis with initial diagnosis by examination of the left ventricular apical "core" excised for insertion of a left ventricular assist device for severe chronic heart failure. *Am J Cardiol.* 2009; 103:110–114.

53. Roberts WC, Waller BF. Cardiac amyloidosis causing cardiac dysfunction: analysis of 54 necropsy patients. *Am J Cardiol.* 1983; 52:137–146.

54. Roberts WC. Defining idiopathic dilated cardiomyopathy: A courtroom discussion. *Am J Cardiol.* 1989; 63:893–896.

55. Ross EM, Roberts WC. Severe atherosclerotic coronary arterial narrowing and chronic congestive heart failure without myocardial infarction; analysis of 18 patients studied at necropsy. *Am J Cardiol.* 1986; 57:51–56.

56. Ross EM, Roberts WC. Severe atherosclerotic coronary artery disease, healed myocardial infarction and chronic congestive heart failure; analysis of 81 patients studied at necropsy. *Am J Cardiol.* 1986; 57:44–50.

57. Rotela Samaniego JA, Castells E, Manito N, et al. Clinical evolution of heart transplantation in patients with previous valvular cardiomyopathy. *Transplant Proc.* 2007; 39:2355–2356.

58. Sagar S, Liu PP, Cooper LT. Myocarditis. *Lancet.* 2012; 379:738–747.

59. Scadding JG. A 'burnt-out' case of sarcoidosis. *Postgrad Med J.* 1968; 4:105–108.

60. Shirani J, Freant LJ, Roberts WC. Gross and semiquantitative histologic findings in mononuclear cell myocarditis causing sudden death, and implications for endomyocardial biopsy. *Am J Cardiol.* 1993; 72:952–957.

61. Shirani J, Maron BJ, Cannon RO, et al. Clinicopathologic features of hypertrophic cardiomyopathy managed by cardiac transplantation. *Am J Cardiol.* 1993; 72:434–440.

62. Shirani J. Subepicardial myocardial lesions. *Am Heart J.* 1993; 125:1346–1352.

63. Siân Pincott E, Burch M. Indications for heart transplantation in congenital heart disease. *Curr Cardiol Rev.* 2011; 7:51–58.

64. Tedford RJ, James C, Judge DP, et al. Cardiac transplantation in arrhythmogenic right ventricular dysplasia/cardiomyopathy. *J Am Coll Cardiol.* 2012; 9:289–290.

65. Theleman KP, Kuiper JJ, Roberts WC. Acute myocarditis (predominately lymphocytic) causing sudden death without heart failure. *Am J Cardiol.* 2001; 88:1078–1083.

66. Tops LF, Prakasa K, Tandri H, et al. Prevalence and pathophysiologic attributes of ventricular dyssynchrony in arrhythmogenic right ventricular dysplasia/cardiomyopathy. *J Am Coll Cardiol.* 2009; 54:445–451.

67. Valantine HA, Tazelaar HD, Macoviak J, et al. Cardiac sarcoidosis: response to steroids and transplantation. *J Heart Transplant.* 1987; 6:244–250.

68. Val-Bernal JF, Nistal JF, Martino M, et al. Isolated non-compaction of the left ventricular myocardium in an adult treated with heart transplantation. *Pathol Int.* 2006; 56:35–39.

69. Varr BC, Liedtke M, Arai S, et al. Heart transplantation and cardiac amyloidosis: approach to screening and novel management strategies. *J Heart Lung Transplant.* 2012; 31:325–331.

70. Waller BF, Smith ER, Blackbourne BD, et al. Congenital hypoplasia of portions of both right and left ventricular myocardial walls. Clinical and necropsy observations in two patients with parchment heart syndrome. *Am J Cardiol.* 1980; 46:885–891.

71. Waller TA, Hiser WL, Capehart JE, et al. Comparison of clinical and morphologic cardiac findings in patients having cardiac transplantation for ischemic cardiomyopathy, idiopathic dilated cardiomyopathy, and dilated hypertrophic cardiomyopathy. *Am J Cardiol.* 1998; 81:884–894.

72. Xu T, Yang Z, Vatta M, et al. Multidisciplinary Study of Right Ventricular Dysplasia Investigators. Compound and digenic heterozygosity contributes to arrhythmogenic right ventricular cardiomyopathy. *J Am Coll Cardiol.* 2010; 55:587–597.

73. Yoda M, Minami K, Fritzsche D, et al. Three cases of orthotopic heart transplantation for arrhythmogenic right ventricular cardiomyopathy. *Ann Thorac Surg.* 2005; 80:2358–2360.

# Secondary Arrhythmogenic Right Ventricular Cardiomyopathy Decades After Operative Repair of Tetralogy of Fallot

Erin E. Donaldson, DO[a], Jong Mi Ko, BA[b], Gonzalo Gonzalez-Stawinski, MD[c], Shelley A. Hall, MD[d], and William C. Roberts, MD[d,e,*]

**We describe a 47-year-old man who underwent heart transplantation (HT) for severe right-sided heart failure and periodic episodes of ventricular tachycardia (VT) 43 years after operative repair of tetralogy of Fallot (T of F). The right-ventricular outflow tract, the site where a patch had been placed 4 decades earlier, was aneurysmal. Such development decades after operative repair of T of F of both aneurysm and episodes of VT is probably more common than previously realized.**  **(Am J Cardiol 2014;114:806−809)**

In July 2011 we reported a 41-year-old man who underwent heart transplantation (HT) because of severe right-sided heart failure and periodic ventricular tachycardia (VT) after operative repair of tetralogy of Fallot (T of F) at age 6.[1] The present report was prompted by studying a similar patient, aged 47, who underwent HT also because of severe right-sided heart failure associated with periodic episodes of VT after operative repair of T of F at age 4. Both patients developed huge right ventricular outflow aneurysms.

## Case Description

A 47-year-old male manual laborer had repair of T of F at 4 years of age. Thereafter, he was asymptomatic until age 33 years, when he had his first symptomatic episode of VT and an intracardiac defibrillator was inserted. Evidence of right-sided failure appeared about the same time and it gradually progressed thereafter. An electrocardiogram before an intracardiac defibrillator was inserted is shown in Figure 1. A computed tomographic image of the heart just before HT is shown in Figure 2. Three months after HT (January 2014) the patient was asymptomatic. Photographs of the explanted heart are shown in Figures 3 and 4.

[a]Department of Family Medicine, Methodist Charlton Medical Center, Dallas, Texas and [b]Baylor Heart and Vascular Institute, [c]Department of Cardiothoracic Surgery, [d]Division of Cardiology, Department of Internal Medicine, and [e]Department of Pathology, Baylor University Medical Center, Dallas, Texas. Manuscript received May 7, 2014; revised manuscript received and accepted May 29, 2014.

The study was funded by the Baylor Health Care System Foundation, Dallas, Texas.

See page 806 for disclosure information.

*Corresponding author: Tel: (214) 820-7911; fax: (214) 820-7533.

*E-mail address:* wc.roberts@baylorhealth.edu (W.C. Roberts).

## Discussion

Described herein is a patient who had HT at age 47 for severe right-sided heart failure and episodic VT occurring several decades after repair of T of F at age 4. The patient described is virtually identical to a patient reported 2 years earlier with a similar scenario (Table 1). The earlier report also described a huge right ventricular outflow tract aneurysm involving the widening patch utilized when eliminating the subvalvular right ventricular outflow tract obstruction. To study 2 similar patients in a 2-year period suggests that aneurysmal formation in the right ventricular outflow tract several decades after repair of T of F may not be an uncommon occurrence but indeed potentially a common late occurrence. The development of episodes of VT with development of the right ventricular outflow aneurysm of course might be described as secondary or acquired arrhythmogenic right ventricular cardiomyopathy/dysplasia.

Shown in Table 2 are selected reports of patients having late follow up after repair of T of F in childhood.[2–9] Of the 1964 patients included none appeared to have a follow up as long as 40 years as did our present patient and our previously described patient (Table 1). Nevertheless, certainly many of the reported patients having pulmonic valve replacement with or without partial excision of the right ventricular outflow tract did have subvalvular aneurysms and some had "arrhythmias" (type not specified).

The other unusual feature here is the use of HT to eliminate both the right-sided severe heart failure and the periodic episodes of ventricular tachycardia. As shown in Table 2, however, HT is infrequently employed for management of late complications after repair of T of F. Only 4 of the previously mentioned 2638 patients (Table 2) underwent HT late after previous "repair" of T of F, and 3 of them previously had homograft replacement of the pulmonic valve.

## Disclosures

The authors have no conflicts of interest to disclose.

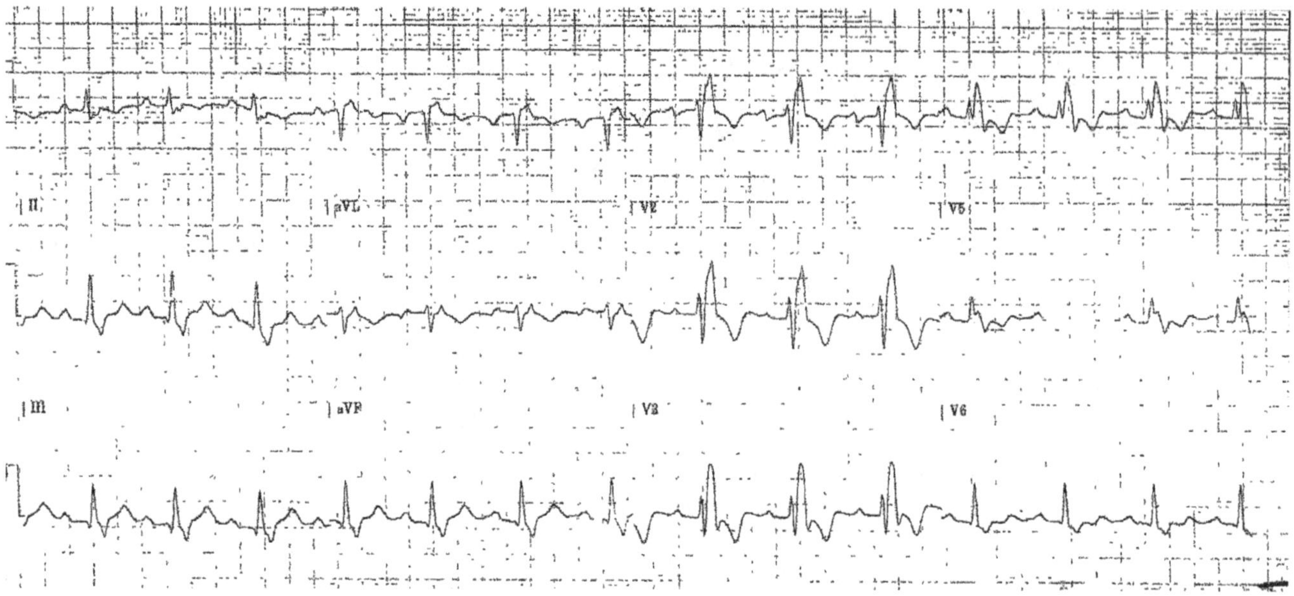


Figure 1. Electrocardiogram in the patient described before an intracardiac defibrillator was inserted. The electrocardiogram discloses a complete left bundle branch block pattern. Shows a complete right bundle branch block pattern. The rhythm is sinus.

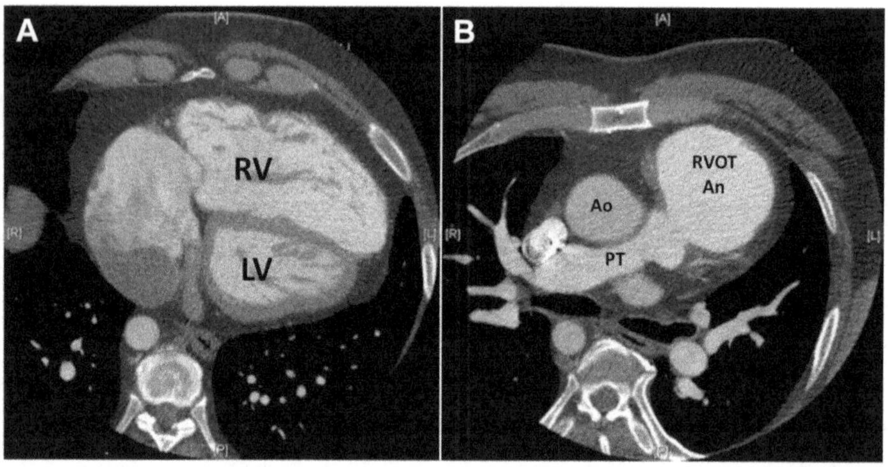


Figure 2. Computed tomographic imaging of the heart in the patient described before cardiac transplantation. *(A)* View showing the right ventricular cavity (inflow portion) and the much smaller left ventricular cavity (LV). The dilated right atrium is also seen as well as the right-sided aortic arch (AO). *(B)* A view showing the marked dilatation of the outflow portion of the right ventricle (RV) just beneath the pulmonic valve (PV). PT = pulmonic trunk; RVOT An = right ventricular outflow tract aneurysm.

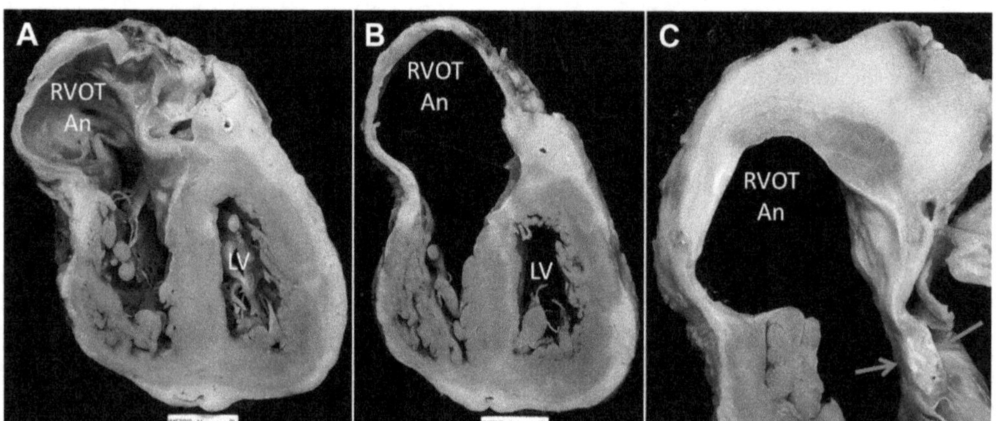


Figure 3. Partial four chamber cuts of the heart in the patient described. *(A)* View of the very dilated right ventricular outflow tract (RVOT), partially destroyed pulmonic valve (PV), left anterior descending coronary artery residing in the excessive subepicardial adipose tissue, right and left ventricular cavities exposing both tricuspid and mitral valves. *(B)* Another view showing the much dilated right ventricular outflow tract and the non-dilated right ventricular inflow tract. The scarring in the cephalad portion of the ventricular septum is the area where the previous ventricular septal defect was closed, approximately 40 years earlier. *(C)* Another view of the right ventricular outflow tract with calcium in the area where a patch *(arrows)* was used to close the ventricular septal defect (CA++). An = aneurysm; LV = left ventricle.

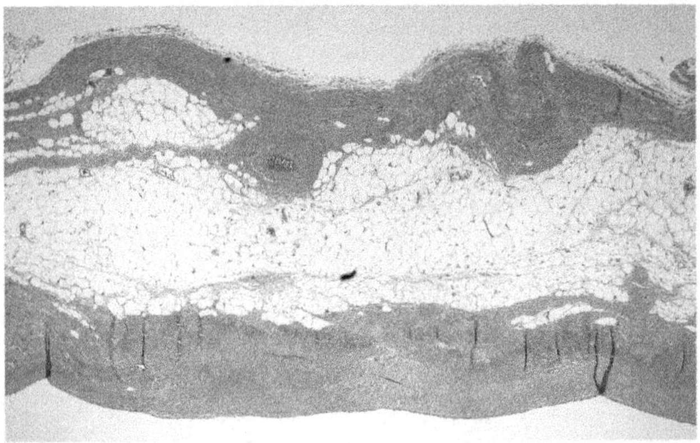

Figure 4. Photomicrograph of a portion of the right ventricular outflow tract showing total absence of myocardial fibers and extensive fibrous deposits in the outer wall and in the inner wall with large deposits of adipose tissue in between. Hematoxylin/eosin stain, ×40.

Table 1
Comparison of certain findings in the 2 men having cardiac transplantation late following repair of tetralogy of Fallot

| Variable | Case 1* | Case 2 |
|---|---|---|
| Age (years) | | |
| At heart transplantation | 41 (November 2010) | 47 (January 2014) |
| At repair of tetralogy of Fallot | 6 | 4 |
| When RV outflow tract aneurysm first noted | 26 | 33 |
| At onset of heart failure | 26 | 33 |
| At onset of ventricular tachycardia | 26 | 33 |
| Right-sided aortic arch | 0 | + |
| Body mass index (kg/m$^2$) | 25 | 32 |
| Heart weight (g) | 653 | 505 |
| Calcium in RV outflow tract aneurysm | + | 0 |
| RV outflow patch | + (calcified) | + |
| Electrophysiology | | |
| Bundle branch block | Left | Right |
| Intracardiac defibrillator | + (age 36) | + (age 33) |
| Radiofrequency ablation | + | 0 |
| Hemodynamics (mm Hg) | | |
| Left ventricle (s/d) | 96/31 | 113/69 (indirect) |
| Pulmonary artery (s/d) | 33/13 | 44/21 |
| Right ventricle (s/d) | 45/19 | 45/8 |
| Lowest LV ejection fraction (%) | 10 | 50 |

LV = left ventricle; RV = right ventricular; s/d = peak systole/end diastole.

* From George BA, Jong MK, Lensing FD, Kuiper JJ, Roberts WC. "Repaired" tetralogy of Fallot mimicking arrhythmogenic right ventricular cardiomyopathy. *Am J Cardiol* 2011;108:326–329.[1]

Table 2
Selected previous publications of patients having repair of tetralogy of Fallot (T of F) early in life with long follow up thereafter

| First Author | Publication Year | Age (Years) at Repair of T of F Mean ± SD [Median] | Number of Patients Having Late Survival | Follow Up (Years) Range (Mean ± SD) | Patients Having Cardiac Transplantation |
|---|---|---|---|---|---|
| Kirklin[2] | 1989 | - [5] | 791 | >2–20 (9 ± 5) | 0 |
| Murphy[3] | 1997 | 10 ± 9 [8] | 163 | 0.08–34 (21 ± 13) | 0 |
| Nollert[4] | 1993 | 12 ± 9 [-] | 490 | 1.06–35 (25 ± -) | 0 |
| Knott-Craig[5] | 1998 | 2 ± 0.2 [-] | 193 | 0.1–26 (11 ± 7) | 0 |
| Norgaard[6] | 1999 | - [13] | 109 | 20–38 (26 ± -) | 1 |
| Gatzoulis[7] | 2000 | 8 ± 8 [6] | 793 | 8–41 (21 ± 9) | 0 |
| Troost[8] | 2007 | - [24] | 68 | 1.3–18 (- ± 8) | 3* |
| Munkhammar[9] | 2013 | - [0.8] | 31 | 2–16 (9 ± 3) | 0 |
| Totals | | | 2638 | | |

\- = no information available.

* All had homograft replacement of the pulmonic valve.

1. George BA, Jong MK, Lensing FD, Kuiper JJ, Roberts WC. "Repaired" tetralogy of Fallot mimicking arrhythmogenic right ventricular cardiomyopathy. *Am J Cardiol* 2011;108:326–329.
2. Kirklin JK, Kirklin JW, Blackstone EH, Milano A, Pacifico AD. Effect of transannular patching on outcome after repair of tetralogy of Fallot. *Ann Thorac Surg* 1989;48:783–791.
3. Murphy JG, Gersh MB, Mair DD, Fuster V, McGoon MD, Ilstrup DM, McGoon DC, Kirklin JW, Danielson GK. Long-term outcome in patients undergoing surgical repair of tetralogy of Fallot. *N Engl J Med* 1993;329:593–599.
4. Nollert G, Fischlein T, Bouterwek S, Bohmer C, Klinner W, Reichart B. Long-term survival in patients with repair of tetralogy of Fallot: 36-year follow-up of 490 survivors of the first year after surgical repair. *J Am Coll Cardiol* 1997;30:1374–1383.
5. Knott-Craig CJ, Elkins RC, Lane MM, Holz J, McCue C, Ward KE. A 26-year experience with surgical management of tetralogy of Fallot: risk analysis for mortality or late reintervention. *Ann Thorac Surg* 1998;66:506–511.
6. Norgaard MA, Lauridsen P, Helvind M, Pettersson G. Twenty-to-thirty-seven year follow-up after repair for tetralogy of Fallot. *Eur J Cardiothorac Surg* 1999;16:125–130.
7. Gatzoulis MA, Balaji S, Webber SA, Siu SC, Hokanson JS, Poile C, Rosenthal M, Nakazawa M, Moller JH, Gillette PC, Webb GD, Redington AN. Risk factors for arrhythmia and sudden cardiac death late after repair of tetralogy of Fallot: a multicentre study. *Lancet* 2000;356:975–981.
8. Troost E, Meyns B, Daenen W, Van de Werf F, Gewillig M, Van Deyk K, Moons P, Budts W. Homograft survival after tetralogy of Fallot repair: determinants of accelerated homograft degeneration. *Eur Heart J* 2007;28:2503–2509.
9. Munkhammar P, Carlsson M, Arheden H, Pesonen E. Restrictive right ventricular physiology after tetralogy of Fallot repair is associated with fibrosis of the right ventricular outflow tract visualized on cardiac magnetic resonance imaging. *Eur Heart J Cardiovasc Imaging* 2013;14:978–985.

# Advanced Heart Failure With Preserved Systolic Function in Nonobstructive Hypertrophic Cardiomyopathy

## Under-Recognized Subset of Candidates for Heart Transplant

Ethan J. Rowin, MD; Barry J. Maron, MD; Michael S. Kiernan, MD; Susan A. Casey, RN; David S. Feldman, MD; Katarzyna M. Hryniewicz, MD; Raymond H. Chan, MD; Kevin M. Harris, MD; James E. Udelson, MD; David DeNofrio, MD; William C. Roberts, MD; Martin S. Maron, MD

***Background*****—**In hypertrophic cardiomyopathy (HCM), heart transplant has been predominantly confined to patients with systolic dysfunction. An underappreciated HCM subset comprises patients with preserved left ventricular (LV) systolic function who may also require consideration for transplantation. Therefore, we sought to define the clinical profile and occurrence of advanced heart failure among patients with nonobstructive HCM and preserved systolic function.

***Methods and Results*****—**Databases from 2 referral centers comprising 2100 HCM patients were interrogated. Forty-six nonobstructive HCM patients (2.2%) either received or were listed for heart transplant, including 20 with normal systolic function (ejection fraction ≥50%). At transplant listing, these 20 patients were 42±13 years old, each in New York Heart Association functional class III/IV with ejection fraction of 62±7%. LV was hypertrophied with maximum wall thickness of 22±4 mm and nondilated (end-diastolic dimension, 39±7 mm). Cardiovascular magnetic resonance in 10 (of 15) patients showed no or minimal fibrosis (≤5% LV mass). Elevated LV end-diastolic or pulmonary capillary wedge pressure, consistent with diastolic dysfunction, was present in 15 patients (75%). LV filling was impaired by echocardiographic measures in all patients, including a restrictive inflow pattern in 8 (40%). In 2 patients, traditional criteria for transplant were absent, including peak $V_{O_2}$ >14 mL/kg/min. Heart transplantation was performed in 12 patients with each alive and without cardiovascular symptoms, 2.3±1.7 years later.

***Conclusions*****—**A previously under-recognized segment of the broad HCM clinical spectrum consists of nonobstructive patients with advanced heart failure, in the presence of preserved systolic function, for whom heart transplant is the sole definitive therapeutic option. **(*Circ Heart Fail*. 2014;7:967-975.)**

**Key Words:** diastolic dysfunction ■ heart transplantation ■ hypertrophic cardiomyopathy

Sudden death has perhaps been the most visible adverse consequence of hypertrophic cardiomyopathy (HCM).[1–4] However, with the increased use of the implantable cardioverter defibrillator for primary prevention,[5–8] heart failure progression and death are emerging prominently within the natural history of HCM and with regard to strategies for disease management.[9–12] In this regard, heart transplantation has, by convention, been confined predominantly to those HCM patients evolving into the end-stage phase, characterized by left ventricular (LV) systolic dysfunction (ejection fraction [EF] <50%).[13–17] However, within the diverse HCM phenotypic spectrum, we have recently recognized a subgroup of nonobstructive patients with severe drug-refractory heart failure symptoms, but nevertheless have preserved LV systolic function; without other therapeutic options, these patients become candidates for heart transplant. Therefore, we take this opportunity to characterize the presentation, clinical profile, and outcome of this largely under-recognized subset within the HCM patient population.

**Clinical Perspective on p 975**

## Methods

### Patient Selection

HCM patient databases of 2 referral centers, Minneapolis Heart Institute Foundation (Minneapolis, MN) and Tufts Medical Center (Boston, MA), were accessed. Patients with HCM who had undergone heart transplant or were listed for transplant (2004–2013) were included. Patients who met the following criteria constitute the preserved LV systolic function study population: (1) EF ≥50%; (2) New York Heart Association (NYHA) functional class III/IV, refractory to maximum medical management; (3) LV outflow gradient <30 mm Hg

Received April 7, 2014; accepted September 15, 2014.

From the Department of Medicine, Hypertrophic Cardiomyopathy Center, Division of Cardiology, Tufts Medical Center, Boston, MA (E.J.R., M.S.K., J.E.U., D.D., M.S.M.); Department of Medicine, the Hypertrophic Cardiomyopathy Center, Minneapolis Heart Institute Foundation, Minneapolis, MN (B.J.M., S.A.C., D.S.F., K.M.H., K.M.H.); Departments of Medicine (Cardiovascular Division) and Radiology, Beth Israel Deaconess Medical Center, Boston, MA (R.H.C.); and Department of Pathology and Medicine, Baylor University Medical Center, Dallas, TX (W.C.R.).

Guest Editor for this article was Douglas L. Mann, MD.

**The Data Supplement is available at http://circheartfailure.ahajournals.org/lookup/suppl/doi:10.1161/CIRCHEARTFAILURE.114.001435/-/DC1.**

Correspondence to Martin S. Maron, MD, Tufts Medical Center, No. 70, 800 Washington St, Boston, MA 02111. E-mail mmaron@tuftsmedicalcenter.org at rest and with physiological (exercise) provocation. Patients with LV outflow obstruction who underwent septal reduction therapy and subsequently developed advanced heart failure were excluded (n=7).

Initial clinical evaluation was the first clinical assessment obtained at either participating institution. Transplant listing was defined as date of acceptance on the UNOS (united network for organ sharing) heart transplant list.[18] Most recent evaluation was obtained during clinic visit or by telephone interview. This study has been reviewed and approved by Institutional Review Boards of the participating institutions, Allina Health Systems and Tufts Medical Center, permitting use of patient medical information for research. All authors had full access and took responsibility for integrity of the data and agreed to the article as written.

## Definitions

### *HCM Diagnosis*

HCM diagnosis was made by echocardiographic and cardiovascular magnetic resonance (CMR) documentation of a hypertrophied and nondilated left ventricle (wall thickness ≥15 mm in adults), at some time during their clinical course, in the absence of another cardiac or systemic disease capable of producing a similar magnitude of hypertrophy.[1]

### *Heart Failure*

Advanced heart failure was defined as symptom limitation to New York Heart Association (NYHA) functional class III or IV, characterized predominately by exertional dyspnea (with or without chest pain). Global LV systolic dysfunction (by convention, end-stage HCM) was arbitrarily defined by EF <50% at rest.[2,15] Patients with EF ≥50% were designated as preserved LV systolic function.[2]

## Echocardiography

Transthoracic echocardiographic studies were performed with commercially available instruments 2.3±6.1 months before transplant listing. Magnitude of LV hypertrophy, left-atrial, and LV end-diastolic dimensions were obtained as previously described.[19] Mitral regurgitation was graded as mild, moderate, or severe by combined analysis of jet area, width, and spectral Doppler intensity. EF was calculated from 2-dimensional echocardiographic images with the modified Simpson rule formula or area-length method.

LV outflow tract obstruction because of systolic anterior motion of the mitral valve with septal contact was imaged in the apical views with continuous wave Doppler. Patients without an LV outflow gradient under basal conditions underwent exercise echocardiography performed with symptom-limited Bruce protocol. LV outflow tract gradient was reassessed immediately after exercise.[19]

Mitral inflow velocity and annular tissue Doppler indices signals were obtained, as previously described.[20] Peak pulsed Doppler velocities were assessed to determine early (E) and late (A) diastolic flow across the mitral valve. Tissue Doppler index of the mitral annulus was obtained from the apical 4-chamber view, and peak early tissue Doppler velocities of the septal mitral annulus (e′) were analyzed. Diastolic dysfunction was classified according to previous consensus recommendations.[20] Echocardiographic measures of diastolic function were not assessed in 2 patients because of presence of atrial fibrillation at the time of study.

## Cardiovascular Magnetic Resonance

CMR studies were performed with a 1.5 Tesla clinical CMR scanner in 15 patients, while 5 patients did not undergo CMR examination because of a previously implanted implantable cardioverter defibrillator. Breath-hold cine steady state free precession sequences were performed in horizontal long axis, vertical long axis, and contiguous short axis slices with full coverage of LV and slice thickness of 10 mm with no gap. Short-axis cine stack was obtained parallel to atrioventricular groove, covering the entire LV chamber.

Late gadolinium enhancement (LGE) images were acquired 10 to 15 minutes after intravenous administration of 0.2 mmol/kg gadolinium-DTPA (Magnevist, Schering;Berlin Germany) using breath-held segmented inversion recovery sequence acquired in same orientations as the cine images. The LV short-axis stack of LGE images was first assessed visually for presence of LGE. Quantification of LGE was then performed on all LGE-positive studies by manually adjusting a grayscale threshold to define areas of visually identified LGE. These areas were then summed to generate a total volume of LGE and expressed as a proportion of total LV myocardium (%LGE).

## Cardiopulmonary Stress Test

Cardiopulmonary stress testing was performed in 17 patients with symptom-limited erect treadmill exercise testing using a standard ramp protocol with simultaneous respiratory gas analysis. Peak oxygen consumption ($Vo_2$) was defined as the maximum $Vo_2$ achieved during exercise, expressed in ml/min/kg. Predicted % $Vo_2$ relative to patient age and sex was calculated according to established guidelines.[18]

## Invasive Hemodynamics

Hemodynamic studies were performed on cardioactive medications, 1.9±3.1 months before transplant listing. Right atrial, pulmonary artery, pulmonary capillary pressures, and LV end-diastolic pressures were measured at end expiration and taken as the average of ≥3 beats. Cardiac output was determined by the Fick method using directly measured saturations and oxygen consumption and indexed to body surface area (cardiac index). Hemodynamic measurements were obtained with exercise in 3 patients in whom LV filling pressures were normal under resting conditions (mean PA pressure ≤25 mm Hg and PCWP ≤15 mm Hg), and peak $Vo_2$ was >14 mL/min/kg. An exercise protocol was performed by outstretched arm adduction lifting of 4 pound weights until fatigue, with hemodynamic parameters measured after peak exercise and at 1 minute recovery.

## Statistical Analysis

Data are displayed as mean± SD for continuous variables and as proportions for categorical variables. Student's *t* test or Wilcoxon rank-sum test assessed statistical significance for continuous variables and $\chi^2$ or Fisher's exact tests for categorical variables. *P* values <0.05 were considered significant and 2-sided where appropriate. Statistical analyses were performed with SAS for Windows version 9.3 (SAS Institute Inc, Cary, NC).

# Results

## Prevalence, Demographics, and Clinical Profile

Of the 2100 HCM patients in the cohort, 46 (2.2%) had been transplanted, listed for transplant, or died while awaiting transplantation. Of these 46 patients, 26 (1.2%) had systolic dysfunction (EF <50%) and were considered to be in the end-stage phase of HCM, while the other 20 patients (1.0%) had preserved EF ≥50% and constitute the study group (prevalence, 9.5 per 1000 HCM patients; Figure 1 and Table 1).

Among the 20 study patients (11 men), initial HCM diagnosis was at 32±15 years of age (range 12–61) and onset of heart failure symptoms at 35±16 years (Figure 2). Patients were listed for transplant at 42±13 years (range 16–66; Tables 2 and 3). Duration between symptom onset and listing was 8.0±8.9 years, including 6 patients listed <2 years after symptom onset and 9 patients ≥5 years after symptoms developed.

Among the 20 nonobstructive HCM patients with preserved LV systolic function, 12 underwent transplant at a mean age of 42±16 years (220±181 days after listing), including 4 patients <30 years of age, 5 patients between 40 and 49 years, and 3 patients >50 years. Time on the waiting list before transplantation ranged from 21 to 615 days (mean, 0.6±0.5 years).

In 14 of the 20 patients, ≥1 family member was known to have HCM, including 5 (25%) with a first-degree relative who developed end-stage HCM (EF=34±2%). Two of the family

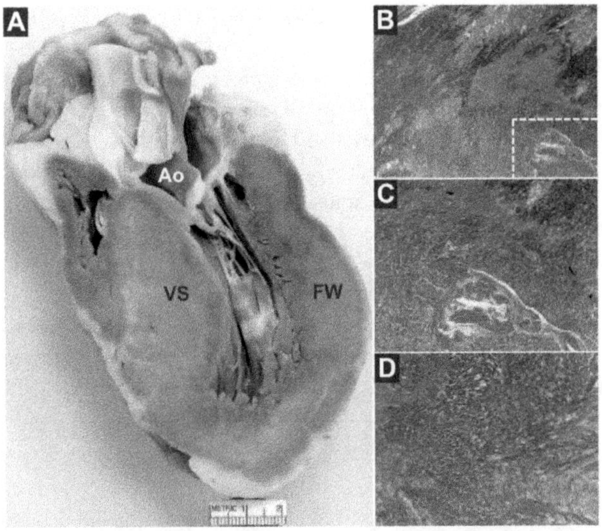


**Figure 1.** Explanted gross heart sectioned longitudinally (**A**) and histopathology (**B–D**) from a 50-year-old woman who underwent transplant for progressive severe heart failure refractory to pharmacological therapy in the presence of preserved left ventricular systolic function (EF=65%; No. 15 in Table 2). **A**, Ventricular septal thickness is marked (30 mm), left ventricular cavity is small, and distribution of hypertrophy is asymmetrical. Heart weight is 450 g. Patchy scarring (white areas) is visible in the septum, left ventricular free wall near the apex and in both papillary muscles. **B**, Area of myocardial scar (stained blue) in ventricular septum adjacent to an abnormal intramural coronary artery evident in the box at lower right. Original magnification 20×. **C**, A higher power micrograph of intramural coronary artery with thickened wall (media) and narrowed lumen, shown in panel B. Original magnification 40×. **D**, Area of viable myocardium (stained red) with cardiac muscle cells arranged in disorganized patterns. Original magnification 40×. Ao indicates aorta; FW, free wall; and VS, ventricular septum. Masson trichome stain for **B–D**.

members in the end-stage (mothers of patients Nos. 6 and 8) required heart transplant at 51 and 58 years of age, respectively, whereas the remaining 3 relatives in end-stage are alive, symptomatic, but without transplant.

A variety of pathogenic sarcomeric protein mutations were identified in 6 of 9 patients who underwent genetic testing: MYH7 (n=3), ACTC1 (n=1), TNNI (n=1), and TPM1 (n=1; Tables 2 and 3), including 1 patient with a family member in the end stage with the identical mutation (MYH7 Arg723Cys; patient No. 1).

## Phenotypic Expression

Based on echocardiography, CMR, and pathological examination of explanted hearts (n=8), each patient had a hypertrophied, thick-walled LV in the presence of a nondilated ventricular cavity. Maximum LV wall thickness (usually in ventricular septum) was 22±4 mm (range, 15–34 mm) by echocardiography, including 4 patients with 25 to 29 mm and 2 patients with massive hypertrophy, that is, ≥30 mm (Figures 1 and 3). LV cavity size was small, 39±7-mm end-diastolic dimension (range, 29–52 mm, and ≤40 mm in 10 patients). Left atrial diameter was 46±8 (range, 31–57 mm). EF was 62±7% (range, 55–70%), including 6 patients with an EF of 70% and 5 with EF of 55%.

Coronary artery patency was examined by arteriogram or CT angiography in 18 of 20 patients and by examination of the explanted heart in the other 2. Atherosclerotic coronary artery disease (ie., ≥50% luminal narrowing in ≥1 epicardial vessels) was absent in each patient. Three patients had a history of angina responsible for functional limitation, considered to be HCM-related.

**Table 1. Demographic and Clinical Variables of 20 HCM Patients with Preserved Systolic Function and 26 End-Stage HCM Patients With or Considered for Heart Transplantation**

| Variable | Preserved LV Systolic Function, EF ≥50% (n=20) | End-stage HCM, EF <50% (n=26) | *P* Value |
|---|---|---|---|
| Male, n (%) | 11 (55%) | 15 (58%) | 0.86 |
| Age at HCM diagnosis, y | 32±15 | 28±15 | 0.44 |
| Age at development of NYHA III/IV symptoms, y | 35±16 | 33±16 | 0.78 |
| Age at transplant listing, y | 42±13 | 42±13 | 0.98 |
| Family history of HCM, n (%) | 14 (70%) | 16 (62%) | 0.56 |
| Family history of end-stage HCM, n (%) | 5 (25%) | 5 (19%) | 0.88 |
| EF, % | 62±7 | 39±12 | 0.0001‡ |
| LVED, mm | 39±7 | 50±9 | 0.0001‡ |
| LA dimension, mm | 46±8 | 49±11 | 0.30 |
| Maximal LV wall thickness, mm | 22±4 | 18±4 | 0.003‡ |
| Diastolic dysfunction* | | | |
| Grade I (impaired relaxation) | 4 (22%) | 3 (19%) | 0.81 |
| Grade II (pseudonormal) | 6 (33%) | 8 (50%) | 0.32 |
| Grade III (restrictive) | 8 (45%) | 5 (31%) | 0.43 |
| E/e′ | 12±4 | 13±5 | 0.64 |
| Peak $Vo_2$, ml/kg/min | 14.6±5.6 | 12.2±3.3 | 0.12 |
| Presence of LGE on CMR, n (%) | 10/15 (66%)† | 5/6 (83%)† | 0.47 |
| Extent of LGE on CMR, % | 9±8 | 18±10 | 0.07 |
| Invasive hemodynamics | | | |
| RA pressure, mm Hg | 12±9 | 12±7 | 0.95 |
| Mean PA pressure, mm Hg | 31±11 | 28±9 | 0.27 |
| PCWP, mm Hg | 22±7 | 19±9 | 0.33 |
| Cardiac index, L/min/m² (Fick Method) | 2.2±0.7 | 2.1±0.5 | 0.71 |
| Outcome | | | |
| Heart transplant | 12 (60%) | 15 (58%) | 0.88 |
| Death awaiting transplant | 2 (10%) | 6 (23%) | 0.26 |
| Active on transplant list | 6 (30%) | 5 (19%) | 0.41 |

Values as mean±standard deviation, or number (% of subjects), when applicable.

CMR indicates cardiac MRI; EF, ejection fraction; HCM, hypertrophic cardiomyopathy; LA, left atrium; LGE, late gadolinium enhancement; LV, left ventricular; LVED, left ventricular end-diastolic dimension; NYHA, New York Heart Association; PA, pulmonary artery; PCWP, pulmonary capillary wedge pressure; RA, right atrium; and $VO_2$, peak oxygen consumption.

*Diastolic function available in 18 patients with preserved systolic function and 16 patients in the end stage.

†Out of 15 patients with preserved LV systolic function and 6 patients in the end-stage phase who underwent cardiovascular magnetic resonance.

‡indicates $P$<0.01.

## Hemodynamics

Evidence of increased LV filling pressure, consistent with diastolic dysfunction, was present at cardiac catheterization

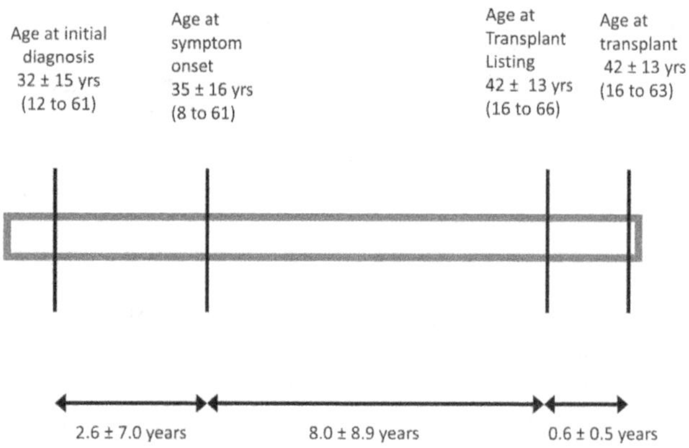


**Figure 2.** Timeline representing the clinical course of patients with nonobstructive hypertrophic cardiomyopathy, preserved left ventricular systolic function, and progression to advanced heart failure symptoms.

under basal conditions in 15 patients (75%), including LV end-diastolic pressure >15 mmHg in 5 patients (range, 20–30) and pulmonary capillary wedge pressure >15 mmHg in 8 patients without left heart catheterization (>25 mmHg in 6; Tables 2 and 3). In 2 patients, pressures were normal at rest, but increased substantially at peak exertion (wedge pressure, 26 and 28 mmHg). With echocardiography, diastolic dysfunction was assessed in 13 patients in sinus rhythm, each with impaired LV filling patterns: restrictive (Grade III) in 8, pseudonormal (Grade II) in 3, and impaired relaxation (Grade I) in 2.

Of the 5 remaining study patients, each had normal LV filling pressures at rest. Invasive hemodynamic assessment with exercise was not performed in 4 (because of particularly severe functional limitation), and in 1 patient, LV filling pressures were normal at rest and with exercise. However, in each of these 5 patients, there was evidence of diastolic dysfunction by echocardiography (Grade I in 2 and Grade II in 3).

## Pathology/Myocardial Fibrosis

### *Explanted Hearts*

Native explanted hearts were available for gross and histological examination in 8 patients (Figure 1). Heart weight was increased in each (508±94 g in males and 418±61 g in females), including two >500 g. In each, histopathology showed cardiac muscle cell disorganization and abnormal

**Table 2. Clinical and Demographic Data From 20 Patients With HCM and Preserved Systolic Function Listed for Heart Transplant**

| Patient | Gender | Age at TP Listing, y | Age at Dx, y | Age at 1st HF Symptoms, y | Time From Listing to TP, y | History of Atrial Fibrillation | Family Hx HCM | NSVT | Genetic Testing | LVED, mm | LA Dimension, mm | Max LV Thickness, mm | EF, % | Mitral Regurgitation (0–4+) |
|---|---|---|---|---|---|---|---|---|---|---|---|---|---|---|
| 1 | F | 16 | 12 | 12 | 0.64 | N | Y; ES | N | MYH7* Arg723Cys | 30 | 36 | 20 | 60 | 1+ |
| 2 | M | 20 | 20 | 19 | 1.13 | Ch-AF | N | N | … | 47 | 55 | 18 | 55 | 1+ |
| 3 | M | 22 | 12 | 22 | 1.68 | N | N | Y | MYH7 Arg719Trp | 49 | 49 | 21 | 55 | 1+ |
| 4 | F | 28 | 12 | 12 | 0.44 | P-AF | Y | N | MYH7† | 29 | 42 | 23 | 60 | 0 |
| 5 | F | 33 | 25 | 32 | … | N | N | N | TNNI3 Ala157Val | 39 | 34 | 18 | 60 | 1+ |
| 6 | F | 40 | 24 | 8 | 0.29 | Ch-AF | Y: ES, TP | N | … | 35 | 54 | 25 | 70 | 1+ |
| 7 | M | 41 | 27 | 29 | … | P-AF | N | N | TPM1 Glu96Asp | 29 | 42 | 24 | 70 | 1+ |
| 8 | M | 41 | 25 | 37 | … | N | Y: ES, TP | N | … | 41 | 47 | 34 | 60 | 1+ |
| 9 | F | 41 | 23 | 22 | 0.44 | P-AF | N | N | … | 38 | 53 | 27 | 70 | 1+ |
| 10 | F | 43 | 41 | 42 | … | N | Y: SD | N | … | 33 | 39 | 26 | 70 | 1+ |
| 11 | M | 44 | 39 | 38 | … | N | Y | Y | … | 45 | 44 | 23 | 70 | 0 |
| 12 | M | 45 | 37 | 42 | 0.21 | Ch-AF | Y | N | … | 31 | 49 | 21 | 55 | 1+ |
| 13 | M | 46 | 43 | 44 | 1.21 | P-AF | Y | Y | … | 44 | 52 | 21 | 65 | 1+ |
| 14 | M | 48 | 47 | 48 | 0.69 | P-AF | Y: ES | N | … | 52 | 48 | 17 | 60 | 0 |
| 15 | F | 50 | 39 | 49 | 0.17 | N | Y: SD | N | ACTC Ala323Val | 47 | 36 | 30 | 65 | 0 |
| 16 | F | 51 | 20 | 28 | … | P-AF | Y | N | … | 42 | 57 | 21 | 65 | 2+ |
| 17 | M | 54 | 44 | 46 | … | P-AF | Y | N | … | 41 | 46 | 15 | 55 | 1+ |
| 18 | F | 57 | 29 | 48 | 0.28 | P-AF | Y | N | … | 29 | 53 | 16 | 65 | 1+ |
| 19 | M | 63 | 58 | 58 | 0.06 | N | Y: ES, SD | Y | … | 35 | 31 | 21 | 70 | 1+ |
| 20 | M | 66 | 61 | 61 | … | Ch-AF | N | Y | … | 46 | 56 | 26 | 55 | 2+ |

ACTC indicates α cardiac actin 1; Ch-AF, chronic atrial fibrillation; Dx, diagnosis; EF, ejection fraction; ES, end stage HCM; HCM, hypertrophic cardiomyopathy; HF, heart failure; LA, left atrium; LV, left ventricular; LVED, left ventricular end-diastolic dimension; MYH7, β myosin heavy chain; NSVT, nonsustained ventricular tachycardia; SD, sudden cardiac death; TNNI3, cardiac troponin I; TPM1, tropomyosin 1 α; and TP, transplant.

*Identical disease causing mutation identified in the patient's father with end-stage HCM.

†Double mutation in MYH7:Arg719Trp, His581Arg (1 inherited from father, 1 from mother).

**Table 3. Clinical and Outcome Data for 20 Patients With HCM and Preserved Systolic Function Listed for Heart Transplant**

| Patient | E/A | E/E′ | Deceleration Time, ms | Diastolic Filling Pattern, Grade | Peak $Vo_2$, ml/min/kg | LGE on CMR, % | RA Pressure, mmHg | PA Pressure S/D (mean), mmHg | PCWP Pressure, mmHg | LV end Diastolic Pressure, mmHg | Fick CO; CI, L/min; L/min/m[2] | Inotrope as Bridge to Transplant | Outcome |
|---|---|---|---|---|---|---|---|---|---|---|---|---|---|
| 1 | 1.3 | 9.8 | 170 | II | 20.1* | 0 | 4 | 29/13 (20) | 14‖ | ... | 3.1;2.4 | Mil | TP;Alive |
| 2 | 2.8 | 10.7 | 140 | III | 22.8* | 0 | 34 | 60/40 (47) | 30 | ... | 2.4;1.3 | Mil | TP; Alive |
| 3 | 2.0 | 7.8 | 160 | II | 12.5 | ... | 4 | 46/21 (31) | 23 | ... | 8.0;4.0 | Mil | TP; Alive |
| 4 | 2.7 | 6.1 | 166 | III | 9.6 | 0 | 11 | 43/23 (30) | 21 | 30 | 1.4;0.9 | ... | TP; Alive† |
| 5 | 0.8 | 8.6 | 180 | I | 24.6 | 0 | 7 | 26/13 (18) | 15‡ | ... | 4.0;2.3 | ... | TL: Status 2 |
| 6 | 1.7 | 8.6 | 200 | II | ... | 4.4 | 8 | 50/21 (32) | 20 | ... | 3.6;1.9 | ... | TP; Alive§ |
| 7 | 1.8 | 13.5 | 140 | III | 18.6* | 1.1 | 11 | 38/23 (30) | 20 | ... | 4.0;1.8 | ... | TL: Status 2 |
| 8 | 1.8 | 13.7 | 160 | II | 14.0 | ... | 7 | 34/3 (25) | 15‖ | 10 | 3.4;1.9 | ... | Died on TL |
| 9 | ... | 24 | 167 | ... | 16.1 | 2.0 | 7 | 54/22 (36) | 26 | ... | 4.2;2.7 | Mil | TP; alive |
| 10 | 0.8 | 12.6 | 240 | I | 16.2 | 4.7 | 12 | 32/18 (22) | 14¶ | ... | 5.4;2.8 | ... | TL: Status 2 |
| 11 | 3.1 | 10.6 | 94 | III | ... | 2.5 | 31 | 69/36 (50) | 31 | 26 | 7.0;2.9 | ... | Died on TL# |
| 12 | 3.1 | 17.4 | 100 | III | 10.1 | 21.0 | 11 | 51/27 (35) | 23 | ... | 4.4;2.1 | Mil | TP; Alive |
| 13 | 0.7 | 9.0 | 210 | I | 10.0 | 1.8 | 5 | 29/13 (20) | 11‖ | 9 | 5.9;2.7 | ... | TP: Alive† |
| 14 | 1.4 | 14.0 | 271 | II | 9.5 | 7.9 | 7 | 50/24 (41) | 26 | 30 | 2.9;1.4 | ... | TP; Alive† |
| 15 | 1.5 | 9.2 | 184 | II | ... | ... | 5 | 23/12 (16) | 11‖ | 15 | 4.5;2.7 | Mil+Dob | TP; Alive |
| 16 | 3.5 | 16.7 | 132 | III | 9.3 | ... | 10 | 40/20 (27) | 25 | 20 | 3.2;1.6 | ... | TL: Status 2 |
| 17 | 2.0 | 16.8 | 120 | III | 8.6 | ... | 15 | 71/39 (50) | 35 | ... | 2.6;1.6 | Mil | TL: Status 1b |
| 18 | 2.7 | 13.0 | 140 | III | 6.7 | 0 | 22 | 47/30 (35) | 30 | ... | 3.1;1.4 | Mil | TP; Alive** |
| 19 | 1.0 | 11.4 | 221 | I | 19.3 | 7.2 | 5 | 26/12 (16) | 15‡ | ... | 5.7;2.7 | Mil+Dob | TP; Alive |
| 20 | ... | 14.2 | 120 | ... | 20.4 | 18 | 17 | 52/26 (35) | 26 | 20 | 4.0/2.0 | ... | TL: Status 2 |

CI indicates cardiac Index; CMR, cardiac MRI; CO, cardiac output; Dob, dobutamine; HCM, hypertrophic cardiomyopathy; LGE, late gadolinium enhancement; LV, left ventricular; LVED, left ventricular end-diastolic dimension; Mil, milrinone; PA, pulmonary artery; PCWP, pulmonary capillary wedge pressure; RA, right atrium; S/D, peak systolic/end diastolic; TL, transplant list; TP, transplant; and $VO_2$, peak oxygen consumption.

*<50% predicted for age.

†Received transplant as exception status.

‡Normal resting LV filling pressures but abnormal exercise hemodynamic (mean PA pressure >30, WP >25).

§Nipride used to optimize hemodynamics as bridge to transplant.

‖Normal resting LV filling pressures, invasive exercise hemodynamic not obtained.

¶Normal resting and exercise LV filling pressures (mean PA ≤30, WP ≤25).

#VAD placed as bridge to transplant.

**Intra-aortic balloon pump placed as bridge to transplant.

intramural coronary arteries typical of HCM.[1] With gross and histopathologic examination, fibrosis was absent or minimal in 5 hearts (Figure 1), whereas moderate-to-extensive diffuse amounts of patchy nontransmural myocardial fibrosis was evident in ventricular septum and lateral wall of 3 hearts.

### *Percent LGE*

Myocardial fibrosis was assessed by contrast-enhanced CMR in 15 patients (Figure 3). LGE was absent in 5 and present in 10 occupying 9±8% of LV mass (range 1.8%–21%), with 5 minimal and focal (<5% of LV mass) and 3 extensive/diffuse (≥15% of LV mass).

## Atrial Fibrillation

Atrial fibrillation was present in 12 patients, paroxysmal in 8 and persistent in 4. Attempts to restore and maintain sinus rhythm were unsuccessful with both electric cardioversion and antiarrhythmic drugs (ie, amiodarone [n=8], dofetilide [n=3], disopyramide [n=3], dronedarone [n=1], and sotalol [n=1]). In 7 patients, isolated pulmonary vein radiofrequency ablation was unsuccessful in restoring and maintaining sinus rhythm. Although heart failure symptoms were exacerbated in atrial fibrillation, all patients were in NYHA functional class III heart failure even when in sinus rhythm.

## Pharmacological and Mechanical Support

Efforts to control heart failure symptoms and chest pain with drug treatment were unsuccessful in all patients, including administration of β-blockers and calcium channel blockers (n=20), diuretics (n=14), angiotensin-converting enzyme inhibitor or angiotension receptor blocker (n=7), aldosterone inhibitor (n=2), or ranolazine/nitrates (n=2). In addition, inotropic therapy (milrinone, n=7; combination milirinone and dobutamine, n=2) was administered to 9 patients. In-hospital support was necessary in 2 patients because of particularly unstable hemodynamic profiles using an LV-assist device in 1 (Thoratec Percutaneous Ventricular Assist Device, Pleasanton, CA) for management of refractory cardiogenic shock with end-organ dysfunction[21] and an intra-aortic balloon pump for persistently low cardiac index (despite inotropic therapy) in 1.

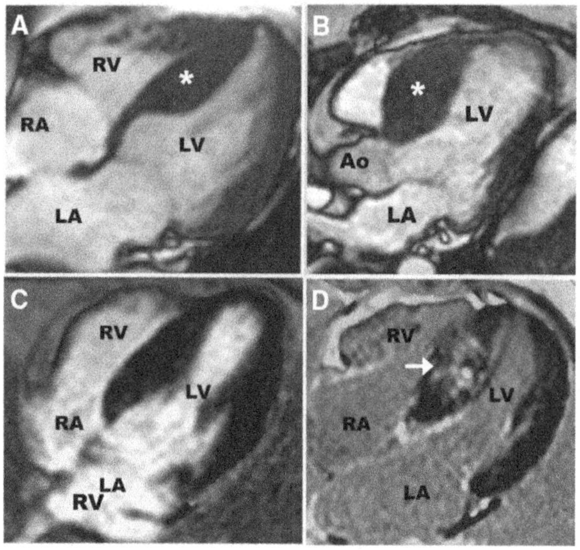


**Figure 3.** Cardiac MRI images of 3 nonobstructive hypertrophic cardiomyopathy patients with preserved systolic function and 1 patient in the end-stage phase with systolic dysfunction (EF<50%), each of whom either received heart transplant or are currently listed for transplant. **A**, Four-chamber long-axis image from a 41-year-old man genotyped to a pathogenic sarcomere mutation (TPM1 Glu 96 Asp) with normal systolic function (EF=70%), small LV cavity (end-diastolic diameter=29 mm), and septal thickness of 24 mm (asterisk; patient No. 7, Tables 2 and 3). **B**, Three-chamber long-axis image in a 63-year-old man with EF of 60% and ventricular septal hypertrophy (21 mm; asterisk) who required inotropic support with intravenous milrinone and dobutamine before heart transplant (patient No. 19). **C**, Four-chamber long-axis contrast-enhanced image demonstrating absence of late gadolinium enhancement (LGE; ie.,fibrosis) in a 33-year-old woman with New York Heart Association functional class IV symptoms, currently status II listed for heart transplant (patient No. 5); **D**, Contrast-enhanced 4-chamber long-axis image in a 23-year-old man with end-stage hypertrophic cardiomyopathy: ejection fraction of 30%, LV end-diastolic cavity dimension of 53 mm, and extensive transmural LGE (arrow) occupying 21% of LV myocardial mass. Ao indicates aorta; LA, left atrium; LV, left ventricle; RA, right atrium; and RV, right ventricle.

### Clinical Determinants of Heart Transplant Listing

In each of the 20 patients, the primary indication for transplant listing was a clinical history of disabling heart failure symptoms of exertional dyspnea (with or without chest pain), consistent with NYHA III/IV and refractory to optimal medical therapy. At least 1 additional clinical criteria supporting the need for transplantation was present in 18 patients, including (1) peak $V_{O_2}$ ≤14 mL/min/kg or <50% predicted for age in 12 patients (Nos. 1–4, 7, 8, 12–14, and 16–18 in Tables 2 and 3); (2) unfavorable resting hemodynamic profile, including elevated LV filling pressures or impaired cardiac index, in 14 patients (Nos. 2–4, 6–9, 11, 12, 14, 16–18, and 20); and (3) acute hemodynamic deterioration requiring inotropic therapy or mechanical support in 10 patients (Nos. 1–3, 9, 11, 12, 15, and 17–19). Therefore, 5 patients had 1 additional supporting criteria for transplant, 8 patients had 2 criteria, and 5 had 3 supporting criteria.

In the remaining 2 patients, inotropic therapy or mechanical support was not required and other traditional criteria for transplant listing were absent, including peak $V_{O_2}$ >14 mL/min/kg or ≥50% predicted for age and normal resting hemodynamic profile (patient Nos. 5 and 10). These patients were listed for transplant solely because of refractory disabling symptoms by history, judged secondary to HCM. In addition, 3 patients (No. 4, 13, and 14) were allowed exceptions by the regional transplant committee to obtain an advanced transplant status (ie., 1Ae or 1Be) than would otherwise be granted, given that traditional therapies that allow 1A or 1B listing criteria are generally not indicated in patients with HCM and preserved LV systolic function.[2]

### Outcome

Twelve patients received a heart transplant and each is currently alive, without cardiovascular symptoms (NYHA functional class I), after 0.5 to 6.3 years (mean 2.3±1.7; Table I in the Data Supplement). In addition, after transplant, invasive hemodynamics parameters were significantly improved, including pulmonary capillary wedge pressure and cardiac index ($P$<0.001), without a significant change in EF (63±6% versus 62±4%; $P$=0.82; Table I in the Data Supplement). Six patients remain active on the transplant list as status 1B (n=1) or status 2 (n=5). Two patients died of unrelenting heart failure awaiting transplant.

### Comparison of Patients With Preserved LV Systolic Function and End Stage

Compared with the study patients with preserved systolic function, those with EF <50% (end-stage) demonstrated evidence of adverse LV remodeling with increased cavity size (50±9 versus 39±7 mm; $P$<0.001), lesser degree of hypertrophy (wall thickness, 18±4 versus 22±4 mm; $P$=0.006), and a trend toward more extensive myocardial fibrosis on contrast-enhanced CMR (% LGE of LV myocardium, 18±10 versus 9±8; $P$=0.07; Table 1 and Figure 3). Particularly extensive fibrosis (LGE ≥15%) was present in 4 of 6 (67%) end-stage HCM patients compared with only 3 of 15 (20%) with preserved systolic function. Several relevant clinical variables were similar between the 2 subgroups, including peak $V_{O_2}$, LV filling pressures, age at heart failure symptom onset, and time from onset of symptoms to transplant listing (Table 1).

## Discussion

Advanced heart failure has become increasingly important among patients with HCM, given the capability of sudden death prevention afforded by the implantable cardioverter defibrillator.[4–8] This evolving recognition underscores the importance of reliably identifying those HCM patients who may be candidates for major life prolonging heart failure therapies. Heart transplantation has traditionally been reserved largely for patients in the end stage of HCM, arbitrarily defined by EF <50%.[2,9,15] In this regard, we have recently recognized a subset of nonobstructive HCM patients eligible for heart transplant because of severe, unrelenting heart failure symptoms refractory to pharmacological treatment, despite evidence of preserved LV systolic function. Therefore, we describe here the clinical profile and natural history of this under-recognized patient subset within the broad disease spectrum of HCM.

By interrogating the databases of 2 major HCM referral cohorts, we found that 2% of patients were listed for heart transplantation, and among these, more than 40% demonstrated a disease phenotype distinctly different from those nonobstructive patients eligible for heart transplant in the end-stage phase, characterized by impaired systolic function and often associated with LV remodeling with regression of hypertrophy and ventricular chamber enlargement.[15,16] In contrast, the novel subgroup reported here experienced progressive and advanced heart failure refractory to maximal medical management, despite demonstrating little or no evidence of LV chamber remodeling. For example, average LV wall thickness was 22 mm (up to 34 mm), and LV cavity dimensions were normal or small, typical of that encountered in the overall HCM disease spectrum.[2] In addition, HCM transplant candidates with systolic dysfunction characteristically show diffuse (and often transmural) LV myocardial scarring grossly visible by examination of the explanted heart and also identifiable by contrast-enhanced CMR (ie, occupying on average almost 20% of total LV mass).[9,15,22] However, in contrast, most of our patients with advanced heart failure and preserved systolic function showed no or minimal myocardial fibrosis.

However, despite these substantial differences in phenotypic expression, our study patients with normal systolic function became transplant candidates in the absence of any other available therapeutic option capable of restoring reasonable expectation for an improved and acceptable quality of life with increased functional capacity. Indeed, each transplanted patient has survived without significant transplant-related complications over a 6-year period and without residual cardiovascular symptoms. Indeed, survival after heart transplant for HCM patients has been shown to be similar (if not better)[23–26] than that for patients with other cardiac diseases, with 75% and 61% survival 5- and 10-years post-transplant.[25] This experience underscores the principle that nonobstructive HCM patients with advanced heart failure symptoms, refractory to medical therapies, can (and should be) considered for cardiac transplantation as a final therapeutic option, even in the presence of normal or hyperdynamic LV systolic function and substantial increase in LV mass.

We found no relevant clinical or imaging marker that adequately predicted risk for advanced heart failure in this subset of HCM patients. Nevertheless, a disproportionate number of probands (ie, 25%) reported here with preserved systolic function had a family history of end-stage HCM with reduced EF and LV remodeling, including 2 relatives who required heart transplant. That relatives within the same HCM family (and presumably with the same disease-causing mutation) progressed to transplant with distinctly different phenotypic expressions[15,27,28] supports the principle that no definitive relationship has been established in HCM between individual sarcomere mutations and cardiac phenotype.[29–31]

The predominant mechanism responsible for the progressive symptoms of heart failure experienced by the HCM patients reported here seems to be LV diastolic dysfunction. This view is supported by evidence of abnormal LV filling at rest (or with exercise) at cardiac catheterization and with echocardiography in each patient, and in the absence of other mechanisms known to produce heart failure in HCM, for example, LV outflow tract obstruction,[10] marked mitral regurgitation,[32] and associated atherosclerotic coronary artery disease.[33] Notably, almost one half of our patients demonstrated a restrictive filling by echocardiography, previously shown to identify HCM patients at increased risk for progressive heart failure and transplant, independent of LV systolic function.[34]

Nevertheless, we recognize that the decision to pursue transplant in this subset of HCM patients is complex and challenging and ultimately requires taking into account the individual clinical profile of the patient, with the greatest weight given to the clinical history and symptom profile. Indeed, 10% of our patients with preserved systolic function were considered for transplant even in the absence of traditional parameters, such as peak $Vo_2$ consumption ≤14 mL/kg/min,[18] after recognition that transplant was the only therapeutic option with the capacity to restore an acceptable quality of life.

Our observations also have implications for current transplant listing criteria, which are based largely on an experience in patients with systolic heart failure and diseases other than HCM, principally ischemic and dilated cardiomyopathies.[18] This underscores the need for clinicians familiar with HCM to participate closely with multidisciplinary heart failure/transplant team to ensure optimal treatment strategies are implemented for this unique subset of HCM patients, including appropriate candidacy for heart transplant.[35]

Notably, the clinical course of HCM patients with advanced heart failure and preserved systolic function proved to be variable, and becoming transplant candidates at a broad range of ages (16–63 years), and at an average age of only 41 years. Furthermore, there were relatively modest time periods between onset of symptoms and listing for transplant (average, 8 years) and particularly between listing and the transplant itself (average, only 0.6 years). Therefore, these data underscore the importance of close longitudinal follow-up for nonobstructive HCM patients with limiting heart failure symptoms and a relatively high index of suspicion and low threshold to pursue cardiovascular evaluation for heart transplantation.[2,13,14]

Several clinical studies and expert consensus guidelines in HCM have, by convention, arbitrarily considered an EF ≥50% to represent preserved systolic function,[1,2,9,14,15,17] which served as the justification for choosing this specific EF cut point to identify our study cohort. However, most importantly, we recognize that HCM encompasses a broad range in EF (ie, from hyperdynamic to systolic dysfunction)[22] expressing a continuum of cardiac systolic function and advanced heart failure because (1) some patients with preserved LV systolic function have relatives with HCM and systolic dysfunction, including transplant candidates;[27,28] (2) several objective measures of advanced heart failure were similar between the 2 groups, including invasive measures of elevated LV filling pressures and level of functional limitation by cardiopulmonary exercise testing; and (3) a variability in the extent of myocardial fibrosis (LGE) evident by some patients with preserved LV systolic function showing substantial LGE and others with systolic dysfunction having minimal or no LGE.[15]

The number of HCM patients considered for transplant with preserved LV systolic function in this study is small (n=20). This limitation is unavoidable given the infrequency in which this subset of patient occurs in this disease. Therefore, it is unlikely that prospective studies with substantially greater numbers of these particular patients will emerge in the near future.

In conclusion, we report a novel subgroup of patients with nonobstructive HCM, who developed advanced progressive heart failure and become transplant candidates, despite preserved systolic function and in the absence of significant LV remodeling. This emerging subgroup expands the spectrum of heart failure requiring transplant in HCM and includes patients with normal LV systolic function. The pathophysiologic determinant of this novel clinical course seems to be LV diastolic dysfunction. However, the severity of symptoms was not always supported by traditional heart transplant testing criteria, and the decision to offer transplant as a final therapeutic option should be made on an individual patient basis in the presence of advanced and refractory heart failure.

## Disclosures

None.

## References


1. Maron BJ, Maron MS. Hypertrophic cardiomyopathy. *Lancet*. 2013;381:242–255.
2. Gersh BJ, Maron BJ, Bonow RO, Dearani JA, Fifer MA, Link MS, Naidu SS, Nishimura RA, Ommen SR, Rakowski H, Seidman CE, Towbin JA, Udelson JE, Yancy CW; American College of Cardiology Foundation/American Heart Association Task Force on Practice Guidelines; American Association for Thoracic Surgery; American Society of Echocardiography; American Society of Nuclear Cardiology; Heart Failure Society of America; Heart Rhythm Society; Society for Cardiovascular Angiography and Interventions; Society of Thoracic Surgeons. 2011 ACCF/AHA guideline for the diagnosis and treatment of hypertrophic cardiomyopathy: a report of the American College of Cardiology Foundation/American Heart Association Task Force on Practice Guidelines. *Circulation*. 2011;124:e783–e831.
3. Elliott PM, Poloniecki J, Dickie S, Sharma S, Monserrat L, Varnava A, Mahon NG, McKenna WJ. Sudden death in hypertrophic cardiomyopathy: identification of high risk patients. *J Am Coll Cardiol*. 2000;36:2212–2218.
4. O'Mahony C, Jichi F, Pavlou M, Monserrat L, Anastasakis A, Rapezzi C, Biagini E, Gimeno JR, Limongelli G, McKenna WJ, Omar RZ, Elliott PM; Hypertrophic Cardiomyopathy Outcomes Investigators. A novel clinical risk prediction model for sudden cardiac death in hypertrophic cardiomyopathy (HCM Risk-SCD). *Eur Heart J*. 2014;35:2010–2020.
5. Maron BJ, Spirito P, Shen WK, Haas TS, Formisano F, Link MS, Epstein AE, Almquist AK, Daubert JP, Lawrenz T, Boriani G, Estes NA III, Favale S, Piccininno M, Winters SL, Santini M, Betocchi S, Arribas F, Sherrid MV, Buja G, Semsarian C, Bruzzi P. Implantable cardioverter-defibrillators and prevention of sudden cardiac death in hypertrophic cardiomyopathy. *JAMA*. 2007;298:405–412.
6. Maron BJ, Spirito P, Ackerman MJ, Casey SA, Semsarian C, Estes NA III, Shannon KM, Ashley EA, Day SM, Pacileo G, Formisano F, Devoto E, Anastasakis A, Bos JM, Woo A, Autore C, Pass RH, Boriani G, Garberich RF, Almquist AK, Russell MW, Boni L, Berger S, Maron MS, Link MS. Prevention of sudden cardiac death with implantable cardioverter-defibrillators in children and adolescents with hypertrophic cardiomyopathy. *J Am Coll Cardiol*. 2013;61:1527–1535.
7. Vriesendorp PA, Schinkel AF, Van Cleemput J, Willems R, Jordaens LJ, Theuns DA, van Slegtenhorst MA, de Ravel TJ, ten Cate FJ, Michels M. Implantable cardioverter-defibrillators in hypertrophic cardiomyopathy: patient outcomes, rate of appropriate and inappropriate interventions, and complications. *Am Heart J*. 2013;166:496–502.
8. Olde Nordkamp LR, Wilde AA, Tijssen JG, Knops RE, van Dessel PF, de Groot JR. The ICD for primary prevention in patients with inherited cardiac diseases: indications, use, and outcome: a comparison with secondary prevention. *Circ Arrhythm Electrophysiol*. 2013;6:91–100.
9. Melacini P, Basso C, Angelini A, Calore C, Bobbo F, Tokajuk B, Bellini N, Smaniotto G, Zucchetto M, Iliceto S, Thiene G, Maron BJ. Clinicopathological profiles of progressive heart failure in hypertrophic cardiomyopathy. *Eur Heart J*. 2010;31:2111–2123.
10. Maron MS, Olivotto I, Betocchi S, Casey SA, Lesser JR, Losi MA, Cecchi F, Maron BJ. Effect of left ventricular outflow tract obstruction on clinical outcome in hypertrophic cardiomyopathy. *N Engl J Med*. 2003;348:295–303.
11. Ommen SR, Maron BJ, Olivotto I, Maron MS, Cecchi F, Betocchi S, Gersh BJ, Ackerman MJ, McCully RB, Dearani JA, Schaff HV, Danielson GK, Tajik AJ, Nishimura RA. Long-term effects of surgical septal myectomy on survival in patients with obstructive hypertrophic cardiomyopathy. *J Am Coll Cardiol*. 2005;46:470–476.
12. Sorajja P, Ommen SR, Holmes DR Jr, Dearani JA, Rihal CS, Gersh BJ, Lennon RJ, Nishimura RA. Survival after alcohol septal ablation for obstructive hypertrophic cardiomyopathy. *Circulation*. 2012;126:2374–2380.
13. Kato TS, Takayama H, Yoshizawa S, Marboe C, Schulze PC, Farr M, Naka Y, Mancini D, Maurer MS. Cardiac transplantation in patients with hypertrophic cardiomyopathy. *Am J Cardiol*. 2012;110:568–574.
14. Biagini E, Spirito P, Leone O, Picchio FM, Coccolo F, Ragni L, Lofiego C, Grigioni F, Potena L, Rocchi G, Bacchi-Reggiani L, Boriani G, Prandstraller D, Arbustini E, Branzi A, Rapezzi C. Heart transplantation in hypertrophic cardiomyopathy. *Am J Cardiol*. 2008;101:387–392.
15. Harris KM, Spirito P, Maron MS, Zenovich AG, Formisano F, Lesser JR, Mackey-Bojack S, Manning WJ, Udelson JE, Maron BJ. Prevalence, clinical profile, and significance of left ventricular remodeling in the end-stage phase of hypertrophic cardiomyopathy. *Circulation*. 2006;114:216–225.
16. Fernández A, Vigliano CA, Casabé JH, Diez M, Favaloro LE, Guevara E, Favaloro RR, Laguens RP. Comparison of prevalence, clinical course, and pathological findings of left ventricular systolic impairment versus normal systolic function in patients with hypertrophic cardiomyopathy. *Am J Cardiol*. 2011;108:548–555.
17. Maron BJ, McKenna WJ, Danielson GK, Kappenberger LJ, Kuhn HJ, Seidman CE, Shah PM, Spencer WH III, Spirito P, Ten Cate FJ, Wigle ED; Task Force on Clinical Expert Consensus Documents. American College of Cardiology; Committee for Practice Guidelines. European Society of Cardiology. American College of Cardiology/European Society of Cardiology clinical expert consensus document on hypertrophic cardiomyopathy. A report of the American College of Cardiology Foundation Task Force on Clinical Expert Consensus Documents and the European Society of Cardiology Committee for Practice Guidelines. *J Am Coll Cardiol*. 2003;42:1687–1713.
18. Mehra MR, Kobashigawa J, Starling R, Russell S, Uber PA, Parameshwar J, Mohacsi P, Augustine S, Aaronson K, Barr M. Listing criteria for heart transplantation: International Society for Heart and Lung Transplantation guidelines for the care of cardiac transplant candidates–2006. *J Heart Lung Transplant*. 2006;25:1024–1042.
19. Maron MS, Olivotto I, Zenovich AG, Link MS, Pandian NG, Kuvin JT, Nistri S, Cecchi F, Udelson JE, Maron BJ. Hypertrophic cardiomyopathy is predominantly a disease of left ventricular outflow tract obstruction. *Circulation*. 2006;114:2232–2239.
20. Nagueh SF, Appleton CP, Gillebert TC, Marino PN, Oh JK, Smiseth OA, Waggoner AD, Flachskampf FA, Pellikka PA, Evangelista A. Recommendations for the evaluation of left ventricular diastolic function by echocardiography. *J Am Soc Echocardiogr*. 2009;22:107–133.
21. Muthiah K, Phan J, Robson D, Macdonald PS, Keogh AM, Kotlyar E, Granger E, Dhital K, Spratt P, Jansz P, Hayward CS. Centrifugal continuous-flow left ventricular assist device in patients with hypertrophic cardiomyopathy: a case series. *ASAIO J*. 2013;59:183–187.
22. Olivotto I, Maron BJ, Appelbaum E, Harrigan CJ, Salton C, Gibson CM, Udelson JE, O'Donnell C, Lesser JR, Manning WJ, Maron MS. Spectrum and clinical significance of systolic function and myocardial fibrosis assessed by cardiovascular magnetic resonance in hypertrophic cardiomyopathy. *Am J Cardiol*. 2010;106:261–267.
23. Coutu M, Perrault LP, White M, Pelletier GB, Racine N, Poirier NC, Carrier M. Cardiac transplantation for hypertrophic cardiomyopathy: a valid therapeutic option. *J Heart Lung Transplant*. 2004;23:413–417.
24. Gajarski R, Naftel DC, Pahl E, Alejos J, Pearce FB, Kirklin JK, Zamberlan M, Dipchand AI; Pediatric Heart Transplant Study Investigators. Outcomes of pediatric patients with hypertrophic cardiomyopathy listed for transplant. *J Heart Lung Transplant*. 2009;28:1329–1334.
25. Maron MS, Kalsmith BM, Udelson JE, Li W, DeNofrio D. Survival after cardiac transplantation in patients with hypertrophic cardiomyopathy. *Circ Heart Fail*. 2010;3:574–579.
26. Warren SE, Cohn LH, Schoen FJ, Mudge GH, Lorell BH. Advanced diatolic heart failure in familial hypertrophic cardiomyopathy managed with cardiac transplant. *J Appl Cardiol* 1988;3:415–422.
27. Roberts WC, Roberts CC, Ko JM, Grayburn PA, Tandon A, Kuiper JJ, Capehart JE, Hall SA. Dramatically different phenotypic expressions of hypertrophic cardiomyopathy in male cousins undergoing cardiac transplantation with identical disease-causing gene mutation. *Am J Cardiol*. 2013;111:1818–1822.
28. Rowin EJ, Maron MS. The ever expanding spectrum of phenotypic diversity in hypertrophic cardiomyopathy. *Am J Cardiol*. 2013;112:463–464.
29. Landstrom AP, Ackerman MJ. Mutation type is not clinically useful in predicting prognosis in hypertrophic cardiomyopathy. *Circulation*. 2010;122:2441–2449; discussion 2450.

30. Maron BJ, Maron MS, Semsarian C. Genetics of hypertrophic cardiomyopathy after 20 years: clinical perspectives. *J Am Coll Cardiol.* 2012;60:705–715.
31. Garcia-Pavia P, Vázquez ME, Segovia J, Salas C, Avellana P, Gómez-Bueno M, Vilches C, Gallardo ME, Garesse R, Molano J, Bornstein B, Alonso-Pulpon L. Genetic basis of end-stage hypertrophic cardiomyopathy. *Eur J Heart Fail.* 2011;13:1193–1201.
32. Yu EH, Omran AS, Wigle ED, Williams WG, Siu SC, Rakowski H. Mitral regurgitation in hypertrophic obstructive cardiomyopathy: relationship to obstruction and relief with myectomy. *J Am Coll Cardiol.* 2000;36:2219–2225.
33. Sorajja P, Ommen SR, Nishimura RA, Gersh BJ, Berger PB, Tajik AJ. Adverse prognosis of patients with hypertrophic cardiomyopathy who have epicardial coronary artery disease. *Circulation.* 2003;108:2342–2348.
34. Biagini E, Spirito P, Rocchi G, Ferlito M, Rosmini S, Lai F, Lorenzini M, Terzi F, Bacchi-Reggiani L, Boriani G, Branzi A, Boni L, Rapezzi C. Prognostic implications of the Doppler restrictive filling pattern in hypertrophic cardiomyopathy. *Am J Cardiol.* 2009;104:1727–1731.
35. Maron BJ, Rastegar H, Udelson JE, Dearani JA, Maron MS. Contemporary surgical management of hypertrophic cardiomyopathy, the need for more myectomy surgeons and disease-specific centers, and the Tufts initiative. *Am J Cardiol.* 2013;112:1512–1515.

## CLINICAL PERSPECTIVE

Heart transplantation in hypertrophic cardiomyopathy (HCM) has traditionally been reserved for patients in the end-stage phase of this disease, arbitrarily defined by ejection fraction <50%. However, a novel subset of nonobstructive HCM patients become candidates for heart transplantation with severe, unrelenting heart failure symptoms refractory to pharmacological treatment, despite evidence of preserved left ventricular systolic function (ejection fraction ≥50%). We describe the clinical profile and natural history of this under-recognized patient subset within the broad disease spectrum of HCM, by assembling 20 such patients (1% of the general HCM cohort). We found no relevant clinical or imaging marker that adequately predicted risk for advanced heart failure with unrelenting symptoms in these patients, given their typical features indistinguishable from the general HCM population: left ventricular wall thickness 22±4 mm, left ventricular cavity nondilated (39±7 mm), and no or minimal fibrosis (≤5% of left ventricular mass by cardiovascular magnetic resonance) in the majority of patients. Additionally, 10% of patients were considered for transplant even in the absence of other traditional transplant parameters, including peak $Vo_2$>14 mL/kg/min, because transplant was the only therapeutic option with the capacity to restore an acceptable quality of life. These findings underscore the need for clinicians familiar with HCM to participate closely with multidisciplinary heart failure teams to ensure that optimal treatment strategies are implemented in this unique subset of HCM patients, including, when appropriate, heart transplantation.

# The Two Extremes of Cardiac Sarcoidosis and the Effect of Prednisone Therapy

Danielle Armstrong, DO[a], Gonzalo V. Gonzalez-Stawinski, MD[b], Jong Mi Ko, BA[c], Shelley A. Hall, MD[d], and William C. Roberts, MD[a,c,d,*]

**Described herein are clinical and morphologic findings in 2 patients who underwent heart transplantation because of severe heart failure resulting from cardiac sarcoidosis. Although the explanted hearts in each patient had characteristic gross changes of cardiac sarcoidosis, one patient who had been treated with prednisone, had no residual sarcoid granulomas in the myocardium, whereas the other patient, in whom diagnosis was not made until heart transplantation, had innumerable sarcoid granulomas in her heart. This report suggests that prednisone can eliminate sarcoid granulomas in the heart but that their replacement is by dense fibrous tissue, something also likely the result of the granulomas themselves, creating a situation where the treated (prednisone) and the non-treated sarcoid heart may appear similar by gross examination.**  **(Am J Cardiol 2015;115:150−153)**

Although it is a systemic disease, sarcoidosis uncommonly affects the heart and when it does the non-cardiac organs are usually minimally affected and they function normally.[1−6] On occasion, cardiac sarcoidosis may lead to such severe heart failure that heart transplantation (HT) is the only reasonable therapy.[3−5] In such situations, diagnosis of cardiac sarcoidosis is usually not made until HT, the usual pre-HT diagnosis being "non-ischemic cardiomyopathy".[5] Recently, 2 patients underwent HT at Baylor University Medical Center (BUMC) in the same month and examination of the explanted heart in one disclosed innumerable myocardial sarcoid granulomas (not diagnosed clinically) and, in the other patient, despite some similar gross findings in the heart, no myocardial granulomas were seen (diagnosed clinically by an earlier biopsy). This report describes findings in these 2 patients to point out the huge spectrum of myocardial changes in patients with cardiac sarcoidosis, and the potential effect of long term prednisone therapy in this condition.

## Patients Studied

Pertinent findings in each of the 2 patients are detailed in Table 1. Both patients were in their 50s; both were white; both had severe (4+/4+) heart failure; both had evidence of cardiac dysfunction for approximately 4 years; both had periodic runs of non-sustained ventricular tachycardia; both had some type of heart block (complete in case #1, and right bundle branch block in case #2); neither had dysfunction of a non-cardiac body organ, and neither patient had narrowing of the epicardial coronary arteries. Diagnosis of sarcoidosis before HT was made in patient #1 by biopsy of a mediastinal lymph node 21 months before HT although 2 years earlier a cardiac biopsy had shown "granulomas". Patient #1, who had no granulomas in his explanted heart, was placed on prednisone after the granulomas were seen in the lymph node and he received this drug for 21 months, at very high doses for 10 months before dose-tapering

Table 1
Clinical and morphologic findings in the 2 patients

| Variable | Case | |
|---|---|---|
| | #1 | #2 |
| Gender | Man | Woman |
| Age (years) | | |
| At heart transplantation | 53 | 57 |
| Onset of symptoms | 49 | 53 |
| Electrophysiology | | |
| Heart block | Complete | RBBB |
| Ventricular tachycardia | + | + |
| Pacemaker | + | 0 |
| Intracardiac defibrillator | + | + |
| Systemic hypertension | + | 0 |
| Body mass index (Kg/m$^2$) | 31.8 | 29.9 |
| Hemodynamic data | | |
| Lowest left ventricular EF (%) | 20 | 15 |
| Cardiac index (L/min/m$^2$) | 2.01 | 1.36 |
| Pressures (mm Hg) | | |
| Blood pressure, indirect (s/d) | 100/85 | 85/40 |
| Right atrial mean | 6 | 2 |
| Right ventricle (s/d) | 26/10 | 48/6 |
| Pulmonary artery (s/d) | 26/14 | 44/11 |
| Pulmonary artery wedge mean | 11 | 14 |
| Prednisone therapy (months) | + (21) | 0 |
| Heart weight (g) | 535 | 380 |
| Cardiac granuloma (0-4+) | 0 | 4+ |
| Left ventricular cavity (cm) | 7.5 | 5.5 |

EF = ejection fraction; RBBB = right bundle branch block; s/d = peak systole/end diastole.

Departments of [a]Pathology, [b]Cardiothoracic Surgery, and [d]Internal Medicine (Division of Cardiology), Baylor University Medical Center, Dallas, Texas and [c]Baylor Heart and Vascular Institute, Baylor University Medical Center, Dallas, Texas. Manuscript received September 2, 2014; revised manuscript received and accepted October 5, 2014.

Support for this investigation was provided by the Baylor Health Care System Foundation.

See page 153 for disclosure information.

*Corresponding author: Tel: 214-820-7911; fax: 214-820-7533.
*E-mail address:* wc.roberts@baylorhealth.edu (W.C. Roberts).

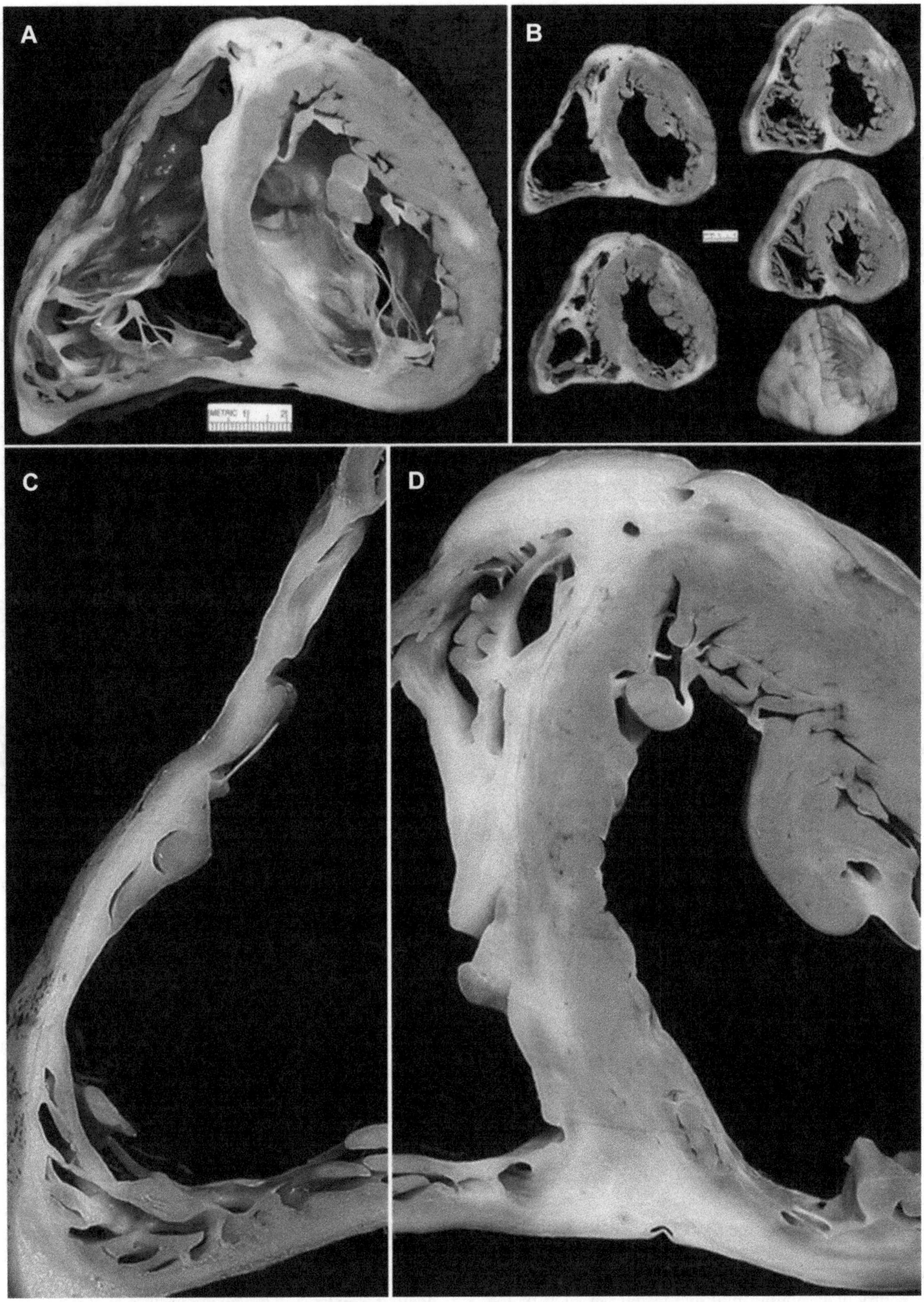


Figure 1. Heart in patient #1. *(A)* View of the base of the heart showing marked dilatation of both right and left ventricular cavities and focal scars in the left and right ventricular free walls and ventricular septum. *(B)* Transverse cuts of the cardiac ventricles caudal to the view shown in *(A)*. *(C)* Close up view of the wall of right ventricle showing extensive scarring and marked thinning of the wall (simulating arrhythmogenic right ventricular dysplasia/cardiomyopathy). *(D)* View of the ventricular septum showing the scarring primarily on the right side of the septum. Because the biotome to biopsy the heart extracts tissue from the right side of the ventricular septum that probably was the reason the biopsy was positive in this patient early in his course.

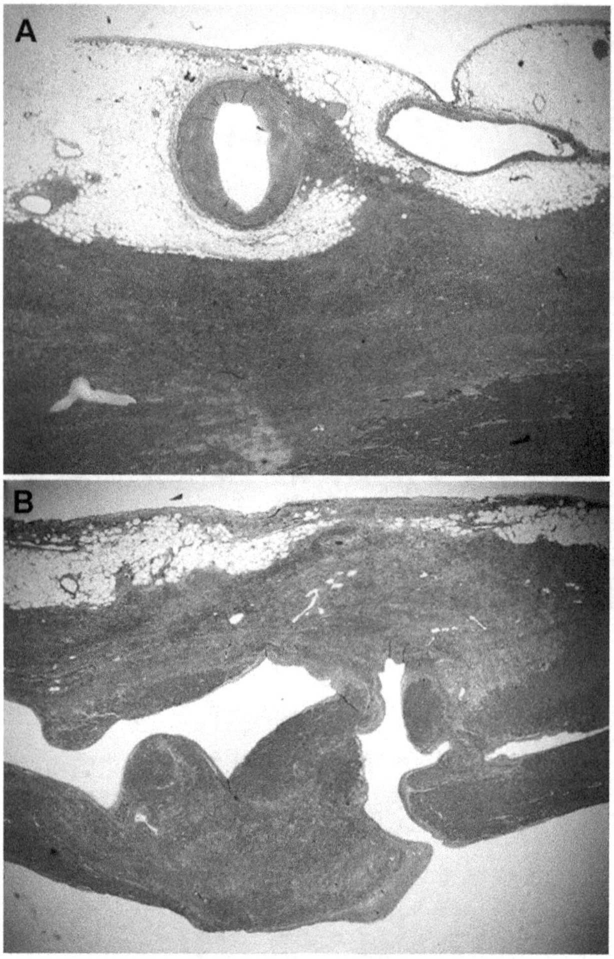

Figure 2. Photomicrographs of portions of the heart in patient #1. *(A)* View of the epicardium, subepicardium, and outer myocardial wall in the anterior portion of left ventricle. The left anterior descending coronary artery and also a coronary vein are shown. The deep blue color represents scar tissue which is located primarily in the subepicardial region rather than the sub-endocardial region. No granulomas were found in the dense fibrous tissue despite examining numerous sections of myocardium. The coronary vessels are surrounded by mainly adipose tissue. *(B)* View of the right ventricular free wall also showing extensive scarring again involving the subepicardial portion more than the subendocardial portion. Trichrome stains, each ×20.

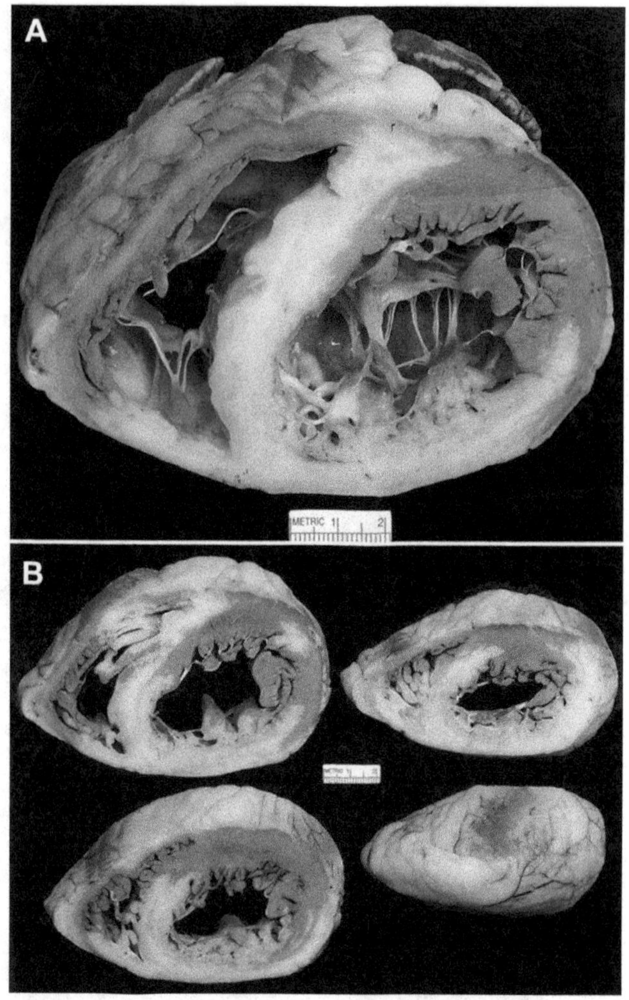

Figure 3. Views of the heart in case #2. *(A)* View of the opened basal portion of the heart showing considerable dilatation of both ventricular cavities and severe scarring of the ventricular septum, posterolateral left ventricular free wall, and posterior wall of right ventricle. Numerous sarcoid granulomas were present in the dense fibrous tissue. *(B)* One-cm thick slices of the ventricles caudal to the upper view. Much of the left ventricular free wall, ventricular septum and right ventricular free wall are replaced by sarcoid granulomas with their surrounding fibrous tissue.

began. Patient #2, whose sarcoidosis was not diagnosed until HT, never received corticosteroid therapy before HT and her explanted heart contained innumerable granulomas typical of sarcoidosis. Photographs of the heart in each patient are shown in Figures 1 to 4.

## Discussion

The explanted hearts in each of the 2 hitherto described patients had gross features characteristic of cardiac sarcoidosis: involvement of the walls of both right and left ventricles and the ventricular septum; multiple lesions in each of the cardiac walls; a tendency for the gross lesions to involve the subepicardial half of the left ventricular free wall and the right ventricular half of the ventricular septum, dilation of both ventricular cavities, and absence of narrowing of the epicardial coronary arteries. Yet one patient, who previously by both cardiac and lymph node biopsies showed sarcoidosis, had no granulomas in his explanted heart; the other patient had innumerable sarcoid granulomas in her heart and diagnosis of sarcoidosis was not made until examination of the explanted heart. Patient #1 who had no granulomas in his explanted heart had received prednisone therapy for 21 months, high doses during 10 of those months. The quantity of scar tissue in both patients' hearts suggests that the sarcoid granulomas and their adjacent lymphocytes are strong fibrous-tissue stimulants, and, moreover, that prednisone therapy is a strong eliminator of sarcoid granulomas but the residue of that healing is extensive replacement fibrosis. (Sarcoidosis in the lung is also a strong fibrosis stimulator.[7]) It seems reasonable to believe that the heart in patient #1 earlier had been loaded with sarcoid granulomas as found in patient #2 but that the prednisone treatment likely played a role in eliminating the sarcoid granuloma by replacing them with dense fibrous

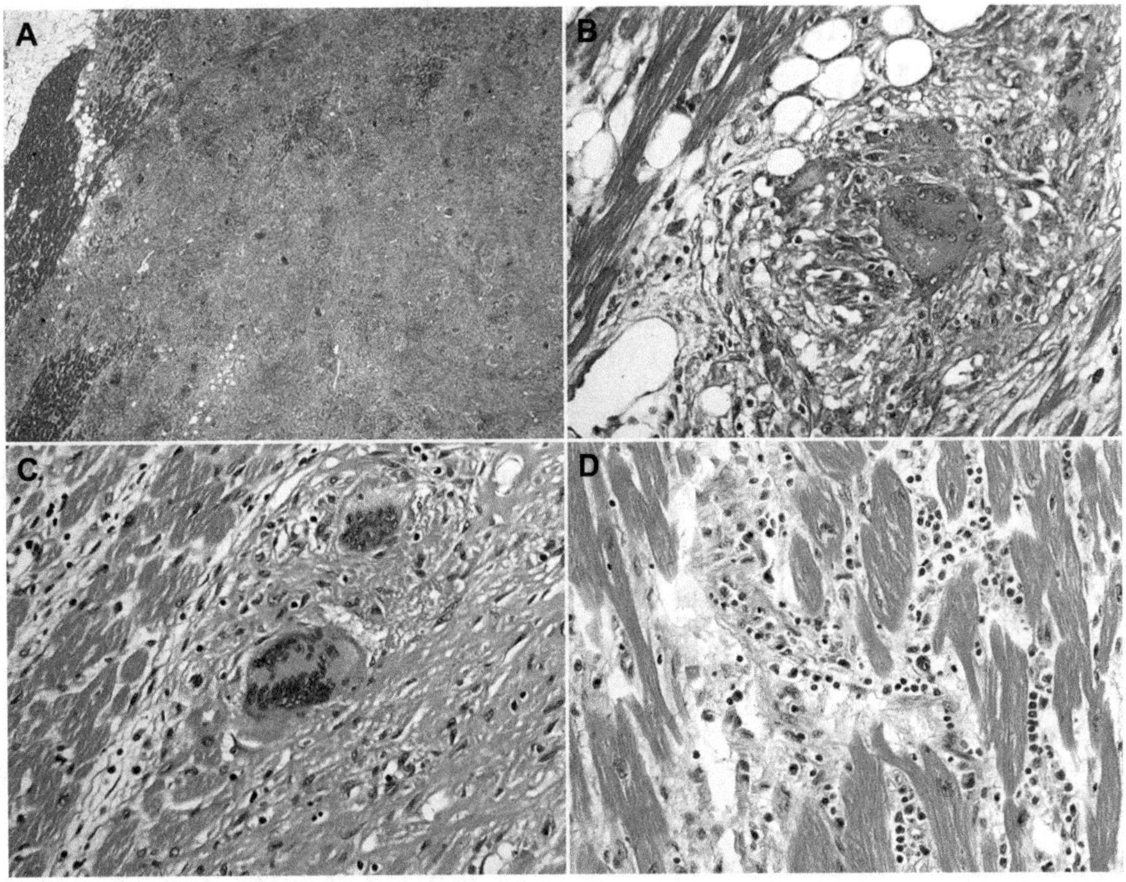

Figure 4. Photomicrographs in patient #2. *(A)* View of a portion of left ventricular free wall showing numerous granulomas surrounded by dense fibrous tissue. *(B)* Close-up view of a single sarcoid granuloma. *(C)* Another view of sarcoid granulomas showing numerous nuclei in each of the giant cells. *(D)* Infiltration between myocardial fibers of lymphocytes typical of sarcoid myocarditis. Trichrome stain, ×40 *(A)*; trichrome stain, ×400 *(B)*; hematoxylin/eosin stain, ×400 *(C)*, and hematoxylin/eosin stain, ×400 *(D)*.

tissue. Such a demonstration to our knowledge has not been provided previous to this report. Earlier we described a patient with typical gross lesions of cardiac sarcoidosis but study of numerous sections of the heart histologically failed to reveal any granulomas.[6] This earlier patient had never received corticosteroid therapy,[6] but earlier histologic examination of a portion of the left ventricular free wall excised to insert a left ventricular assist device did disclose sarcoid granulomas.

## Disclosures

The authors have no conflicts of interest to disclose.


1. Roberts WC, McAllister HA Jr, Ferrans VJ. Sarcoidosis of the heart. A clinicopathologic study of 35 necropsy patients (Group I) and review of 78 previously described necropsy patients (Group II). *Am J Med* 1977;63:86–108.
2. Virmani R, Bures JC, Roberts WC. Cardiac sarcoidosis: a major cause of sudden death in young individuals. *Chest* 1980;77:423–428.
3. Donsky AS, Escobar J, Capehart J, Roberts WC. Heart Transplantation for undiagnosed cardiac sarcoidosis. *Am J Cardiol* 2002;89:1447–1450.
4. Roberts WC, Vowels TJ, Ko JM, Capehard JE, Hall SA. Cardiac transplantation for cardiac sarcoidosis with initial diagnosis by examination of the left ventricular apical "core" excised for insertion of a left ventricular assist device for severe chronic heart failure. *Am J Cardiol* 2009;103:110–114.
5. Sharma PS, Lubahn JG, Donsky AS, Yoon AD, Carry MM, Grayburn PA, Wood PB, Ko JM, Burton EC, Roberts WC. Diagnosing cardiac sarcoidosis clinically without tissue confirmation. *Proc (Bayl Univ Med Cent)* 2009;22:236–238.
6. Roberts WC, Chung MS, Ko JM, Capehart JE, Hall SA. Morphologic features of cardiac sarcoidosis in native hearts of patients having cardiac transplantation. *Am J Cardiol* 2014;113:706–712.
7. Crystal RG, Roberts WC, Hunninghake GW, Gadek JE, Fulmer JD, Line BR. Pulmonary sarcoidosis: a disease characterized and perpetuated by activated lung T-lymphocytes. *Ann Intern Med* 1981;94:73–94.

# Surviving Malignant Hypertrophic Cardiomyopathy With all Major Complications in a Single Patient

Barry J. Maron, MD[a,*], Henry L. Weiner, MD[b], Martin S. Maron, MD[c], and William C. Roberts, MD[d]

The natural history and clinical course of hypertrophic cardiomyopathy (HC) is diverse, ranging from benign forms compatible with normal or extended longevity to adverse consequences requiring major interventions: surgical myectomy (or selectively alcohol septal ablation) for left ventricular (LV) outflow obstruction producing progressive heart failure; defibrillation and therapeutic hypothermia for cardiac arrest; implantable cardioverter-defibrillators (ICD) for prevention of sudden death; and heart transplant for refractory progressive heart failure in the absence of obstruction.[1,2] Patients with HC may have their clinical course importantly influenced by either of these 3 major disease complications,[1,2] but the occurrence of all 3 sequentially in a single patient over a 38 year period represents a notable and unusually aggressive form of HC. We present such a patient, prospectively followed and evaluated, who not only has incurred all major adverse consequences of HC but most importantly has survived due to effective treatment modalities available to patients with this disease.

## Case Description

This patient was initially diagnosed with obstructive HC after a precordial murmur was detected at age 3 (Figure 1). Her father had experienced a resuscitated cardiac arrest from HC and one brother (age 40) has HC with an uneventful course. Surgical myectomy was performed at age 11 years to relieve outflow tract obstruction (gradient, 100 mm Hg) and heart failure symptoms, associated with massive ventricular septal hypertrophy (wall thickness, 35 mm). Symptomatic improvement ensued briefly, but at age 19, the patient was successfully resuscitated from an out-of-hospital cardiac arrest, and a secondary prevention implantable cardioverter-defibrillator (ICD) was placed and subsequently replaced at ages 24, 27 (with biventricular pacing), and 33 years. A lead extraction at age 26 was complicated by a tear in the superior vena cavae which was repaired surgically.

Appropriate ICD interventions for sustained ventricular tachycardia (VT) or ventricular fibrillation (VF) occurred at ages 25 (during tennis), 26, and 32 (sitting at beach) and 34 years. In addition, 25 episodes of monomorphic VT terminated by anti-tachycardia pacing were tabulated, as well as hundreds of spontaneously aborted runs of nonsustained VT evident on ICD interrogation.

At age 26, the patient developed progressive heart failure in NYHA class III associated with adverse LV remodeling: maximum LV wall thickness = 11 mm; LV end-diastolic cavity dimension = 56 mm, and ejection fraction = 20%. Advanced heart failure symptoms persisted for the next 12 years refractory to a variety of pharmacologic agents, including beta-blockers, verapamil, angiotensin-converting enzyme inhibitors, sotalol, mexiletine, digoxin and spironolactone. Despite her significant functional limitation, the patient held sedentary jobs and performed treadmill exercise and yoga.

During this time period, LV remodeling progressed with cavity dimension increasing to 68 mm, and ejection fraction decreasing to only 15%. Peak oxygen consumption ranged from 19 to 21 ml/kg/min; cardiac index was 2.1 L/min/m$^2$; pulmonary capillary wedge pressure was 18 mm Hg, and brain natriuretic peptide was 3500 pg/ml. At age 38, the patient consented to heart transplant listing, and the operation was performed at Hospital of University of Pennsylvania. Postoperative recovery has been uneventful. Genetic testing documented a pathogenic mutation in the MYBPC3 gene (c. 2441_2443 delAGA).

The explanted heart weighed 440 g. Ventricular septum was 14 mm in thickness, and the LV free wall was 16 mm (Figure 2). The LV cavity was markedly dilated, but the right ventricle was normal-sized. Extensive areas of grossly visible scarring were present involving the ventricular septum and LV free wall. The mural endocardium of ventricular septum in apposition to the anterior mitral leaflet was severely thickened by fibrous tissue, extending distally and resulting (at least in part) from the myectomy performed 27 years earlier. The LV wall at the apex was thinned, aneurysmal, and fibrotic. The epicardial coronary arteries were free of atherosclerotic plaque, and the right and left main coronary arteries arose from the aorta in normal position.

Extensive scarring of the LV wall was confirmed histologically. In addition, many myocytes in the subendocardial regions were vacuolated and enlarged. Disorganized patterns of myocyte arrangement were present in ventricular septum, associated with numerous intramural coronary arteries, increased in size with thickened walls and luminal narrowing (Figure 3), both histopathologic hallmarks of HC.

## Comments

The patient presented here illustrates the most extreme example of HC and its deleterious consequences through the first 38 years of life, but nevertheless represents an important principle for this complex genetic disease. Once regarded as a disease with uniformly grim prognosis largely without effective management strategies,[2] this patient underscores the new paradigm in which HC has become

[a]Hypertrophic Cardiomyopathy Center, Minneapolis Heart Institute Foundation, Minneapolis, Minnesota; [b]Care Cardiology Consultants, Newark, New Jersey; [c]Hypertrophic Cardiomyopathy Center, Tufts Medical Center, Boston, Massachusetts; and [d]Baylor University Medical Center, Dallas, Texas. Manuscript received October 29, 2014; revised manuscript received and accepted November 3, 2014.

See page 404 for disclosure information.

*Corresponding author: Tel: +612-863-3996; fax: +612-863-3875.

*E-mail address:* hcm.maron@mhif.org (B.J. Maron).

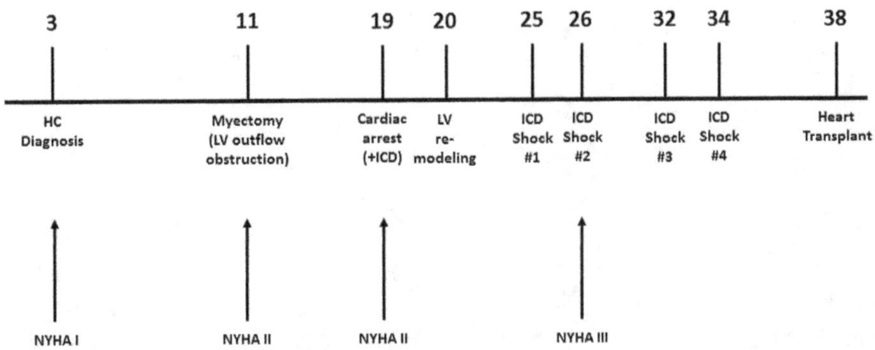


Figure 1. Time-line of cardiac events in our 38-year-old patient. The numbers at the top represent the ages when the events occurred. HC = hypertrophic cardiomyopathy; ICD = intracardiac defibrillator; LV = left ventricular; NYHA = New York Heart Association.

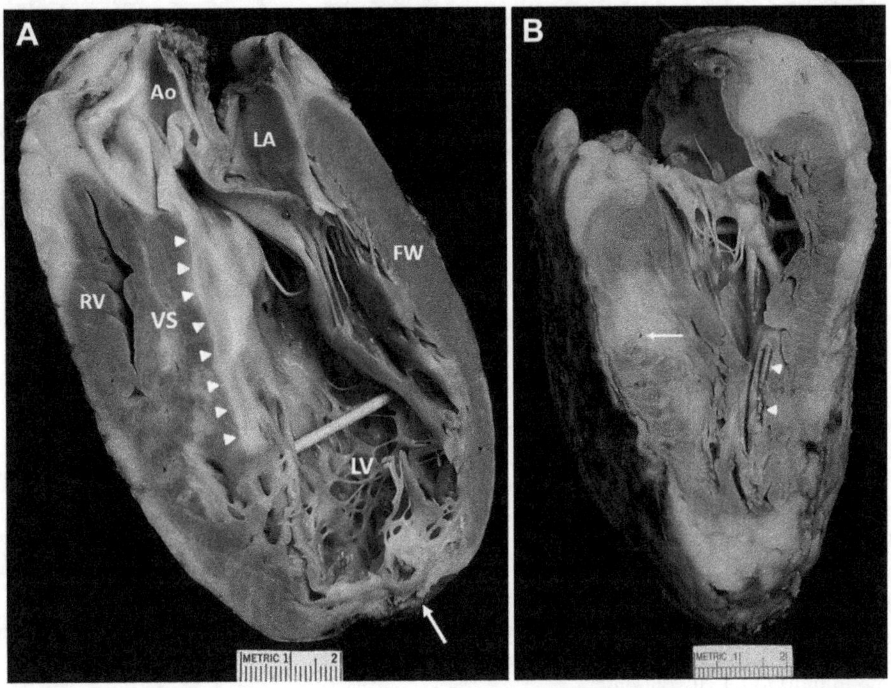


Figure 2. Parasagittal views of the heart from the left side *(A)* and from the right side *(B)*. *(A)* The left ventricle (LV) is greatly dilated, ventricular septum (VS) is focally scarred, and the apex (*white arrow*) is severely scarred, and with pressure would bulge externally (i.e., aneurysmal). The *white arrowheads* point to the mural endocardium of the septum, which is quite thickened by fibrous tissue and represents the extent of the ventricular septal myectomy performed during childhood (at age 11). The left atrium (LA) does not appear to be dilated. *(B)* View from the right side. The wall to the left represents ventricular septum which contains a large scar within which there is a large intramural coronary artery (*arrow*). Defibrillator lead is embedded in white fibrous tissue, extending from the apex into the tricuspid valve orifice (*arrowheads*). Ao = aorta; FW = free wall of left ventricle; RV = right ventricle.

a treatable cardiac disease,[3] with management options now available to target each adverse complication and prolong life, that is, surgical septal myectomy (or alcohol ablation) for limiting symptoms caused by LV outflow obstruction;[1,4,5] external defibrillation for cardiac arrest, often with therapeutic hypothermia;[6] ICD therapy to terminate potentially lethal ventricular tachyarrhythmias (VT/VF) and prevent sudden death;[7] and ultimately heart transplant only in the event that progressive end-stage heart failure intervenes associated with extreme LV remodeling (and in the absence of outflow obstruction).[8,9]

Implementation of these interventions permits most HC patients to achieve extended longevity with good quality of life, and for the present patient the prolongation of life.[1] Notably, this patient endured NYHA class III heart failure symptoms and limitations for at least 12 years before consenting to heart transplantation. Finally, despite the fact that atrial fibrillation is common in HC (in about 20% of patients), and is also linked to end-stage heart failure, our patient showed no evidence of left atrial dilatation (or atrial fibrillation).[1]

Typical of the HC end-stage there was substantial LV remodeling with striking regression from massive hypertrophy (in childhood) to virtually normal wall thickness, associated with LV chamber dilatation. The basis for the LV wall thinning was the development of extensive, diffuse and transmural myocardial scarring, presumably resulting from microvascular ischemia, and also involving the most distal LV segment where early aneurysm formation is evident.[10]

Two additional issues related to the natural history of HC are underscored by the findings in this informative patient.

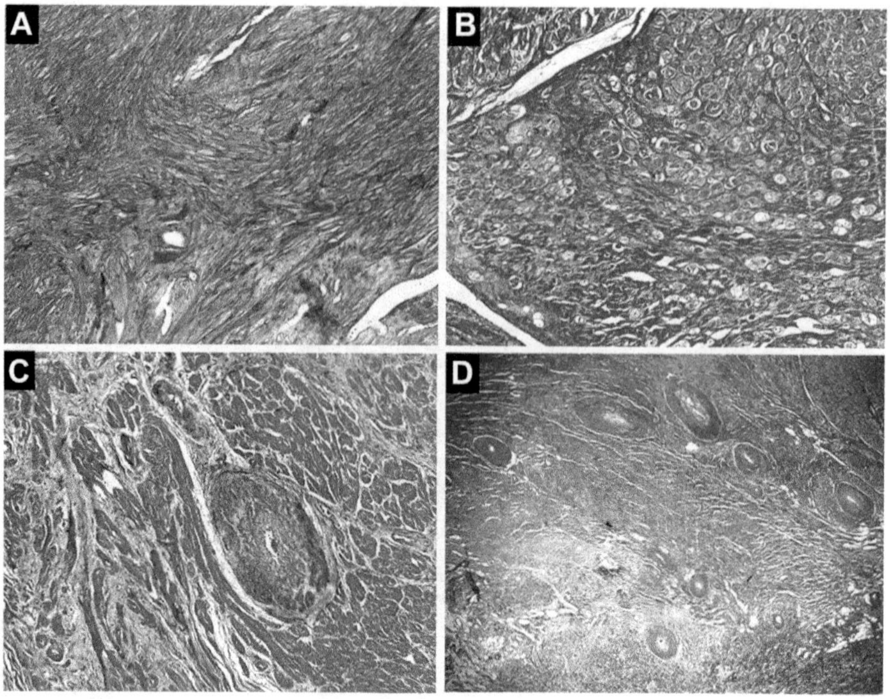


Figure 3. Histologic sections of portions of the ventricular septum *(A, C, D)* and left ventricular papillary muscle *(B)*, all stained with Masson's trichrome. *(A)* Disordered arrangement of myocytes interwoven with scar tissue (*blue*) (x20). *(B)* Large scar in the anterolateral papillary muscle; myofibers are enlarged (x20). *(C)* High power view of a single large and narrowed intramural coronary artery (x40). *(D)* Multiple large and narrowed intramural coronary arteries (*arrows*) embedded within a large scar in ventricular septum (x20).

First, the characteristic heterogeneity of disease expression and clinical course is evident in the diverse disease pathways taken by our patient's malignant course in comparison to that of her asymptomatic 40-year-old brother, with HC and the same pathogenic mutation and genetic substrate. Second, the mutation in the sarcomere MYBPC3 gene responsible for HC in our patient with highly aggressive HC has been previously regarded as benign.[11] Therefore, this patient's clinical profile is consistent with the principle that specific mutations cannot predict future outcome in individual HC patients.[11]

## Disclosures

The authors have no conflicts of interest to disclose.


1. Maron BJ, Ommen SR, Semsarian C, Spirito P, Olivotto I, Maron MS. Hypertrophic cardiomyopathy: present and future, with translation into contemporary cardiovascular medicine. *J Am Coll Cardiol* 2014;64: 83–99.
2. Maron BJ, Braunwald E. Evolution of hypertrophic cardiomyopathy to a contemporary treatable disease. *Circulation* 2012;126:1640–1644.
3. Maron BJ. Recognition of hypertrophic cardiomyopathy as a contemporary, relatively common and treatable disease: International Summit V. *Am J Cardiol* 2014;113:739–744.
4. Ommen SR, Maron BJ, Olivotto I, Maron MS, Cecchi F, Betocchi S, Gersh BJ, Ackerman MJ, McCully RB, Dearani JA, Schaff HV, Danielson GK, Tajik AJ, Nishimura RA. Long-term effects of surgical septal myectomy on survival in patients with obstructive hypertrophic cardiomyopathy. *J Am Coll Cardiol* 2005;46:470–476.
5. Maron MS, Olivotto I, Betocchi S, Casey SA, Lesser JR, Losi MA, Cecchi F, Maron BJ. Effect of left ventricular outflow tract obstruction on clinical outcome in hypertrophic cardiomyopathy. *N Engl J Med* 2003;348:295–303.
6. Maron BJ, Maron MS, Maron BA, Haas TS, Altman RK, Smalley SJ, Doerer JJ, Link MS, Mooney MR. Successful therapeutic hypothermia in patients with hypertrophic cardiomyopathy. *J Am Coll Cardiol* 2011;57:2454–2456.
7. Maron BJ, Spirito P, Shen WK, Haas TS, Formisano F, Link MS, Epstein AE, Almquist AK, Daubert JP, Lawrenz T, Boriani G, Estes NA 3rd, Favale S, Piccininno M, Winters SL, Santini M, Betocchi S, Arribas F, Sherrid MV, Buja G, Semsarian C, Bruzzi P. Implantable cardioverter-defibrillators and prevention of sudden cardiac death in hypertrophic cardiomyopathy. *JAMA* 2007;298:405–412.
8. Harris KM, Spirito P, Maron MS, Zenovich AG, Formisano F, Lesser JR, Mackey-Bojack S, Manning WJ, Udelson JE, Maron BJ. Prevalence, clinical profile and significance of left ventricular remodeling in the end-stage phase of hypertrophic cardiomyopathy. *Circulation* 2006;114:216–225.
9. Rowin EJ, Maron BJ, Kiernan MS, Casey SA, Feldman DS, Hryniewicz KM, Chan RHM, Harris KM, Udelson JE, DeNofrio D, Roberts WC, Maron MS. Advanced heart failure with preserved systolic function in nonobstructive hypertrophic cardiomyopathy: under-recognized subset of candidates for heart transplant. *Circ Heart Fail* 2014;7:967–975.
10. Maron MS, Finley JJ, Bos JM, Hauser TH, Manning WJ, Haas TS, Lesser JR, Udelson JE, Ackerman MJ, Maron BJ. Prevalence, clinical significance, and natural history of left ventricular apical aneurysms in hypertrophic cardiomyopathy. *Circulation* 2008;118:1541–1549.
11. Maron BJ, Maron MS, Semsarian C. Genetics of hypertrophic cardiomyopathy after 20 years: Clinical perspectives. (State-of-the-art). *J Am Coll Cardiol* 2012;60:705–715.

# Atrophy of the Heart After Insertion of a Left Ventricular Assist Device and Closure of the Aortic Valve

William C. Roberts, MD[a,b,c,*], Shelley A. Hall, MD[b], Jong M. Ko, BA[a], Peter A. McCullough, MD, MPH[a,b], and Brian Lima, MD[d]

**Described are findings in a 70-year-old man who had heart transplantation 4 years after treatment with a left ventricular assist device, and surgical closure of his previously replaced aortic valve. The result was a totally nonfunctioning left ventricle resulting in severe atrophy.**  **(Am J Cardiol 2016;117:878–879)**

Exercise enlarges our noncardiac striated muscles and disuse atrophies them. The same would appear to be the case with cardiac muscle. We recently studied a very small heart of a very large man who 4 years earlier had undergone insertion of a left ventricular assist device (LVAD) with surgical closure of his previously replaced aortic valve. This report describes findings in this patient in whom the LVAD totally replaced his left ventricular (LV) function.

### Description of Patient

This 70-year-old man, who was born in June 1945, underwent heart transplantation (HT) because of severe heart failure in July 2015. His symptoms of heart failure began when he was aged 45 years. At age 55 years, he underwent aortic valve replacement with a St. Jude Medical prosthesis for aortic stenosis involving a congenitally bicuspid aortic valve. Because of worsening heart failure when he was aged 65 years (2011), an HeartMate 2 LVAD was inserted, and an occluding patch was placed on the aortic aspect of the prosthesis in the aortic valve position preventing blood flow into the aorta through the prosthetic valve (Figure 1). These endeavors resulted in some improvement in symptoms. Because of chronic atrial fibrillation, he underwent an ablation procedure on 3 occasions. Because of severe heart failure, HT was performed at age 70 years. By 2 months postoperatively, he had resumed near-normal activities. He was 78-inch tall, and his maximum weight was 250 pounds (body mass index 28 kg/m$^2$).

The operatively excised native heart weighed 280 g and contained several scars in the posterolateral LV wall despite a wide-open dominant right coronary artery (Figure 2). In contrast, the left anterior descending and left circumflex coronary arteries were severely narrowed by plaque. Histologic study of sections of the LV wall showed thinning of numerous myofibers (Figure 3).

[a]Baylor Heart and Vascular Institute, Department of Internal Medicine, Dallas, Texas; and Divisions of [b]Cardiology, [c]Pathology, and [d]Cardiothoracic Surgery, Baylor University Medical Center, Dallas, Texas. Manuscript received November 19, 2015; revised manuscript received and accepted December 3, 2015.

Funding: This study was funded by the Baylor Health Care System Foundation.

See page 879 for disclosure information.

*Corresponding author: Tel: (214) 820-7911; fax: (214) 820-7533.

*E-mail address:* wc.roberts@baylorhealth.edu (W.C. Roberts).

### Comments

The extremely small heart (280 g) in this very large man (220 pounds) just before HT and the total lack of functioning of his left ventricle during the 4 years before HT strongly suggest that his LV wall atrophied and scarred during the 4-year total nonuse period. Total dependence on the LVAD for such a long period (4 years) due to the operative closure of the aortic valve distinguishes this patient from earlier studies of patients with a LVAD and normally functioning aortic valves. The LV cavity was small in contrast to the right ventricular cavity which was dilated. Histologic study of the LV myocardium showed the myocytes to be much thinner than normal. The subepicardial adipose tissue in our patients did not appear to be affected by the myocardial atrophy.

Previous reports have described alterations of the LV wall, cavity, and function after insertion of a LVAD. An early report was by Altemose et al.[1] who examined LV cavity size and mass by echocardiography in 8 patients with idiopathic dilated cardiomyopathy. Each had had a LVAD device in place for 17 to 56 days (mean 42 days) before HT. The LV mass during this short period decreased from 505 to 297 g and myocyte diameter from 28 to 22 μm; the LV end-diastolic diameter decreased from 78 to 55 mm, and pulmonary arterial wedge pressure from 29 to 17 mm Hg. These 8 patients of course had normal aortic valve function during the short LVAD support period in contrast to our patient.

Any condition associated with lack of physical activity can result in skeletal muscle atrophy (muscle wasting) and probably also some cardiac muscle atrophy. Commonly recognized conditions causing skeletal muscle atrophy are diseases or injuries making it difficult or impossible to move, for example, an arm or leg. Examples include peripheral neuropathy, poliomyelitis, multiple sclerosis, anorexia nervosa, AIDS, osteomalacia, osteoarthritis, herniated disk, stroke, hypercalcemia, burns, Creutzfeldt-Jakob, bovine spongiform encephalopathy (mad cow disease), Kwashiorkor, axillary nerve dysfunction, amyotrophic lateral sclerosis, Guillain–Barre syndrome, necrotizing vasculitis, abetalipoproteinemia, malabsorption syndrome, Legg-Calve-Perthes disease, Becker muscular dystrophy,

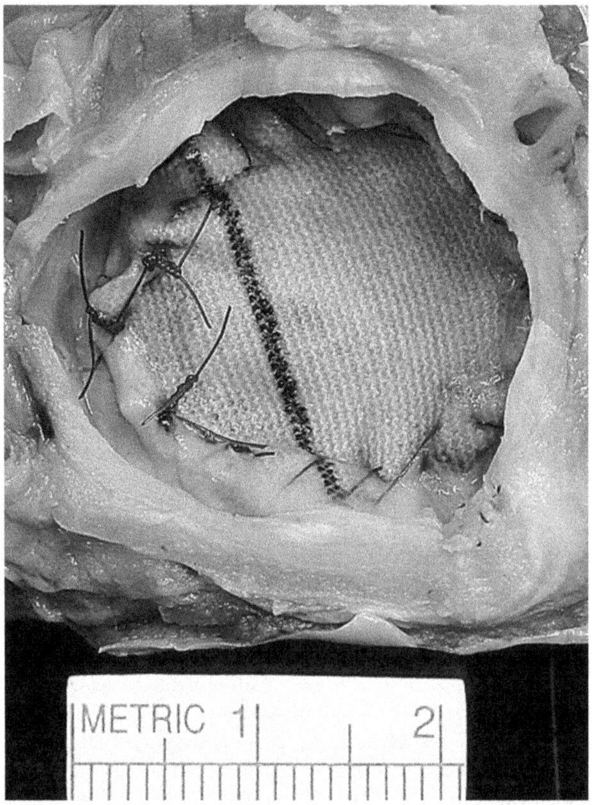


Figure 1. View of the base of the aorta showing a cloth patch used to close off the aorta from the left ventricle.

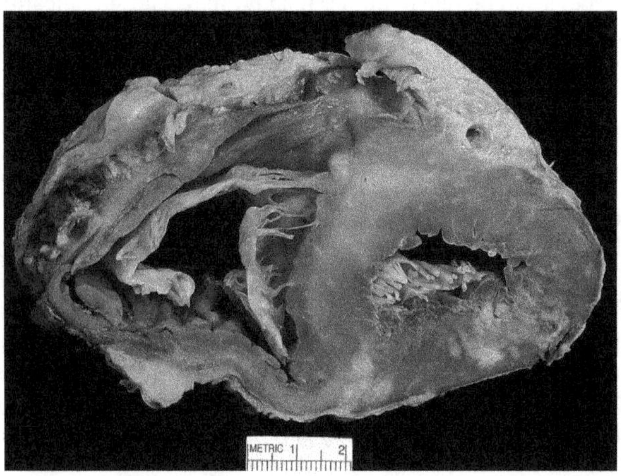

Figure 2. View of the base of the heart showing the nondilated LV cavity and the dilated right ventricular cavity portions of both tricuspid and mitral valves and the focal scars in the posterior and lateral walls of the left ventricle. The subepicardial fat is increased in quantity.

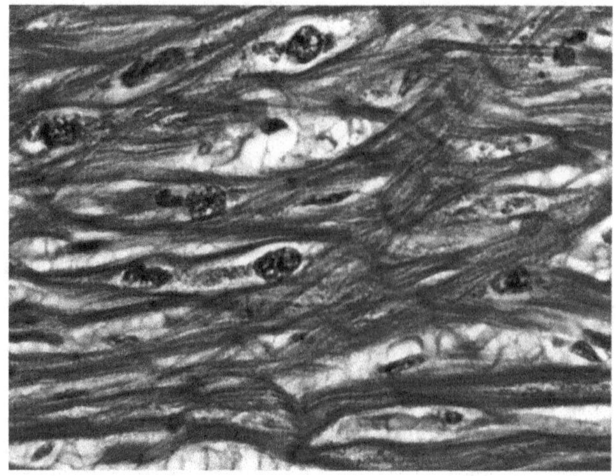

Figure 3. Photomicrograph of LV wall showing attenuated myofibers. Trichrome stain, ×1000.

long-term corticosteroid therapy, rheumatoid arthritis, and diabetes mellitus.

During the 1970s, avid dieters using the liquid-protein-modified-fast diet occasionally died suddenly. Isner et al.[2] studied at necropsy in 17 such subjects (average age 37 years; 16 women). They lost an average of 41 kg or 35% of their pre-diet weight over a 5-month average period. Histologic study of their LV myocardium (14 patients) disclosed attenuated myocardial fibers in 12 and increased lipofuscin pigment in 11 (not observed in the present patient) patients. The heart weights in the women (available in 14) ranged from 260 to 325 g (mean 296), strongly suggesting that myocardial atrophy and skeletal muscle atrophy occurred in these cachexic sudden-death victims.

Thus, the determinate of myocardial atrophy appears to be both hemodynamic and nutritional. Our patient exemplifies what can happen when the left ventricle is completely rested for a prolonged period.

### Disclosures

The authors have no conflicts of interest to disclose.

1. Altemose GT, Gritsus V, Jeevanadam V, Goldman B, Marguilies KB. Altered myocardial phenotype after mechanical support in human beings with advanced cardiomyopathy. *J Heart Lung Transpl* 1997;16: 765–773.
2. Isner JM, Sours HE, Paris AL, Ferrans VJ, Roberts WC. Sudden, unexpected death in avid dieters using the liquid-protein-modified-fast diet: observations in 17 patients and the role of the prolonged QT Interval. *Circulation* 1979;60:1401–1412.

# Frequency of Massive Cardiac Adiposity (Floating Heart) in the Native Hearts of Patients Having Heart Transplantation at a Single Texas Hospital (2013 to 2015) and Comparison of Various Clinical and Morphologic Variables in the Patients With Massive Versus Nonmassive Cardiac Adiposity

William C. Roberts, MD[a,b,c,*], Vera S. Won, BS[a], Anupama Vasudevan, BDS, MPH, PhD[a], Jong Mi Ko, BA[a], Shelley A. Hall, MD[b], and Gonzalo V. Gonzalez-Stawinski, MD[d]

**Body weight continues to increase worldwide due primarily to the increase in body fat. This study analyzes the frequency of massive adiposity at hearts of patients who underwent heart transplantation (HT) determined by the ability of the heart to float in a container of 10% formaldehyde (because adipose tissue is lighter than myocardium) and compares certain characteristics of those patients with and without floating hearts. The hearts studied at HT during a 3-year period (2013 to 2015) at Baylor University Medical Center were carefully "cleaned" and weighed by the same individual and tested as to their ability to float in a container of formaldehyde, an indication of severe cardiac adiposity. Of the 220 hearts studied, 84 (38%) floated in a container of formaldehyde and 136 (62%) did not. Comparison of the 84 patients with floating hearts to the 136 with nonfloating hearts showed a significant difference in ages, but a nonsignificant difference in gender, body mass index, frequency of systemic hypertension, or diabetes mellitus. The odds of a heart being a floating one was increased in patients with a diagnosis of ischemic cardiomyopathy (unadjusted odds ratio 2.12, 95% CI 1.21 to 3.70). The frequency of massive cardiac adiposity in the native hearts of patients having HT (38%) is striking and appears to have increased in frequency in the recent decades.**  **(Am J Cardiol 2016;117:1375−1380)**

Because overweightness including obesity is now a worldwide problem, it is reasonable to believe that hearts of patients who underwent heart transplantation (HT) would possess considerable quantities of adipose tissues. We studied the native hearts of 220 patients having HT at Baylor University Medical Center in a 3-year period (2013 to 2015) and compared various clinical and morphologic variables in those with massive (floating hearts) versus nonmassive quantities of cardiac adipose tissue.

## Methods

All cardiovascular specimens removed at operation at the Baylor University Medical Center since April 1993 have been described by one of us (W.C.R.) and most have been photographed by one of us (J.M.K.). After removing all extraneous tissues after fixation for 2 to 4 days, the hearts were tested for floating in a container of 10% formaldehyde. If the heart floated in the container after asserting that all air had been removed from the cardiac chambers, it was considered "a floating heart," which indicated that the heart contained a "massive" amount of adipose tissue[1] because adipose tissue is lighter than myocardial tissue. If the heart did not float in the container, it was considered "a nonfloating heart," which indicates that the quantity of cardiac adipose tissue is usually less than that present in the floating heart. After excising all extraneous tissues, the hearts were weighed (by W.C.R.) after opening the cardiac chambers, removing all intrachamber clot and gently drying all exposed portions of the heart with paper towels. The scales used were accurate to 0.1 g (Ohaus Scout Pro Scale) or to 1.0 g (Acculab Vicon Digital Scale).

The clinical records were then obtained on all 220 patients through the Baylor Health Care System's electronic medical record (Allscripts Sunrise Enterprise).

Statistical analysis was done using STATA 14.0 (StataCorp. 2015. Stata Statistical Software: Release 14, College Station, TX: StataCorp LP). The baseline characteristics of patients with floating and nonfloating hearts were compared using chi-square/Fisher's exact tests for proportions and *t*-test/Wilcoxon rank-sum test for continuous variables

[a]Department of Baylor Heart and Vascular Institute, [b]Division of Cardiology, Department of Internal Medicine, [c]Department of Pathology, and [d]Department of Cardiothoracic Surgery, Baylor University Medical Center, Dallas, Texas. Manuscript received January 15, 2016; revised manuscript received and accepted January 20, 2016.

This study was funded by the Baylor Health Care System Foundation through the Cardiovascular Research Review Committee and in cooperation with the Baylor Heart and Vascular Institute.

See page 1380 for disclosure information.

*Corresponding author: Tel: +(214) 820-7911; fax: +(214) 820-7533.
*E-mail address:* wc.roberts@baylorhealth.edu (W.C. Roberts).

Table 1
Clinical and morphologic finding in the 220 patients who underwent cardiac transplantation at Baylor University Medical Center from January 2013 to November 2015 comparing the finding in the patients with floating and nonfloating hearts

| Variable | Total (n = 220) | Transplant (n = 220) | | p-Value | Unadjusted OR (95%CI) |
|---|---|---|---|---|---|
| | | Float (n = 84 [38%]) | Nonfloat (n = 136 [62%]) | | |
| Sex | | | | | |
| Men | 160 (73%) | 66 (41%) | 94 (59%) | | |
| Women | 60 (27%) | 18 (30%) | 42 (70%) | 0.13 | 0.61 (0.32-1.15) |
| Age (years) (Mean±SD) | 56±11 | 59±9 | 54±12 | | |
| Range [median] | 20-76 [58] | 32-76 [62] | 20-71 [57] | 0.01 | 1.03 (1.01-1.07) |
| Men | | | | | |
| Mean±SD | 57±11 | 59±9 | 56±12 | | |
| Range [median] | 20-76 [60] | 32-76 [62] | 20-71 [59] | 0.1 | |
| 20-40 | 14 (9%) | 3 (21%) | 11 (79%) | | |
| 41-60 | 70 (44%) | 26 (37%) | 44 (63%) | | |
| 61-80 | 76 (48%) | 37 (49%) | 39 (51%) | 0.11 | |
| Women | | | | | |
| Mean±SD | 53±11 | 57±10 | 51±12 | | |
| Range [median] | 26-69 [55] | 34-69 [56] | 26-69 [54] | 0.09 | |
| 20-40 | 10 (17%) | 1 (10%) | 9 (90%) | | |
| 41-60 | 31 (51%) | 9 (29%) | 22 (71%) | | |
| 61-80 | 19 (32%) | 8 (42%) | 11 (58%) | | |
| Coronary Artery Disease | 93 (42%) | 40 (43%) | 53 (57%) | 0.21 | 1.42 (0.82-2.47) |
| Healed myocardial infarct | 73 (33%) | 35 (48%) | 38 (52%) | 0.04 | 1.84 (1.04-3.27) |
| Acute myocardial infarct | 1 (0.5%) | 1 (100%) | 0 | 0.38 | NA |
| Both | 2 (1%) | 1 (50%) | 1 (50%) | | |
| Neither | 17 (8%) | 3 (18%) | 14 (82%) | | |
| Diabetes Mellitus | 82 (37%) | 32 (39%) | 50 (61%) | 0.84 | 1.05 (0.60-1.86) |
| Hypertension (by history) | 132 (60%) | 47 (36%) | 85 (64%) | 0.34 | 0.76 (0.44-1.33) |
| Body Mass Index (kg/m$^2$) (Mean±SD) | 29.1±5 | 29.6±5 | 28.9±5 | | |
| Range [median] | 17.8-42.3 [28.9] | 20.3-39.1 [29.8] | 17.8-42.3 [28.4] | 0.18 | 1.03 (0.97-1.08) |
| 16-20 | 5 (2%) | 0 | 5 (100%) | | |
| 21-25 | 48 (22%) | 15 (31%) | 33 (69%) | | |
| 26-30 | 78 (36%) | 32 (41%) | 46 (59%) | | |
| 31-35 | 60 (27%) | 27 (45%) | 33 (55%) | | |
| 36-40 | 26 (12%) | 10 (38%) | 16 (62%) | | |
| 41-45 | 3 (1%) | 0 | 3 (100%) | 0.23 | |
| Men | | | | | |
| Mean±SD | 29.1±5 | 29.5±4 | 28.9±5 | | |
| BMI Range [median] | 19-41.4 [28.8] | 20.7-37.8 [29.7] | 19-41.4 [28.4] | 0.25 | |
| Women | | | | | |
| Mean±SD | 29.2±6 | 29.9±5 | 28.9±6 | | |
| BMI Range [median] | 17.8-42.3 [29.0] | 20.3-39.1 [30.6] | 17.8-42.3 [28.5] | 0.46 | |
| Diagnosis | | | | | |
| Ischemic Cardiomyopathy | 88 (40%) | 43 (49%) | 45 (51%) | 0.008 | 2.12 (1.21-3.70) |
| Men | 74 (47%) | 39 (53%) | 35 (47%) | 0.006 | |
| Women | 14 (24%) | 4 (29%) | 10 (71%) | 1.00 | |
| Idiopathic Dilated Cardiomyopathy | 88 (40%) | 29 (33%) | 59 (67%) | 0.19 | 0.69 (0.39-1.21) |
| Men | 53 (33%) | 17 (32%) | 36 (68%) | 0.13 | |
| Women | 35 (58%) | 12 (34%) | 23 (66%) | 0.57 | |
| Other* | 44 (20%) | 12 (27%) | 32 (73%) | 0.09 | 0.54 (0.26-1.12) |
| Men | 33 (21%) | 10 (30%) | 23 (70%) | 0.15 | |
| Women | 11 (19%) | 2 (18%) | 9 (82%) | 0.48 | |
| Heart Weight (g)(Mean±SD)† | 486±119 | 490±103 | 483±128 | | |
| Range [median] | 215-883 [480] | 285-755 [490] | 215-883 [478] | 0.47 | 1.004 (0.99-1.003) |
| Men | | | | | |
| Mean±SD | 509±119 | 508±94 | 509±135 | | |
| Range [median] | 215-883 [502] | 285-695 [508] | 215-883 [494] | 0.71 | |
| >400g | 130 (82%) | 53 (41%) | 77 (59%) | 0.95 | |
| Women | | | | | |
| Mean±SD | 423±93 | 420±107 | 425±88 | | |
| Range [median] | 235-755 [425] | 290-755 [420] | 235-599 [429] | 0.49 | |
| >350g | 46 (78%) | 12 (26%) | 34 (74%) | 0.38 | |
| Left Ventricular Assist Device | 43 (20%) | 16 (37%) | 27 (63%) | 0.88 | 0.95 (0.48-1.89) |

* See Table 2.

† Two patients' heart weights were not available to obtain.

Table 2
Cardiac condition included in the category labeled "other" in Table 1

| Cardiac Condition | Number of Patients | Age (years) mean ± SD | BMI (kg/m2) mean ± SD | M/F | Floating/ Nonfloating |
|---|---|---|---|---|---|
| Amyloidosis | 8 | 56±13 | 27.4±4 | 7/1 | 2/6 |
| Hypertrophic cardiomyopathy | 6 | 48±10 | 29±5 | 4/2 | 3/3 |
| Congential heart disease | 8 | 53±11 | 29±7 | 7/1 | 4/4 |
| Sarcoidosis | 6 | 58±4 | 27.3±5 | 5/1 | 2/4 |
| Arrhythmogenic right ventricular cardiomyopathy | 3 | 46±12 | 27.4±5 | 2/1 | 0/3 |
| Valvular heart disease | 3 | 55±9 | 32.4±5 | 2/1 | 0/3 |
| Radiation heart disease | 3 | 50±13 | 30±6 | 2/1 | 0/3 |
| Pericardial heart disease (constriction)* | 1 | 55 | 22.3 | 1/0 | 0/1 |
| Primary pulmonary hypertension | 1 | 33 | 24.0 | 0/1 | 0/1 |
| Chagas disease | 1 | 28 | 19.2 | 0/1 | 0/1 |
| Toxic cardiomyopathy (adriamycin) | 1 | 27 | 26.3 | 1/0 | 0/1 |
| Ehlers-Danlos Syndrome | 1 | 31 | 17.8 | 0/1 | 0/1 |
| Anthracycline cardiomyopathy | 1 | 57 | 26 | 1/0 | 1/0 |
| Multivessel disease | 1 | 66 | 31.1 | 1/0 | 0/1 |
| Totals | 44 | 52±12 | 27.9±5 | 33/11 | 12/32 (38%) |

BMI = body mass index; F = female; M = male.
* Two previous operations for relief of calcific pericardial constriction of uncertain cause had been performed.

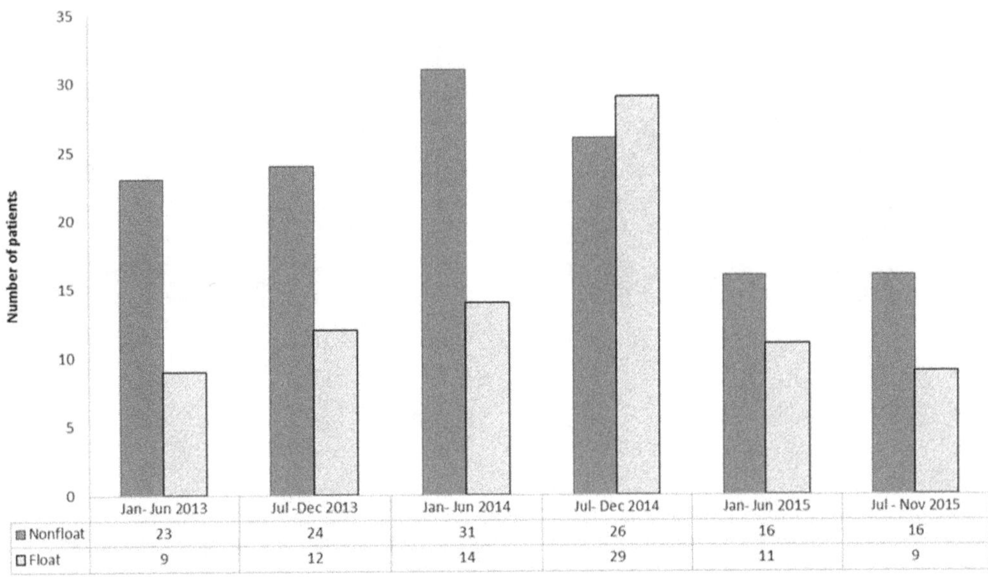

Figure 1. Distribution of floating and nonfloating hearts during the study period (2013 to 2015).

where applicable. In addition, comparisons were repeated separately for men and women. Unadjusted odds ratios with 95% CI were obtained for these variables of interest by logistic regression analysis.

The study was approved by an institutional review board.

## Results

The major findings are summarized in Tables 1 and 2. Of the 220 hearts, 84 (38%) contained such a large quantity of adipose tissue that they floated in a container of 10% formaldehyde, and 136 (62%) did not float. The proportion of the hearts that floated in the container increased from 30% in 2013 to 40% in 2014 (Figure 1). The distribution of age, body mass index, and heart weight in the patients with floating and nonfloating hearts are shown in Figure 2. Comparison of the 84 patients with floating hearts to the 136 with nonfloating hearts showed a significant difference in mean ages, but a nonsignificanct difference in gender, body mass index, frequency of systemic hypertension, and diabetes mellitus. The odds of a heart floating in formaldehyde increased with age (unadjusted odds ratio 1.04, 95% CI 1.01 to 1.07) and ischemic cardiomyopathy (unadjusted odds ratio 2.12, 95% CI 1.21 to 3.70). The median body mass index increased over the years in those with floating hearts, whereas it decreased in those patients with nonfloating hearts (Figure 3). Photographs of 2 floating hearts are shown in Figures 4 and 5.

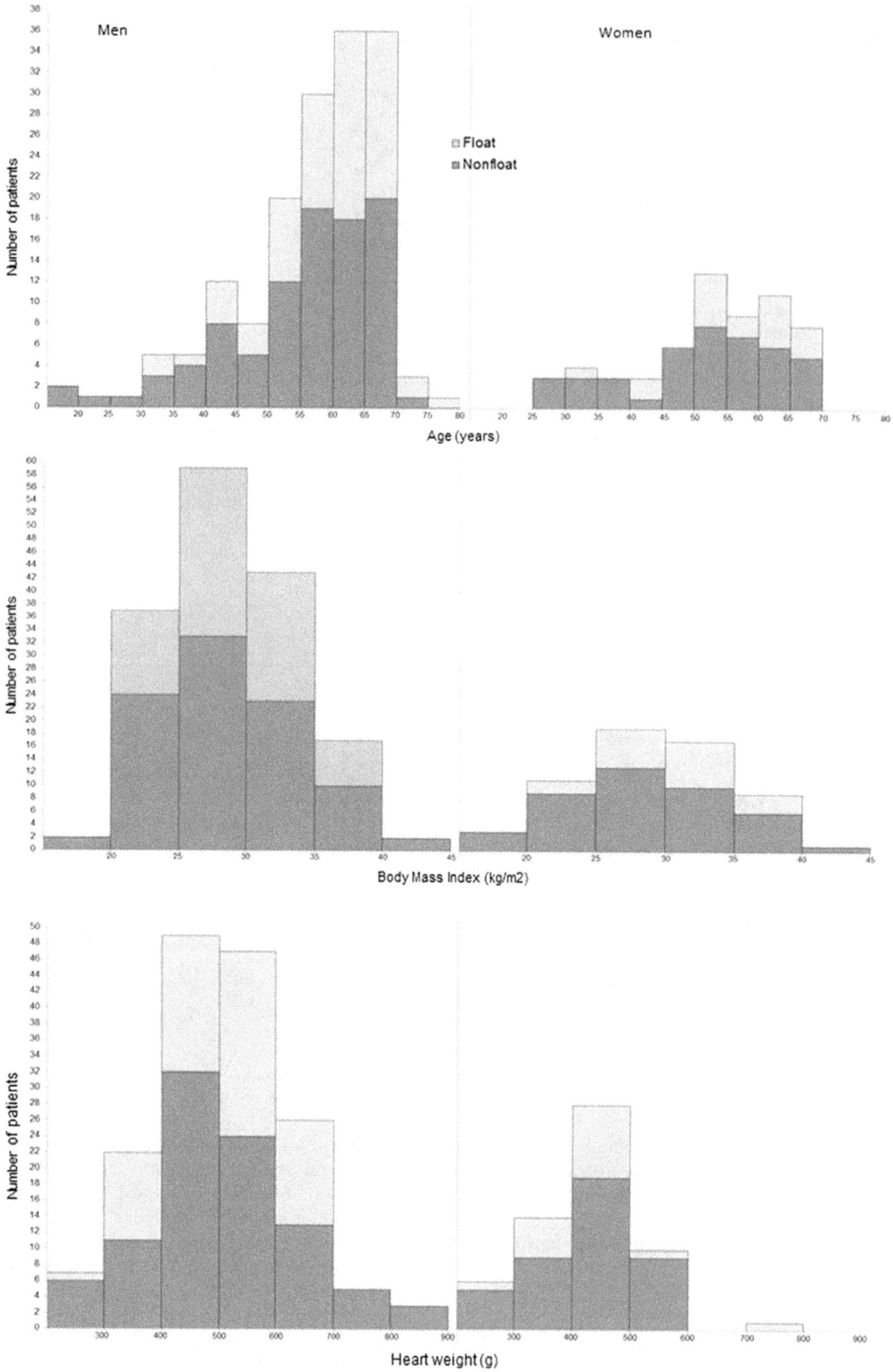


Figure 2. Stacked bar graphs showing ages, body mass indexes, and heart weight of the men and women sorted by numbers of those with and without floating hearts.

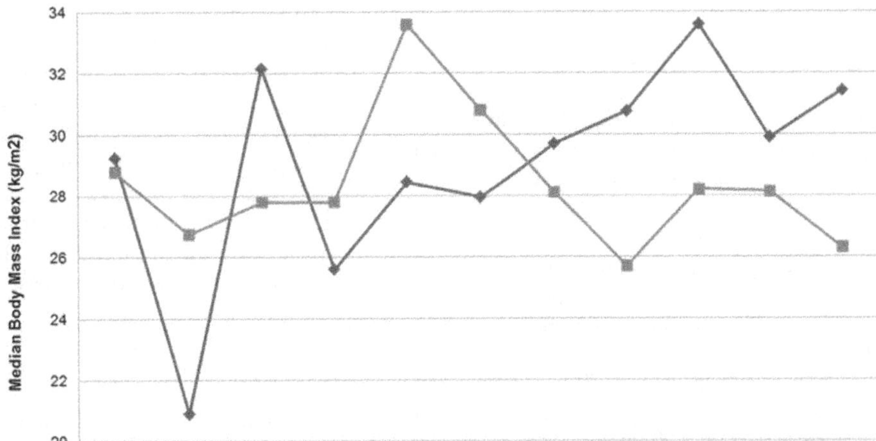


| | Q1 2013 | Q2 2013 | Q3 2013 | Q4 2013 | Q1 2014 | Q2 2014 | Q3 2014 | Q4 2014 | Q1 2015 | Q2 2015 | Q3 2015 |
|---|---|---|---|---|---|---|---|---|---|---|---|
| Float (Median BMI) | 29.25 | 20.9 | 32.15 | 25.6 | 28.45 | 27.95 | 29.7 | 30.75 | 33.6 | 29.9 | 31.42 |
| Non float (Median BMI) | 28.8 | 26.75 | 27.8 | 27.8 | 33.6 | 30.8 | 28.1 | 25.7 | 28.2 | 28.13 | 26.3 |

Figure 3. Body mass index (BMI) in floating and nonfloating patients during the study period. The median BMI increased over the years in those with floating hearts, whereas it decreased in those patients with nonfloating hearts.

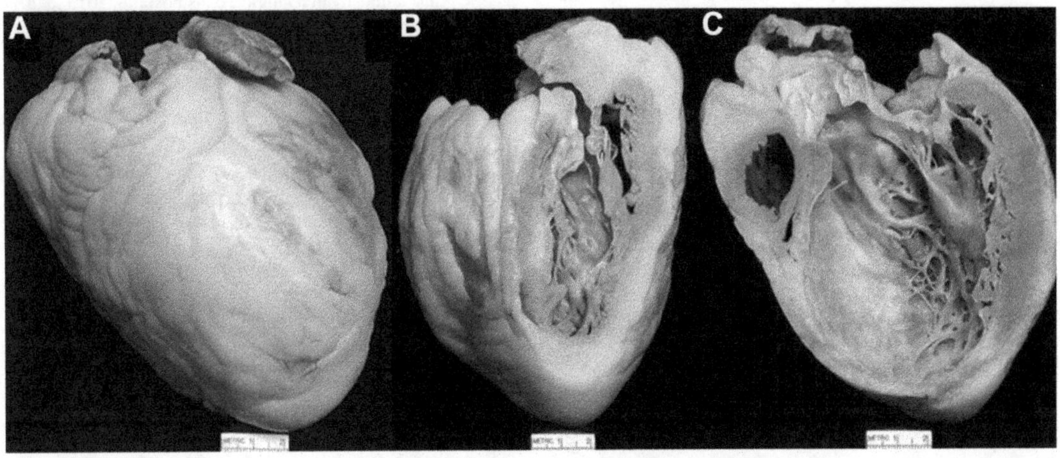


Figure 4. Floating heart in a 59-year-old woman who had had a large acute myocardial infarction at age 37 years and heart failure and periodic ventricular tachycardia subsequently shown here in the external view of the 405-g heart nearly covered with adipose tissue *(A)*; a left parasagittal view showing a huge anteroseptal scar and marked left ventricular dilation *(B)*; and a right parasagittal view exposing the tricuspid valve and right ventricular inflow portion and the excessive subepicardial adipose tissue.

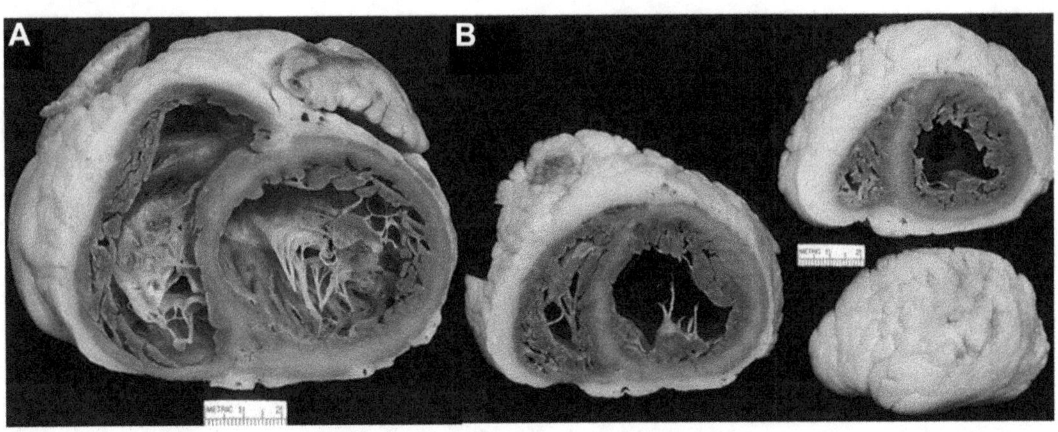


Figure 5. Floating heart in a 63-year-old woman with heart failure some age 43 years. Angiography disclosed no luminal narrowing, and examination of the heart conformed the diagnosis of idiopathic dilated cardiomyopathy shown in *(A)* is the basal portion of the heart exposing the extremely dilated ventricle, the tricuspid and mitral valves, the wide-open coronary artery, the absence of grossly visible myocardial lesion, and the excess subepicardial adipose tissue. Shown in *(B)* are more apical cuts of the ventricular wall, nearly all of which are covered by adipose tissue.

## Discussion

The major finding in this study is the high frequency (38%) of massive cardiac adiposity (floating hearts) in the patients having HT, an observation not reported previously. The second important finding was the lack of significant differences between the patients with floating versus those with nonfloating hearts in age, gender, body mass index, and use of a left ventricular assist device.

The concept of "floating heart" was presented initially in an article by Roberts and Roberts[1] in 1983 who described a 5% frequency of floating hearts in 55 necropsy patients included in a 2.5-year period in the early 1980s. A more recent study by Roberts et al[2] at a single Texas hospital in 2013 to 2014 showed a 52% frequency of floating hearts in 146 "necropsy" patients. Thus, a dramatic increase in the frequency of the floating heart, that is, massive cardiac adiposity, during the 32-year interval.

The present study of course has limitations. That a heart floats in formaldehyde or water indicates that the heart contains a huge quantity of adipose tissue. If, however, the myocardial mass is considerable and even though the quantity of adipose tissue is also considerable, the heart may not float because the myocardial mass, by weighing more than the fatty mass, prevents the heart from floating. Although the present study focuses on HT patients with floating hearts, indicating massive cardiac adiposity, the nonfloating hearts, with few exceptions, also had a considerably increased quantity of cardiac adipose tissue, just not quite enough to allow the heart to float. The latter fact may explain the lack of significant clinical differences between the floating and nonfloating cases.

## Disclosures

The authors have no conflicts of interest to disclose.

1. Roberts WC, Roberts JD. The floating heart or the heart too fat to sink: analysis of 55 necropsy patients. *Am J Cardiol* 1983;52:1286–1289.
2. Roberts WC, Won VS, Vasudevan A, Ko JM, Guileyardo JM. Frequency of massive cardiac adiposity (floating heart) at necropsy and comparison of clinical and morphologic variables with nonmassive cardiac adiposity at a single Texas hospital, 2013 to 2014. *Am J Cardiol*, http://dx.doi.org/10.1016/j.amjcard.2015.12.039, 2016;117.

# Comparison of Characteristics of Patients Undergoing Heart Transplantation at the Same Hospital in Two Different Time Periods (1997-2012 and 2013-2015)

William C. Roberts, MD[a,b,c,*], Vera S. Won, BS[a], Anupama Vasudevan, BDS, MPH, PhD[a], Pranav Kapoor[a], Jong Mi Ko, BA[a], Dan M. Meyer, MD[d], Shelley A. Hall, MD[b], and Gonzalo V. Gonzalez-Stawinski, MD[d]

**Heart transplantation (HT) increases at some centers each year and decreases at others. We examined characteristics of patients having HT at the same hospital in 2 different time periods (1997−2012 and 2013−2015) by 2 different surgical groups. We compared certain clinical and morphological finding in 291 patients having HT 1997 to 2012 to finding in 228 other patients having HT from 2013 to 2015. Several significant (p <0.05) differences were found: in the most recent time period (2013−2015) compared to the earlier time period (1997−2012), the mean ages of the men were older (57 years -vs- 55 years); diabetes mellitus was more frequent (37% -vs- 21%); systemic hypertension (by history) was more frequent (59% -vs- 32%); the mean body mass index was higher (29.2 kg/m$^2$ -vs- 26.5 kg/m$^2$), and mean heart weight was lower in both men (509 g -vs- 549 g) and women (422 g -vs- 454 g). There were insignificant (p >0.05) differences in gender, frequency of massive cardiac adiposity, underlying cardiac condition, frequency of coronary heart disease, and frequency of previous insertion of a left ventricular assist device. In conclusion, certain characteristics of patients having HT at one Texas hospital changed in several respects in 2 time periods corresponding to changes in surgeons doing the HTs.** 
**(Am J Cardiol 2016;118:288−291)**

The number of heart transplantations (HTs) at Baylor University Medical Center (BUMC) at Dallas from 1997 through 2012 averaged 18 for each of the 16 years; the number of HTs from 2013 through 2015 averaged 76 for each of the 3 years (Figure 1). This report compares various clinical and morphologic characteristics of the patients undergoing HT in each of the 2 time periods.

## Methods

Since March 1993 all cardiac specimens received in the surgical pathology division of the department of pathology of BUMC have been described by WCR and most have been photographed by JMK. All hearts were cleaned of extraneous tissues, fixed in 10% formaldehyde for 2 to 4 days, determined if the specimen floated in a container of formaldehyde, opened, and then weighed after gently patting each surface to remove extraneous fluid (water or formaldehyde). The scales used were accurate to 1.0 g.

The clinical records were then obtained in all 519 patients via the Baylor Health Care System's electronic medical record (Allscripts Sunrise Enterprise, Chicago, IL). All 519 patients included in this study had a single HT. Patients having > 1 HT were excluded.

Statistical analyses were conducted using STATA 14.1 (StataCorp. 2015. Stata Statistical Software: Release 14. College Station, TX: StataCorp LP). Baseline characteristics were presented as means/medians for continuous variables and proportions for categorical variables. Comparisons were done using chi-square/fisher exact test for proportions and wilcoxon rank-sum/student t-test for continuous variables where applicable. A p value of < 0.05 was deemed to be statistically significant.

The study was approved by the institutional review board.

## Results

The major findings are summarized in Table 1. Several significant differences were found among the patients in the 2 time periods: in the recent time period (2013−2015) compared to the first time period (1997−2012), the men were older (57 years -vs- 55 years); diabetes mellitus was more frequent (37% -vs- 21%); systemic hypertension (by history) was more frequent (59% -vs- 32%); mean body mass index (BMI) was higher (29.2 kg/m$^2$ -vs- 26.5 kg/m$^2$), and mean heart weight was lower in both men (509 g -vs- 549 g) and women (422 g -vs- 454 g) (Figure 2). There were insignificant differences in gender, frequency of massive cardiac adiposity (floating heart[1]), reason for HT, frequency

[a]Baylor Heart and Vascular Institute, [b]Department of Internal Medicine (Division of Cardiology), [c]Department of Pathology, and [d]Department of Cardiothoracic Surgery, Baylor University Medical Center, Dallas, Texas. Manuscript received March 23, 2016; revised manuscript received and accepted April 20, 2016.

This study was funded by the Baylor Health Care System Foundation, Dallas, Texas through the Cardiovascular Research Review Committee and in cooperation with the Baylor Heart and Vascular Institute.

See page 291 for disclosure information.

*Corresponding author: Tel: (+1) 214-820-7911; fax: (+1) 214-820-7533.

*E-mail address:* wc.roberts@baylorhealth.edu (W.C. Roberts).

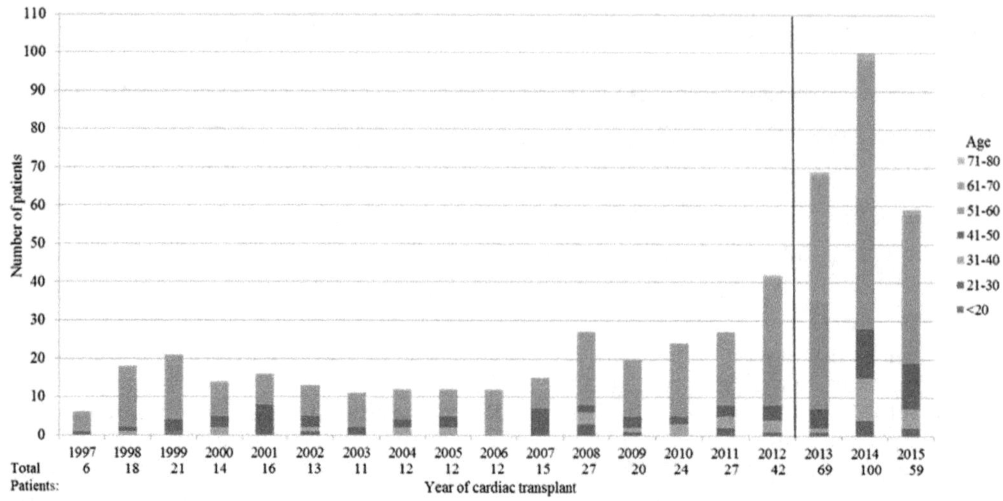


Figure 1. Bar graph showing numbers of heart transplants performed at Baylor University Medical Center Dallas from 1997 through 2015 subdivided by age groups in years.

Table 1
Comparison of certain variables among patients having cardiac transplantation at Baylor University Medical Center in 2 time periods: 1997-2012 -vs- 2013-2015

| Variable | TOTAL (N=519) | Transplant (n=519) 1997-2012 (n=291[56%]) | 2013-2015 (n=228[44%]) | P Value |
|---|---|---|---|---|
| Age (years) (Mean ±SD) | 55±11 | 55±11 | 56±11 | |
| Range [median] | 19-76 [57] | 19-73 [57] | 20-76 [58] | 0.06 |
| Men | | | | |
| Mean ±SD | 56±11 | 55±11 | 57±11 | |
| Range [median] | 19-76 [59] | 19-73 [58] | 20-76 [60] | 0.04 |
| Women | | | | |
| Mean ±SD | 53±11 | 53±11 | 53±11 | |
| Range [median] | 26-69 [55] | 26-69 [55] | 26-69 [55] | 0.69 |
| Sex | | | | |
| Men | 385 (74%) | 219 (75%) | 166 (73%) | |
| Women | 134 (26%) | 72 (25%) | 62 (27%) | 0.53 |
| Diabetes Mellitus | 147 (28%) | 62 (21%) | 85 (37%) | <0.001 |
| Hypertension (by history) | 227 (44%) | 92 (32%) | 135 (59%) | <0.001 |
| Body Mass Index (kg/m2) (Mean ±SD) | 27.7±5 | 26.5±4 | 29.2±5 | <0.001 |
| Range [median] | 16.9-42.3 [27.5] | 16.9-38 [26.9] | 17.8-42.3 [28.9] | |
| Men | | | | |
| Mean ±SD | 27.9±5 | 26.9±4.2 | 29.1±5 | <0.001 |
| Range [median] | 16.9-41.4 [27.8] | 16.9-38 [27.2] | 19-41.4 [28.8] | |
| Women | | | | |
| Mean ±SD | 27.0±5 | 25.1±4 | 29.1±6 | <0.001 |
| Range [median] | 17.4-42.3 [26.5] | 17.4-33.8 [25.3] | 17.8-42.3 [29.0] | |
| Floating Heart | 202 (39%) | 113 (39%) | 89 (39%) | 0.96 |
| Heart Weight (g) (Mean ±SD) | 508±119 | 526±117 | 485±118 | |
| Range [median] | 215-940 [495] | 232-940 [513] | 215-883 [480] | 0.0001 |
| Men | | | | |
| Mean ±SD | 532±115 | 549±110 | 509±118 | |
| Range [median] | 215-940 [515] | 312-940 [540] | 215-883 [501] | 0.0008 |
| >400g | 345 (90%) | 207 (95%) | 137 (83%) | <0.001 |
| Women | | | | |
| Mean ±SD | 439±100 | 454±106 | 422±91 | |
| Range [median] | 232-755 [428] | 232-726 [441] | 235-755 [423] | 0.08 |
| >350g | 112 (84%) | 63 (88%) | 49 (79%) | 0.19 |
| Diagnosis | | | | |
| Ischemic Cardiomyopathy | 228 (44%) | 137 (47%) | 91 (40%) | 0.10 |
| Idiopathic Dilated Cardiomyopathy | 190 (37%) | 99 (34%) | 91 (40%) | 0.17 |
| Others | 101 (19%) | 55 (19%) | 46 (20%) | 0.72 |
| Coronary Artery Disease | 233 (45%) | 136 (47%) | 97 (43%) | 0.34 |
| Healed myocardial infarct | 191 (37%) | 115 (40%) | 76 (33%) | 0.15 |
| Acute myocardial infarct | 3 (0.6%) | 2 (0.7%) | 1 (0.4%) | NA |
| Both | 3 (0.6%) | 1 (0.3%) | 2 (0.9%) | 0.59 |
| Neither | 47 (9%) | 28 (10%) | 19 (8%) | 0.65 |
| Left Ventricular Assist Device | 96 (18%) | 50 (17%) | 46 (20%) | 0.38 |

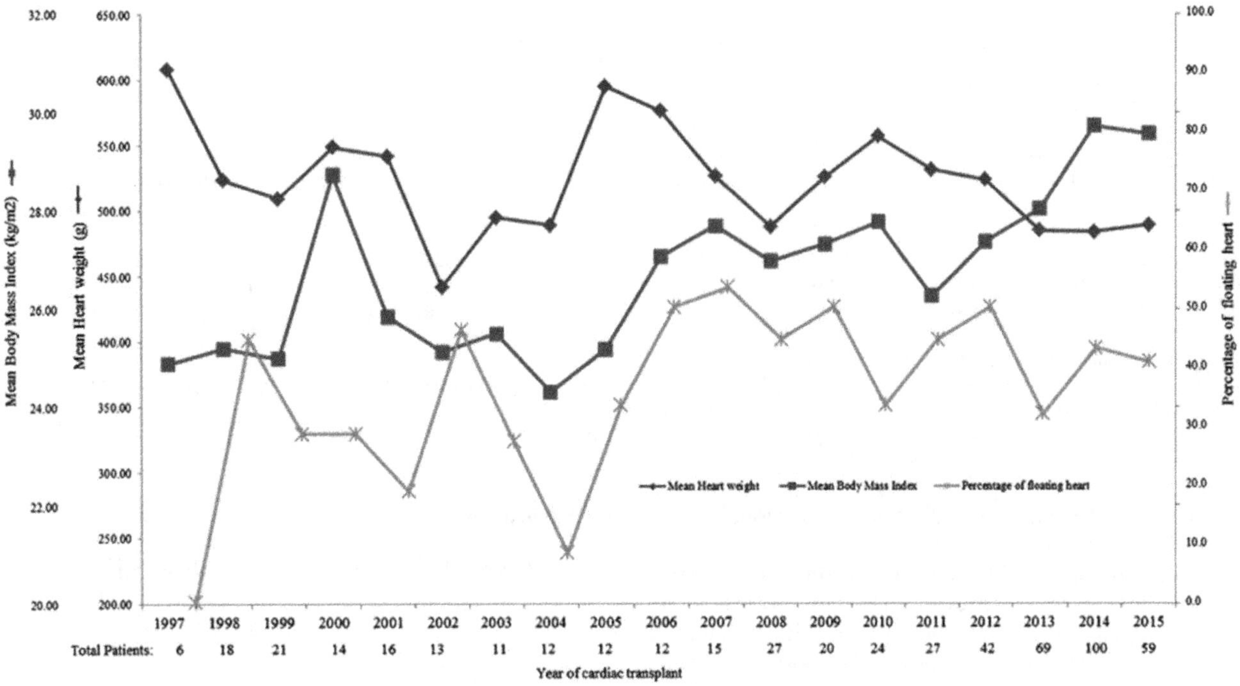


Figure 2. Graph showing mean heart weight, mean body mass index, and percent of hearts floating in formaldehyde after excision (a measure of cardiac adiposity since adipose tissue is lighter than myocardial tissue) in the 519 patients having heart transplantation at Baylor University Medical Center Dallas from 1997 through 2015.

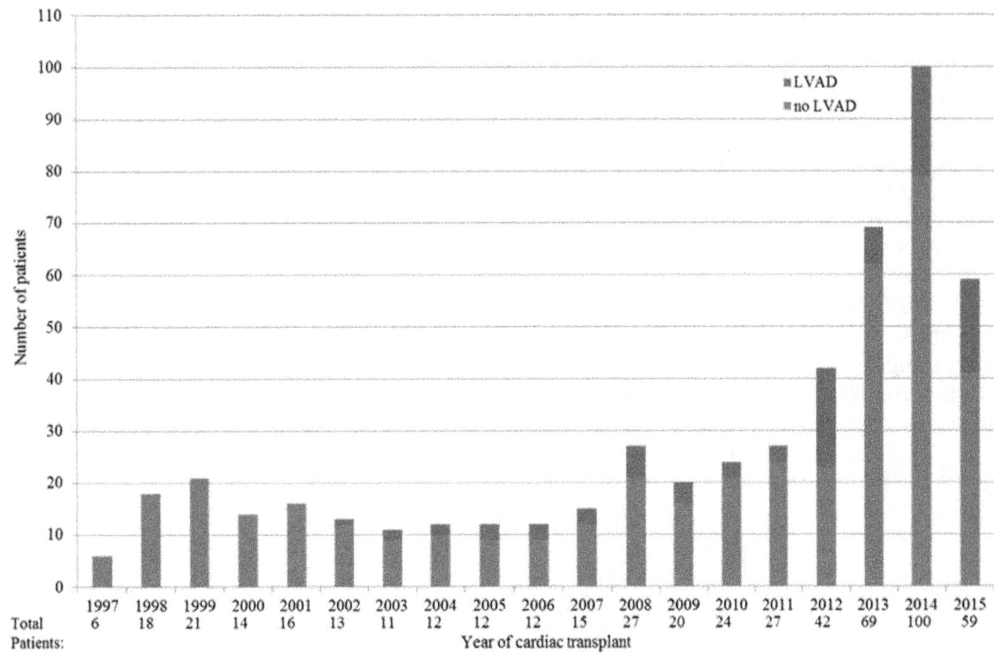


Figure 3. Bar graph showing numbers of heart transplants at Baylor University Medical Center Dallas each year from 1997 through 2015 subdivided by patients having or not having a left ventricular assist device previously inserted.

of coronary heart disease, and frequency of previous insertion of a left ventricular assist device.

## Discussion

What the hitherto described findings indicate are that some patient characteristics were different in the 2 time periods. The patients having HT in the later time period (2013–2015) compared to the patients in the earlier time period (1997–2012) had a higher frequency of diabetes mellitus and systemic hypertension, larger mean BMIs, and lower mean heart weights. Additionally, the more recent HT patients received more left ventricular assist devices than the patients in the earlier time period (Figure 3), but the percent

Table 2
Previously published studies of body mass index before cardiac transplantation and comparison to each of the 2 study periods in the present study

| First Author | Years Patients Studied | Year of Publication | Number of Patients | Body Mass Index (Kg/m$^2$) 15-20 | 21-25 | 26-30 | 31-35 | 36-40 | >40 |
|---|---|---|---|---|---|---|---|---|---|
| Carrier* | 1981-1992 | 1998 | 778 | 91 (12%) | 347 (45%) | | 340 (44%) | | |
| Grady† | 1990-1995 | 1999 | 4,515 | 527 (12%) | 2,869 (64%) | 799 (18%) | | 320 (7%) | |
| Clark‡ | 1984-1999 | 2007 | 1,902 | | 944 (50%) | 824 (43%) | | 134 (7%) | |
| Russo§ | 1995-2005 | 2010 | 19,593 | 741 (4%) | 7,883 (40%) | 7,280 (37%) | 3,005 (15%) | 684 (4%) | |
| Roberts | 1997-2012 | 2016 | 291 | 34 (12%) | 92 (32%) | 121 (42%) | 39 (13%) | 5 (2%) | 0 |
| Roberts | 2013-2015 | 2016 | 228 | 9 (4%) | 57 (25%) | 81 (36%) | 56 (25%) | 22 (10%) | 3 (1%) |

* Original body mass index category: <20, 20-24, and ≥25.
† Original body mass index category for men: <20.7, 20.7-27.7, 27.8-31.0, and ≥31.1; for women: <19.1, 19.1-27.2, 27.3-32.2, and ≥32.3.
‡ Original body mass index category: <21, <24, <28, <30, and ≥30.
§ Original body mass index category: <18.5, 18.5-25, 25-30, 30-35, and 35-40.

increase was not significantly different proportional to the total number of HTs/year.

The reasons for the differences in patient characteristics during the 2 time periods are several. The most prominent one is that the surgeons performing the HTs were different in each time period. Whether the surgeons in the most recent time period were too aggressive or the surgeons in the earlier time period were too conservative is as yet unclear became long-term follow-up data is not available for patients in the latter time period. Some follow-up data are available for the patients having HT at the earlier time period.[2]

The BMIs of patients having HT appear to have increased progressively in the last 30 years as have the BMIs of the general population. As shown in Table 2,[3–6] the BMI was >30 kg/m$^2$ in only 7% of the 4,515 patients reported by Grady and associates,[4] having HT from 1990 to 1995; in 7% of the 1,902 patients reported by Clark and colleagues[5] having HT from 1984 to 1999; in 19% the 19,593 patients reported by Russo and associates[6] having HT from 1995 to 2005, and in 35% of the 228 patients having HT at BUMC from 2013 to 2015.

The major strength of the present study is that it is the first to compare characteristics of patients having HT at the same institution during 2 time periods by 2 entirely different surgical groups. The major limitation is the lack of outcome data of the patients in the most recent time period.

## Disclosures

The authors have no conflicts of interest to disclose.

1. Roberts WC, Won VS, Vasudevan A, Ko JM, Guileyardo JM. Frequency of massive cardiac adiposity (floating heart) at necropsy and comparison of clinical and morphologic variables to cases with non-massive cardiac adiposity at a single Texas hospital 2013-2014. *Am J Cardiol* 2016;117:1006–1013.
2. Roberts WC, Roberts CC, Ko JM, Filardo G, Capehart JE, Hall SA. Morphologic features of the recipient heart in patients having cardiac transplantation and analysis of the congruence or incongruence between the clinical and morphologic diagnoses. *Medicine* 2014;93:211–235.
3. Carrier M, Rivard M, Latter D, Kostuk W. Predictors of early mortality after heart transplantation: the Canadian transplant experience from 1981 to 1992. The CASCADE investigators. Canadian study of cardiac transplant atherosclerosis determinants. *Can J Cardiol* 1998;14:703–707.
4. Grady KL, White-Williams C, Naftel D, Costanzo MR, Pitts D, Rayburn B, Vanbakel A, Jaski B, Bourge R, Kirklin J. Are preoperative obesity and cachexia risk factors for post heart transplant morbidity and mortality: a multi-institutional study of preoperative weight-height indices. *J Heart Lung Transplant* 1999;18:750–763.
5. Clark AL, Knosalla C, Birks E, Loebe M, Davos CH, Tsang S, Negassa A, Yacoub M, Hetzer R, Coats AJ, Anker SD. Heart transplantation in heart failure: the prognostic importance of body mass index at time of surgery and subsequent weight changes. *Eur J Heart Fail* 2007;9:839–844.
6. Russo MJ, Hong KN, Davies RR, Chen JM, Mancini DM, Oz MC, Rose EA, Gelijns A, Naka Y. The effect of body mass index on survival following heart transplantation: do outcomes support consensus guidelines? *Ann Surg* 2010;251:144–152.

## Patient acceptance of the Heart-to-Heart program: Using patients' native hearts to promote post-transplant health

Megan C. Reynolds, MS,[a]
Sandra A. Carey, PhD,[b] Simon Driver, PhD,[a]
Jong Ko, BA,[c] Joost Felius, PhD,[d]
William C. Roberts, MD,[c] and
Shelley A. Hall, MD[b]

*From the [a]Baylor Institute for Rehabilitation, Dallas, Texas; [b]Center for Advanced Heart and Lung Disease, Baylor University Medical Center, Dallas, Texas; [c]Baylor Heart and Vascular Institute, Baylor University Medical Center, Dallas, Texas; and the [d]Annette C. and Harold C. Simmons Transplant Institute, Baylor University Medical Center, Dallas, Texas*

There is limited research examining patients' adherence to medical recommendations after organ transplant. One way of improving non-adherence to a health behavior is enhancing patients' education. Consequently, the Heart-to-Heart program, introduced here, was based on the tenets of behavior change using the health belief model[1] to promote post-transplant health and to improve patient adherence to post-operative management strategies. Here we report qualitative feedback from participants in a pilot program to guide future clinical and research efforts.

After heart transplantation, all explanted native hearts are routinely sent to the surgical pathology department for examination by the program's pathologist and then are stored indefinitely at the cardiovascular laboratory. The Heart-to-Heart program started in January 2014. Patients receiving a heart transplant are invited by the clinical team to participate. Patients who are interested in participating

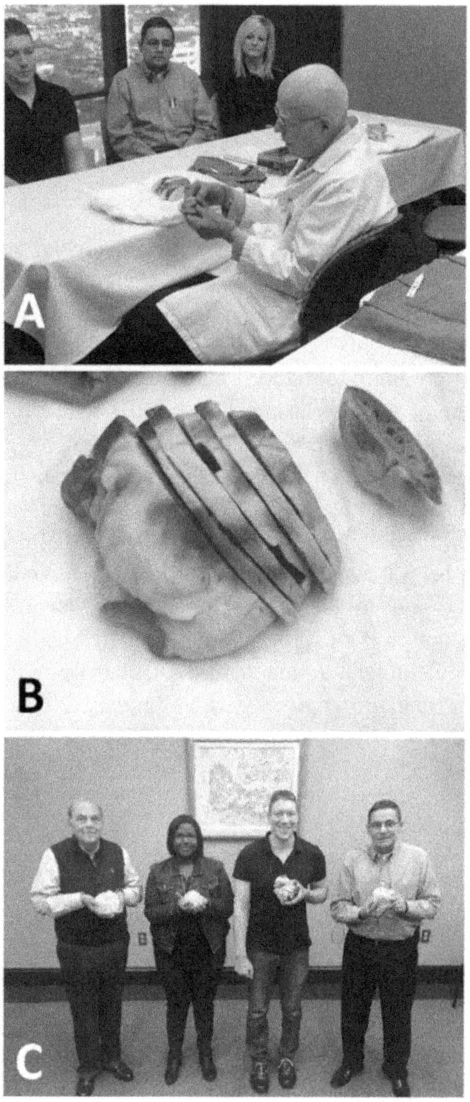

**Figure 1** (A) Participant with family in a Heart-to-Heart program session led by the investigator. (B) Preserved and sliced native heart used for educational purposes in the Heart-to-Heart program. (C) Participants in the Heart-to-Heart pilot program at a participant reunion on February 14, 2016. They each hold their native heart. All individuals depicted granted permission to the authors for reproduction of these photographs.

sign a written informed consent and are referred to a laboratory coordinator who schedules their session, which usually takes place before or after one of their routine follow-up appointments at the transplant center. During each session, led by 1 investigator (W.C.R.), cardiac health is discussed using the patient's preserved native heart as an educational tool. The Heart-to-Heart program and consent form were approved by the Baylor University Medical Center Institutional Review Board, Dallas.

The first 13 heart transplant recipients were invited and agreed to participate in a separate pilot program. They were contacted by telephone after the program to rate the educational value and the effect on their post-transplant health behaviors. Twelve participants provided feedback (Figure 1); the remaining patient withdrew from participation because of illness. Participants were a mean age of 52 years, 91.6% were male, 75% were non-Hispanic, and 41.6% were diagnosed with ischemic cardiomyopathy.

Feedback sessions lasted approximately 10 minutes with each individual. A numeric rating scale of 0 to 10 (with 10 best) was used. Participants were asked, "How comfortable were you with the experience [of participating in this program] as a whole?" and responded with a mean of 9.6 (range, 8–10). All participants were then asked, "On a scale of 0 to 10, how meaningful was this as a learning experience?" and "On a scale of 0 to 10, would you recommend this experience to other patients?" All participants responded to both questions with a score of 10.

Further, 9 participants stated that their health behaviors "changed to a great degree" as a result of the program because, as one individual stated, "It will change the way you treat yourself, what you eat, how you work." When describing their overall impression of their experience in the program, individuals frequently characterized the Heart-to-Heart program as "undoubtedly one of the most remarkable experiences of my life" and that it was a "rare opportunity for patients." In addition, most patients described similar feelings, such as "a sense of closure," that "allowed them to say goodbye" to their native heart and "recognize the sacrifice that someone else made."

All individuals who provided feedback brought family members (e.g., spouses, children, siblings, cousins, grandchildren) to participate in the Heart-to-Heart program and stated that this social support provided "help with the process." Two individuals stated that they wished to schedule additional appointments in the Heart-to-Heart program to include more family members in the experience.

When discussing how individuals would modify the program in the future, participants requested more time with their native heart and a larger room for the session to take place in to accommodate guests of the participant as well as medical residents and fellows observing the session.

Although it is recognized that there is inherent self-selection bias in the experiences reported by the participants, the feedback from the participants will lend itself to other novel interventions that could lead to lifestyle changes among heart transplant recipients in an effort to reduce the mortality and morbidity related to behavior choices in this patient population. The results and feedback from this first series of patients have meanwhile led to a wider implementation of the program at our site, and 65 patients have participated to date.

## Disclosure statement

None of the authors has a financial relationship with a commercial entity that has an interest in the subject of the presented manuscript or other conflicts of interest to disclose.

## References

1. Hochbaum G, Rosenstock I, Kegels S. Health belief model. Hyattsville, MD: United States Public Health Service; 1952.

# Coronary arterial aneurysms in previously transplanted (donor) hearts

Nitin Kondapalli, MBBS, and William C. Roberts, MD

Described herein is a 57-year-old man who had had a cardiac transplant 5 years earlier (at age 52) and died of a ruptured abdominal aortic aneurysm. The donor heart was found to have a fusiform aneurysm, each filled with thrombus, in 2 major epicardial coronary arteries.

The occurrence of aneurysm involving the aorta is fairly common. In contrast, aneurysm involving one or more epicardial coronary arteries is extremely uncommon. In a 24-year period, Roberts (1) collected at necropsy the native hearts of 20 adults who had large aneurysms of one or more major epicardial coronary arteries. Those 20 cases were found from examining approximately 12,000 hearts during that time. Recently, we observed coronary aneurysms in a donor heart that had been transplanted 5 years earlier. A description of this unusual finding is the purpose of this report.

## CASE STUDY

A 57-year-old white man who had had a heart transplant at age 52 died suddenly from a ruptured abdominal aortic aneurysm. The transplanted heart contained huge quantities of adipose tissue and floated in a container of formaldehyde. The left anterior descending and ramus intermedius coronary arteries each had a fusiform aneurysm filled with thrombus *(Figure)*. All of the major epicardial coronary arteries contained considerable quantities of atherosclerotic plaque that narrowed their lumens. Despite this narrowing, there were no grossly visible myocardial lesions, and neither ventricular cavity was dilated. The heart weighed 570 grams and the patient's body mass index was 36 kg/m$^2$.

## DISCUSSION

The cause of aneurysmal formation in epicardial coronary arteries in native hearts is entirely unclear. The aneurysms in this location, with rare exception, are fusiform and contain thrombus superimposed on atherosclerotic plaque (1). Their rarity in coronary arteries in contrast to their relative frequency in the aorta may in part be related to their exposure to only a systemic diastolic pressure rather than to a peak systolic pressure, as occurs in the aorta. The aneurysms in native coronary arteries are not the consequence of an underlying arteritis.

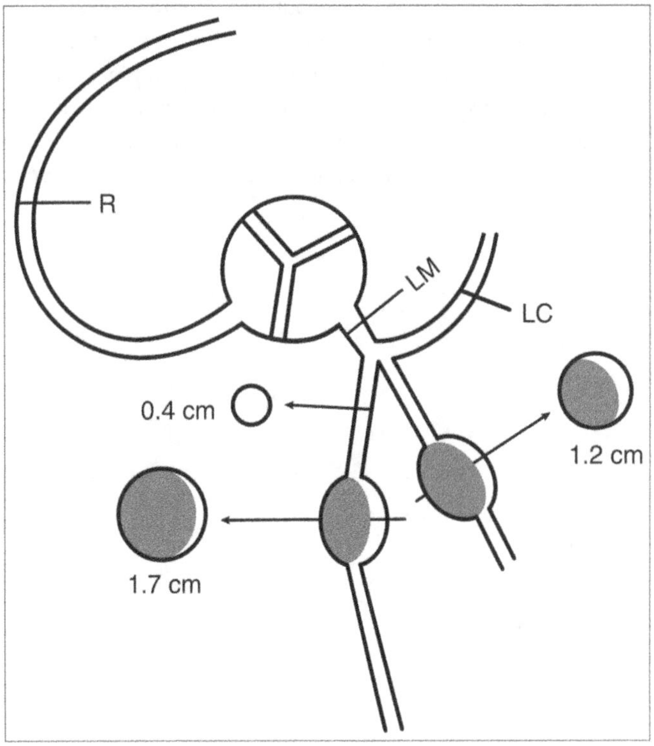


**Figure.** Diagram showing the aneurysms in the left anterior descending and ramus intermedius coronary arteries. Thrombus, shown in red, is present in each aneurysm. A cross-section is also shown of each aneurysm demonstrating that the thrombus does not involve all surfaces of the artery, thereby making the lumen at the site of the aneurysm eccentric. The largest diameter of each aneurysm was approximately 4 times that of the adjacent normal coronary artery. Heavy atherosclerotic plaque was present diffusely in all epicardial coronary arteries. LM indicates left main; R, right coronary artery.

The occurrence of aneurysm in one or more epicardial coronary arteries in donor hearts must be exceedingly uncommon. We have encountered coronary aneurysm in only one of 79 donor hearts studied at necropsy. (The longest interval from

From the Baylor Heart and Vascular Institute and the Departments of Internal Medicine (Cardiology) and Pathology, Baylor University Medical Center, Dallas, Texas.

**Corresponding author:** William C. Roberts, MD, Baylor Heart and Vascular Institute, 621 N. Hall Street, Suite H030, Dallas, TX 75226 (e-mail: william.roberts1@bswhealth.org).

heart transplant to death was 17 years.) Haddad and colleagues (2) described by computed tomography an aneurysm involving the left main and proximal left anterior descending artery in a 75-year-old woman who had had a heart transplant 18 years earlier; they also described a patient (age not given) who had a single aneurysm involving the right coronary artery also found by computed tomography 22 years after the heart transplant. These authors believed that the aneurysms in both patients contained thrombus. They speculated that the aneurysms in both patients were examples of "cardiac allograft vasculopathy." These 2 patients underwent heart transplantation nearly 2 decades earlier, and few patients have computed tomography that long after a heart transplant. In other words, the occurrence of coronary aneurysm after heart transplant may be much higher than presently recognized. Additionally, the autopsy rate in persons having earlier heart transplant is exceedingly low, a fact that might prevent recognition of coronary aneurysm if indeed it was present. Even if recognized, however, proper therapy is debated (3). Anticoagulation, because of the presence of intra-aneurysmal thrombus, certainly appears to be reasonable in patients with coronary arterial aneurysm.

1. Roberts WC. Natural history, clinical consequences, and morphologic features of coronary arterial aneurysms in adults. *Am J Cardiol* 2011; 108(6):814–821.
2. Haddad F, Perez M, Fleischmann D, Valantine H, Hunt SA. Giant coronary aneurysms in heart transplantation: an unusual presentation of cardiac allograft vasculopathy. *J Heart Lung Transplant* 2006;25(11):1367–1370.
3. Harandi S, Johnston SB, Wood RE, Roberts WC. Operative therapy of coronary arterial aneurysm. *Am J Cardiol* 1999;83(8):1290–1293.

# Usefulness of Total 12-Lead QRS Voltage as a Clue to Diagnosis of Patients With Cardiac Sarcoidosis Severe Enough to Warrant Orthotopic Heart Transplant

William C. Roberts, MD; Tiffany M. Becker, BS; Shelley A. Hall, MD

**IMPORTANCE** Severe heart failure caused by cardiac sarcoidosis is difficult to diagnosis without biopsy.

**OBJECTIVE** To assess whether total electrocardiographic 12-lead QRS voltage may be a clue to diagnosis.

**DESIGN, SETTING, PARTICIPANTS** Case-series study with cases collected at Baylor University Medical Center at Dallas, Dallas, Texas, from January 13, 2005, to January 24, 2017. The clinical records of 16 patients with severe heart failure caused by cardiac sarcoidosis were studied. Examination of total 12-lead electrocardiographic QRS voltage (peak of the R wave to the nadir of either the Q or S wave, whichever was deeper) was performed prior to orthotopic heart transplant (OHT). Gross and microscopic pathologic specimens of the native hearts were studied.

**MAIN OUTCOMES AND MEASURES** The primary outcome was to correlate the total 12-lead QRS voltage measurement with various morphologic features in the native diseased heart.

**RESULTS** The 16-patient study group consisted of 8 men and 8 women; 12 (75%) were white and 4 (25%) were black. At the time of OHT, patient age ranged from 50 to 67 years (mean, 57 years). Cardiac sarcoidosis was diagnosed by pre-OHT biopsy results in 2 (13%) patients and by examination of the native heart after OHT in 14 (87%) patients. Total nonpaced 12-lead QRS voltage mean was 117 mm (range, 52-155 mm) for 8 patients and total paced 12-lead QRS voltage was 90 mm (range, 67-161 mm) for 12 patients. These low mean values were similar to those of patients with carcinoid heart disease (mean [SD], 105 [40] mm), cardiac amyloidosis (104 [35] mm), and severe cardiac adiposity (120 [31] mm) studied at necropsy or after OHT. In contrast, mean (SD) values were 323 (109) mm in patients with massive cardiomegaly, 257 mm in patients with severe aortic stenosis, 272 (86) mm in patients with severe pure aortic regurgitation, 220 (67) mm in patients with severe pure mitral regurgitation, 197 (64) mm in patients with hypertrophic cardiomyopathy, and 153 (40) mm in patients with idiopathic dilated cardiomyopathy.

**CONCLUSIONS AND RELEVANCE** Most patients diagnosed with cardiac sarcoidosis causing severe heart failure and warranting OHT had low total 12-lead QRS voltage measurements despite having native hearts of increased weight. This finding may provide a clue to the diagnosis of this disease.

*JAMA Cardiol*. 2018;3(1):64-68. doi:10.1001/jamacardio.2017.4172
Published online November 15, 2017.

**Author Affiliations:** Baylor Heart and Vascular Institute, Baylor University Medical Center at Dallas, Dallas, Texas (Roberts, Becker, Hall); Department of Pathology, Baylor University Medical Center, Dallas, Texas (Roberts, Becker, Hall); Department of Internal Medicine, Baylor University Medical Center, Dallas, Texas (Roberts, Becker, Hall).

**Corresponding Author:** William C. Roberts, MD, Baylor Heart and Vascular Institute, 621 N Hall St, Ste H030, Dallas, TX 75226 (william.roberts1@bswhealth.org).

The first study of the utility of total 12-lead electrocardiographic QRS voltage was published in 1982 and reported findings for patients with aortic valve stenosis.[1] Subsequently, total 12-lead QRS voltage has been reported in a number of other conditions.[2] In each of those studies, the total 12-lead QRS voltage was compared with the weight of the native diseased heart at necropsy or after orthotopic heart transplant (OHT). The present report describes total 12-lead QRS voltage of 16 patients undergoing OHT because of severe heart failure due to cardiac sarcoidosis.

**Key Points**

**Question** Is total 12-lead electrocardiographic QRS voltage a diagnostic clue for patients with cardiac sarcoidosis severe enough to warrant orthotopic heart transplant?

**Findings** In this case-series study, the mean total 12-lead QRS voltage in 16 patients with severe heart failure caused by extensive cardiac sarcoidosis (101 mm) was similar to that determined in patients with cardiac amyloidosis, carcinoid heart disease, and severe cardiac adiposity. In contrast, patients with fatal idiopathic dilated cardiomyopathy had a mean total 12-lead QRS voltage (153 mm).

**Meaning** The low total 12-lead QRS voltage measurement on electrocardiogram in patients with cardiac sarcoidosis, despite increased weight of the native heart, may be a clue to its correct diagnosis before orthotopic heart transplant.

## Methods

From January 13, 2005, through January 24, 2017, 16 patients at Baylor University Medical Center at Dallas (BUMC), Dallas, Texas, had OHT because of cardiac sarcoidosis. The study was approved by the Baylor Research Institute Institutional Review Board, which also waived the need for informed patient consent.

Each patient's native heart was examined by one of us (W.C.R.), and he prepared the final report. Accurate scales were used to weigh the native heart after fixation in formaldehyde for several days. The aorta and pulmonary trunk were excised about 2 cm above the sinotubular junction; all extraneous tissue was removed before weighing. Prior to weighing, the heart was opened and excessive water or formaldehyde was removed from its surfaces by gentle patting with paper towels. Clinical records and all electrocardiograms recorded at BUMC were reviewed and examined. The total 12-lead QRS voltage (defined as the distance in millimeters from the peak of the R wave to the nadir of either the Q or S wave, whichever was deeper) was measured by 2 of us (W.C.R. and T.M.B.). The statistics performed were limited to the calculation of the mean and SD. No statistical package or system was required for these calculations.

## Results

The 16-patient study group consisted of 8 men and 8 women; 12 were white and 4 were black. Pertinent morphologic and electrocardiographic findings for the 16 patients are detailed in the **Table** and illustrated in **Figure 1** and **Figure 2**. At the time of OHT, the patient age ranged from 50 to 67 (mean, 57) years. Cardiac sarcoidosis was diagnosed by biopsy in 2 patients (13%) and by examination of the native heart after OHT in 14 patients (87%). The body mass index (calculated as the weight in kilograms divided by height in meters squared) ranged from 18.8 to 32.9 (mean, 27.1). Before OHT, 6 of the 16 patients (37%) had atrial fibrillation; 12 (75%) had bundle branch block (4 with left bundle branch block and 8 with right bundle branch block), and 7 (44%) had complete heart block. The low-density lipoprotein cholesterol levels before OHT ranged from 52 to 147 mg/dL (mean, 93 mg/dL) (to convert to millimoles per liter, multiply by 0.0259). Only patient 12 (Table) had greater than 75% in cross-sectional area narrowing of 1 or more major epicardial coronary arteries (defined as the right, left main, left anterior descending, and left circumflex).

The native heart weighed from 420 to 605 g (mean, 509 g) for the 8 men and from 370 to 600 g (mean, 442 g) for the 8 women. The quantity of cardiac adipose tissue was excessive such that the heart floated in a container of formaldehyde in 7 of the 11 hearts (64%) in which that determination was made. (Cardiac adipose tissue weighs less than myocardium.) Typical sarcoid granulomas were found in the walls of the right and left ventricles and in the ventricular spectrum in all patients. In 1 patient, however, granulomas were seen in the left ventricular wall ("button") removed for insertion of a left ventricular assist device but were not seen in the heart specimen after OHT. The number of granulomas and extent of ventricular wall scarring were subjectively quantified on a scale of 1+ (mild scarring) to 3+ (severe scarring). The distribution of sarcoid lesions is shown in the gross pathologic heart specimens for 3 of the 16 patients (Figure 2).

QRS voltage was measured using a 10-mm standard scale (10 mm = 1 mV) in all 12 leads of an electrocardiogram for all 16 patients. Mean total nonpaced 12-lead QRS voltage was 117 mm (range, 52-155 mm) for 8 patients: 3 men (mean, 137 mm [range, 121-155 mm]) and 5 women (mean, 105 mm [range, 52-144 mm]). Mean total paced 12-lead QRS voltage was 90 mm (range, 67-161 mm) for 12 patients: 6 men (mean, 81 mm [range, 47-103 mm]) and 6 women (mean, 98 mm [range, 67-161 mm]).

## Discussion

Described herein are findings from measurement of total 12-lead electrocardiographic QRS voltage and findings from the examination of the native heart in 16 patients who underwent OHT because of severe heart failure due to cardiac sarcoidosis. These low total 12-lead nonpaced (mean, 117 mm) and paced (mean, 90 mm) QRS voltage values are similar to those values previously reported in patients with a variety of other conditions after OHT or necropsy.[2] The mean (SD) total 12-lead QRS voltage for several cardiac diseases is as follows: 105 (40) mm in 19 patients with carcinoid heart disease,[3] 104 (35) mm in 30 patients with cardiac amyloidosis,[4] and 120 (31) mm in 30 patients with severe cardiac adiposity.[5] In contrast, mean (SD) total 12-lead QRS voltage was 323 (109) mm in 17 patients with massive cardiomegaly (weight of native heart, >1000 g),[6] 257 mm in 50 patients with

Table. Pertinent Clinical and Morphological Findings in 16 Patients Who Underwent Heart Transplant for Cardiac Sarcoidosis

| Patient No. | Age at HT, y | ECG Paced[a] | QRS Amplitude in Each ECG Lead: I | II | III | aVR | aVL | aVF | $V_1$ | $V_2$ | $V_3$ | $V_4$ | $V_5$ | $V_6$ | Total 12-Lead QRS Voltage, mm | Interval to ECG and HT, mo | BBB (Side)[b] | CHB[b] | LDL-C, mg/dL | SA Pressure, s/d, mm Hg | CI, L/min/$m^2$ | HW, g | Location of Granulomas and Scar: RV | VS | LV | Heart Floated[c] |
|---|---|---|---|---|---|---|---|---|---|---|---|---|---|---|---|---|---|---|---|---|---|---|---|---|---|---|
| **Men** | | | | | | | | | | | | | | | | | | | | | | | | | | |
| 1 | 50 | 0 | 7 | 11 | 14 | 5 | 9 | 12 | 6 | 14 | 19 | 7 | 10 | 7 | 121 | 31 | + (L) | 0 | 119 | 130/89 | 1.7 | 605 | 0 | 1+ | 3+ | NA |
| 2 | 52 | 0 | 14 | 12 | 8 | 13 | 11 | 7 | 12 | 8 | 8 | 18 | 22 | 22 | 155 | 32 | + (R) | 0 | 108 | 98/58 (I) | 1.6 | 440 | 1+ | 2+ | 1+ | NA |
| 3 | 53 | + | 7 | 7 | 10 | 4 | 8 | 9 | 5 | 7 | 5 | 6 | 7 | 6 | 81 | 5 | 0 | + | 120 | 116/66 (I) | 1.9 | 535 | 3+ | 3+ | 3+ | NA |
| 4 | 53 | + | 4 | 12 | 9 | 6 | 3 | 9 | 7 | 7 | 3 | 7 | 10 | 9 | 86 | 0.1 | + (R) | + | 112 | 104/70 (I) | 1.6 | 555 | 3+ | 3+ | 3+ | + |
| 5 | 58 | + | 9 | 9 | 6 | 4 | 4 | 6 | 5 | 3 | 8 | 8 | 8 | 7 | 77 | 1 | + (L) | 0 | 64 | 88/55 (I) | 1.2 | 420 | 3+ | 3+ | 3+ | 0 |
| 6 | 63 | + | 5 | 12 | 8 | 8 | 5 | 10 | 8 | 9 | 14 | 10 | 9 | 5 | 103 | 9 | + (L) | + | 52 | 126/78 | 1.6 | 470 | 3+ | 3+ | 3+ | + |
| 7 | 63 | 0 | 8 | 6 | 3 | 6 | 6 | 4 | 9 | 10 | 13 | 18 | 22 | 29 | 134 | 34 | + (R) | 0 | 86 | 120/84 (I) | 1.7 | 540 | 3+ | 3+ | 3+ | + |
| | | + | 5 | 8 | 11 | 5 | 6 | 11 | 2 | 4 | 12 | 17 | 11 | 3 | 95 | 2 | | | | | | | | | | |
| 8 | 67 | + | 4 | 5 | 7 | 2 | 5 | 5 | 2 | 2 | 6 | 5 | 3 | 1 | 47 | 3 | 0 | + | 70 | 96/59 | 1.6 | 510 | 3+ | 3+ | 3+ | + |
| **Women** | | | | | | | | | | | | | | | | | | | | | | | | | | |
| 9 | 50 | 0 | 6 | 15 | 7 | 9 | 3 | 10 | 7 | 10 | 16 | 16 | 17 | 16 | 132 | 40 | 0 | + | 74 | 100/60 (I) | – | 440 | 1+ | 3+ | 3+ | 0 |
| | | + | 2 | 23 | 13 | 6 | 7 | 28 | 4 | 12 | 16 | 20 | 18 | 12 | 161 | 1 | | | | | | | | | | |
| 10 | 52 | + | 5 | 5 | 5 | 5 | 2 | 8 | 6 | 7 | 7 | 5 | 5 | 7 | 67 | 3 | + (L) | 0 | 64 | 115/79 | 2.3 | 440 | 1+ | 3+ | 2+ | 0 |
| 11 | 56 | + | 4 | 7 | 8 | 5 | 6 | 8 | 4 | 8 | 4 | 5 | 7 | 7 | 73 | 0.5 | 0 | 0 | 118 | 92/64 | – | 450 | 1+ | 3+ | 3+ | + |
| 12 | 57 | 0 | 5 | 1 | 6 | 3 | 6 | 4 | 5 | 9 | 5 | 4 | 2 | 2 | 52 | 18 | + (R) | 0 | 94 | 101/58 (I) | 1.4 | 380 | 3+ | 3+ | 3+ | NA |
| 13 | 58 | 0 | 8 | 8 | 15 | 3 | 11 | 12 | 5 | 7 | 4 | 4 | 6 | 6 | 89 | 49 | + (R) | 0 | 147 | 102/57 (I) | 2.2 | 560 | 3+ | 3+ | 3+ | + |
| | | + | 3 | 3 | 4 | 2 | 3 | 3 | 3 | 7 | 3 | 3 | 4 | 4 | 69 | 2 | | | | | | | | | | |
| 14 | 59 | 0 | 11 | 11 | 17 | 8 | 14 | 13 | 9 | 5 | 9 | 12 | 16 | 19 | 144 | 36 | + (R) | + | 69 | 124/92 | 1.3 | 370 | 1+ | 2+ | 1+ | NA |
| | | + | 10 | 12 | 19 | 8 | 14 | 15 | 8 | 9 | 10 | 13 | 15 | 14 | 147 | 35 | | | | | | | | | | |
| 15 | 61 | + | 4 | 4 | 5 | 3 | 6 | 4 | 4 | 10 | 5 | 7 | 7 | 8 | 72 | 0.5 | + (R) | + | 60 | 95/61 (I) | 1.2 | 300 | 3+ | 3+ | 3+ | + |
| 16 | 62 | 0 | 10 | 11 | 10 | 7 | 7 | 7 | 10 | 9 | 7 | 9 | 10 | 10 | 107 | 1 | + (R) | 0 | 129 | 109/68 (I) | 1.5 | 600 | 1+ | 1+ | 3+ | 0 |

Abbreviations: a, augmented; BBB, bundle branch block; CHB, complete heart block; CI, cardiac index; ECG, electrocardiogram; HT, heart transplant; HW, weight of native heart; I, indirect; L, left (or left arm for ECG leads); LDL-C, low-density lipoprotein cholesterol; LV, left ventricle; NA, no information available; R, right (or right arm for ECG leads); RV, right ventricle; SA, systemic artery; s/d, systolic/diastolic; V, voltage; VS, ventricular septum.

SI conversion factor: To convert LDL-C to millimoles per liter, multiply by 0.0259.

[a] + Indicates paced; 0, nonpaced.

[b] + Indicates present; 0, not present.

[c] + Indicates present; 0, not present; and NA, no information available.

Figure 1. 12-Lead Electrocardiograms

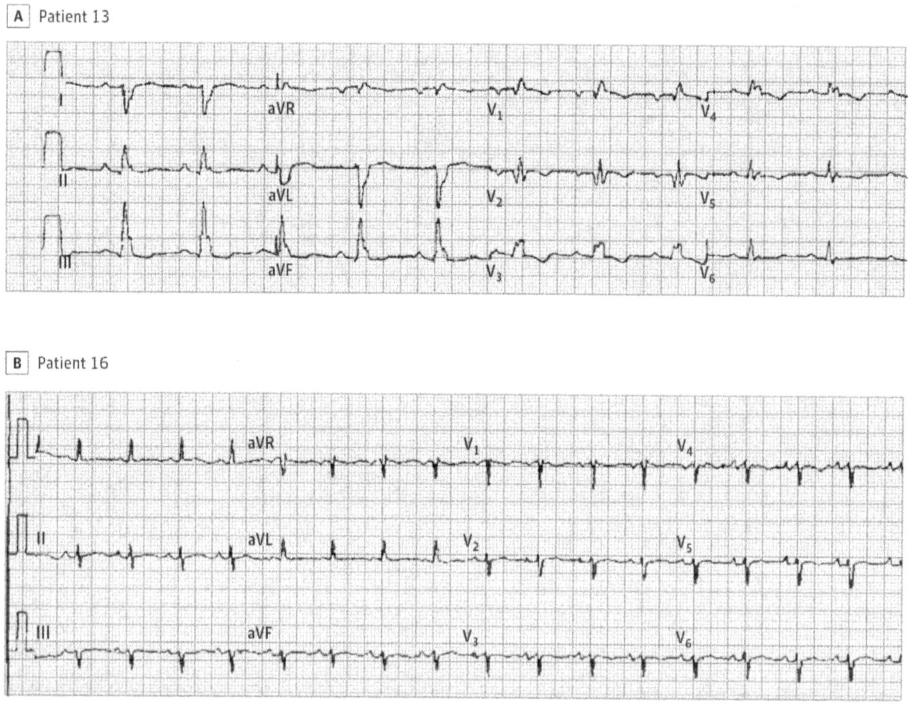


A, Patient 13: total 12-lead QRS voltage is 89 mm; weight of native heart, 560 g. B, Patient 16: total 12-lead QRS voltage is 107 mm; weight of native heart = 600 g. Leads (recording electrodes) are designated as follows: standard (bipolar) leads, I, II, and III; precordial (unipolar) leads, $V_1$, $V_2$, $V_3$, $V_4$, $V_5$, and $V_6$; and augmented limb leads/unipolar extremity leads, aVR, aVL, and aVF (a, augmented; V, voltage; R, right arm; L, left arm; and F, foot).

severe aortic stenosis,[1] 272 (86) mm in 30 patients with severe pure aortic regurgitation,[7] 220 (67) mm in 24 patients with pure mitral regurgitation,[8] 197 (64) mm in 57 patients with hypertrophic cardiomyopathy,[9,10] and 153 (40) mm in 49 patients with idiopathic dilated cardiomyopathy.[11] Thus, most of our patients (15 of 16 [94%]) with severe cardiac sarcoidosis, despite having native hearts of increased weight (>350 g in women and >400 g in men), had low total 12-lead QRS voltages.

### Limitations and Strengths

A limitation of the present report is that the time interval between the recording of the electrocardiogram tracing and the OHT procedure was rather long for some patients. It is likely, however, as described previously in patients with idiopathic dilated cardiomyopathy,[12] that the total 12-lead QRS voltage would decrease as the time interval increases between initially developing cardiac sarcoidosis and OHT procedure.[12]

The strong features of the present report are that both the weight of the native heart and the extent of the cardiac sarcoid lesions were known for all 16 patients. To our knowledge, electrocardiographic QRS voltage has not been described previously in patients with cardiac sarcoidosis.[12]

## Conclusions

Most patients diagnosed with cardiac sarcoidosis causing severe heart failure and warranting OHT had low total 12-lead QRS voltage measurements despite having native hearts of increased weight. This finding may provide a clue to the diagnosis of this disease.

ARTICLE INFORMATION

**Accepted for Publication:** September 19, 2017.

**Published Online:** November 15, 2017. doi:10.1001/jamacardio.2017.4172

**Author Contributions:** Dr Roberts and Ms Becker had full access to all of the data in the study and take responsibility for the integrity of the data and the accuracy of the data analysis.
*Study concept and design:* Roberts, Becker.
*Acquisition, analysis, or interpretation of data:* All authors.
*Drafting of the manuscript:* Roberts.
*Critical revision of the manuscript for important intellectual content:* Roberts.
*Administrative, technical, or material support:* Hall.
*Study supervision:* Roberts.

**Conflict of Interest Disclosures:** All authors have completed and submitted the ICMJE Form for Disclosure of Potential Conflicts of Interest and none were reported.

REFERENCES

1. Siegel RJ, Roberts WC. Electrocardiographic observations in severe aortic valve stenosis: correlative necropsy study to clinical, hemodynamic, and ECG variables demonstrating relation of 12-lead QRS amplitude to peak systolic transaortic pressure gradient. *Am Heart J*. 1982;103(2):210-221.

2. Roberts WC, Filardo G, Ko JM, et al. Comparison of total 12-lead QRS voltage in a variety of cardiac conditions and its usefulness in predicting increased cardiac mass. *Am J Cardiol*. 2013;112(6):904-909.

3. Ross EM, Roberts WC. The carcinoid syndrome: comparison of 21 necropsy subjects with carcinoid heart disease to 15 necropsy subjects without carcinoid heart disease. *Am J Med*. 1985;79(3):339-354.

Figure 2. Basal Portions of Native Heart and Photomicrograph of Myocardial Wall in Patients Who Underwent Cardiac Transplant Because of Cardiac Sarcoidosis

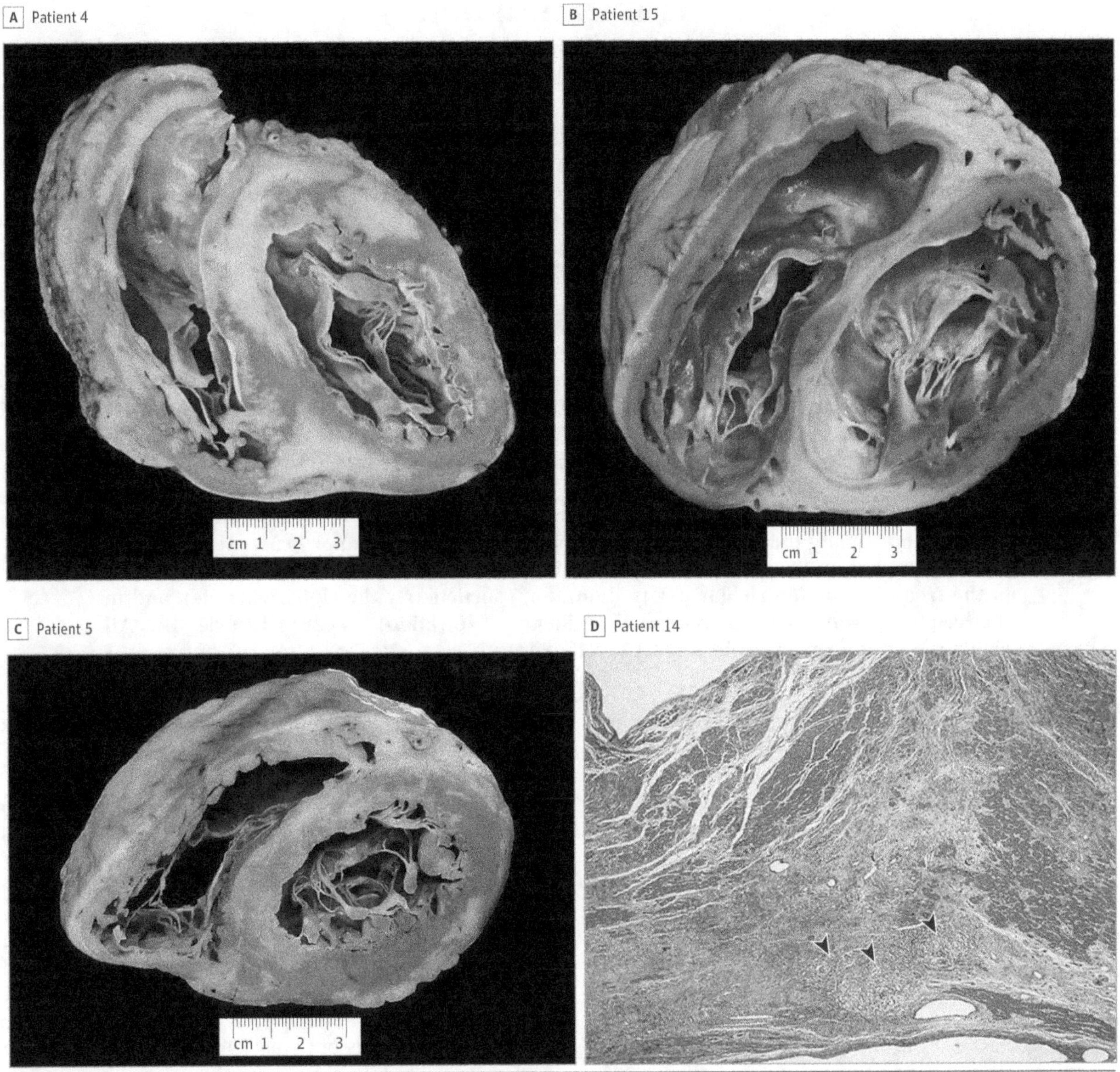


Basal portions of the heart exposing the tricuspid and mitral values. The ventricular septal and left ventricular free wall and a portion of right ventricular free wall contain white lesions; these represent scar tissue within which are sarcoid granulomas. All ventricular cavities are largely dilated. D, Photomicrograph of a portion of the left ventricular free wall of patient 14. The myocardial wall is partially, but extensively replaced by dense fibrous tissue that stains blue and contains several sarcoid granulomas (arrowheads) (trichrome stain, original magnification ×100). Scale bars in A through C are in centimeters.


4. Roberts WC, Waller BF. Cardiac amyloidosis causing cardiac dysfunction: analysis of 54 necropsy patients. *Am J Cardiol*. 1983;52(1):137-146.

5. Shirani J, Roberts WC. Clinical, electrocardiographic and morphologic features of massive fatty deposits ("lipomatous hypertrophy") in the atrial septum. *J Am Coll Cardiol*. 1993;22(1):226-238.

6. Roberts WC, Podolak MJ. The king of hearts: analysis of 23 patients with hearts weighing 1,000 grams or more. *Am J Cardiol*. 1985;55(4):485-494.

7. Roberts WC, Day PJ. Electrocardiographic observations in clinically isolated, pure, chronic, severe aortic regurgitation: analysis of 30 necropsy patients aged 19 to 65 years. *Am J Cardiol*. 1985;55(4):432-438.

8. Glick BN, Roberts WC. Usefulness of total 12-lead QRS voltage in diagnosing left ventricular hypertrophy in clinically isolated, pure, chronic, severe mitral regurgitation. *Am J Cardiol*. 1992;70(11):1088-1092.

9. Dollar AL, Roberts WC. Usefulness of total 12-lead QRS voltage compared with other criteria for determining left ventricular hypertrophy in hypertrophic cardiomyopathy: analysis of 57 patients studied at necropsy. *Am J Med*. 1989;87(4):377-381.

10. Shirani J, Maron BJ, Cannon RO III, Shahin S, Roberts WC. Clinicopathologic features of hypertrophic cardiomyopathy managed by cardiac transplantation. *Am J Cardiol*. 1993;72(5):434-440.

11. Roberts WC, Siegel RJ, McManus BM. Idiopathic dilated cardiomyopathy: analysis of 152 necropsy patients. *Am J Cardiol*. 1987;60(16):1340-1355.

12. Wilensky RL, Yudelman P, Cohen AI, et al. Serial electrocardiographic changes in idiopathic dilated cardiomyopathy confirmed at necropsy. *Am J Cardiol*. 1988;62(4):276-283.

# Morphologic Findings in Donor (Transplanted) Hearts at Necropsy Early and Late After Orthotopic Heart Transplantation

William C. Roberts, MD*, Nitin Kondapalli, MBBS, and Joseph M. Guileyardo, MD

**Little necropsy information is available on donor hearts in place in recipients for varying periods. Necropsy studies were performed in 79 patients who had survived from 1 day to 17 years after orthotopic heart transplantation (OHT). At OHT, the 79 patients ranged in age from 3 to 70 years (mean 51), and at death, from 20 to 76 years (mean 54). The native hearts tended to be larger than the donor hearts in the 22 patients surviving ≤60 days and the donor hearts tended to be larger in the 57 patients surviving >60 days, suggesting that the donor hearts increased in weight with time. Cardiac adiposity increased with time. Grossly visible myocardial lesions were seen in 24 (30%) of the 79 cases: necrosis only in 20; fibrosis only in 2, and both in 2. One or more epicardial coronary arteries were narrowed >75% in cross-sectional area in 25 (32%), 1 of whom was in the group surviving ≤60 days. The right ventricular cavity was dilated in 73 cases (92%) and the left ventricular cavity in 39 cases. Evidence of graft rejection (lymphocytic infiltrates) was found in 50 patients (63%); in 8 (36%) of the 22 patients surviving ≤60 days, and in 42 (74%) of the 57 surviving >60 days. The lymphocytic infiltrates were largest in the subepicardial adipose tissue, next in myocardium, and least in endocardium. The quantity of the cellular infiltrates varied considerably among the patients. In conclusion, with time, the donor hearts tended to increase in weight, in the quantity of adipose tissue, in the amounts of coronary narrowing, in the frequency of ventricular cavity dilatation (particularly the right ventricle), and in the frequency of lymphocytic infiltrates (evidence of rejection).**  **(Am J Cardiol 2018;121:217–240)**

In 2014, Roberts and colleagues[1] described certain clinical and morphologic findings in 314 patients who had undergone orthotopic heart transplantation (OHT) at Baylor University Medical Center at Dallas from 1993 to 2012. The present study focuses on 79 patients who had OHT from 1989 to 2017, and it focuses on findings in the donor hearts. Surprisingly, essentially no studies have been reported describing or illustrating findings in donor (transplanted) hearts having been in place for varying periods after OHT. Such is the purpose of this report.

## Methods

A total of 79 donor hearts were studied at necropsy (Tables 1 and 2). These included 70 cases studied at Baylor University Medical Center from August 1993 through March 2017 (23 years) and 9 cases submitted to one of us (WCR) from 1989 to 2015. Most autopsies were performed by JMG. All 79 hearts were examined by WCR who prepared the final descriptive reports in all but a few cases. Nearly all hearts were photographed. All histologic sections were examined by NK and WCR and photomicrographs were made by WCR.

Baylor Heart and Vascular Institute, the Departments of Pathology and Internal Medicine (Division of Cardiology), Baylor University Medical Center, Baylor Scott & White Health, Dallas, Texas. Manuscript received September 29, 2017; revised manuscript received and accepted October 4, 2017.

See page 239 for disclosure information.

*Corresponding author:

*E-mail address:* William.Roberts1@bswhealth.org (W.C. Roberts).

The clinical records were retrieved in all patients and examined by NK and WCR. The sections of hearts submitted for preparation of histologic sections included the walls of both ventricles and were through-and-through from endocardium to epicardium. Additionally, one or more sections of epicardial coronary arteries were prepared and examined in each patient. Most hearts were weighed by WCR after removal of the parietal pericardium and extraneous tissues. The ascending aorta and pulmonary trunk were excised approximately 2 cm above their sinotubular junctions. The weights of the hearts were those after the heart had been fixed in 10% formaldehyde for several days (all <1 week). Whether the heart floated in a container of formaldehyde was determined in many patients. All histologic sections were stained by hematoxylin/eosin and also either by trichrome or Movat methods.

## Results

Of the 79 patients, 22 (28%) survived ≤60 days, and 57 (72%) >60 days (Tables 1 and 2): 57 (72%) were men and 22 (28%) were women. The ages at OHT ranged from 3 to 70 years (mean 51 ± 13) and at death, from 20 to 76 years (mean 54 ± 12). The primary cause of death is summarized in Table 3. The weights of the native and donor hearts in the men surviving ≤60 days ranged from 280 to 835 g (mean 579 ± 150) and 355 to 480 g (mean 460 ± 200), respectively, and in the women surviving ≤60 days from 240 to 755 g (mean 454 ± 200) and 330 to 445 g (mean 400 ± 42), respectively; the weights of the native and donor hearts in the men surviving >60 days ranged from 310 to 755 g (mean 519 ± 120)

Table 1

Clinical and morphological findings in the 22 patients who survived ≤60 days after heart transplantation

| Pt. No. | Age at OHT (yrs) | Age at Death (yrs) | Interval from OHT to Death (days) | Sex | BMI Before OHT (kg/m$^2$) | Weight of Native Heart (g) | Weight of Donor Heart (g) | Native Heart Floats | Donor Heart Floats | Reason for OHT | Necropsy Findings in the Donor Heart: RV Cavity Dilated | LV Cavity Dilated | Grossly Visible Myocardial Lesion: N | F | Coronary Artery Narrowing by Plaque | Microscopic Sized Necrosis | Microscopic Sized Fibrosis | Lymphocytes in Left Ventricle (0–3$^+$): Epi | Myo | Endo |
|---|---|---|---|---|---|---|---|---|---|---|---|---|---|---|---|---|---|---|---|---|
| 1 | 28 | 28 | 1 | Female | – | 280 | 415 | – | 0 | IDC | + | + | + | 0 | 0 | + | 0 | 3+ | 3+ | 2+ |
| 2 | 64 | 64 | 1 | Female | – | 310 | 435 | + | 0 | IDC | + | + | + | 0 | 0 | + | 0 | 0 | 0 | 0 |
| 3 | 67 | 67 | 2 | Male | 26 | 660 | 465 | 0 | + | IC* | ++ | 0 | 0 | 0 | 0 | 0 | + | 0 | 0 | 0 |
| 4 | 57 | 57 | 3 | Male | 25 | 600 | 480 | 0 | 0 | IDC | ++ | ++ | 0 | 0 | 0† | + | 0 | 0 | 0 | 0 |
| 5 | 28 | 28 | 4 | Female | – | 240 | 330 | 0 | 0 | LM | ++ | ++ | 0 | 0 | 0 | 0 | + | 1+ | 3+ | 0 |
| 6 | 39 | 39 | 6 | Male | 32 | 600 | 490 | 0 | 0 | IDC | + | 0 | 0 | 0 | 0 | + | 0 | 0 | 0 | 0 |
| 7 | 51 | 51 | 7 | Male | 32 | 335 | 435 | 0 | 0 | IC | ++ | 0 | 0 | 0 | 0 | + | 0 | 0 | 2+ | 0 |
| 8 | 58 | 58 | 9 | Male | 24 | 355 | – | + | 0 | IDC | + | 0 | 0 | 0 | 0 | 0 | 0 | 0 | 0 | 0 |
| 9 | 44 | 44 | 9 | Female | 29 | 755 | 370 | + | + | CHD | 0 | 0 | + | 0 | 0 | + | 0 | 3+ | 3+ | 3+ |
| 10 | 56 | 56 | 13 | Female | – | 385 | 440 | + | + | IC | 0 | 0 | 0 | 0 | + | 0 | 0 | 0 | 0 | 0 |
| 11 | 62 | 62 | 16 | Male | 24 | 475 | 430 | 0 | 0 | IDC | + | 0 | 0 | 0 | 0 | 0 | 0 | 0 | 0 | 0 |
| 12 | 66 | 66 | 16 | Male | 28 | 545 | 480 | 0 | 0 | IC* | 0 | 0 | 0 | 0 | 0 | 0 | 0 | 0 | 0 | 0 |
| 13 | 65 | 65 | 19 | Male | 36 | 780 | 355 | + | 0 | IC* | + | 0 | 0 | 0 | 0 | + | 0 | 0 | 0 | 0 |
| 14 | 60 | 60 | 23 | Male | – | 835 | 480 | – | + | IC | + | 0 | + | 0 | 0 | + | 0 | 0 | 0 | 0 |
| 15 | 56 | 56 | 27 | Female | 32 | 630 | 365 | + | 0 | IC* | + | 0 | 0 | 0 | 0 | 0 | 0 | 0 | 0 | 0 |
| 16 | 52 | 52 | 28 | Female | 29 | – | 445 | – | 0 | IC | + | 0 | 0 | 0 | 0 | 0 | 0 | 1+ | 1+ | 0 |
| 17 | 45 | 45 | 30 | Male | 39 | 760 | 455 | + | + | IDC | ++ | + | 0 | 0 | 0 | + | + | 1+ | 1+ | 1+ |
| 18 | 53 | 53 | 35 | Male | 25 | 555 | 480 | + | 0 | Sarcoid* | + | 0 | 0 | 0 | 0 | 0 | 0 | 0 | 0 | 0 |
| 19 | 51 | 51 | 45 | Male | 39 | 645 | 480 | 0 | 0 | IDC | +++ | + | +‡ | 0 | 0 | 0 | + | 3+ | 3+ | 1+ |
| 20 | 47 | 47 | 51 | Male | – | 450 | 480 | 0 | 0 | IDC | ++ | 0 | 0 | 0 | 0 | + | 0 | 1+ | 3+ | 1+ |
| 21 | 52 | 52 | 54 | Male | – | 510 | 475 | – | 0 | IC* | ++ | ++ | 0 | 0 | 0 | + | + | 0 | 0 | 0 |
| 22 | 53 | 53 | 58 | Female | – | 580 | 410 | + | 0 | IDC | + | 0 | 0 | 0 | 0 | + | 0 | 0 | 0 | 0 |

AMI = Acute Myocardial Infarction; BMI = Body Mass Index; CHD = Congenital Heart Disease; CABG = Coronary Artery Bypass Grafting; CAD = Coronary Artery Disease; CSA = Cross-Sectional Area; Endo = Endocardium; Epi = Epicardium; F = Fibrosis; g = gram(s); IDC = Idiopathic Dilated Cardiomyopathy; IC = Ischemic Cardiomyopathy; LM = Lymphocytic Myocarditis; m = month(s); Myo = Myocardium; N = Necrosis; OHT = Orthotopic Heart Transplantation.

* CABG in the native heart.

† Thrombus in coronary artery.

‡ Abscess in the myocardium.

Table 2
Clinical and morphological findings in the 57 patients who survived ≥60 days after orthotopic heart transplantation

| Pt. No. | Age at OHT (yrs) | Age at Death (yrs) | Interval from HT to Death (months) | Sex | BMI Before OHT (kg/m$^2$) | Weight of Native Heart (g) | Weight of Donor Heart (g) | Native Heart Floats | Donor Heart Floats | Reason for OHT | Necropsy Findings in the Donor Heart: RV Cavity Dilated | LV Cavity Dilated | Grossly Visible Myocardial Lesion | | Coronary Artery Narrowing by Plaque | Coronary Arteritis | Microscopic Sized Necrosis | Microscopic Sized Fibrosis | Lymphocytes in Left Ventricle (0–3$^+$) | | |
|---|---|---|---|---|---|---|---|---|---|---|---|---|---|---|---|---|---|---|---|---|---|
| | | | | | | | | | | | | | N | F | | | | | Epi | Myo | Endo |
| 23 | 50 | 50 | 2 | Male | – | 570 | 475 | + | – | IC* | + | + | 0 | 0 | 0 | + | + | 0 | 2+ | 2+ | 2+ |
| 24 | 66 | 67 | 2 | Male | 23 | 445 | 390 | 0 | 0 | IC* | + | 0 | +† | 0 | 0 | – | + | 0 | 0 | 0 | 0 |
| 25 | 69 | 69 | 3 | Male | 31 | 310 | 530 | 0 | + | IDC | + | + | 0 | 0 | 0 | 0 | 0 | + | 1+ | 1+ | 0 |
| 26 | 61 | 61 | 3 | Male | 22 | 450 | 420 | + | 0 | IDC | + | 0 | 0 | 0 | + | + | + | 0 | 3+ | 1+ | 3+ |
| 27 | 54 | 54 | 4 | Female | 20 | 220 | 255 | 0 | 0 | IC* | ++ | + | 0 | 0 | 0 | 0 | 0 | + | 0 | 0 | 0 |
| 28 | 70 | 70 | 4 | Female | – | 315 | 420 | + | + | IDC | + | 0 | 0 | 0 | 0 | 0 | 0 | + | 1+ | 1+ | 0 |
| 29 | 50 | 50 | 4 | Male | – | 395 | 515 | + | – | IC | + | + | + | 0 | 0 | 0 | + | + | 1+ | 0 | 0 |
| 30 | 57 | 58 | 7 | Male | 29 | 420 | 430 | 0 | 0 | Amyloid | ++ | + | 0 | 0 | 0 | 0 | 0 | 0 | 0 | 0 | 0 |
| 31 | 57 | 58 | 7 | Female | 25 | 380 | 440 | 0 | 0 | IDC | ++ | + | + | 0 | + | + | + | 0 | 1+ | 1+ | 1+ |
| 32 | 41 | 42 | 8 | Male | 40 | 610 | 650 | 0 | 0 | IDC | ++ | 0 | 0 | 0 | + | + | 0 | + | 3+ | 3+ | 2+ |
| 33 | 33 | 33 | 8 | Male | 36 | 345 | 430 | – | 0 | IDC | 0 | 0 | + | 0 | 0 | 0 | + | 0 | 1+ | 1+ | 1+ |
| 34 | 61 | 62 | 9 | Male | 28 | 510 | 530 | + | 0 | Amyloid | ++ | 0 | + | 0 | 0 | + | + | 0 | 1+ | 1+ | 1+ |
| 35 | 60 | 61 | 10 | Male | – | 365 | 360 | – | 0 | IC | + | 0 | 0 | 0 | 0 | 0 | 0 | 0 | 1+ | 1+ | 0 |
| 36 | 56 | 57 | 10 | Female | 21 | 585 | 620 | 0 | 0 | IDC | + | 0 | 0 | 0 | 0 | + | + | 0 | 3+ | 3+ | 3+ |
| 37 | 52 | 53 | 11 | Male | 32 | 670 | 630 | 0 | 0 | IDC | ++ | ++ | + | 0 | 0 | + | + | 0 | 3+ | 3+ | 2+ |
| 38 | 22 | 23 | 12 | Male | 22 | – | 600 | – | 0 | IDC | + | + | 0 | 0 | 0 | – | + | + | 1+ | 1+ | 1+ |
| 39 | 51 | 52 | 13 | Male | 34 | – | – | – | + | IC* | 0 | 0 | 0 | 0 | 0 | – | 0 | 0 | 0 | 0 | 0 |
| 40 | 60 | 61 | 13 | Male | 26 | 460 | 505 | 0 | 0 | IC* | + | + | + | 0 | 0 | + | + | 0 | 3+ | 2+ | 2+ |
| 41 | 56 | 57 | 14 | Male | 35 | 550 | 550 | + | 0 | IC* | ++ | + | 0 | 0 | 0 | 0 | 0 | + | 3+ | 1+ | 0 |
| 42 | 52 | 53 | 15 | Female | 31 | 440 | 470 | 0 | 0 | Sarcoid | ++ | + | 0 | 0 | 0 | 0 | + | 0 | 3+ | 2+ | 2+ |
| 43 | 28 | 30 | 15 | Male | 23 | – | 465 | – | 0 | IDC | ++ | + | 0 | 0 | + | + | 0 | 0 | 3+ | 1+ | 3+ |
| 44 | 51 | 52 | 16 | Male | – | – | – | – | 0 | IDC | ++ | + | + | + | + | – | + | + | 0 | 0 | 0 |
| 45 | 51 | 53 | 18 | Female | 39 | 440 | 630 | 0 | 0 | IDC | ++ | 0 | + | 0 | 0 | + | + | 0 | 3+ | 3+ | 2+ |
| 46 | 25 | 26 | 20 | Male | – | 450 | 505 | – | 0 | IDC | ++ | ++ | + | 0 | + | + | + | + | 3+ | 2+ | 1+ |
| 47 | 36 | 38 | 22 | Male | – | – | – | – | – | IC | 0 | 0 | 0 | + | + | – | 0 | + | 1+ | 1+ | 1+ |
| 48 | 55 | 57 | 25 | Male | 30 | 495 | 475 | + | 0 | IDC | ++ | + | + | 0 | + | + | + | 0 | 3+ | 3+ | 3+ |
| 49 | 51 | 54 | 32 | Male | – | 565 | 660 | + | 0 | IC | + | + | + | 0 | + | + | + | 0 | 3+ | 1+ | 1+ |
| 50 | 67 | 70 | 33 | Male | – | – | 700 | – | 0 | IC* | ++ | 0 | 0 | 0 | 0 | 0 | 0 | + | 1+ | 1+ | 0 |
| 51 | 39 | 42 | 33 | Male | 29 | 755 | 490 | 0 | 0 | IDC | + | + | 0 | 0 | + | 0 | 0 | 0 | 0 | 0 | 0 |
| 52 | 57 | 60 | 34 | Male | – | – | 550 | – | + | IDC | + | 0 | + | 0 | 0 | 0 | + | 0 | 0 | 0 | 0 |
| 53 | 34 | 37 | 37 | Female | – | – | 440 | – | – | IC | + | + | 0 | 0 | + | + | 0 | + | 2+ | 2+ | 2+ |

(*continued on next page*)

Table 2
*(continued)*

| Pt. No. | Age at OHT (yrs) | Age at Death (yrs) | Interval from HT to Death (months) | Sex | BMI Before OHT (kg/m$^2$) | Weight of Native Heart (g) | Weight of Donor Heart (g) | Native Heart Floats | Donor Heart Floats | Reason for OHT | Necropsy Findings in the Donor Heart: RV Cavity Dilated | LV Cavity Dilated | Grossly Visible Myocardial Lesion | | Coronary Artery Narrowing by Plaque | Coronary Arteritis | Microscopic Sized Necrosis | Microscopic Sized Fibrosis | Lymphocytes in Left Ventricle (0–3+) | | |
|---|---|---|---|---|---|---|---|---|---|---|---|---|---|---|---|---|---|---|---|---|---|
| | | | | | | | | | | | | | N | F | | | | | Epi | Myo | Endo |
| 54 | 52 | 55 | 40 | Male | – | – | 505 | – | 0 | IC* | + | + | + | + | + | – | + | + | 1+ | 1+ | 1+ |
| 55 | 58 | 61 | 40 | Male | – | – | 445 | – | – | IC | + | + | + | 0 | + | 0 | + | 0 | 0 | 0 | 0 |
| 56 | 49 | 53 | 45 | Male | 27 | 735 | 415 | 0 | 0 | IC | ++ | + | 0 | 0 | + | + | 0 | + | 2+ | 2+ | 1+ |
| 57 | 46 | 50 | 55 | Female | – | 380 | 355 | + | 0 | IDC | + | 0 | 0 | 0 | + | + | + | + | 1+ | 2+ | 0 |
| 58 | 54 | 59 | 56 | Female | – | – | 640 | – | + | – | +++ | + | + | 0 | + | + | + | + | 2+ | 1+ | 1+ |
| 59 | 52 | 57 | 60 | Male | 36 | – | 570 | – | + | IC | + | 0 | 0 | 0 | ++ | – | 0 | 0 | 0 | 0 | 0 |
| 60 | 54 | 59 | 60 | Female | 24 | 540 | 385 | + | + | IC* | ++ | + | 0 | 0 | 0 | + | 0 | + | 3+ | 2+ | 1+ |
| 61 | 61 | 66 | 68 | Male | – | 485 | 405 | – | – | Amyloid | + | 0 | 0 | 0 | 0 | 0 | 0 | 0 | 0 | 0 | 0 |
| 62 | 25 | 31 | 77 | Male | – | 475 | 500 | – | – | IDC | + | + | 0 | + | 0 | 0 | + | 3+ | 2+ | 2+ | 2+ |
| 63 | 57 | 64 | 86 | Male | – | – | 575 | – | + | IC | + | 0 | 0 | 0 | 0 | 0 | 0 | 0 | 0 | 0 | 0 |
| 64 | 58 | 66 | 92 | Male | – | 550 | 600 | – | + | IC* | ++ | + | 0 | 0 | 0 | 0 | 0 | + | 0 | 0 | 0 |
| 65 | 54 | 63 | 103 | Male | – | – | 540 | – | 0 | IC | ++ | 0 | 0 | 0 | + | 0 | 0 | + | 1+ | 0 | 1+ |
| 66 | 51 | 60 | 109 | Male | – | – | 520 | – | + | IC | +++ | +++ | + | 0 | +‡ | 0 | + | 3+ | 2+ | 2+ | 1+ |
| 67 | 49 | 58 | 109 | Male | – | – | 530 | – | + | IC* | + | + | 0 | 0 | + | 0 | 0 | 3+ | 2+ | 2+ | 0 |
| 68 | 56 | 66 | 116 | Female | – | – | 355 | – | + | IC | + | + | + | 0 | + | 0 | + | 3+ | 2+ | 2+ | 1+ |
| 69 | 66 | 76 | 118 | Female | 20 | – | 630 | – | + | IC | ++ | + | 0 | 0 | +‡ | 0 | 0 | 3+ | 2+ | 0 | 1+ |
| 70 | 52 | 62 | 119 | Male | 31 | – | 580 | – | + | IDC | ++ | 0 | 0 | 0 | 0 | 0 | 0 | 3+ | 2+ | 1+ | 1+ |
| 71 | 47 | 57 | 119 | Male | 34 | 705 | 660 | – | + | IDC | + | 0 | 0 | 0 | + | 0 | 0 | 2+ | 2+ | 1+ | 0 |
| 72 | 42 | 52 | 120 | Male | – | – | 740 | – | + | IC | ++ | 0 | 0 | 0 | 0 | 0 | 0 | 2+ | 0 | 1+ | 0 |
| 73 | 61 | 71 | 122 | Male | 25 | 465 | 585 | – | + | IC* | ++ | 0 | 0 | 0 | 0 | 0 | 0 | + | 2+ | 1+ | 0 |
| 74 | 53 | 64 | 126 | Female | – | – | 245 | – | + | IDC | ++ | + | 0 | 0 | 0 | 0 | 0 | 3+ | 0 | 0 | 0 |
| 75 | 57 | 68 | 130 | Male | – | 535 | 480 | + | – | IC | + | + | 0 | 0 | 0 | 0 | 0 | 3+ | 1+ | 1+ | 1+ |
| 76 | 61 | 73 | 136 | Male | – | 660 | 545 | + | + | IC* | ++ | 0 | 0 | 0 | 0 | 0 | 0 | + | 0 | 0 | 0 |
| 77 | 18 | 31 | 152 | Male | – | – | 510 | – | 0 | IDC | ++§ | + | 0 | 0 | 0 | 0 | 0 | 3+ | 3+ | 0 | 0 |
| 78 | 57 | 71 | 167 | Male | – | – | 575 | – | + | IC | +++ | 0 | 0 | 0 | 0 | 0 | 0 | 1+ | 0 | 0 | 0 |
| 79 | 3 | 20 | 206 | Female | 31 | – | 275 | – | 0 | CHD | +++ | + | 0 | 0 | + | + | 0 | 3+ | 3+ | 1+ | 0 |

BMI = Body Mass Index; CHD = Congenital Heart Disease; CABG = Coronary Artery Bypass Grafting; CAD = Coronary Artery Disease; CSA = Cross-Sectional Area; Endo = Endocardium; Epi = Epicardium; F = Fibrosis; g = gram(s); IDC = Idiopathic Dilated Cardiomyopathy; IC = Ischemic Cardiomyopathy; Myo = Myocardium; N = Necrosis; OHT = Orthotopic Heart Transplantation.

* CABG in the native heart.

† Abscess in the myocardium.

‡ PCI + Stent in the donor heart.

§ Tricuspid Valve Replacement (bioprosthesis).

Table 3
Causes of death after heart transplantation

| Cause | Length of Survival (Days) | |
|---|---|---|
| | <60 (n = 22) | >60 (n = 59) |
| 1. Rejection | | |
| With pump failure | 9 | 12 |
| Without pump failure | 0 | 4 |
| 2. Pump failure without rejection | 6 | 3 |
| 3. Infection | 1 | 4 |
| 4. Operative problem (technical, bleeding) | 3 | 1 |
| 5. Non-cardiovascular death (cancer, other) | 0 | 4 |
| 6. Non-cardiac death | | |
| Stroke | 3 | 4 |
| Abdominal aortic aneurysm | 0 | 2 |
| Chronic kidney disease | 0 | 6 |
| Pulmonary embolism | 0 | 1 |
| 7. Epicardial coronary artery disease | | |
| With rejection | 0 | 3 |
| Without rejection | 0 | 1 |
| Sudden death outside hospital | 0 | 7 |
| Acute myocardial infarction | 0 | 4 |
| 8. Amyloidosis | 0 | 1 |

and 360 to 750 g (mean 530 ± 86), respectively, and in the women from 220 to 585 g (mean 413 ± 117) and 245 to 630 g (mean 440 ± 142), respectively (Figure 1). Of the patients surviving ≤60 days, 9 (50%) of 18 native hearts and 5 (23%) of 22 donor hearts floated in a container of formaldehyde due to excessive fat (adipose tissue is lighter than myocardium), and of the patients surviving >60 days, 12 (48%) of 25 native hearts and 20 (41%) of 49 donor hearts floated in a container of formaldehyde. (The body mass indexes before OHT varied from 20 to 40 kg ($m^2$) [mean 29].)

The cardiac condition prompting the OHT was ischemic cardiomyopathy in 38 patients (48%), idiopathic dilated cardiomyopathy in 32 patients (41%), and miscellaneous nonischemic conditions in 9 patients (11%) (Tables 1 and 2).

Many findings at necropsy are illustrated in Figures 2–26. Of the 79 patients, the right ventricular cavity was dilated in 73 (92%), and the left ventricular cavity in 40 (51%). Both ventricular cavities were dilated in 40 patients (51%). All of the 40 patients with dilated left ventricles also had dilated right ventricles; 32 (44%) of the 73 patients with dilated right ventricular cavities had no dilatation of the left ventricular cavity.

Grossly visible foci of necrosis (acute myocardial infarcts) were seen in 23 (29%) and 1 or more left ventricular scars, in 4 (5%) of the 79 patients. Histologic evidence of necrosis and/or fibrosis was seen in most patients (Tables 1 and 2). Histologic evidence of myofiber necrosis was found in 6 (27%) of the 22 patients surviving ≤60 days, and in 41 (72%) of the 57 patients surviving >60 days.

## Discussion

Although numerous publications have appeared describing morphologic components of what constitutes evidence of cardiac rejection after OHT,[2–7] only 1 report has described nonrejection features of a donor heart.[8] That report consisted of an 11-page description by Thomson[8] of the heart of the first ever OHT (by Christian N. Barnard). Subsequently,

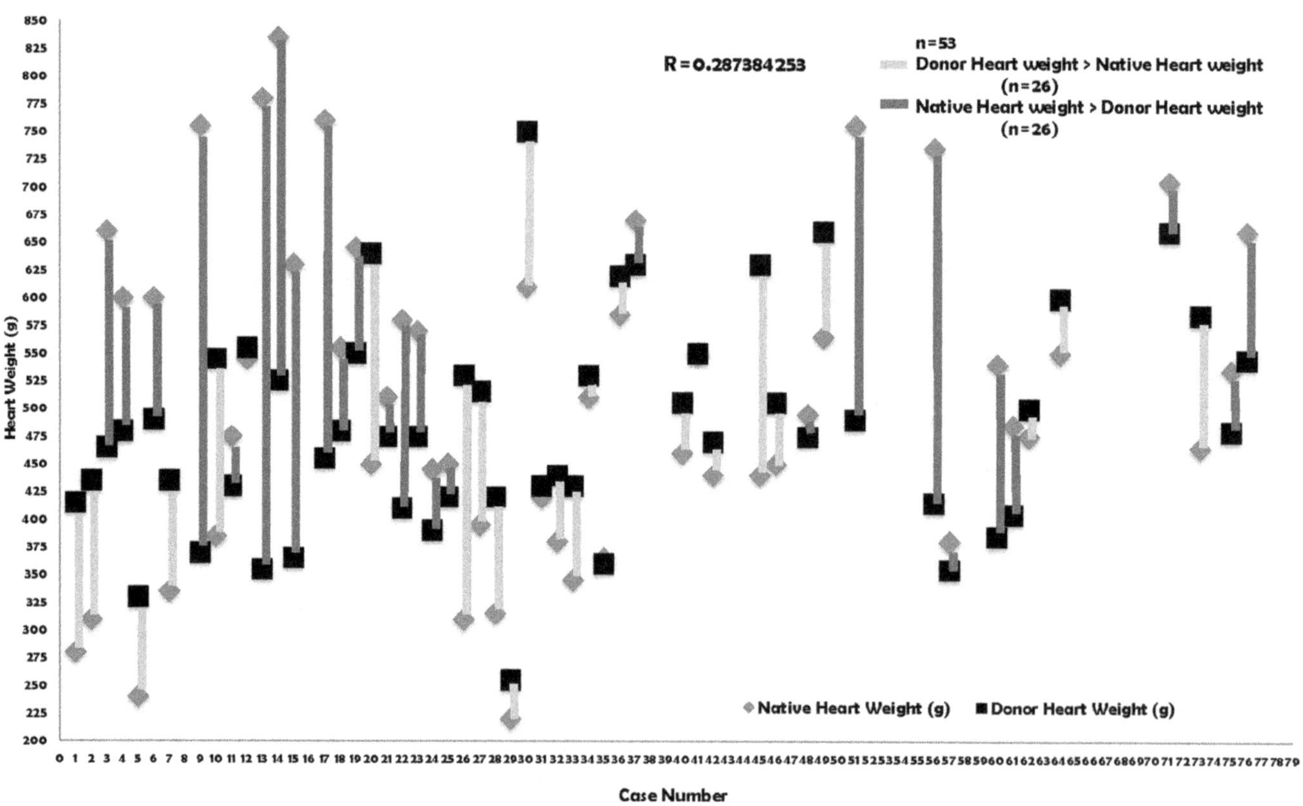


Figure 1. The weights of both native and donor hearts were available in 53 of the 79 patients. This graph shows the hearts of both. The *red lines* show the native hearts in 26 patients to be heavier than the donor hearts, and the *green lines* show the donor hearts in 26 patients to be heavier than the native hearts.

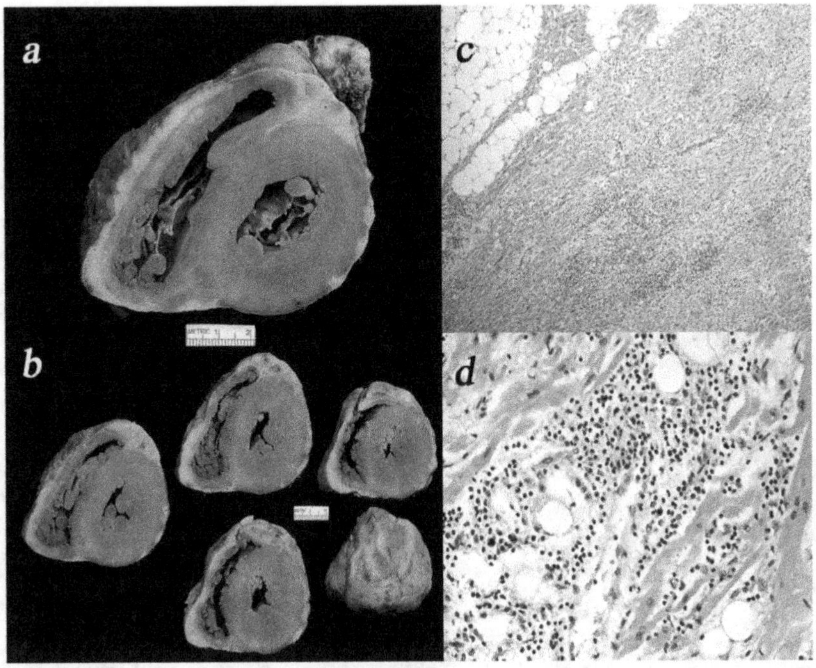


Figure 2. (Patient #9, Table 1). This 44-year-old woman survived 9 days after OHT and died from acute rejection. The native heart weighed 755 g and the donor heart weighed 370 g. Both hearts floated in a container of formaldehyde due to excessive adipose tissue. *(A)* The donor heart near the base exposing the tricuspid and mitral valves. No grossly visible myocardial lesions are seen. The right ventricular cavity is dilated. Brownish-colored deposits are present around the left anterior descending and first diagonal coronary arteries and they represent collections of lymphocytes. *(B)* Cuts of the ventricles more apical to the left upper view. *(C)* A photomicrograph of myocardium at its most subepicardial location. Numerous collections of lymphocytes are seen. *(D)* Close-up of some of the mononuclear cells within the myocardial wall. Hematoxylin/eosin stains ×40 *(C)* and ×100 *(D)*.

no report has described gross findings in the donor heart or provided illustrations of it.[9–15] Nakhleh and colleagues[9] reported findings in 22 donor hearts and focused on causes of death and ability to detect rejection by taking biopsies from 4 different sites. Rose and associates[10] studied 81 donor hearts focusing entirely on the causes of death. Graham[11] studied 44 donor hearts at autopsy, again focusing on the causes of death and frequency of rejection. Luthringer et al[12] studied 11 donor hearts at necropsy focusing on the causes of death, frequency of rejection, and significance of epicardial lymphoid infiltrates. Alexander and Steenbergen[13] studied 39 donor hearts at autopsy, again focusing on the causes of death, particularly that occurring suddenly. Birati and colleagues[14] analyzed causes of death after OHT in 40 patients who died >6 months after OHT. In none of these 5 cited studies were any grossly visible cardiac findings described, and none illustrated any gross features of donor hearts.

The present study describes gross and histologic features in 79 donor hearts collected over a nearly 3-decade period. The cases were divided into those surviving ≤60 days (n = 22), and those surviving >60 days (n = 57). The donor hearts tended to weigh less than the native hearts in those surviving the shorter period (14 of 20 [70%]), and to weigh more than the native hearts in those surviving the longer period (17 of 33 [52%]). In none of the 79 patients was the donor heart weighed before being placed in the recipient. Excessive adipose tissue (floated in formaldehyde) was present in 5 of 22 (23%) patients surviving ≤60 days and in 20 of 49 (41%) surviving >60 days, including 16 of 18 patients (89%) surviving ≥5 years after OHT. The long-term use of prednisone after the OHT probably was a major factor causing the excessive cardiac adiposity.[15]

Right-sided heart failure is a recognized complication of OHT.[16] In 73 (92%) of the 79 patients, the right ventricular cavity by gross inspection was dilated at necropsy and 40 of the 73 also had dilated left ventricular cavities. All 40 patients with dilated left ventricular cavities also had dilated right ventricular cavities.

Narrowing (>75% in cross-sectional area), nearly always by concentric noncalcified fibrous plaque, in 1 or more epicardial coronary arteries was present in 1 (5%) of the 22 patients dying early (≤60 days after OHT), and in 24 (42%) of those surviving >60 days. Grossly visible foci of necrosis or fibrosis or both were found in 5 (23%) of the 22 patients surviving ≤60 days and in 20 (35%) of the 57 patients surviving >60 days.

Most reported morphologic interpretations of cardiac rejection after OHT have been based on examination of biopsies obtained by a percutaneous catheter sampling from the right ventricular aspect of the ventricular septum (hopefully). These samples altogether during each biopsy procedure add up to no more than about 0.1 g and provide a look at endocardium and immediate subendocardial myocardium but not epicardium. Much debate has ensued regarding whether collections of lymphocytes in endocardium (Quilty lesions [5]) actually represent evidence of rejection.[2–7] Similarly, 1 report[12] argued that collections of lymphocytes (follicles) in the subepicardial adipose tissue do not represent evidence of rejection. The present study describes where in the ventricular wall (subepicardial adipose tissue, myocardium, and endocardium)

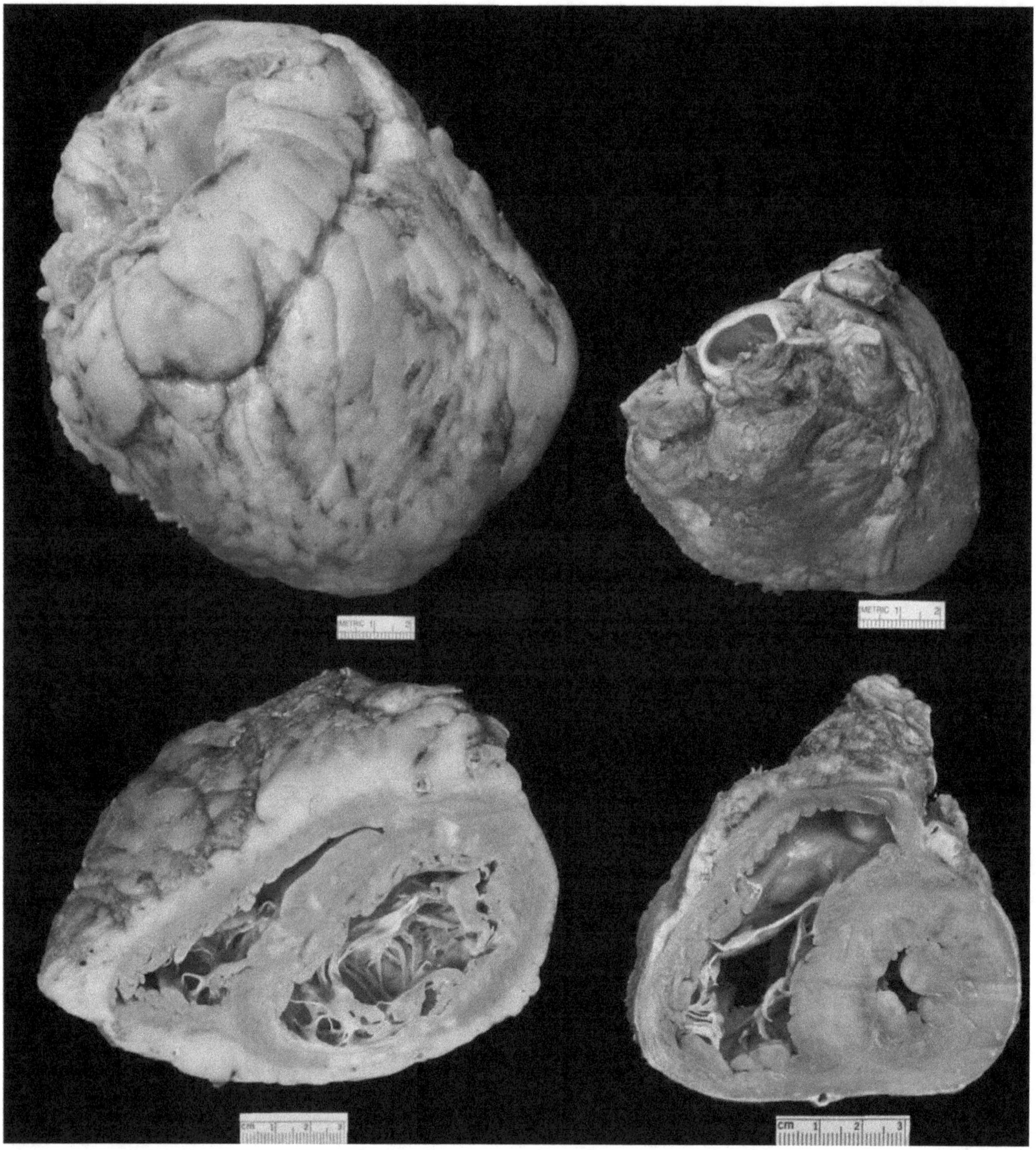

Figure 3. (Patient #13, Table 1). Shown here is the native heart *(left)* and donor heart *(right)* in a 65-year-old man who had an acute myocardial infarction at age 33, coronary bypass at age 49, and OHT at age 65. Considerable bleeding occurred at the OHT operation. The native heart weighed 780 g and contained a huge amount of subepicardial adipose tissue and floated in a container of formaldehyde. In contrast, the donor heart weighed 355 g (45% of what the native heart had weighed). The patient was very obese before the OHT. He died from "pump failure" without rejection 19 days after the OHT. Shown in the *upper* panel is the native heart on the *left* and the donor heart on the *right*. The *lower* panel shows the opened ventricles near their bases. Portions of the tricuspid and mitral valve leaflets and chords are visualized. The native heart has several scars. The large transmural scar is posterior and just beneath the posteromedial papillary muscle. Smaller scars are seen in the ventricular septum and anterior left ventricular free wall. The epicardial coronary arteries were severely narrowed in the native heart. Both ventricular cavities were dilated (ischemic cardiomyopathy). The donor heart *(bottom right)* shows the left ventricular cavity not to be dilated but the right ventricular cavity to be quite dilated. During the patient's 14-day post-OHT course, cardiac arrest occurred on the first postoperative day, and thereafter there was evidence of poor perfusion of all body organs, such that mental capacity was considerably decreased, total bilirubin levels were elevated, and urine output was quite diminished.

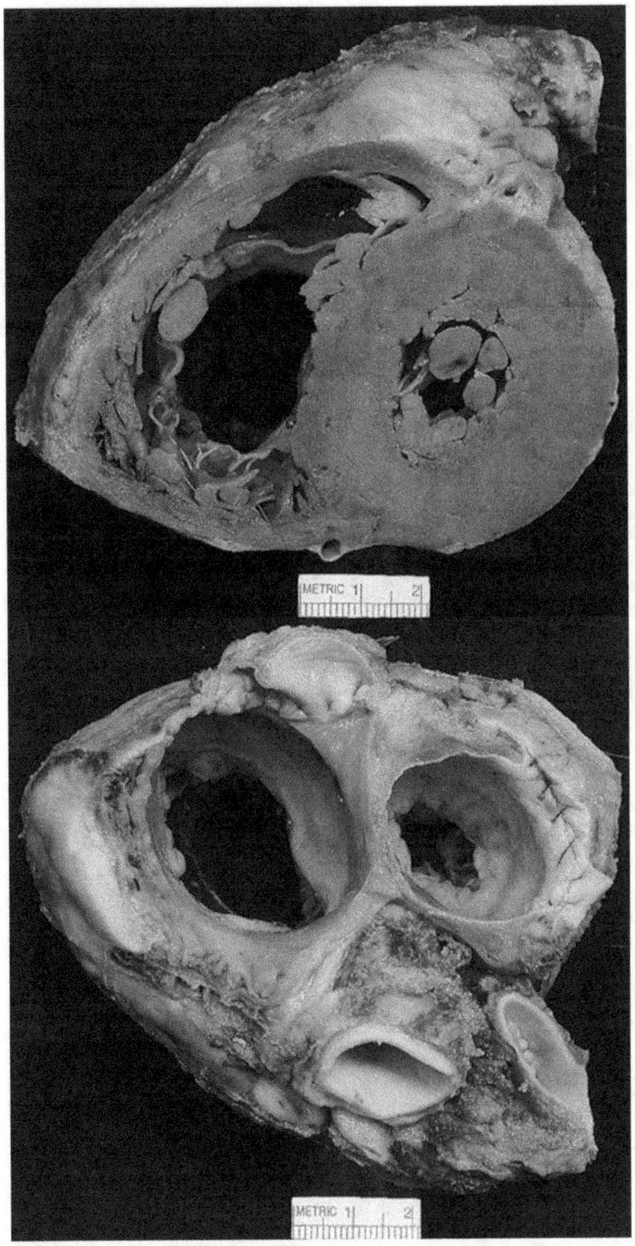


Figure 4. (Patient #15, Table 1). This 56-year-old woman underwent OHT 27 days earlier because of severe coronary artery disease causing ischemic cardiomyopathy. She had undergone coronary bypass grafting sometime before the OHT. She had had an acute myocardial infarction at age 43. She died from pump failure without evidence of rejection. *Upper view*: The basal portion of the donor heart. The right ventricular cavity is greatly dilated and the left ventricular cavity is not dilated at all. The coronary arteries are wide open and there was no histologic evidence of rejection. *Lower view*: Right atrium and left atrium after deroofing. The right atrium is probably twice as large as the left atrium.

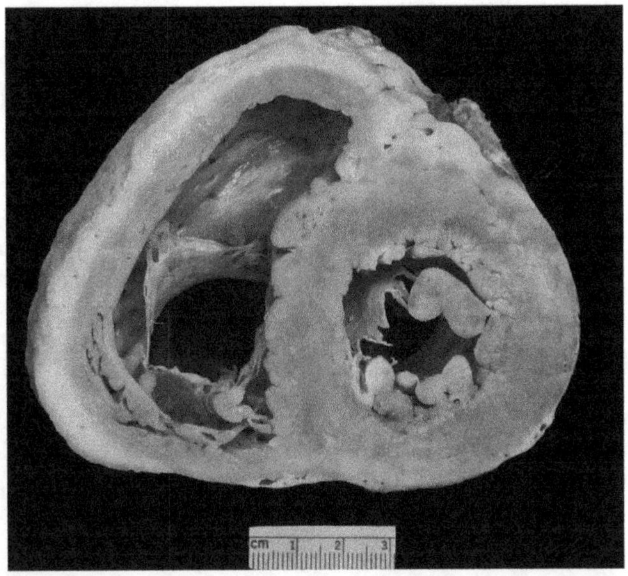


Figure 5. (Patient #19, Table 1). This 51-year-old man whose body mass index was 39 kg/m$^2$ underwent OHT for idiopathic dilated cardiomyopathy 45 days before death. He developed a fatal infection postoperatively associated with evidence of rejection (see Figure 6). View of the most basal portion of his heart showing that the right ventricular cavity is considerably dilated and the left ventricular cavity is only minimally dilated. An abscess is present in the posteromedial papillary muscle *(arrow)*.

collections of lymphocytes (sometimes with other cells) were found. No attempt was made to determine whether these collections of cells accumulated acutely or hyperacutely or chronically, or whether the cells histologically appeared "aggressive" or nonaggressive. Many sections of the entire left and right ventricular walls were examined. These foci of mainly lymphocytes were found in the left ventricular wall in 8 (36%) of the 22 patients surviving ≤60 days, and in 42 (74%) of the 57 patients surviving >60 days after OHT. Thus, 50 (63%) of the 79 patients had foci of lymphocytes in the donor heart: in 32 of the 50 patients (64%) in epicardium, myocardium, and endocardium; in 13 patients (26%) in 2 of these 3 compartments, and in 4 patients (13%) in only 1 of these 3 compartments. The largest collections of these lymphocytes were located in the subepicardial adipose tissue, the site of the largest collections of vascular channels and a site that percutaneous transvenous biopsy does not sample. We believe that these collections of mainly lymphocytes at all 3 locations represent evidence of rejection. The sizes of the foci of lymphocytes in the donor hearts, however, vary considerably from case to case. In our experience, these multilocations of collections of lymphocytes are found only in donor hearts after OHT, and not in any other condition except possibly acute lymphocytic leukemia.[17]

In conclusion, with time, the donor hearts tended to increase in weight, in the quantity of adipose tissue, in the amounts of coronary narrowing, in the frequency of ventricular cavity dilation (particularly the right ventricle), and in the frequency of lymphocytic infiltrates (evidence of rejection). A positive feature of the present study is the fact that all hearts were studied by the same individual. A deficiency is the lack of morphologic information in some of the native hearts. It also would have been helpful if the donor hearts had been weighed before being inserted into the recipient.

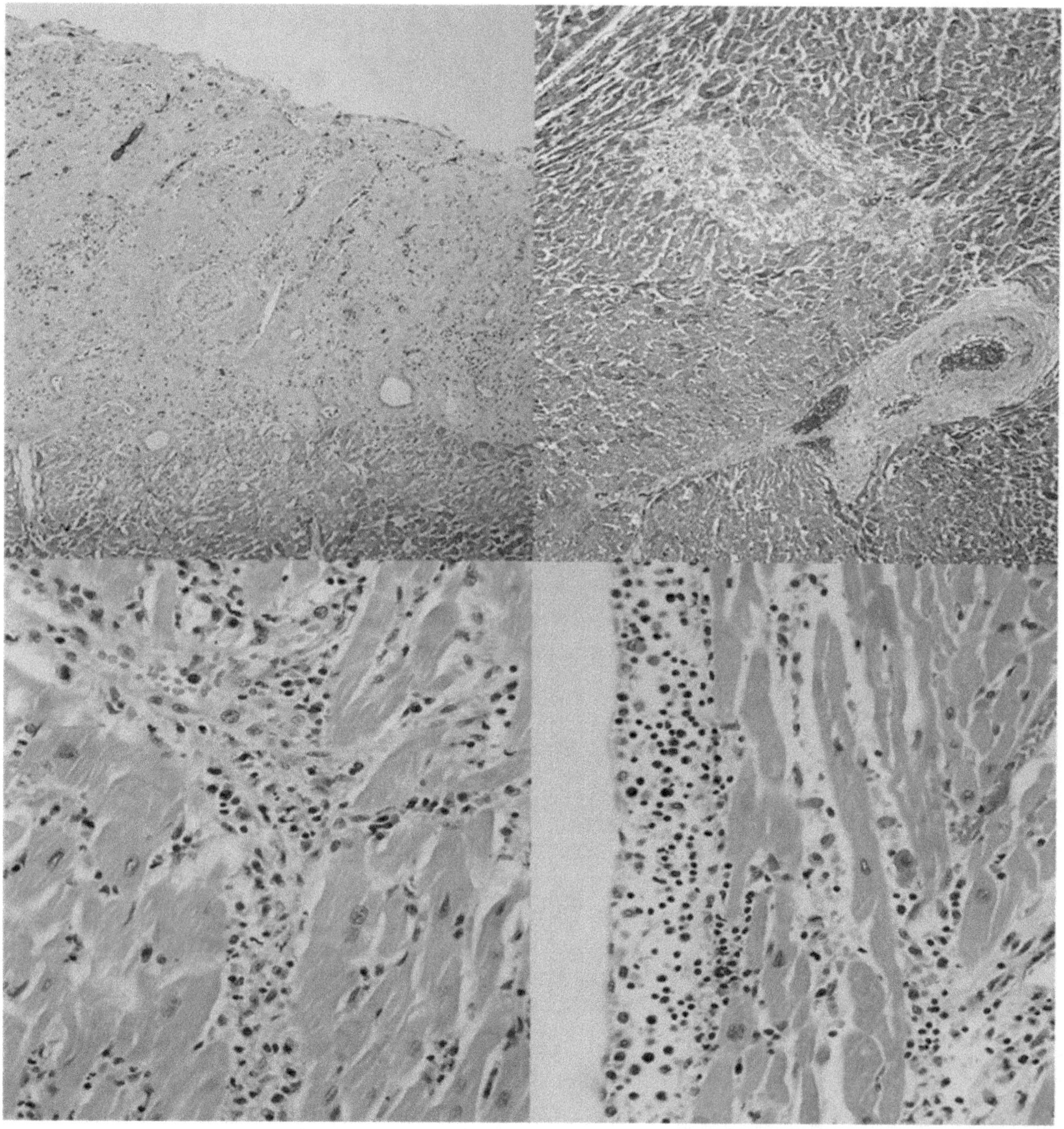

Figure 6. (Patient #19, Table 1). Shown here are 4 photomicrographs of the heart in the patient described in Figure 5. *Upper left*: View mainly of the subepicardial area showing dense fibrous tissue. *Upper right*: An intramural coronary artery is shown and a small focus of myocytolysis. *Lower left*: Some cellular infiltrates in the myocardium. *Lower right*: Endocardium and a portion of subendocardial myocardium both containing a number of monocytes, mainly lymphocytes. Movat stain, *upper left* and *upper right*; hematoxylin/eosin stains, *lower left* and *lower right*. Magnification, ×100, *upper left* and *upper right*; ×400, *lower left* and *lower right*.

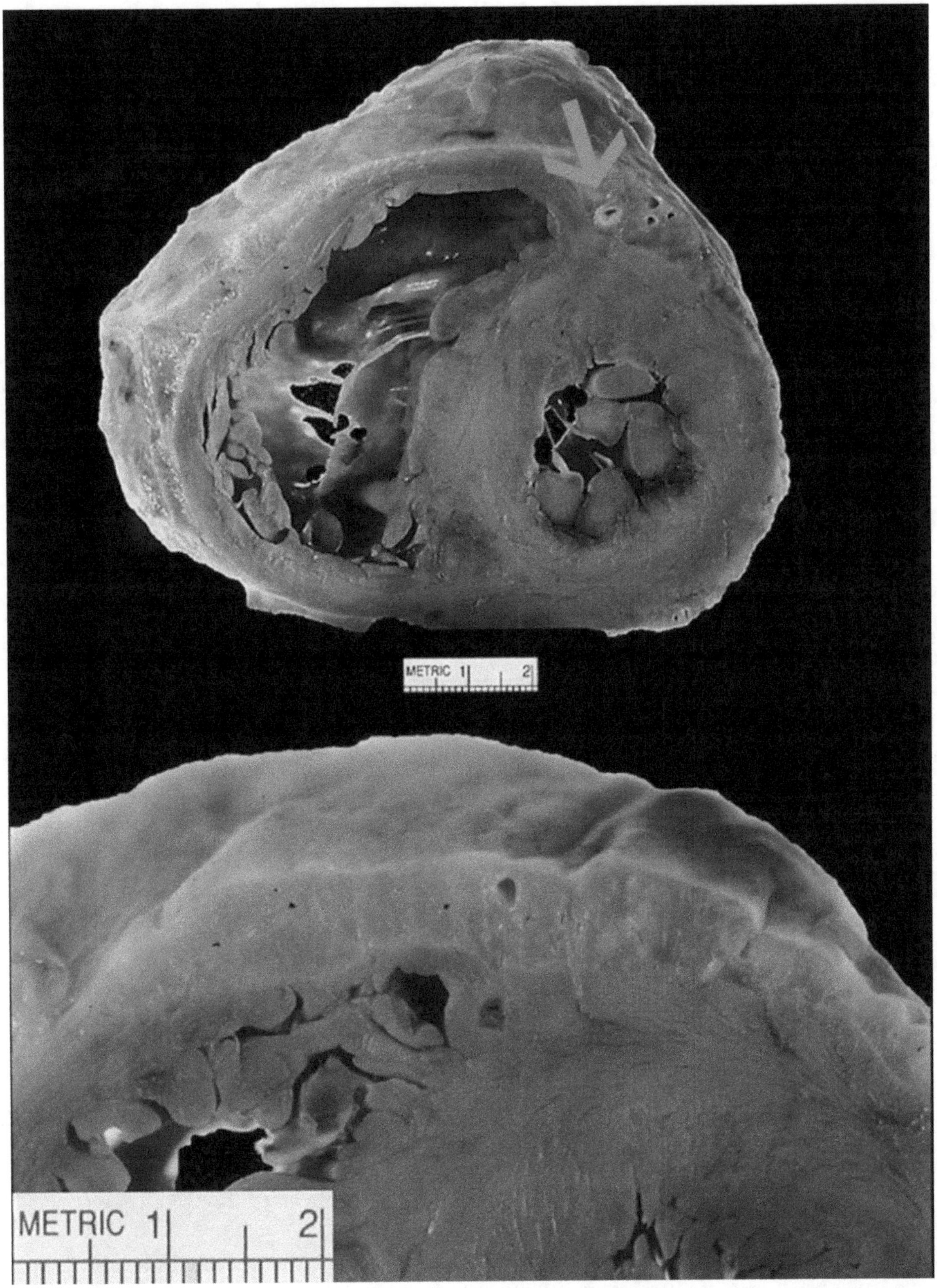


Figure 7. (Patient #25, Table 2). This 61-year-old man died of a stroke 3 months after OHT. Histologic sections showed a large number of lymphocytes in the epicardium, fewer numbers in the myocardium, and quite a few in the endocardium. Monocytes also were seen in the walls of the coronary arteries. *Upper view*: A photograph of the heart exposing the tricuspid and mitral valves. The right ventricle is quite dilated and the left ventricle is not. No grossly visible lesions are noted in the myocardial walls. The left anterior descending coronary artery *(arrow)* is quite narrowed and clumps of lymphocytes are present in the subepicardial adipose tissue surrounding that artery and also the first diagonal coronary artery. *Lower view*: A close-up of the left anterior descending artery and its surroundings showing the adipose tissue to be discolored because of large collections of lymphocytes.

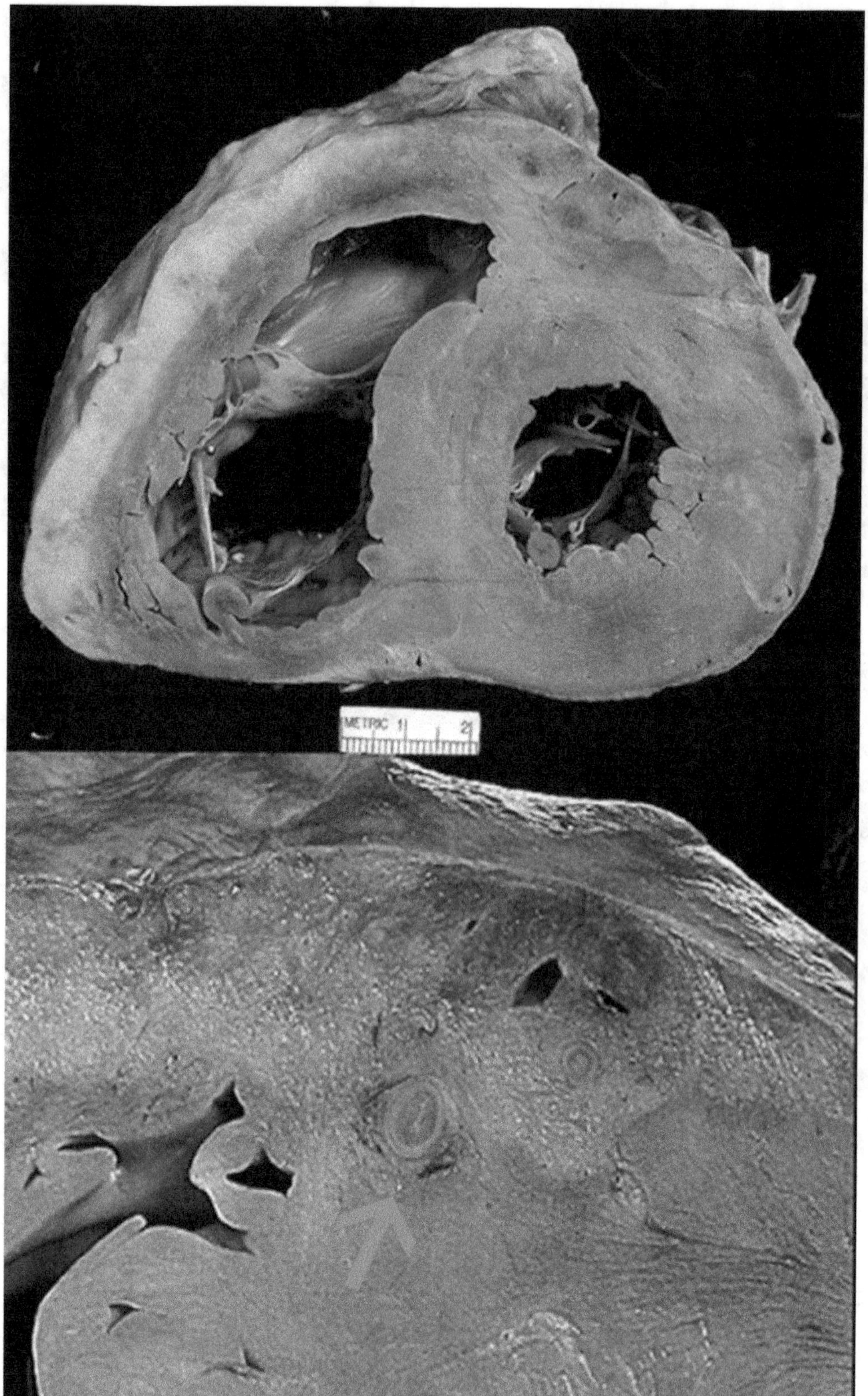


Figure 8. (Patient #30, Table 2). This 42-year-old man underwent OHT for idiopathic dilated cardiomyopathy 8 months before death. His postoperative course was apparently smooth until a blackout spell occurred while at home. He was hospitalized and the next day in the hospital had sudden cardiac arrest. The patient was obese. (At one time his body mass index was 40 kg/m$^2$). Shown here are sections of the heart. *Top*: At the base exposing the tricuspid and mitral valves. The left ventricular cavity is not dilated, but the right ventricular cavity is considerably dilated. In the atrioventricular sulcus the coronary arteries are narrowed and surrounded by dark tissue which represents collections of lymphocytes (rejection cells). The *bottom view* shows large collections of lymphocytes around both coronary arteries and coronary veins. The left anterior descending *(arrow)* is severely narrowed.

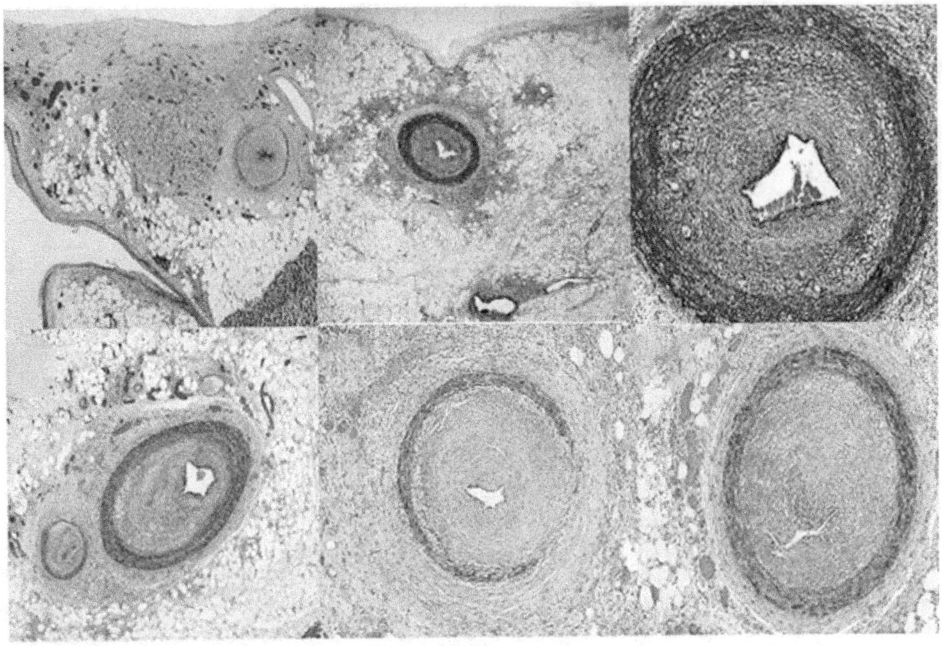

Figure 9. (Patient #30, Table 2). Shown here are photomicrographs of various areas of epicardium showing the coronary arteries to be severely narrowed by fibromuscular tissue typical of rejection. The patient is the same one whose heart is shown in Figure 8. All of the 6 photomicrographs are stained by the Movat method. *Upper left*: Shown is a severely narrowed epicardial coronary artery adjacent to a large follicle of lymphocytes. Focally the medial is destroyed. *Upper middle*: Another epicardial coronary artery surrounded by lymphocytes and within the lumen is a great deal of fibromuscular tissue. A close-up of this artery is shown in the *top right* view. The *bottom left* view shows another epicardial coronary artery and one of its branches which is nearly occluded by fibromuscular tissue. The media of the little artery is partially destroyed. *Middle bottom*: Another epicardial coronary artery severely narrowed and a portion of its medial is entirely destroyed. Lymphocytes are present between the internal elastic membrane and the fibromuscular intimal tissue. The adventitia is severely thickened by dense fibrous tissue. *Bottom right*: Another epicardial coronary artery with some inflammatory cells within the intimal fibrous tissue. The media in this artery is not affected, but the adventitia is thickened by fibrous tissue. Original magnification ×20 *upper left*; ×20 *upper middle*; ×100 *upper right*; ×40 *lower left*; ×100 *lower middle*, and ×100 *lower right*.

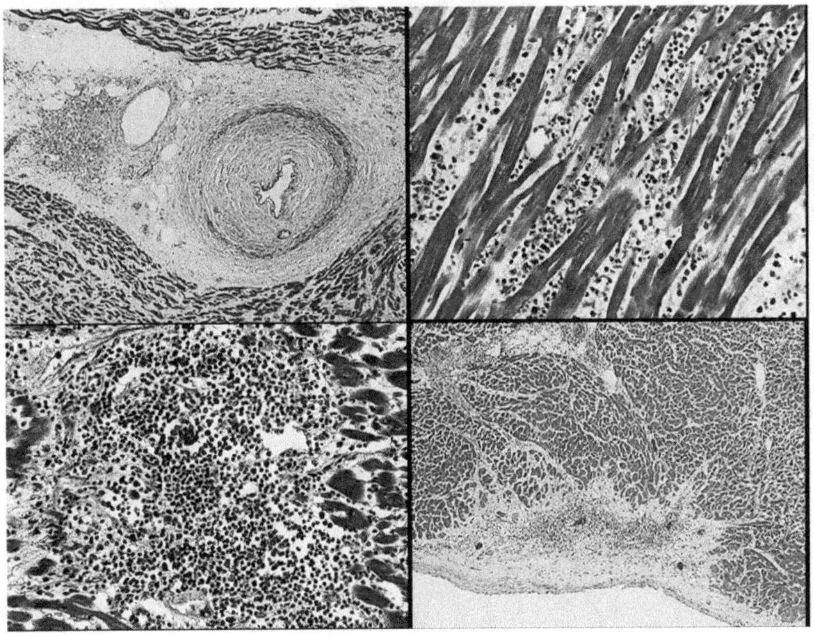

Figure 10. (Patient #30, Table 2). Shown here are photomicrographs in the myocardial wall. The patient is described in the legends of Figures 8 and 9. *Upper left*: An intramural coronary artery containing fibromuscular tissue in the intima with considerably narrowed lumen. A portion of the media is wiped out. A small follicle of lymphocytes is shown toward the left adjacent to a coronary vein, the wall of which is partially infiltrated by lymphocytes. *Top right*: An area of myocardium containing large numbers of lymphocytes between myocardial fibers. *Lower left*: A large follicle of lymphocytes within the myocardial wall. *Lower right*: A portion of endocardium showing lymphocytes within the endocardial tissue. All four of these sections were stained by the Movat method: ×100 *upper left*, *upper right*, and *lower left*; ×40, *lower right*.

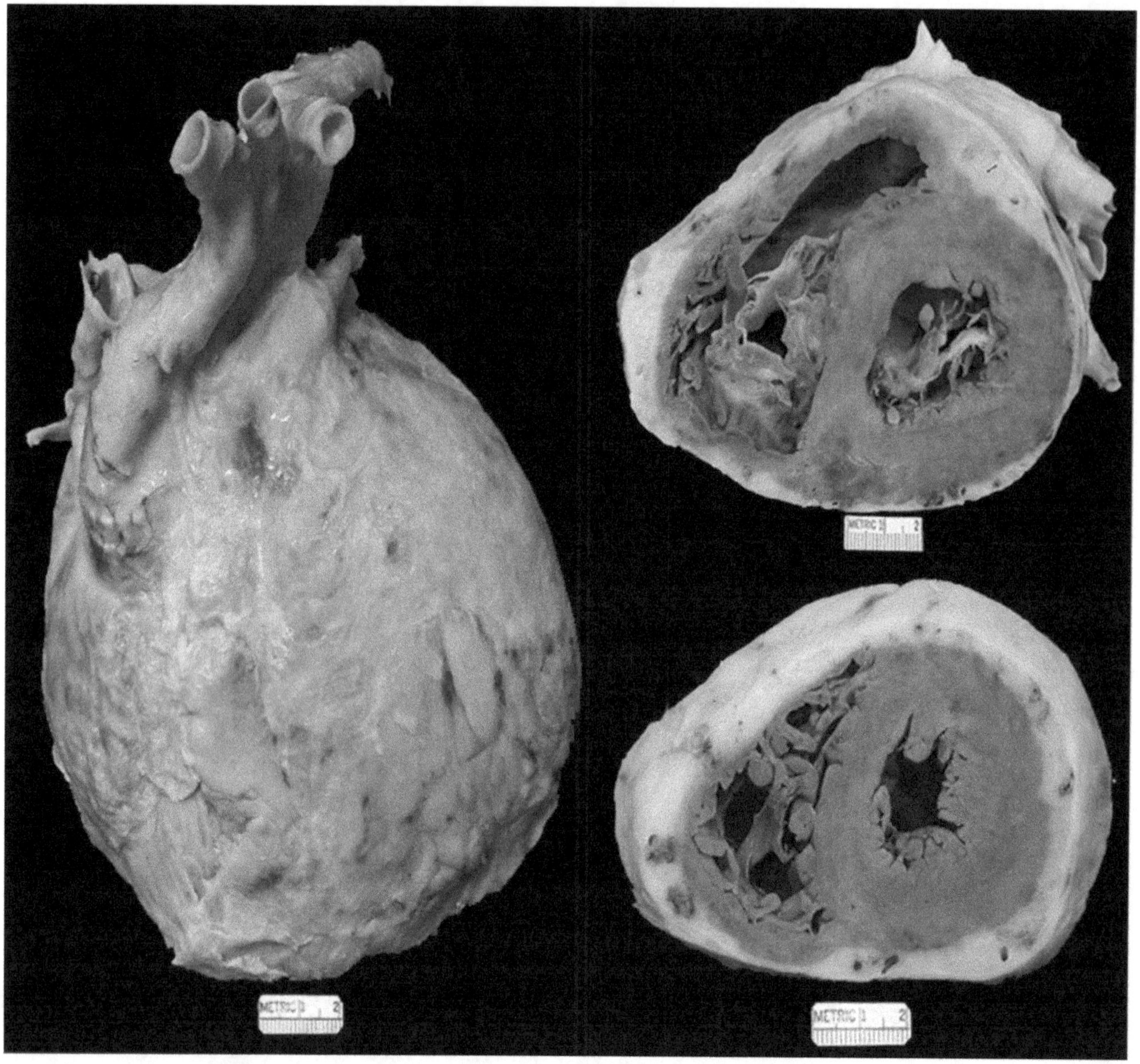

Figure 11. (Patient #34, Table 2). This 62-year-old man died 9 months after OHT of cardiac amyloidosis. No amyloid was seen in the donor heart but foci of lymphocytes and a few plasma cells were present in the subepicardial adipose tissue and the interstitium of the myocardium that contained increased quantities of fibrous tissue focally. Small coronary arteries in the subepicardial adipose tissue had a few lymphocytes in the intima. He probably died from pulmonary embolism and a pulmonary infarct was present. A thrombus was present in the body of the left atrium. Shown on the *left* is the exterior view of the heart, with discoloration of the epicardium and a few deposits of adipose tissue. The *upper right* shows the base of the heart with the tricuspid and mitral valves. The quantity of subepicardial adipose tissue is considerable and the *lower right* shows that the myocardium is totally covered by adipose tissue. The right ventricular cavity is clearly dilated.

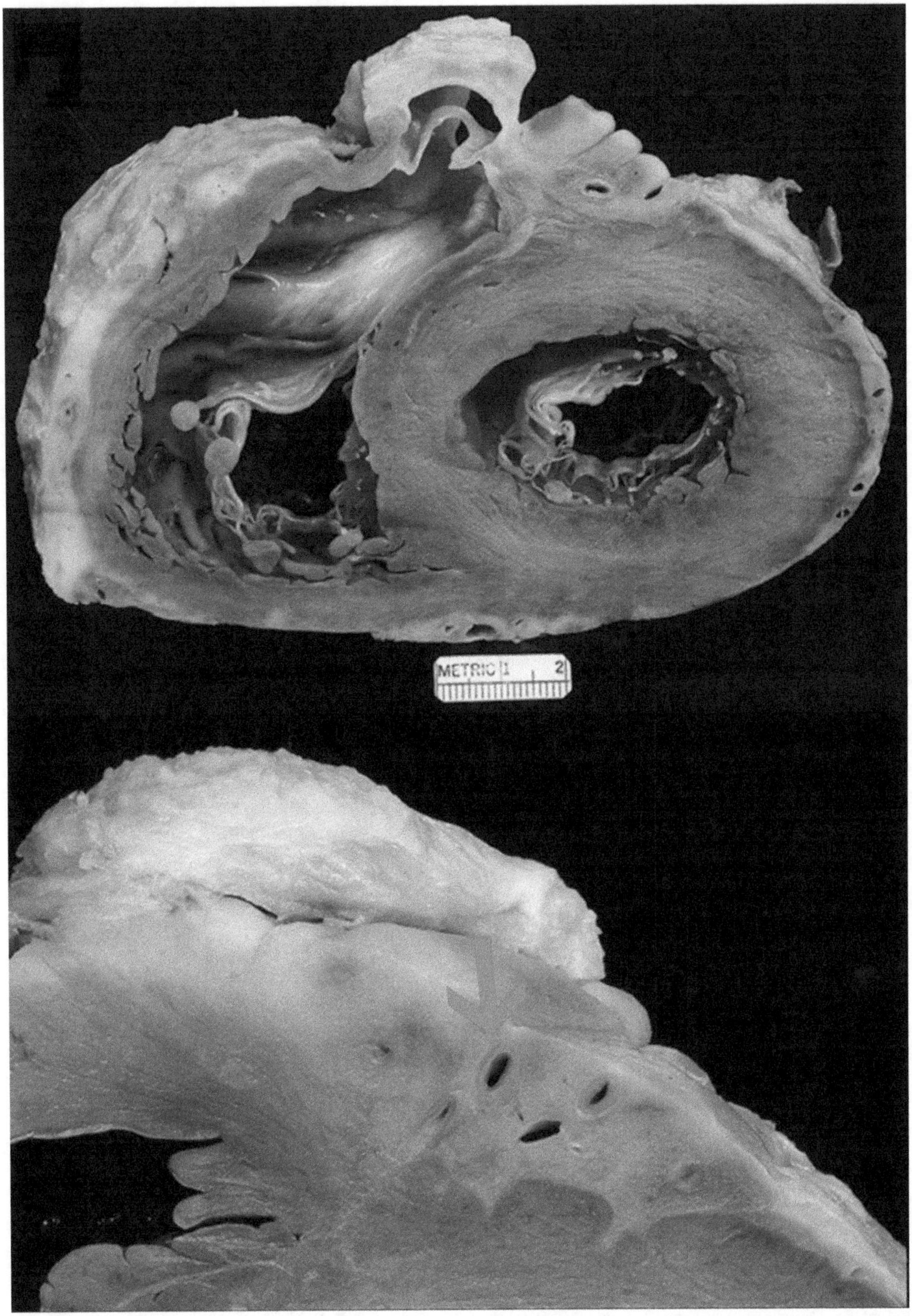


Figure 12. (Patient #41, Table 2). This 57-year-old man underwent OHT for ischemic cardiomyopathy 14 months before his death from pump failure with evidence of rejection. A coronary bypass had been performed on the native heart. *Top*: The donor heart at the base. Both ventricular cavities are dilated, the right considerably more than the left. The left anterior descending artery is surrounded by collections of lymphocytes. There are no grossly visible myocardial lesions. *Bottom*: Close-up of the coronary arteries anteriorly including the left anterior descending *(arrow)*, left diagonal, and first obtuse marginal. The latter artery is severely narrowed by fibrous plaque.

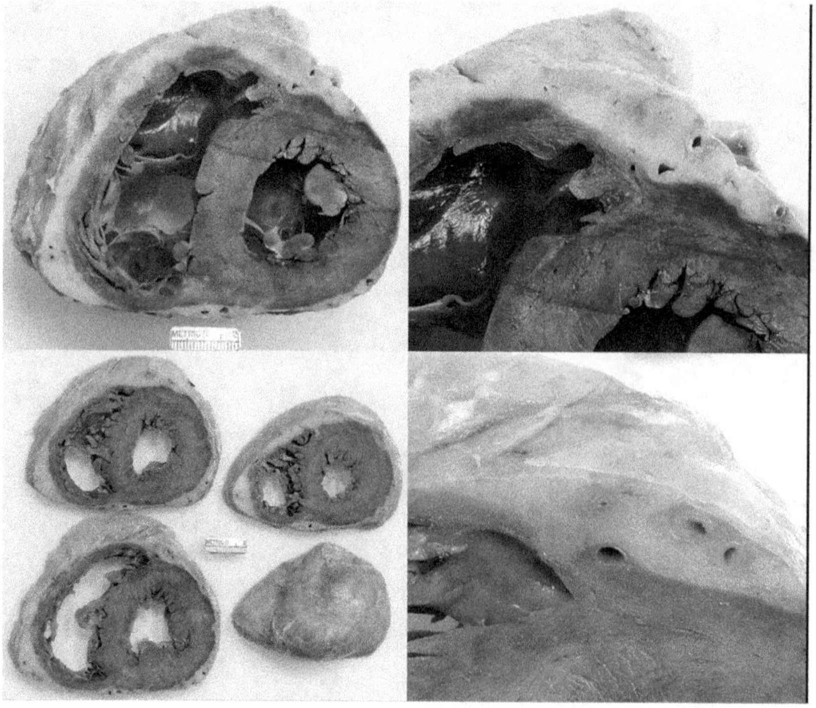

Figure 13. (Patient #42, Table 2). This 53-year-old woman had a heart transplantation 15 months earlier because of cardiac sarcoidosis. During the few months before death heart failure returned. *Top left*: View of the heart exposing both tricuspid and mitral valves. Both ventricular cavities are dilated, the right more than the left. The quantity of subepicardial adipose tissue is considerable. Some brownish discoloration is present around the epicardial coronary arteries, and it represents foci of lymphocytes, a clear evidence of rejection. *Bottom left*: Additional slices of the ventricles toward the apex. *Top right*: Close-up view of the anterior descending and first diagonal coronary arteries surrounded by brownish discoloration representing collections of lymphocytes. *Bottom right*: Another view of epicardial coronary arteries surrounded by brownish discoloration of the adipose tissue representing collections of lymphocytes.

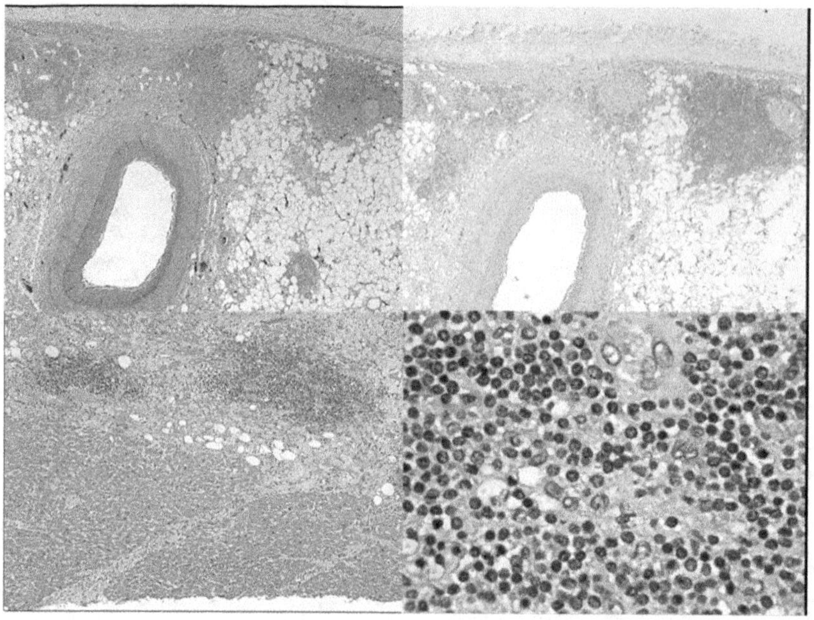

Figure 14. (Patient #42, Table 2). Photomicrographs of subepicardial adipose tissue areas and myocardium in the patient whose gross pictures of the heart are shown in Figure 13. *Top left*: View of an epicardial coronary artery with large collections of lymphocytes in the subepicardial adipose tissue. The adventitia is considerably thickened by fibrous tissue. *Top right*: A similar view but stained with hematoxylin/eosin showing the same coronary artery and large collections of lymphocytes in the subepicardial adipose tissue. *Bottom left*: A view within the myocardial wall showing large collections of lymphocytes. *Bottom right*: Close-up view of mainly lymphocytes within the myocardium. Movat stain, *top left*; hematoxylin/eosin stains, *top right*, *bottom left*, and *bottom right*. Original magnification, ×20, *top left* and *top right*; ×100, *bottom left*, and ×400, *bottom right*.

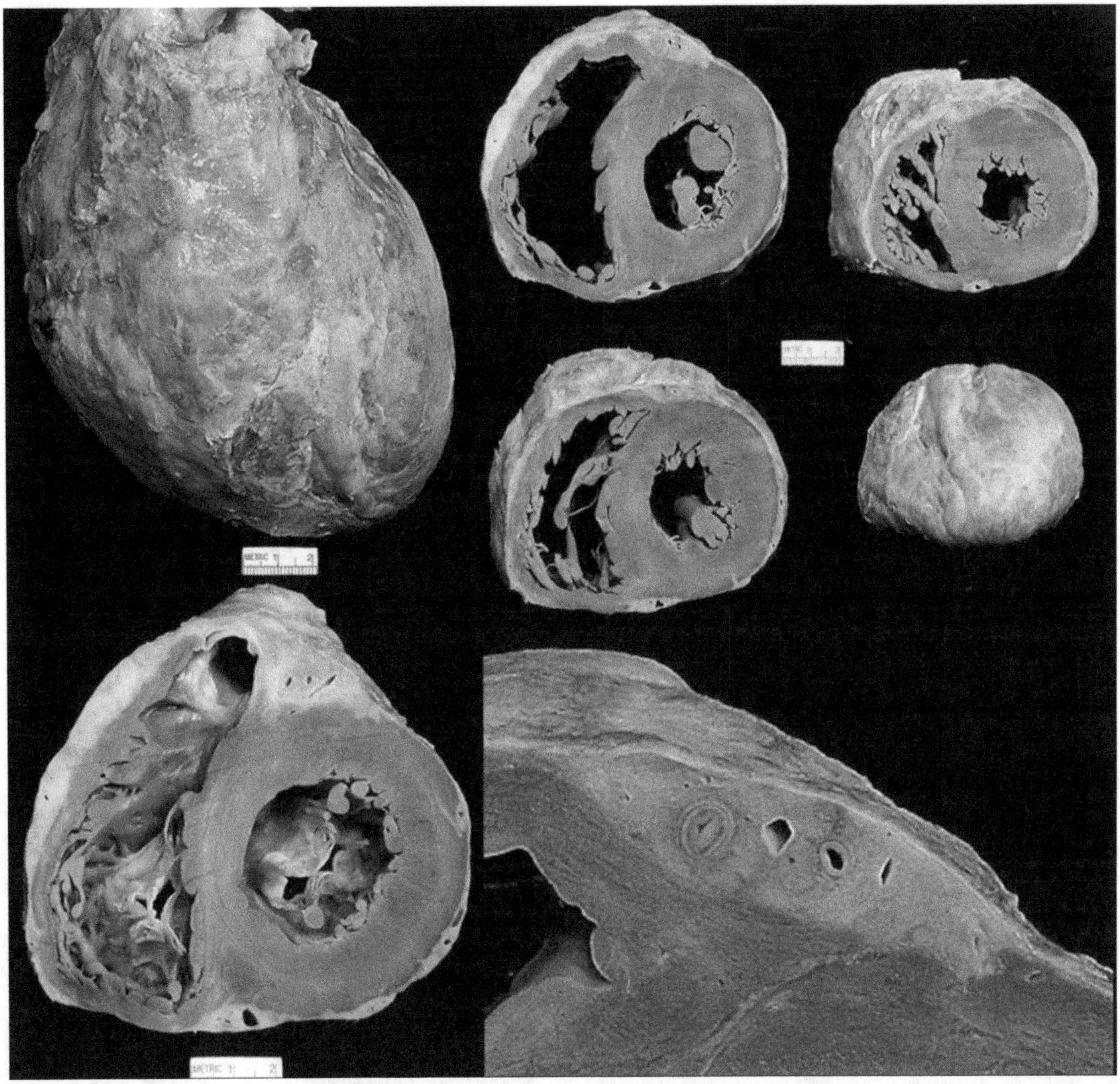

Figure 15. (Patient #43, Table 2). Shown here are various views of the heart in a 30-year-old man who died suddenly at home 15 months after OHT for idiopathic dilated cardiomyopathy. *Top left*: View of the heart from the front showing the scarred epicardium. There were dense fibrous adhesions between the visceral and parietal pericardia. *Bottom left:* View of both right and left ventricles exposing the tricuspid, pulmonic, and mitral valves. Both ventricular cavities are dilated. No myocardial lesions are present. The left anterior descending and first diagonal coronary arteries are shown, and there is a brownish appearance around each, and this brownish appearance represents collections of lymphocytes. *Top right*: Views of the various slices of the ventricles caudal to the view shown in *bottom left*. Again, no myocardial lesions are seen. *Bottom right*: Close-up of the heart slice shown in the *top right* figure. The left anterior descending coronary artery is severely narrowed and in this view the diagonal is not. A coronary vein is between these 2 arteries. Surrounding each artery are collections of lymphocytes.

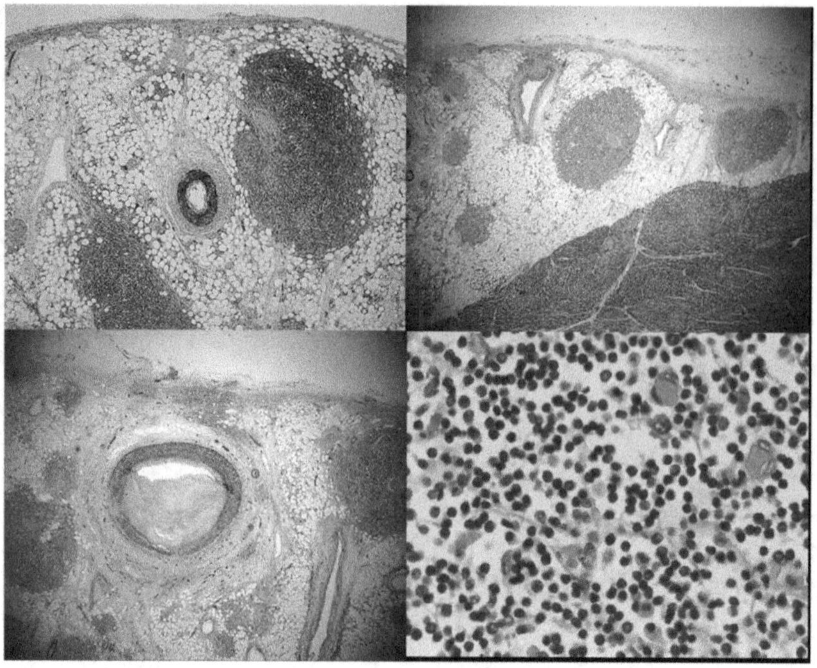

Figure 16. (Patient #43, Table 2). Photomicrographs of various portions of the subepicardial regions in a 30-year-old man whose heart is shown in Figure 15. *Top left*: Shown are 2 huge collections of lymphocytes (follicles) and one small coronary artery surrounded by dense fibrous tissue. Other smaller collections of lymphocytes are seen in other areas of this region. *Top right*: A portion of subepicardial adipose tissue containing 5 large collections of lymphocytes and 2 smaller vessels. The myocardium is located in the bottom portion. *Bottom left:* A coronary artery quite narrowed by fibrocellular fibrous tissue. The adventitia is thickened by fibrous tissue. Other collections of lymphocytes are seen in the epicardial adipose tissue. *Bottom right*: A close-up view of lymphocytes and plasmacytes in the subepicardial adipose tissue. Movat stains (*top left, top right*, and *bottom left*); hematoxylin/eosin stain, *bottom right*; original magnification ×40, *top left,* ×20, *top right*, ×20, *bottom left*, and ×1000, *bottom right*.

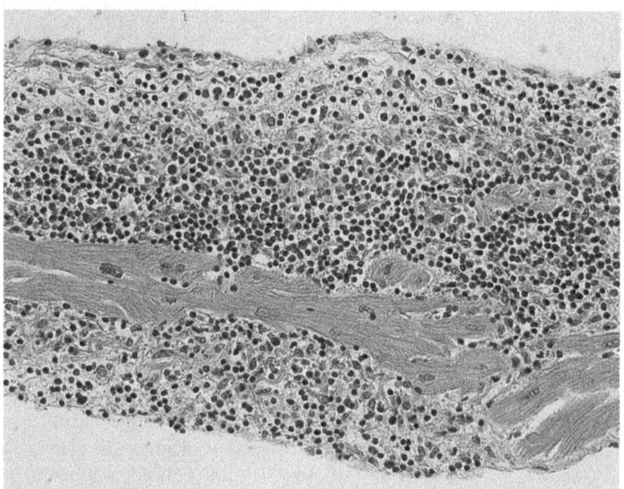

Figure 17. (Patient #43, Table 2). Shown here is a portion of mural endocardium in a small pectinate muscle in the left ventricle in the patient's heart illustrated in Figures 15 and 16. In the central portion are myocardial fibers that are totally surrounded by mainly lymphocytes and some plasma cells. Hematoxylin/eosin stain, ×400.

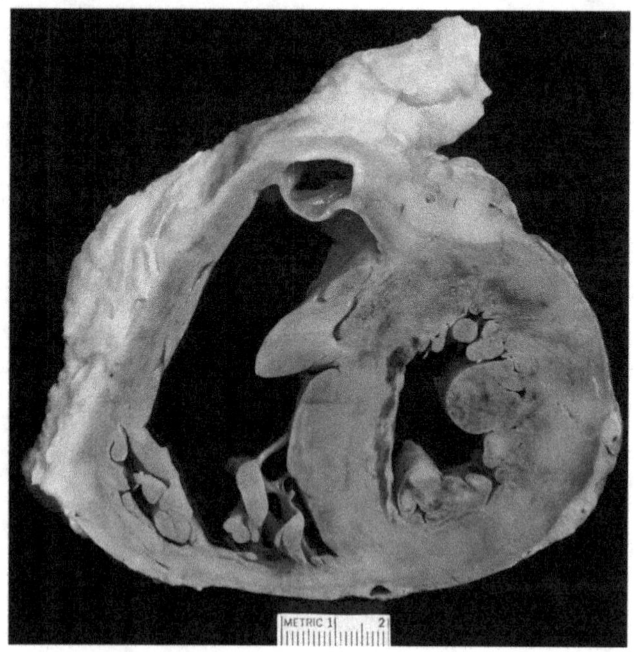

Figure 18. (Patient #48, Table 2). Shown here is the basal portion of heart in a 57-year-old man who had OHT 25 months before death because of idiopathic dilated cardiomyopathy. Thirteen days before death he had cardiac arrest during a hernia repair operation. After his cardiac arrest he developed multiorgan perfusion problems during the subsequent 13 days. The heart shows acute infarcts, mainly subendocardial in the left ventricular free wall and ventricular septum. The right ventricular cavity is much dilated. The left anterior descending coronary artery *(arrow*) is severely narrowed.

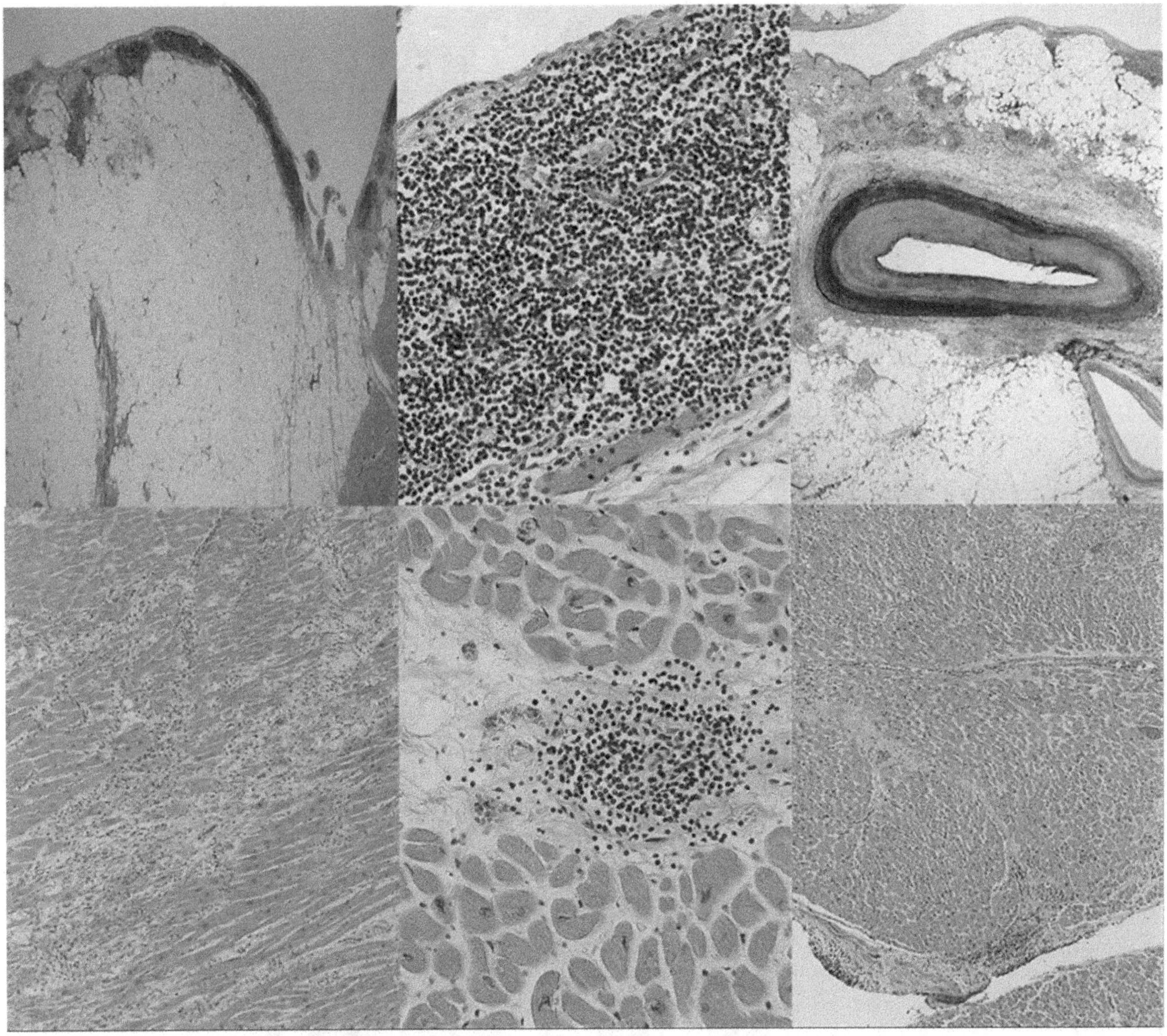

Figure 19. (Patient #48, Table 2). Photomicrographs of sections of the heart in the patient whose heart is shown in Figure 18. *Upper left*: A view of the epicardial fat and the most outer portion of visceral pericardium contains huge collections of mononuclear cells, mainly lymphocytes. *Upper middle:* Close-up view of lymphocytes in the most outer portion of visceral pericardium. *Upper right:* Another view of the subepicardial adipose tissue area showing multifocal collections of lymphocytes and an epicardial artery containing a great deal of intimal fibrous tissue. *Lower left*: Portion of left ventricular myocardium showing large collections of rejection cells and necrosis of adjacent myofibers. *Lower middle*: Another collection of lymphocytes in left ventricular myocardium. *Lower right*: A portion of mural endocardium showing huge collections of lymphocytes in the endocardial region. Hematoxylin/eosin stains: ×20 *upper left, upper middle, lower left, lower middle,* and *lower right*; Movat stain, *upper right.* Original magnification ×20, *upper left, lower left, lower right,* and *upper right*; ×100, *upper middle* and *lower middle*.

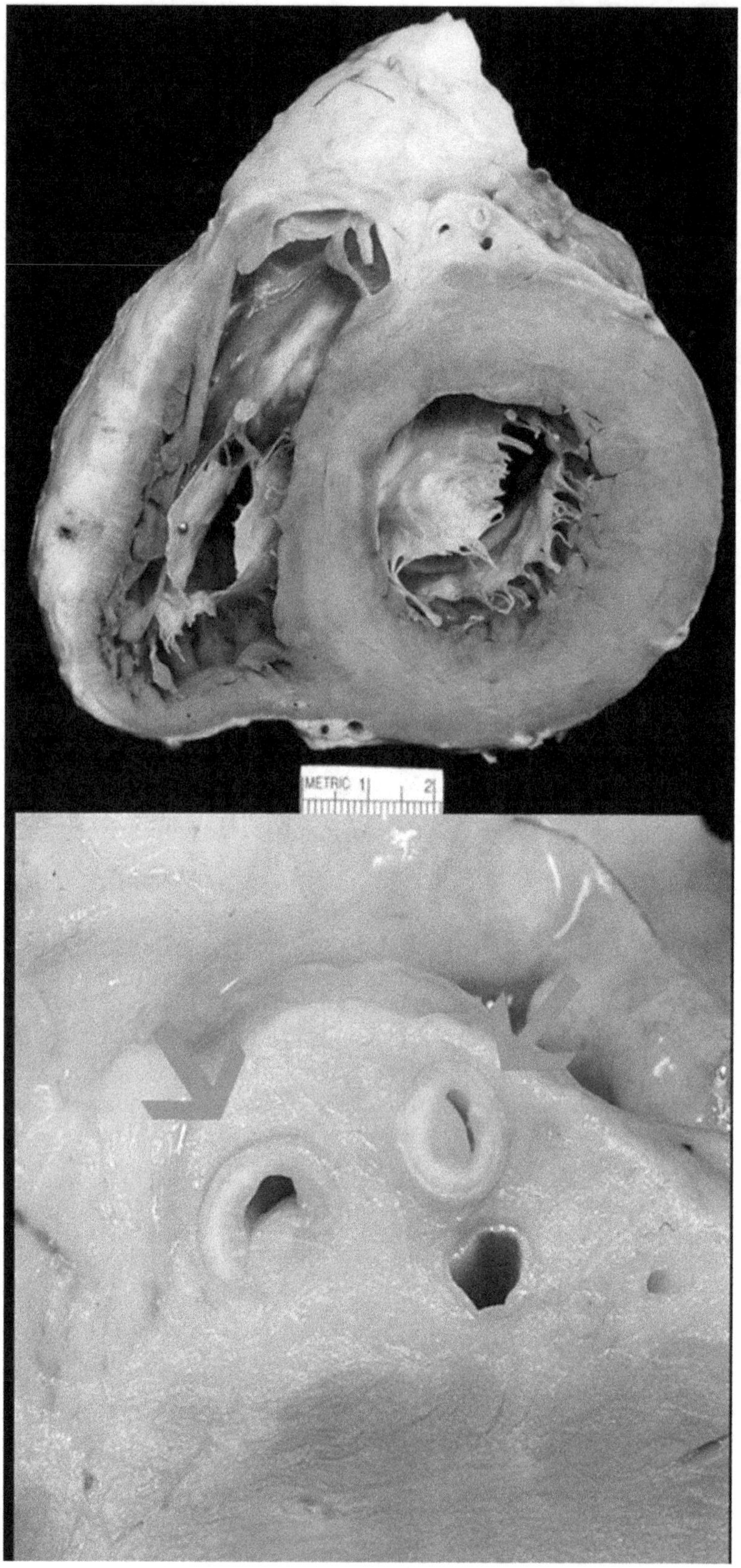


Figure 20. (Patient #51, Table 2). The heart shown here belonged to a 42-year-old man who had an OHT for idiopathic dilated cardiomyopathy when he was 39 years of age. During the 33-month interval between the OHT and death he developed severe kidney disease and was on hemodialysis during his last year of life. *Top*: View of the ventricles showing both tricuspid valve and mitral valve. The ventricles are devoid of grossly visible lesions, the first diagonal coronary artery is severely narrowed and plaque is also present in the left anterior descending artery. Both ventricular cavities are dilated. *Bottom*: Close-up views of the left anterior descending and first diagonal coronary arteries showing uniform plaque in both (arrows). No evidence of rejection was present clinically.

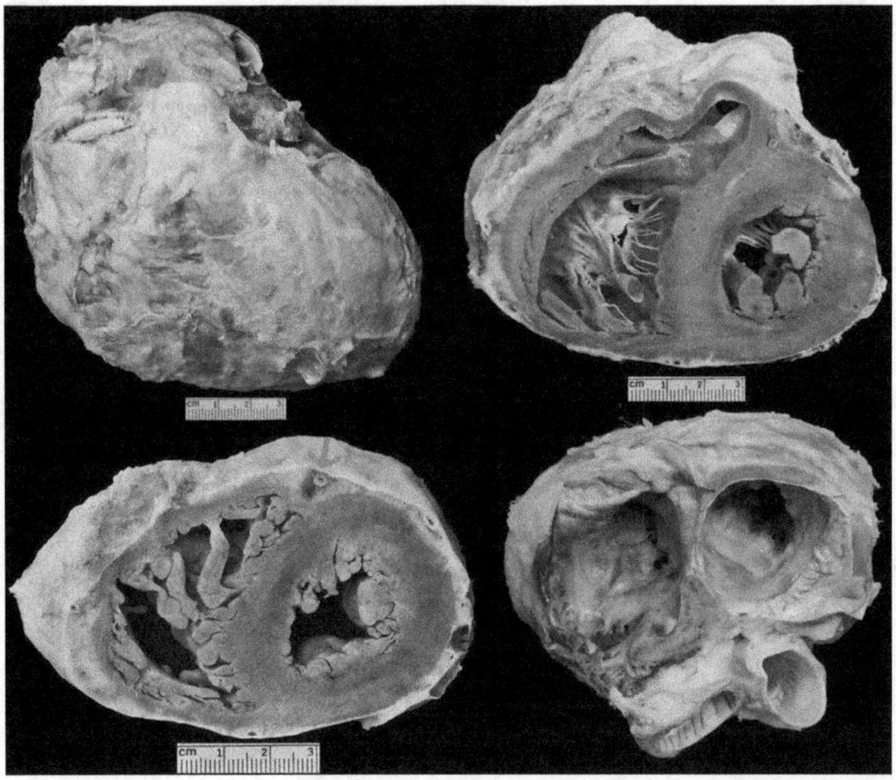

Figure 21. (Patient #56, Table 2). This 53-year-old man underwent OHT because of ischemic cardiomyopathy and died 45 months later because of acute development of heart failure associated with rejection. *Top left*: The anterior surface of the heart showing dense fibrous thickening of the epicardium. *Top right*: The basal portion of the heart showing a much dilated right ventricle. Collections of rejection cells (lymphocytes) surround the coronary arteries. *Bottom left*: Another view more apical of the ventricles showing the left anterior descending coronary artery surrounded by lymphocytes and the artery severely narrowed by plaque (arrow). Other portions of the subendocardial adipose tissue contain large collections of lymphocytes. *Bottom right*: View of the right and left atria after their "deroofing." The right atrium is larger than the left atrium. The wall of the right atrium contains numerous extravasated erythrocytes.

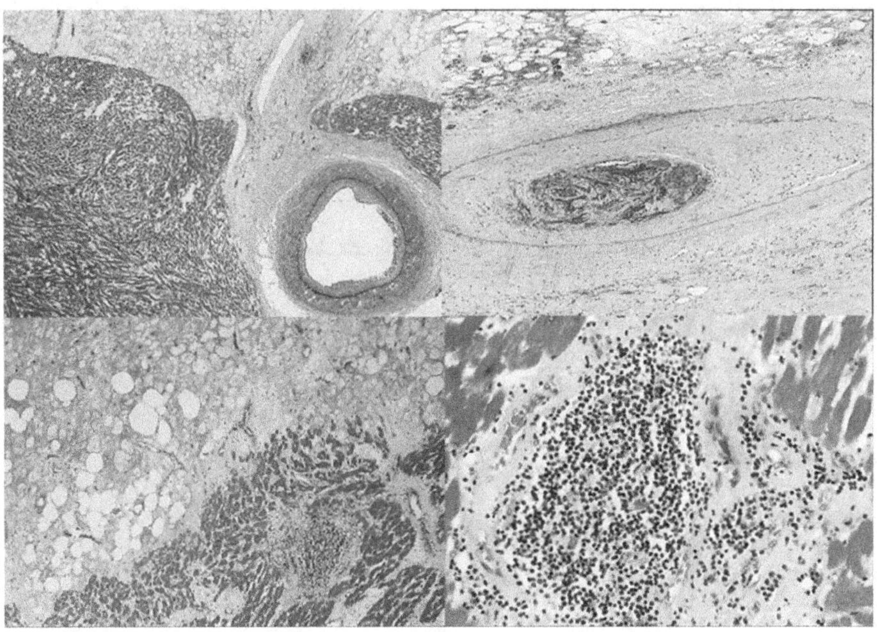

Figure 22. (Patient #56, Table 2). Photomicrographs of various portions of the heart in the patient described in Figure 21. *Upper left*: View of a portion of subepicardial adipose tissue and the subepicardial myocardium. A "tunneled" coronary artery is seen and its intima is mildly thickened by fibrous tissue. A small collection of lymphocytes is present in the subepicardial tissue and also in the myocardium. *Upper right*: A large coronary artery in the epicardium is occluded by a combination thrombus overlying fibromuscular tissue. The thrombus suggests that the underlying fibrous tissue was also the result of thrombosis. The adventitia is densely fibrotic. *Lower left*: A collection of lymphocytes in the subepicardial myocardium. *Lower right*: Close-up of those cells shown in the *lower left* view. All are Movat stains. Original magnification: *upper left*, ×40; *upper right*, ×100; *lower left*, ×40; and *lower right*, ×400.

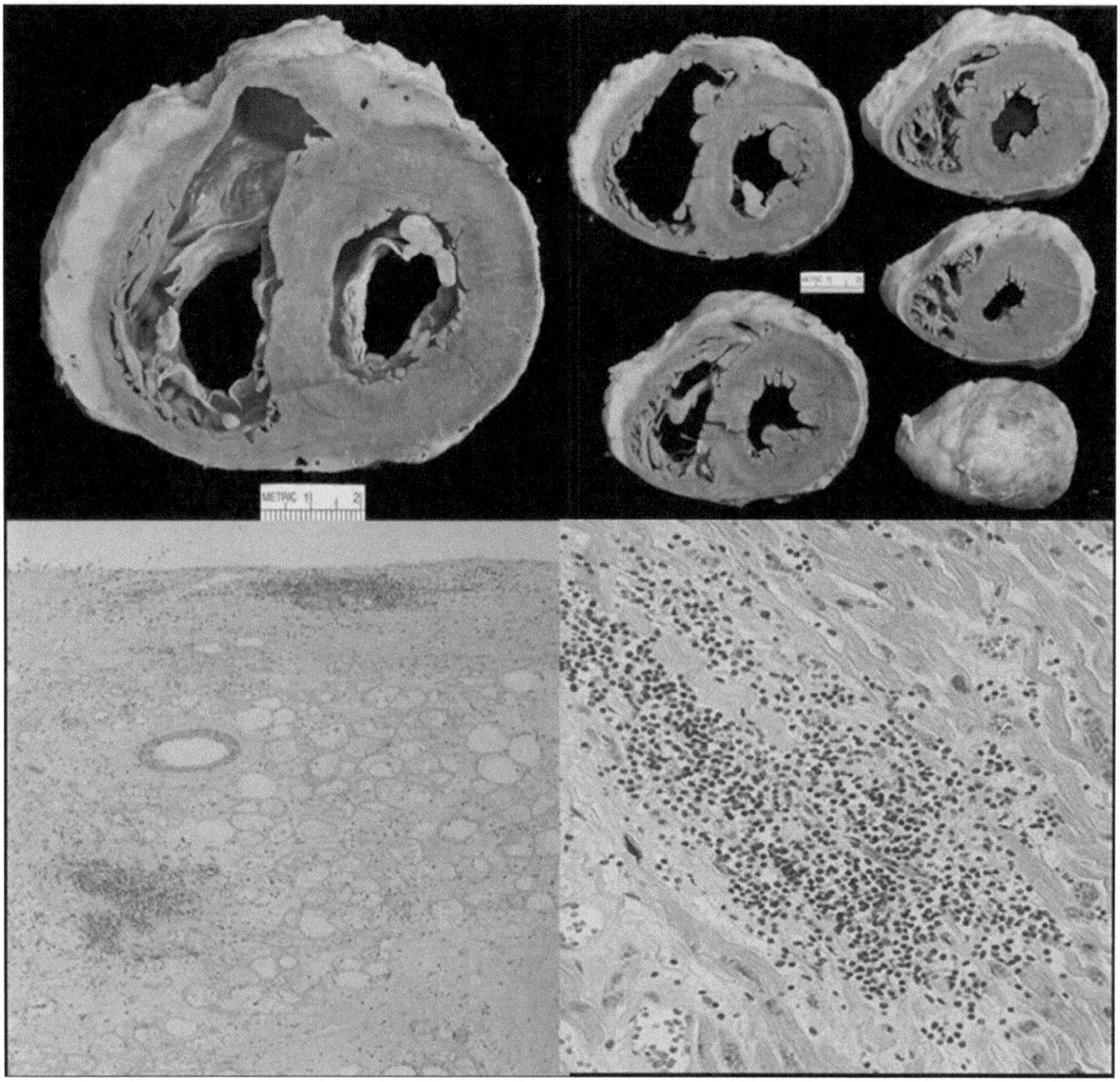

Figure 23. (Patient #60, Table 2). This 59-year-old woman underwent OHT because of ischemic cardiomyopathy 60 months before death. The patient had acute heart failure associated with rejection and it was fatal. Shown in the *upper* panels is the heart; in the *lower* panels, photomicrographs of epicardium, *lower left*, and myocardium, *lower right*. The quantity of adipose tissue is such that the heart floated in a container of formaldehyde. Both ventricular cavities are dilated, the right ventricle much more than the left. The epicardial coronary arteries were wide open. The anterolateral papillary muscle in the *upper left view* is necrotic, and in the slices of the heart shown in the *upper right* view, the posteromedial papillary muscle is shown to be scarred. *Lower left*: Photomicrograph of the epicardium showing collections of lymphocytes in 2 areas and a normal small epicardial coronary artery. *Lower right*: A collection of lymphocytes in myocardium. Hematoxylin/eosin stains: ×40, *lower left* and ×100, *lower right*.

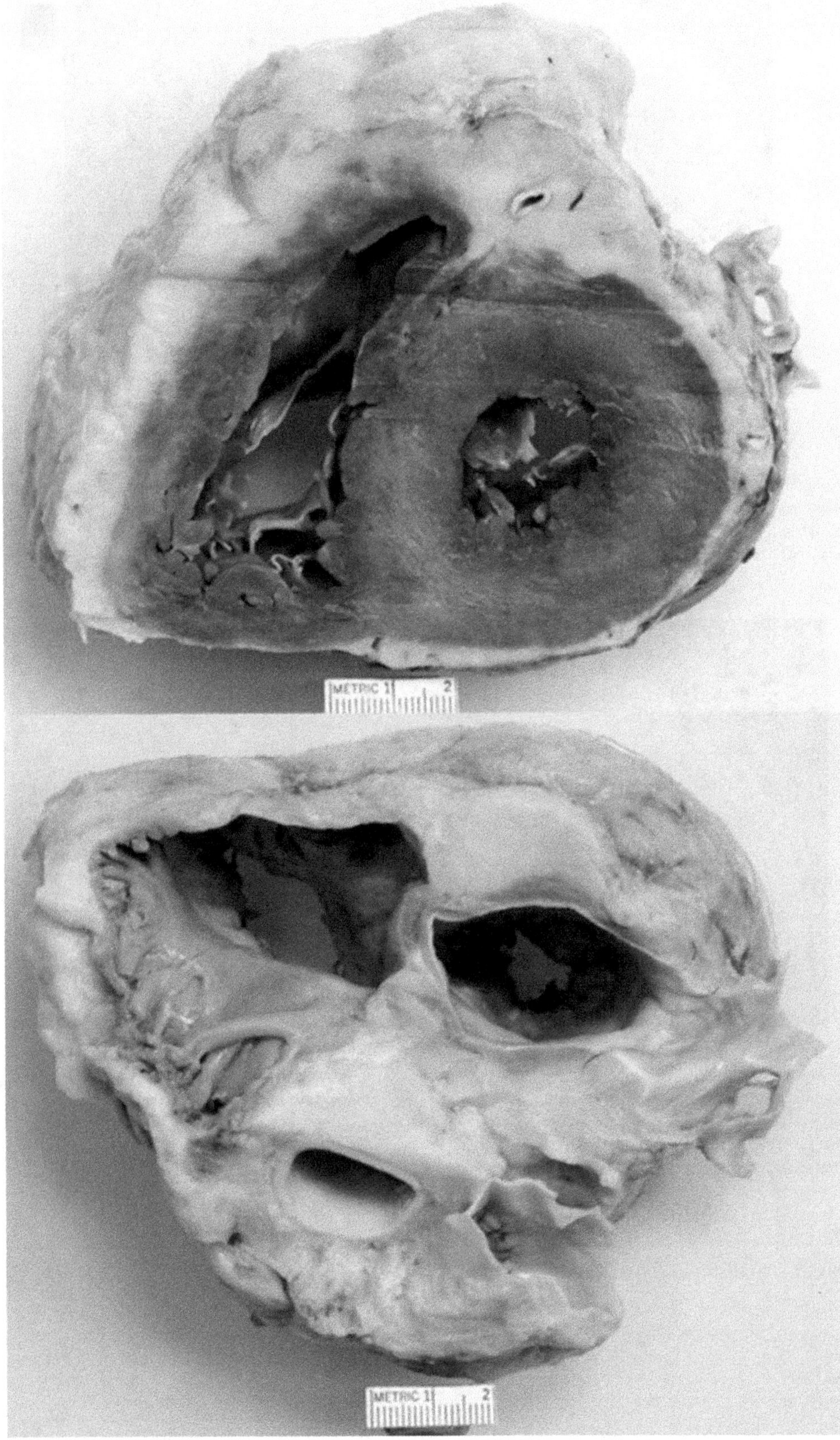

Figure 24. (Patient #71, Table 2). Shown are pictures of the heart in a 57-year-old man who had OHT at age 47 because of idiopathic cardiomyopathy. His post-transplant course was smooth until he developed cancer of the tongue and died 119 months (9.9 years) after the OHT. *Top*: View of the heart at the base showing a huge quantity of subepicardial adipose tissue. The heart floated in a container of formaldehyde. The left ventricular cavity was normal in size, and the right ventricular cavity is dilated. *Bottom*: View of the atria after "deroofing." The quantity of adipose tissue around the great arteries and in the atrial walls is also excessive. The right atrial cavity is quite a bit larger than the left atrial cavity.

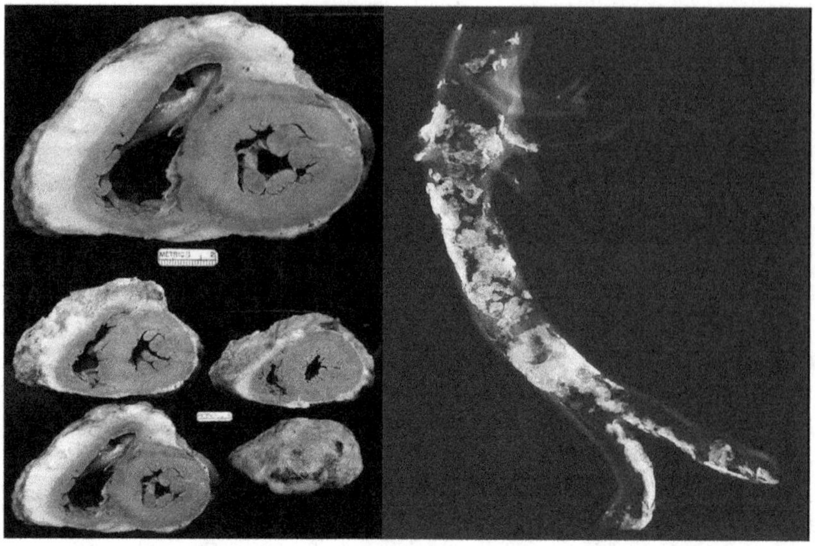

Figure 25. (Patient 73, Table 2). View of the heart (*left*) and radiograph of the abdominal aorta (*right*) in a 71-year-old man who died 10.2 years after OHT from acute aortic dissection with tear in the ascending aorta. The right ventricular cavity is dilated and the left ventricular cavity is of normal size. The quantity of subepicardial adipose tissue is excessive. Although the quantity of calcium in the aorta and its branches is considerable, its lumen is wide open and there is no aortic dilatation.

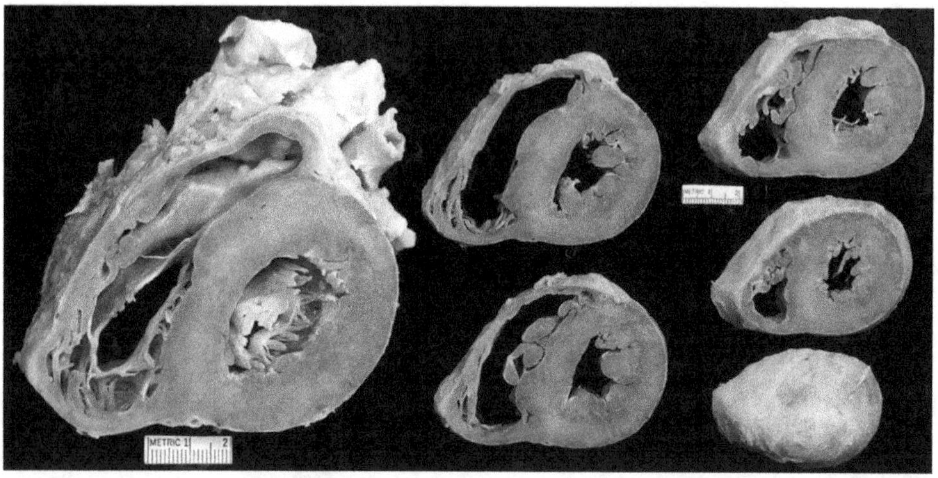

Figure 26. (Patient #79, Table 2). Shown is the heart in a 20-year-old woman who had OHT at age 3 years because of complete transposition of the great arteries. She did well for many years until evidence of heart failure reappeared, primarily right-sided with anasarca. Death was attributed to pump failure with some evidence of rejection. *Left:* View of the ventricles at the base exposing the atrioventricular valves. The right ventricle is considerably dilated; the left ventricle only mildly dilated. *Right*: Views of the ventricles more apical than the view shown on the *left*. The left anterior descending coronary artery and the other major coronary arteries were quite narrowed. The epicardium as shown in the photograph on the *bottom lower right* was densely scarred and the parietal and visceral pericardia were densely attached to one another.

## Disclosures

The authors have no conflicts of interest to disclose.


1. Roberts WC, Roberts CC, Ko JM, Filardo G, Capehart JE, Hall SA. Morphologic features of the recipient heart in patients having cardiac transplantation and analysis of the congruence or incongruence between the clinical and morphologic diagnoses. *Medicine (Baltimore)* 2014;93:211–235.
2. Billingham ME. The pathologic changes in long-term heart and lung transplant survivors. *J Heart Lung Transplant* 1992;11(4 pt 2):S252–S257.
3. Winters GL, Loh E, Schoen FJ. Natural history of focal moderate cardiac allograft rejection. Is treatment warranted? *Circulation* 1995;91:1975–1980.
4. Chu KE, Ho EK, de la Torre L, Vasilescu ER, Marboe CC. The relationship of nodular endocardial infiltrates (Quilty lesions) to survival, patient age, anti-HLA antibodies, and coronary artery disease following heart transplantation. *Cardiovasc Pathol* 2005;14:219–224.
5. Marboe CC, Billingham M, Eisen H, Deng MC, Baron H, Mehra M, Hunt S, Wohlgemuth J, Mahmood I, Prentice J, Berry G. Nodular endocardial infiltrates (Quilty lesions) cause significant variability in diagnosis of ISHLT Grade 2 and 3A rejection in cardiac allograft recipients. *J Heart Lung Transplant* 2005;24(7 suppl):S219–S226.
6. Stewart S, Winters GL, Fishbein MC, Tazelaar HD, Kobashigawa J, Abrams J, Andersen CB, Angelini A, Berry GJ, Burke MM, Demetris AJ, Hammond E, Itescu S, Marboe CC, McManus B, Reed EF, Reinsmoen NL, Rodriguez ER, Rose AG, Rose M, Suciu-Focia N, Zeevi A, Billingham ME. Revision of the 1990 working formulation for the standardization of nomenclature in the diagnosis of heart rejection. *J Heart Lung Transplant* 2005;24:1710–1720.

7. Berry GJ, Burke MM, Andersen C, Bruneval P, Fedrigo M, Fishbein MC, Goddard M, Hammond EH, Leone O, Marboe C, Miller D, Neil D, Rassl D, Revelo MP, Rice A, Rene Rodriguez E, Stewart S, Tan CD, Winters GL, West L, Mehra MR, Angelini A. The 2013 International Society for Heart and Lung Transplantation Working Formulation for the standardization of nomenclature in the pathologic diagnosis of antibody-mediated rejection in heart transplantation. *J Heart Lung Transplant* 2013;32:1147–1162.
8. Thomson JG. Heart transplantation in man—necropsy findings. *Br Med J* 1968;2:511–517.
9. Nakhleh RE, Jones J, Goswitz JJ, Anderson EA, Titus J. Correlation of endomyocardial biopsy findings with autopsy findings in human cardiac allografts. *J Heart Lung Transplant* 1992;11(3 pt 1):479–485.
10. Rose AG, Viviers L, Odell JA. Autopsy-determined causes of death following cardiac transplantation. A study of 81 patients and literature review. *Arch Pathol Lab Med* 1992;116:1137–1141.
11. Graham AR. Autopsy findings in cardiac transplant patients. A 10-year experience. Am *J Clin Pathol* 1992;97:369–375.
12. Luthringer DJ, Yamashita JT, Czer LS, Trento A, Fishbein MC. Nature and significance of epicardial lymphoid infiltrates in cardiac allografts. *J Heart Lung Transplant* 1995;14:537–543.
13. Alexander RT, Steenbergen C. Cause of death and sudden cardiac death after heart transplantation. An autopsy study. *Am J Clin Pathol* 2003;119:740–748.
14. Birati EY, Mathelier H, Molina M, Hanff TC, Mazurek JA, Atluri P, Acker MA, Rame JE, Margulies KB, Goldberg LR, Jessup M. Comparison of causes of death after heart transplantation in patients with left ventricular ejection fractions ≤35% versus >35. *Am J Cardiol* 2016;117:1322–1326.
15. Roberts WC, Won VS, Vasudevan A, Guileyardo JM. Characteristics of hearts at necropsy in patients treated chronically with prednisone (The Corticosteriod Heart). *Am J Cardiol* 2016;118:1935–1940.
16. Chen J, Stein S, Molina M, Owens A, Han Y. Right heart size in orthotopic heart transplant population: influence of donor and recipient gender, race, and body surface area. *Int J Cardiol* 2016;203:105–106.
17. Roberts WC, Bodey GP, Wertlake PT. The heart in acute leukemia. A study of 420 autopsy cases. *Am J Cardiol* 1968;21:388–412.

# Complications of Radiofrequency Ablation for Supraventricular Tachycardia in the Wolff-Parkinson-White Syndrome Associated With Noncompaction Cardiomyopathy

William C. Roberts, MD[a,b,c,*], Paul A. Grayburn, MD[a], and Shelley A. Hall, MD[a]

**Described herein is a 52-year-old man with Wolff-Parkinson-White syndrome and noncompaction cardiomyopathy who underwent 4 sternotomies to correct complications of 3 ablation procedures (2 open) for recurring supraventricular tachycardia, mitral valve repair for a damaged mitral valve during the third radiofrequency ablation procedure, and finally orthotopic heart transplantation.**  **(Am J Cardiol 2018;121:1442–1444)**

Few patients undergo 4 sternotomies. Such was the case, however, in the patient described herein, a 52-year-old man with Wolff-Parkinson-White syndrome and noncompaction cardiomyopathy complicated by periodic supraventricular tachycardia who underwent 3 ablation procedures (2 open), operative repair of a damaged mitral valve (during ablation), and finally orthotopic heart transplantation.

## Case description

A 52-year-old white man had been well until age of 24 years (1989) when he developed supraventricular tachycardia and was found to have the Wolff-Parkinson-White syndrome, and underwent the first of 3 radiofrequency ablation procedures. The first 2 procedures were conducted by sternotomy and the third, was by the percutaneous approach. The 2 subsequent procedures were done at ages 25 and 29 years. During the third ablation procedure, the mitral valve was inadvertently damaged leading to mitral regurgitation. At age 33 (1998), a partial ring (size 30) was placed in the mitral annular position to alleviate the symptomatic mitral regurgitation. The patient was then asymptomatic for the next 7 years when episodes of ventricular tachycardia began and the first of 3 intracardiac defibrillators were inserted. In the next several years, 23 defibrillator shocks occurred. His body weight increased to 310 pounds (height 72 in, body mass index 41 kg/m$^2$) over the years. Diabetes mellitus, systemic hypertension, and obstructive sleep apnea developed. Right-sided cardiac catheterization at age 57 (2017) disclosed the following pressures in mm Hg: pulmonary artery wedge mean 25, A wave 25, and V wave 36; pulmonary artery, 64/23; right ventricle, 66/7, and right atrial mean 3, A wave 6, and V wave 6. The Fick cardiac index was 1.9 L/min/m$^2$. By echocardiogram (Figure 1), the left ventricular ejection fraction was 20%, the left ventricular cavity was mildly dilated, the right ventricular cavity and both atria were severely dilated, and numerous noncompacted trabeculations were present in the left ventricular cavity, which also had been recognized during life. Moderate tricuspid valve regurgitation and trace mitral regurgitation were present. A mean gradient of 6 mm Hg was recorded across the mitral valve, which had an area of 1.4 cm$^2$. Orthotopic heart transplantation was performed in September 2017 for intractable heart failure. In December 2017, when the patient returned to view his excised native heart, he was doing well.

The operatively excised heart weighed 650 g (Figures 2 and 3). The quantity of subepicardial adipose tissue was greatly increased and the heart floated in a container of formaldehyde (fat is lighter than myocardium). A radiograph (Figure 2) of the heart specimen showed a mass in the posterior portion of the atrial septum (not recognized clinically) and its outer border was calcified. Its interior consisted of thrombus. The partial ring in the mitral annular region was calcified and its orifice accepted only the tip of my index finger (2 cm in diameter). In contrast, the tricuspid valve orifice readily accepted 3 of WCR's fingers. The walls of the epicardial coronary arteries were focally but heavily calcified, and their lumens were insignificantly narrowed. The noncompacted portion of the left ventricle is shown in Figure 3.

## Comments

The third ablation procedure described in the patient was complicated by damage to the mitral valve that later led to the insertion of the annular ring. The thrombus in the posterobasal portion of the atrial septum was not recognized until examination of the heart after cardiac transplantation, which appears to have resulted in some way from the ablation procedure. The quantity of calcium in the walls of the patient's major epicardial coronary arteries without significant luminal narrowing was a surprise finding, particularly in view of his very low serum cholesterol numbers (low-density lipoprotein cholesterol, 33 mg/dl while taking atorvastatin 20 mg/day). There were no lesions in the ventricular walls.

[a]Baylor Heart and Vascular Institute, Baylor Scott & White Health, Dallas, Texas; [b]Department of Pathology, Baylor University Medical Center, Baylor Scott & White Health, Dallas, Texas; and [c]Department of Internal Medicine, Baylor University Medical Center, Baylor Scott & White Health, Dallas, Texas. Manuscript received January 6, 2018; revised manuscript received and accepted February 15, 2018.

See page 1444 for disclosure information.

*Corresponding author: Tel: (214) 820-7911.

*E-mail address:* William.Roberts1@bswhealth.org (W.C. Roberts).

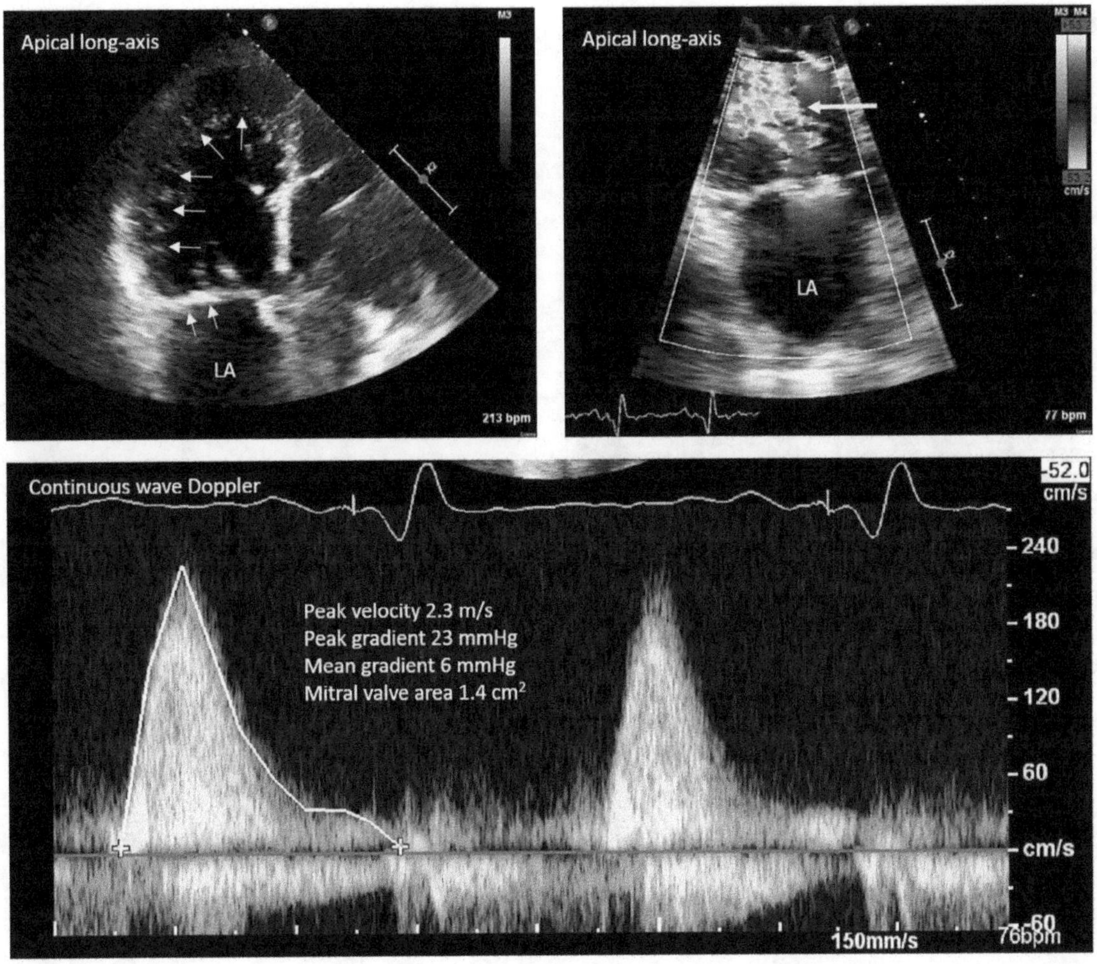


Figure 1. *Top left*. Apical long-axis view showing deep trabeculations in posterolateral wall and apex (*white arrows*), diagnostic of LV noncompaction. An undersized mitral annuloplasty ring is present (*yellow arrows*). *Top right*. Same view, magnified with color Doppler showing turbulent mitral inflow (*yellow arrow*) consistent with mitral stenosis. *Bottom panel*. Continuous wave Doppler confirming mitral stenosis with peak velocity 2.3 m/s, peak gradient 23 mm Hg, mean gradient 6 mm Hg and calculated mitral valve area 1.4 cm$^2$ at a heart rate of 76 beats/min.

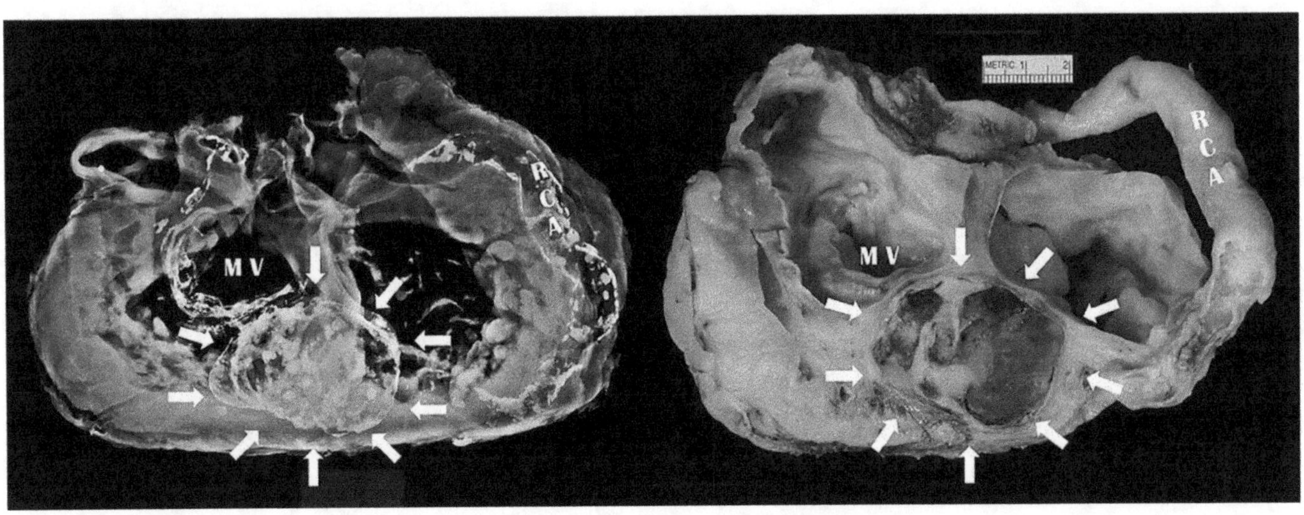


Figure 2. The *left image* shows a radiograph of the heart at autopsy. The *white arrows* indicate a calcified thrombus in the posterior portion of the atrial septum. The wall of this thrombus contains focal calcific deposits. A picture of that thrombus again outlined by *white arrows* is shown in the right part of the figure, which is a photograph of the heart itself. The mitral valve shown in both parts of the figures contains a partial ring, the wall of which is calcified. The orifice of the mitral valve containing the ring is quite narrow whereas the orifice of the tricuspid valve is wide open. Heavy calcific deposits are also present in the right coronary artery, which is quite large but its lumen is adequately patent.

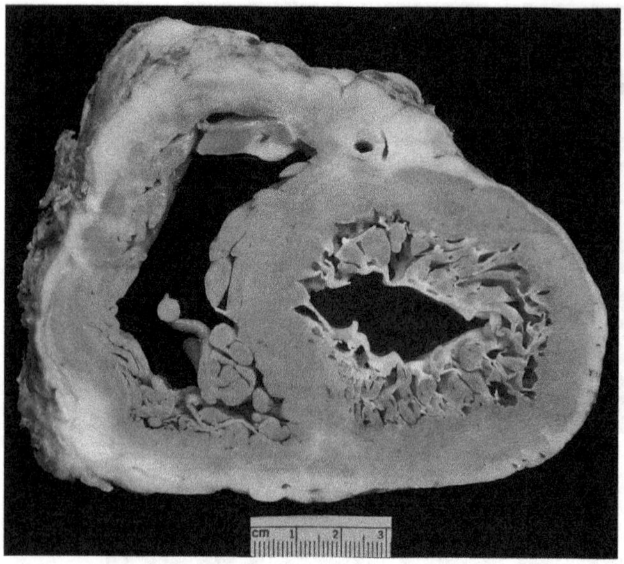


Figure 3. This is a cross-section of the ventricles showing a large noncompacted portion of the left ventricle. The endocardium of most of the trabeculations is thickened by fibrous tissue, which is probably a result of the insertion of the partial ring in the tricuspid position 19 years earlier. The right ventricular wall is quite thickened. Calcium is present in the wall of the left anterior descending coronary artery but its lumen is wide open.

The patient had evidence of mitral stenosis after a partial ring had been inserted into the mitral annular position 19 years before he underwent heart transplantation because of mitral regurgitation resulting from damage during the third ablation procedure. The mitral stenosis led to predominant right-sided cardiac failure and considerable pulmonary hypertension. The case further emphasizes that mitral rings, whether complete (360°) or incomplete (as in the present patient), are not benign interventions and can lead to conversion of a purely regurgitant mitral valve to a stenotic one.[1,2]

## Disclosures

The authors have no conflicts of interest to disclose.

1. Roberts WC, Moore M, Ko JM, Hamman BL. Mitral valve replacement after failed mitral ring insertion with or without leaflet/chordal repair for pure mitral regurgitation. *Am J Cardiol* 2016;117:1790–1807.
2. Becker TM, Grayburn PA, Roberts WC. Mitral valve repair for pure mitral regurgitation followed years later by mitral valve replacement for mitral stenosis. *Am J Cardiol* 2017;120:160–166.

# Usefulness of Total 12-Lead QRS Voltage for Diagnosis of Arrhythmogenic Right Ventricular Cardiomyopathy in Patients With Heart Failure Severe Enough to Warrant Orthotopic Heart Transplantation and Morphologic Illustration of Its Cardiac Diversity

William C. Roberts, MD*, Nitin Kondapalli, MBBS, and Shelley A. Hall, MD

**Although several electrocardiographic features of arrhythmogenic right ventricular cardiomyopathy (ARVC) (also called dysplasia) have been described, total 12-lead QRS voltage is not one of them. This report describes total 12-lead QRS voltage in 11 patients with ARVC who underwent orthotopic heart transplantation (OHT) because of progressively severe heart failure. Additionally, it illustrates the varied morphologic features of ARVC. The total 12-lead nonpaced QRS voltages before OHT ranged from 28 to 118 mm (mean 74 ± 32), and those in the paced tracings, from 33 to 129 mm (62 ± 32). The voltages are the lowest we have encountered among 12 previously reported cardiovascular conditions. The heart weights among the 11 ARVC patients ranged from 285 to 670 g (mean 448 ± 125). Very low 12-lead QRS voltage is characteristic of patients with ARVC with heart failure severe enough to warrant OHT, and thus may serve as a clue to its diagnosis.**  **(Am J Cardiol 2018;122:1051−1061)**

Although recognized by morphologic studies earlier,[1] the present concepts of arrhythmic right ventricular cardiomyopathy (ARVC) were introduced by Marcus et al in 1982.[2] Several reports have described various electrocardiographic features of ARVC but none have described total 12-lead QRS voltage or its potential diagnostic usefulness.[3−13] Such is one purpose of this report. Another is to illustrate several hearts of patients with ARVC to demonstrate the morphologic variability of this condition.

## Methods

From 2009 to 2017, 11 adults at Baylor University Medical Center at Dallas had orthotopic heart transplantation (OHT) because of ARVC. The study was approved by the Baylor Research Institute's Institutional Review Board, which also waived the need for informed patient consent.

One of us (WCR) examined each patient's native heart and also prepared the final report. Accurate scales were used to weigh the native heart after fixation in formaldehyde for several days. The ascending aorta and pulmonary trunk were excised about 2 cm above the sinotubular junction; all extraneous tissues were removed before weighing. Before weighing, the heart was opened and excessive water or formaldehyde was removed from its surfaces by gentle patting with paper towels. Clinical records and all electrocardiograms recorded at Baylor University Medical Center were reviewed and examined. The total 12-lead QRS voltage (defined as the distance in millimeters from the peak of the R wave to the nadir of either the Q or S wave, whichever was deeper, with 10 mm standard [=1 mV]) was measured by 2 of us (WCR and NK). The statistics performed was limited to the calculation of the means and standard deviations.

From the Baylor Scott & White Heart and Vascular Institute, the Departments of Pathology and Internal Medicine (Division of Cardiology), Baylor University Medical Center, Part of Baylor Scott & White Health, Dallas, Texas. Manuscript received May 30, 2018; revised manuscript received and accepted June 6, 2018.

*Corresponding author: Tel: (214) 820-7911; fax: (214) 820-7533.

*E-mail addresses:* ajc@baylorhealth.edu, William.Roberts1@bswhealth.org (W.C. Roberts).

## Results

Pertinent clinical, morphologic, and electrocardiographic data are displayed in Tables 1 and 2. At the time of OHT, the patients' ages ranged from 21 to 70 years (mean 49 ± 17); 8 were men and 3 were women. ARVC was diagnosed before OHT in 3 patients and from examination of the operatively excised heart in the other 8 patients. All 11 patients had clinical evidence of heart failure, especially severe right-sided heart failure; by electrocardiogram, 8 had documented runs of ventricular tachycardia, 3 had epsilon waves (small amplitude distinct potentials between the end of the QRS complex and the beginning of the T wave), and 5 had inverted T waves in 1 or more precordial leads; all 11 had low QRS voltage, and 5 had right bundle branch block; by echocardiogram or computed tomography, all 11 patients had very dilated right ventricular cavities and 10 had dilated, but less so, left ventricular cavities. The body mass indexes ranged from 22 to 37 kg/m$^2$ (mean 29 ± 5). The progression of heart failure to class III or IV prompted the OHT.

The electrocardiographic findings before OHT are tabulated in Table 2. Six nonpaced and 7 paced electrocardiographic tracings were available for analysis. The nonpaced total 12-lead QRS voltages ranged from 28 to 118 mm (mean 74 ± 32), and those in paced tracings, from

Table 1
Arrhythmogenic right ventricular cardiomyopathy—Clinical and morphologic features

| Patient no (figure no) | Age at OHT (yrs) | Family history of SD/VT | BMI (kg/m$^2$) | TC (mg/dl) | LDL-C (mg/dl) | HDL-C (mg/dl) | TG (mg/dl) | LVEF (%) | CI (L/min/m$^2$) | ARVC diagnosed clinically | Pressures (mm Hg) (s/d) SA | RV | PA | HW (g) | Coronary artery narrowing (>75% CSA) by plaque | Heart floated in formalin | LV involvement Scar | Fat | Associated Condition |
|---|---|---|---|---|---|---|---|---|---|---|---|---|---|---|---|---|---|---|---|
| MEN | | | | | | | | | | | | | | | | | | | |
| 1(3) | 21 | 0 | 27 | 147 | 72 | 65 | 62 | 5 | 1.1 | 0 | 144/96* | 21/14 | 17/11 | 490 | 0 | 0 | 0 | 0 | 0 |
| 2 | 26 | 0 | 35 | 204 | 134 | 56 | 149 | 10 | 0.8 | 0 | 180/100* | - | 50/30 | 595 | 0 | 0 | 0 | 0 | Gilbert's syndrome |
| 3(4) | 34 | 0 | 27 | 154 | 73 | 80 | 65 | 3 | 1.3 | 0 | 75/55* | 48/12 | 20/14 | 515 | 0 | 0 | + | 0 | Rheumatoid arthritis |
| 4 | 44 | + | 22 | 175 | 112 | 50 | 87 | 25 | 1.9 | 0 | 95/60* | 19/12 | 22/11 | 315 | 0 | 0 | 0 | 0 | Hypothyroidism |
| 5(5) | 54 | + | 26 | 145 | 68 | 62 | 74 | 30 | 1.5 | + | 75/50* | 31/4 | 25/10 | 670† | + | + | + | + | 0 |
| 6(1&6) | 62 | 0 | 35 | 173 | 86 | 82 | 94 | 20 | 1.4 | 0 | 100/70* | 25/10 | 21/12 | 420 | 0 | + | 0 | 0 | Guillain Barre syndrome |
| 7(7) | 66 | 0 | 29 | 235 | 107 | 94 | 184 | 15 | 1.5 | 0‡ | 80/55* | 18/9 | 16/3 | 450 | 0 | + | + | + | Hypothyroidism |
| 8(8) | 68 | 0 | 28 | 165 | 97 | 32 | 296 | 30 | 1.4 | 0 | 155/80* | 26/7 | 24/16 | 460 | +§ | + | + | 0 | 0 |
| WOMEN | | | | | | | | | | | | | | | | | | | |
| 9(9)¶ | 44 | + | 37 | 204 | 149 | 44 | 119 | 10 | 1.5 | 0 | 125/85* | 40/-1 | 42/13 | 420 | 0 | + | 0 | 0 | Limb-girdle muscular dystrophy |
| 10(10) | 49 | 0 | 27 | 237 | 112 | 100 | 200 | 56 | 1.5 | + | 85/40* | 22/12 | 20/13 | 305 | 0 | + | 0 | 0 | 0 |
| 11(2&11) | 70 | + | 26 | 254 | 149 | 68 | 297 | 55 | 1.7 | + | 185/100* | 17/5 | 17/3 | 285 | 0 | + | 0 | 0 | Hypothyroidism |

ARVC = arrhythmogenic right ventricular cardiomyopathy; BMI = body mass index; CABG = coronary artery bypass grafting; CI = cardiac index; CSA = cross-sectional area; g = gram(s); Hg = hydrargyrum (Mercury); HW = heart weight; ICD = Implantable Cardioverter Defibrillator; kg = kilogram(s); L = Liter(s); LDL-C = low-density lipoprotein cholesterol; LVAD = left ventricular assist device; LVEF = left ventricular ejection fraction; m = meter(s); min = minute(s); OHT = orthotopic heart transplantation; PA = pulmonary artery; RV = right ventricle; s/d = peak systole/end-diastole; SD = sudden death; SA = systemic artery; TC = total cholesterol; VT = ventricular tachycardia; Yrs = year(s).

* Indirect pressure (cuff).

† An LVAD was inserted 34 months before the OHT.

‡ The result of performed biopsy was negative for ARVC changes.

§ Patient had CABG 25 years before the OHT.

¶ Patient died 48 days after the OHT.

Table 2
Electrocardiographic features of arrhythmogenic right ventricular cardiomyopathy

| Patient no. (figure no.) | Age at OHT (yrs) | ECG Paced | QRS amplitude in each electrocardiographic lead(mm) | | | | | | | | | | | | Total 12-lead QRS voltage (mm) | ECG to OHT interval (mos) | HW (g) | ECG changes before OHT | | | | | | | |
|---|---|---|---|---|---|---|---|---|---|---|---|---|---|---|---|---|---|---|---|---|---|---|---|---|---|
| | | | I | II | III | aVR | aVL | aVF | V1 | V2 | V3 | V4 | V5 | V6 | | | | AF | VPCs | VT | Epsilon wave | Inverted T waves | Right BBB | LAFB | CHB |
| MEN | | | | | | | | | | | | | | | | | | | | | | | | | |
| 1(3) | 21 | 0 | 5 | 3 | 3 | 3 | 3 | 2 | 6 | 11 | 14 | 14 | 8 | 19 | 91 | 8.0 | 490 | 0 | + | 0 | 0 | + | 0 | 0 | 0 |
| 2 | 26 | 0 | 3 | 3 | 6 | 2 | 5 | 5 | 4 | 5 | 10 | 8 | 7 | 9 | 67 | 0.2 | 595 | 0 | + | + | 0 | + | + | + | 0 |
| | | + | 4 | 3 | 8 | 2 | 7 | 5 | 4 | 5 | 8 | 8 | 7 | 7 | 68 | 3.0 | | | | | | | | | |
| 3(4) | 34 | + | 3 | 4 | 4 | 3 | 4 | 5 | 6 | 6 | 4 | 7 | 11 | 8 | 65 | 0.7 | 515 | 0 | + | 0 | 0 | 0 | 0 | 0 | + |
| 4 | 44 | + | 1 | 4 | 4 | 3 | 2 | 5 | 2 | 3 | 6 | 8 | 9 | 5 | 52 | 0.5 | 315 | + | 0 | + | 0 | 0 | + | 0 | 0 |
| 5(5) | 54 | + | 3 | 8 | 9 | 5 | 4 | 10 | 8 | 13 | 23 | 20 | 16 | 10 | 129 | 15.5 | 670* | 0 | + | + | 0 | 0 | 0 | 0 | 0 |
| 6(1&6) | 62 | 0 | 6 | 6 | 10 | 5 | 8 | 9 | 7 | 9 | 6 | 7 | 10 | 7 | 90 | 170.0 | 420 | + | + | + | + | + | + | + | 0 |
| | | + | 3 | 3 | 5 | 2 | 4 | 4 | 2 | 6 | 2 | 3 | 3 | 4 | 41 | 5.0 | | | | | | | | | |
| 7(7) | 66 | + | 3 | 2 | 3 | 1 | 3 | 3 | 1 | 3 | 3 | 5 | 4 | 2 | 33 | 0.3 | 450 | + | 0 | + | 0 | 0 | 0 | 0 | 0 |
| 8(8) | 68 | + | 3 | 3 | 2 | 3 | 2 | 1 | 2 | 9 | 7 | 6 | 5 | 4 | 47 | 0.3 | 460 | + | + | + | 0 | 0 | 0 | 0 | 0 |
| WOMEN | | | | | | | | | | | | | | | | | | | | | | | | | |
| 9(9) | 44 | 0 | 10 | 10 | 10 | 10 | 8 | 9 | 11 | 12 | 10 | 10 | 9 | 9 | 118 | 23.0 | 420 | + | + | + | 0 | + | + | 0 | 0 |
| 10(10) | 49 | 0 | 2 | 3 | 3 | 2 | 2 | 3 | 2 | 2 | 3 | 2 | 2 | 2 | 28 | 3.5 | 305 | + | + | 0 | + | 0 | + | 0 | 0 |
| 11(2&11) | 70 | 0 | 8 | 3 | 7 | 4 | 7 | 3 | 2 | 5 | 2 | 2 | 4 | 5 | 52 | 1.0 | 285 | + | + | + | + | + | 0 | + | 0 |

AF = atrial fibrillation; BBB = bundle branch block; CHB = complete heart block; ECG = electrocardiogram; LAFB = left anterior fascicular block; mm = millimeter(s); OHT = orthotopic heart transplantation; VPCs = ventricular premature complexes; VT = ventricular tachycardia; Yrs = year(s).

* A left ventricular assist device was inserted 34 months before the OHT.

Table 3
Total 12-lead QRS voltage in different cardiovascular conditions*

| Condition | Gender | No. of cases | Age in years (mean) | Total 12-Lead QRS voltage in mm (mean) | Patients with 12-Lead QRS voltage >175mm | Heart weight (g) | Total 12-lead QRS voltage (mm)/heart weight (g) | Year of Publication | Authors (reference Number) |
|---|---|---|---|---|---|---|---|---|---|
| Hearts weigh >1000 g | M | 16 | 29-64 (42) | 140-414 (306) | 16 (94%) | 1005-1360 (1102) | 0.28 | 1985 | Roberts and Podolak[14] |
| | F | 1 | 20 | 601 | | 1250 | 0.48 | | |
| Aortic valve stenosis | M | 36 | 16-64 (48) | 144-417 (249) | 47 (94%) | 440-880 (639) | 0.39 | 1982 | Siegel and Roberts[15] |
| | F | 14 | 16-65 (47) | 193-376 (277) | | 380-700 (521) | 0.53 | | |
| Aortic regurgitation | M | 22 | 19-59 (44) | 109-428 (271) | 27 (90%) | 430-1100 (717) | 0.38 | 1985 | Roberts and Day[16] |
| | F | 8 | 35-56 (48) | 169-384 (275) | | 375-950 (638) | 0.43 | | |
| Mitral regurgitation | M | 11 | 24-84 (47) | 111-364 (245) | 17 (71%) | 400-775 (629) | 0.39 | 1992 | Glick and Roberts[17] |
| | F | 13 | 21-64 (37) | 114-290 (199) | | 350-675 (472) | 0.42 | | |
| Hypertrophic cardiomyopathy without cardiac transplantation | M | 21 | 14-68 (46) | 107-339 (190) | 30 (53%) | 325-1070 (671) | 0.28 | 1989 | Dollar and Roberts[18] |
| | F | 36 | 19-87 (51) | 68-327 (201) | | 290-1230 (547) | 0.38 | | |
| Hypertrophic cardiomyopathy with cardiac transplantation | M | 6 | 19-46 (35) | 109-201 (142) | 4 (40%) | 310-480 (393) | 0.36 | 1993 | Shirani et al[19] |
| | F | 4 | 24-45 (35) | 172-378 (241) | | 290-650 (408) | 0.59 | | |
| Idiopathic dilated cardiomyopathy | M | 35 | 19-73 (46) | 74-281 (147) | 20 (41%) | 400-940 (620) | 0.24 | 1987 | Roberts et al[20] |
| | F | 14 | 22-75 (54) | 75-243 (167) | | 400-860 (602) | 0.28 | | |
| Lipomatous hypertrophy of the atrial septum | M | 12 | 48-84 (67) | 93-241 (140) | 3 (11%) | 410-795 (576) | 0.24 | 1993 | Shirani and Roberts[21] |
| | F | 16 | 59-83 (74) | 59-266 (124) | | 330-680 (502) | 0.25 | | |
| Carcinoid syndrome with carcinoid heart disease | M | 11 | 39-72 (56) | 58-227 (120) | 2 (11%) | 220-480 (350) | 0.34 | 1985 | Ross and Roberts[22] |
| | F | 8 | 28-64 (54) | 58-128 (84) | | 200-290 (245) | 0.34 | | |
| Carcinoid syndrome without carcinoid heart disease | M | 10 | 42-75 (55) | 89-129 (137) | 2 (13%) | 240-570 (350) | 0.39 | | |
| | F | 5 | 28-67 (50) | 102-135 (121) | | 150-270 (230) | 0.53 | | |
| Aortic syphilis | M | 11 | 33-84 (28) | 57-161 (120) | 0 | - | - | 2015 | Roberts et al[23] |
| | F | 13 | 58-83 (28) | 64-146 (106) | | - | - | | |
| Cardiac adiposity | M | 13 | 51-73 (64) | 73-159 (114) | 1 (3%) | 320-795 (485) | 0.24 | 1995 | Shirani et al[24] |
| | F | 17 | 40-85 (70) | 77-210 (124) | | 250-575 (395) | 0.31 | | |
| Cardiac amyloidosis | M | 15 | 32-69 (52) | 60-197 (99) | 2 (7%) | 410-850 (570) | 0.17 | 1983 | Roberts and Waller[25] |
| | F | 15 | 21-93 (69) | 58-199 (109) | | 370-900 (494) | 0.22 | | |
| Cardiac sarcoidosis (Nonpaced) | M | 3 | 50,52,63 (55) | 121,155,134 (137) | 0 | 605,440,540 (528) | 0.26 | 2018 | Roberts et al[26] |
| | F | 5 | 50-62 (57) | 52-144 (105) | | 370-600 (470) | 0.22 | | |
| Cardiac sarcoidosis (Paced) | M | 6 | 53-67 (59) | 47-103 (82) | 0 | 420-555 (505) | 0.16 | | |
| | F | 6 | 50-61 (56) | 67-161 (98) | | 300-560 (427) | 0.23 | | |
| Arrhythmogenic right ventricular cardiomyopathy (Nonpaced) | M | 3 | 21,26,62 (36) | 91,67,90 (83) | 0 | 490,595,420 (502) | 0.17 | 2018 | Roberts et al |
| | F | 3 | 44,49,70 (54) | 28,61,118 (69) | | 420,305,285 (337) | 0.2 | | |
| Arrhythmogenic right ventricular cardiomyopathy (Paced) | M | 7 | 26-68 (51) | 33-129 (62) | 0 | 315-670 (489) | 0.13 | | |
| | F | 0 | - | - | | - | - | | |

* Parts of this table have been published previously in the following reports: Roberts WC, Filardo G, Ko JM, Siegel RJ, Dollar AL, Ross EM, Shirani J. Comparison of total 12-lead QRS voltage in a variety of cardiac conditions and its usefulness in predicting increased cardiac mass. *Am J Cardiol* 2013; 112(6):904-909. Permission to republish this updated table is granted by the authors and the publisher, Elsevier.

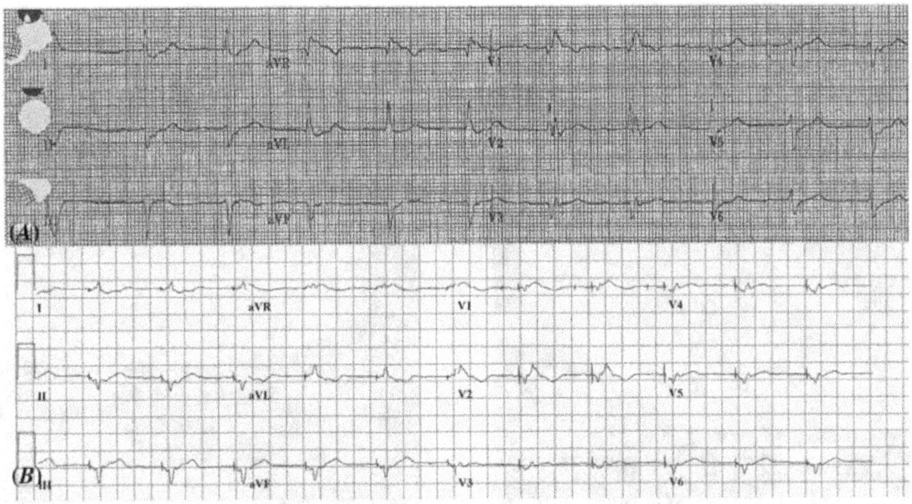


Figure 1. Case #6, Tables 1 and 2. Electrocardiograms nonpaced *(upper)* and paced *(lower)*. The total 12-lead QRS voltage in the upper tracing is 90 mm and in the lower tracing, 41 mm with 10 mm standard. Prominent epsilon waves are present in 1 or more precordial leads in the two patients.

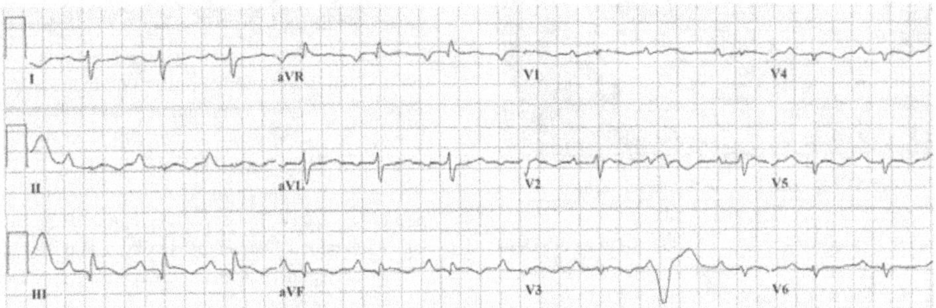


Figure 2. Case #11, Tables 1 and 2. Nonpaced electrocardiogram with total 12-lead QRS voltage of 52 mm. The PR interval is prolonged (236 ms), many T waves are inverted, and an occasional ventricular premature complex is present.

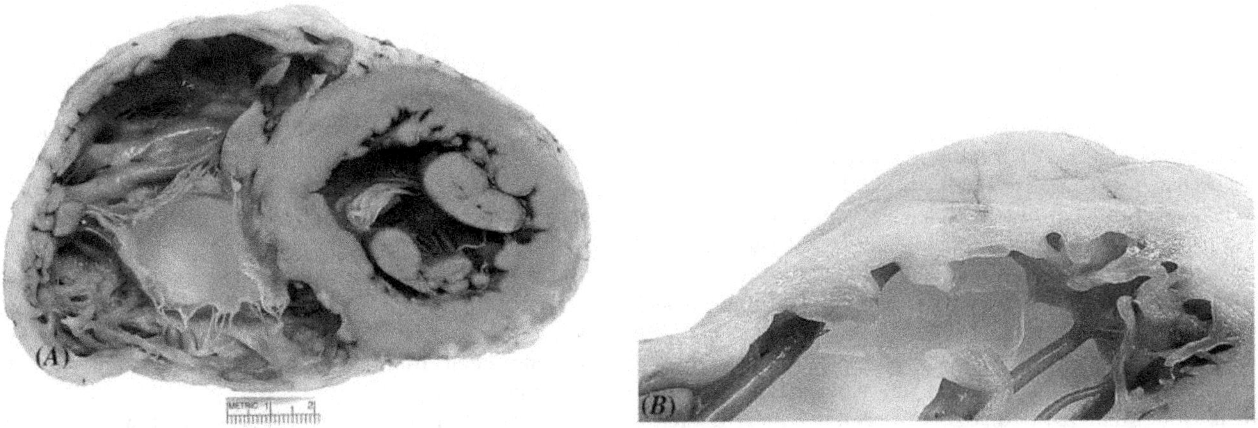


Figure 3. Case #1, Tables 1 and 2. Shown here are 2 photographs of the heart in a 21-year-old man. (*A*) Shown here is the basal portion of the heart showing marked dilatation of the right ventricular cavity and dilatation but less so of the left ventricular cavity. Most of the right ventricular wall is replaced by adipose tissue. There is some infiltration of fat in the subepicardial portion of left ventricular wall and some small scars in the subepicardial portion of left ventricular wall. (*B*) A close-up of the right ventricular outflow tract showing the right ventricular wall to be focally replaced by adipose tissue. Total nonpaced 12-lead QRS voltage in this patient was 91 mm and the heart weighed 490 g.

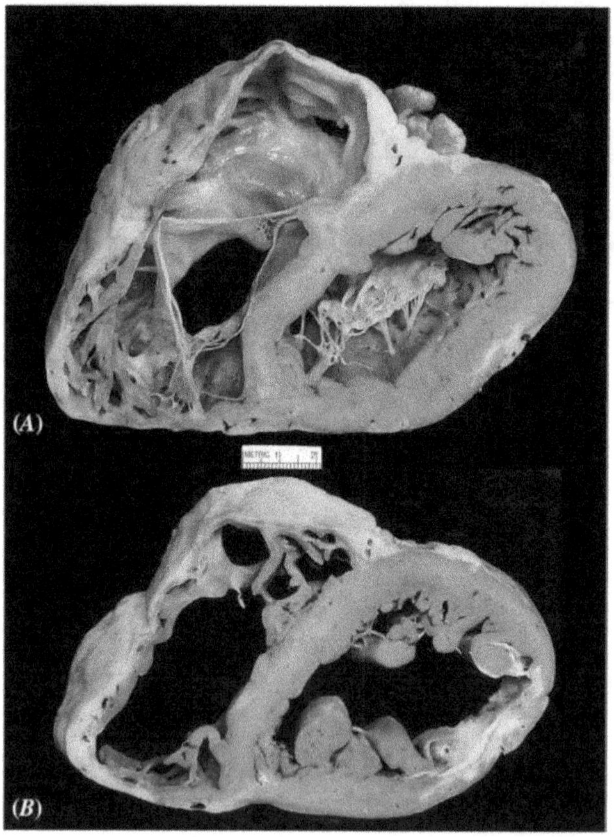

Figure 4. Case #3, Tables 1 and 2. Shown here is the basal portion of the ventricular walls in a 34-year-old man. The two ventricular cavities are dilated but the right one far more than the left. (*A*) The right ventricular free wall is replaced focally by either adipose tissue or fibrous tissue or both. (*B*) This cut of the ventricular walls not only shows the thinning of the right ventricular free wall focally but also a scar in the lateral wall of left ventricular between the two papillary muscles. The epicardial coronary arteries were wide open. Total paced 12-lead QRS voltage was 65 mm, and the heart weighed 515 g.

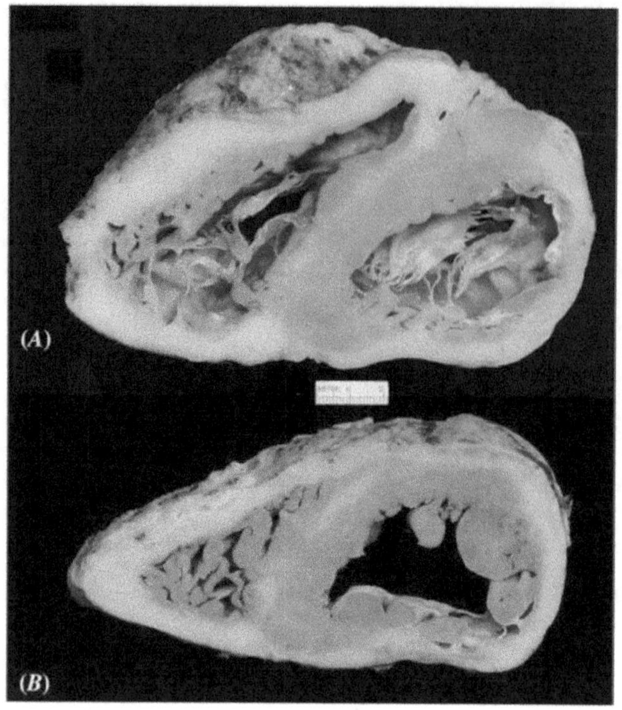

Figure 5. Case #5, Tables 1 and 2. Shown here is the basal portion of the ventricles in *A* and another portion more apically located in *B*. (*A*) The two ventricular cavities are dilated. Most of the right ventricular wall is replaced by adipose tissue. (*B*) Much of the entire left ventricular free wall, particularly the subepicardial region, is replaced by adipose tissue making the wall much thinner than the ventricular septum. The lumen of the right coronary artery was considerably narrowed by atherosclerotic plaque. Total paced 12-lead QRS voltage was 129 mm and the heart weighed 670 g. This patient had a left ventricular assist device in place for 34 months before the OHT.

33 to 129 mm (mean 62 ± 32). Before OHT, atrial fibrillation was present in 7 patients, and occasional ventricular premature complexes in 9 patients, 5 of whom also had runs of ventricular tachycardia.

The hearts of the 8 men ranged in weight from 315 to 670 g (mean 489 ± 108), and in the 3 women, from 285 to 420 g (mean 337 ± 73). The quantity of adipose tissue in the heart was huge in 7 of 11 patients causing their hearts to float in a container of formaldehyde (adipose tissue is lighter than myocardium). Two patients had narrowing of 1 or more major epicardial coronary arteries, one of whom had undergone coronary arterial bypass grafting 25 years before the OHT. All patients had dilated right ventricular cavities and all but 1 also had dilated left ventricular cavities but in all cases the right ventricular cavity was much more dilated than the left one. The right ventricular wall was focally replaced mainly by adipose tissue in which some scar tissue usually also was present. Focal scars replaced portions of the left ventricular free wall and/or ventricular septum in 4 patients, 2 of whom had narrowing >75% in cross-sectional area by plaques of 1 or more major epicardial coronary arteries. Two of 4 patients with left ventricular scars also had focal fatty replacement of these walls by adipose tissue.

## Discussion

Described herein are findings from measurement of total 12-lead QRS voltage and findings from the examination of the native hearts in 11 patients who underwent OHT because of severe heart failure due to ARVC. These total 12-lead nonpaced QRS voltages (mean 74 ± 32) and paced (mean 62 ± 32) are the lowest found in any of the 12 previously reported conditions we have studied (summarized in Table 3).[14–26] The total 12-lead QRS voltage was lower in the 7 paced electrocardiograms than in the 6 nonpaced electrocardiograms.

A limitation of the present report is that the time interval between the recording of the electrocardiogram and the OHT procedure was rather long in 3 of 11 patients. It is likely, however, as described previously in patients with idiopathic dilated cardiomyopathy that the total 12-lead QRS voltage would decrease as the time interval increased

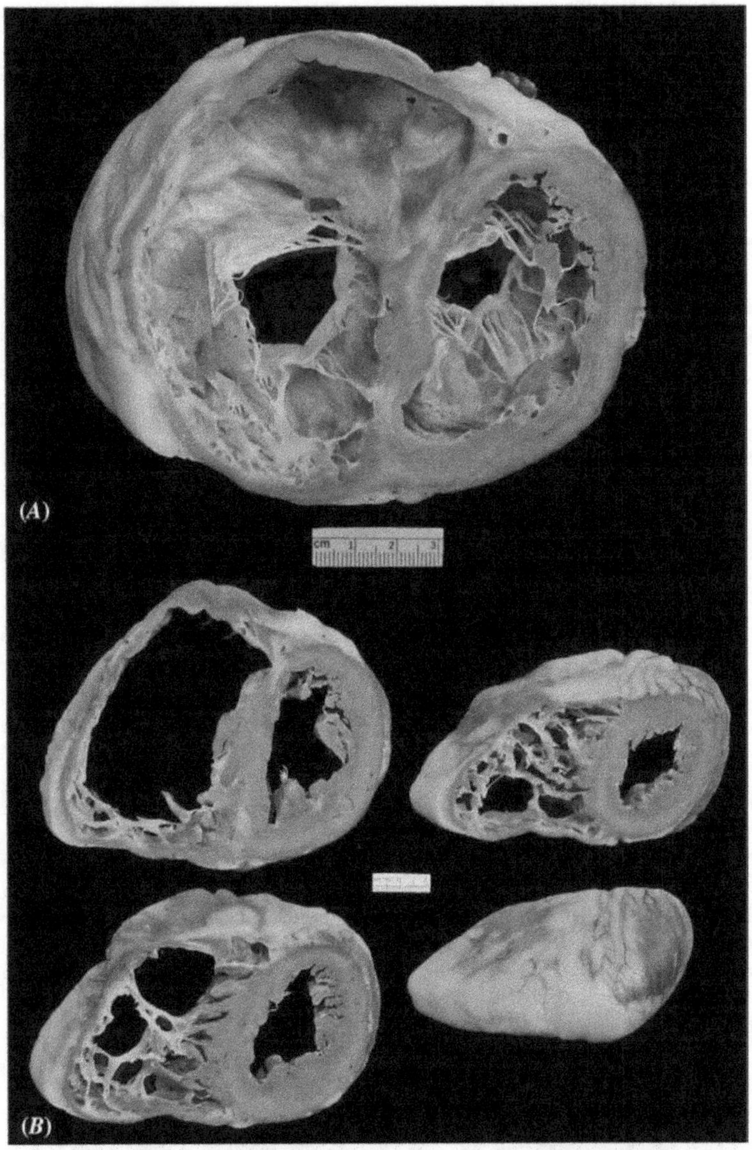


Figure 6. Case #6, Tables 1 and 2. Shown here are portions of a heart in a 63-year-old man. (*A*) The two ventricular cavities are greatly dilated, the right much more than the left. The right ventricular free wall is focally replaced, mainly by adipose tissue. Focal scars are also present in the ventricular septum. (*B*) These are transverse cuts of the ventricles caudal to the view shown in *A*. These views show scarring in the right ventricular pectinate muscles as well as focally in the ventricular septum. The right ventricular cavity is much larger than the left. Total nonpaced 12-lead QRS voltage was 90 mm and paced, 41 mm, and the heart weighed 420 g.

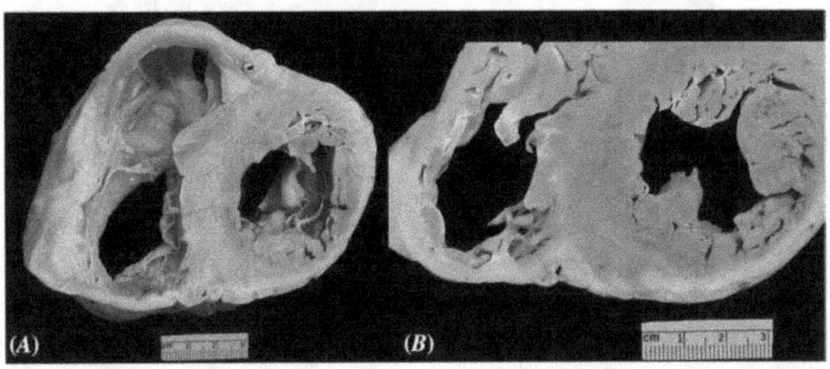


Figure 7. Case #7, Tables 1 and 2. Shown in *A* is the basal portion of the heart showing replacement of much of the walls of the two ventricles by adipose tissue. The lateral wall of the left ventricle is much thinner than the ventricular septum due to replacement of myocardium by both adipose tissue and fibrous tissue. (*B*) A closer view more apically better showing the fatty infiltration of the myocardial walls. The quantity of fat was such that the heart floated in a container of formaldehyde (adipose tissue is lighter than myocardium). The total paced 12-lead QRS voltage was only 33 mm, and the heart weighed 450 g.

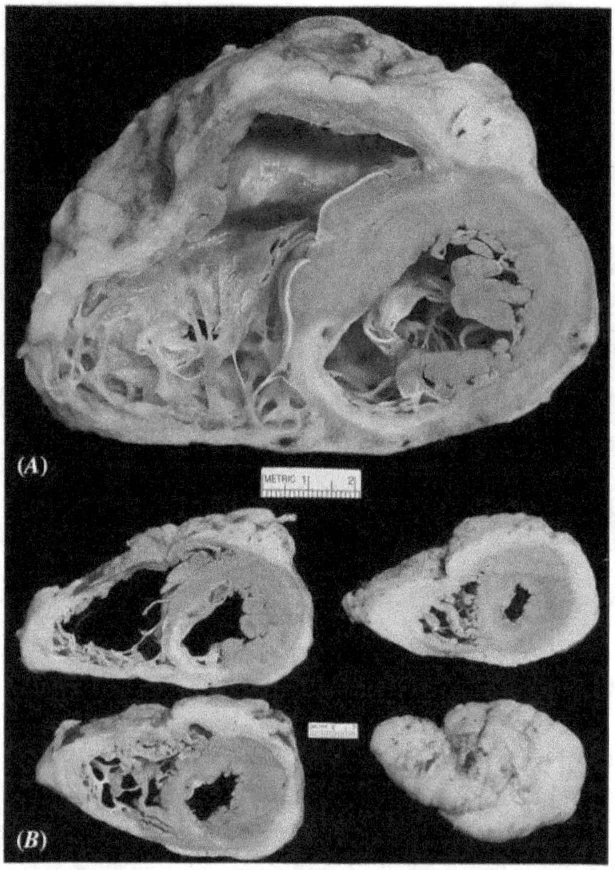


Figure 8. Case #8, Tables 1 and 2. Shown here are views of the cardiac ventricles on various levels in a 68-year-old man. The two ventricular cavities are dilated but the right far more than the left. The right ventricular cavity posteriorly and laterally is replaced by mainly adipose tissue but some scar tissue is present. The posterior portion of the ventricular septum and the posterior left ventricular free wall is replaced by scar tissue. (*B*) Photographs of the ventricular slices caudal to the view shown in *A*. The quantity of subepicardial adipose tissue is excessive such that the heart floated in a container of formaldehyde. Total paced 12-lead QRS voltage was 47 mm, and the heart weighed 460 g.

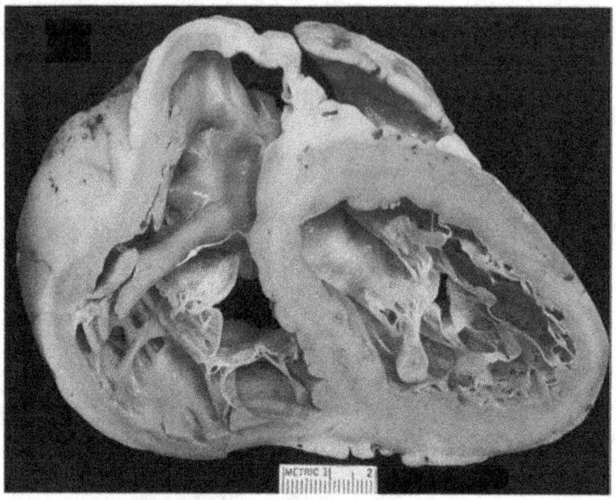

Figure 9. Case #9, Tables 1 and 2. Shown here is the basal portion of the heart in a 44-year-old woman who had limb-girdle muscular dystrophy. This photograph shows marked dilatation of the two ventricular cavities. The right ventricular free wall anteriorly adjacent to the septum is replaced by adipose tissue. The lateral wall of left ventricle between the two papillary muscles is thinner than other portions of the left ventricular free wall. Total nonpaced 12-lead QRS voltage in this patient was 118 mm, and the heart weighed 420 g.

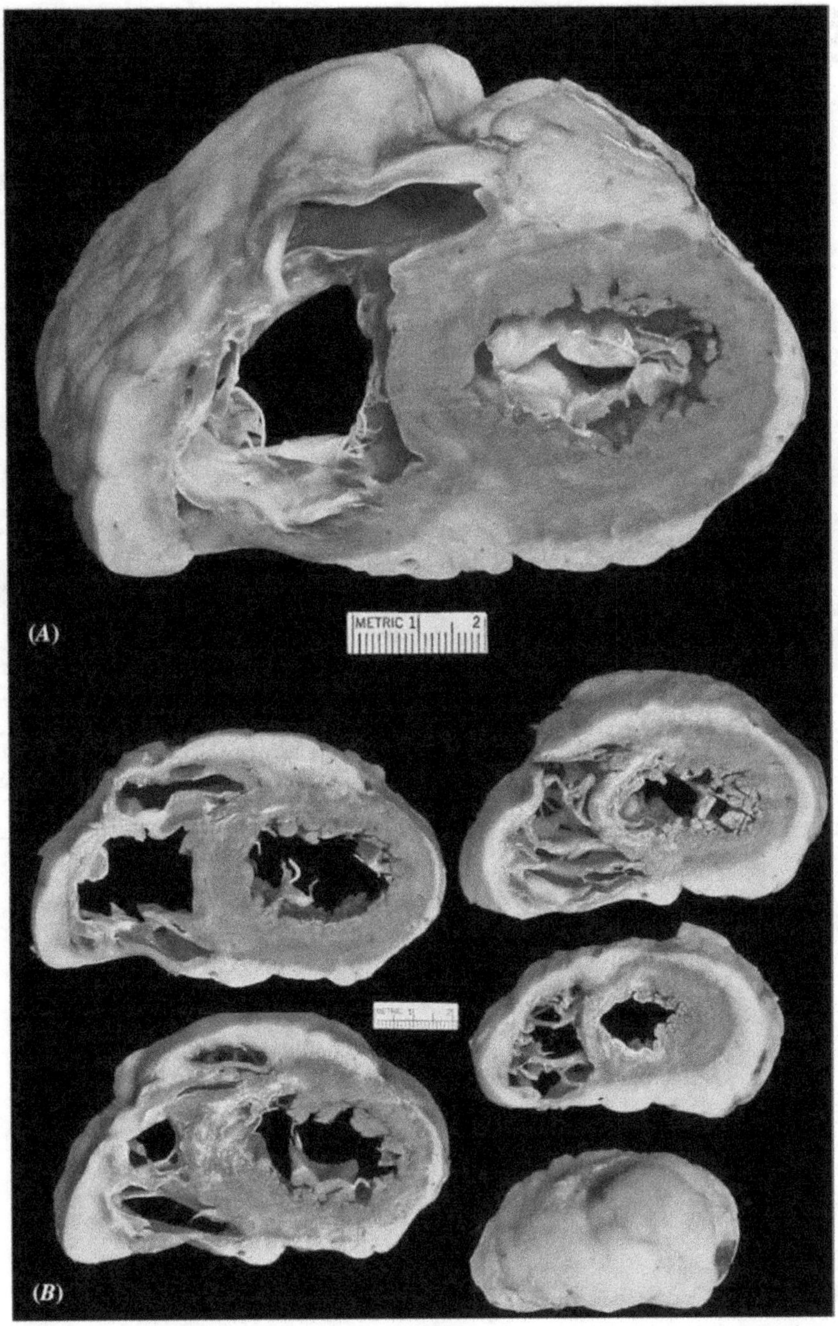


Figure 10. Case #10, Tables 1 and 2. Shown here is the heart in a 49-year-old woman. (*A*) Shown is the basal portion of the ventricles. The right ventricular cavity is considerably dilated and the left, minimally so. Portions of the endocardium of right ventricle are thickened by fibrous tissue and portions of the right ventricular free wall are replaced by fibrous tissue. No definite lesions are noted in the left ventricular free wall at the base. (*B*) Shown here are more apical cuts of the ventricular wall. The ventricular septum and the right ventricular free wall are extensively scarred. The epicardial coronary arteries were wide open. The total nonpaced 12-lead QRS voltage was 118 mm, and the heart weighed only 305 g. The heart floated in a container of formaldehyde.

between initially developing ARVC and the OHT procedure.[27] Strong features of the present report are that both the weight of the native heart and the extent of the cardiac lesions were known in all 11 patients. To our knowledge, total 12-lead electrocardiographic QRS voltage has not been described previously in patients with ARVC, and gross differing features of the hearts have not been well illustrated previously. The electrocardiographic findings may provide a clue to the diagnosis of ARVC (Figures 1–11).

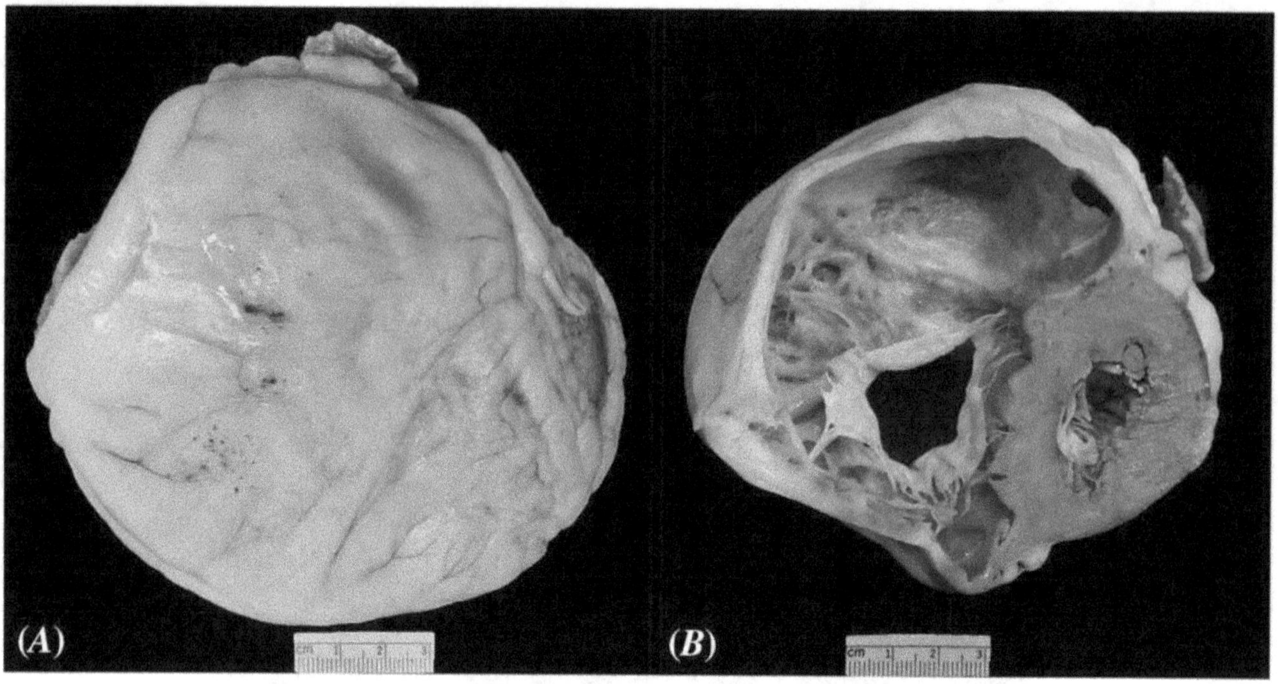


Figure 11. Case #11, Tables 1 and 2. Shown in *A* is the outside of the heart anteriorly. The right ventricular cavity is greatly dilated and totally covered by adipose tissue. (*B*) A photograph of the basal portion of the ventricles showing the enormously dilated right ventricular cavity and a normal-sized left ventricular cavity. About 90% of the right ventricular free wall is replaced by adipose tissue. The tricuspid valve annulus is greatly dilated. In contrast, no lesions are noted in the left ventricular free wall or in the ventricular septum. This patient was 70 years of age at the time of the OHT. ARVC was diagnosed clinically and the patient was found to have the nonsense mutation PKP2 c.235 C ->T (p.Arg79*), one of the mutations specific for ARVC. The same mutation was found in the patient's son and grandson, but neither had signs or symptoms of ARVC. The total nonpaced 12-lead QRS voltage was 52 mm, and the heart, which floated in formaldehyde, weighed only 285 g.


1. Roberts WC, Ko JM, Kuiper JJ, Hall SA, Meyer DM. Some previously neglected examples of arrhythmic right ventricular dysplasia/cardiomyopathy and frequency of its various reported manifestations. *Am J Cardiol* 2010;106:268–2074.
2. Marcus FI, Fontaine GH, Guiraudon G, Frank R, Laurenceau JL, Malergue C, Grosgogeat Y. Right ventricular dysplasia: a report of 24 adult cases. *Circulation* 1982;65:384–398.
3. Blomström-Lundqvist C, Sabel KG, Olsson SB. A long-term follow-up of 15 patients with arrhythmogenic right ventricular dysplasia. *Br Heart J* 1987;58:477–488.
4. Lemery R, Brugada P, Janssen J, Cheriex E, Dugernier T, Wellens HJ. Nonischemic sustained ventricular tachycardia: clinical outcome in 12 patients with arrhythmogenic right ventricular dysplasia. *J Am Coll Cardiol* 1989;14:96–105.
5. Pinamonti B, Sinagra G, Salvi A, Di Lenarda A, Morgera T, Silvestri F, Bussani R, Camerini F. Left ventricular involvement in right ventricular dysplasia. *Am Heart J* 1992;12:711–724.
6. Corrado D, Basso C, Thiene G, McKenna WJ, Davies MJ, Fontaliran F, Nava A, Silvestri F, Blomstrom-Lundqvist C, Wlodarska EK, Fontaine G, Camerini F. Spectrum of clinicopathologic manifestations of arrhythmogenic right ventricular cardiomyopathy/dysplasia: a multicenter study. *J Am Coll Cardiol* 1997;30:1512–1520.
7. Hulot JS, Jouven X, Empana JP, Frank R, Fontaine G. Natural history and risk stratification of arrhythmogenic right ventricular dysplasia/cardiomyopathy. *Circulation* 2004;110:1879–1884.
8. Dalal D, Nasir K, Bomma C, Prakasa K, Tandri H, Piccini J, Roguin A, Tichnell C, James C, Russell SD, Judge DP, Abraham T, Spevak PJ, Bluemke DA, Calkins H. Arrhythmogenic right ventricular dysplasia: a United States experience. *Circulation* 2005;112:3823–3832.
9. Marcus FI, Zareba W. The electrocardiogram in right ventricular cardiomyopathy/dysplasia. How can the electrocardiogram assist in understanding the pathologic and functional changes of the heart in this disease? *J Electrocardiol* 2009;42. 136.e1-136.e5.
10. Marcus FI, McKenna WJ, Sherrill D, Basso C, Bauce B, Bluemke DA, Calkins H, Corrado D, Cox MG, Daubert JP, Fontaine G, Gear K, Hauer R, Nava A, Picard MH, Protonotarios N, Saffitz JE, Sanborn DM, Steinberg JS, Tandri H, Thiene G, Towbin JA, Tsatsopoulou A, Wichter T, Zareba W. Diagnosis of arrhythmogenic right ventricular cardiomyopathy/dysplasia: proposed modification of the task force criteria. *Circulation* 2010;121:1533–1541.
11. Hauer RN, Cox MG, Groeneweg JA. Impact of new electrocardiographic criteria in arrhythmogenic cardiomyopathy. *Front Physiol* 2012;3:352.
12. Mast TP, James CA, Calkins H, Teske AJ, Tichnell C, Murray B, Loh PI, Russell SD, Velthuis BK, Judge DP, Dooijes D, Tedford RJ, van der Heijden JF, Tandri H, Hauer RN, Abraham TP, Doevendans PA, Te Riele AS, Cramer MJ. Evaluation of structural progression in arrhythmogenic right ventricular dysplasia/cardiomyopathy. *JAMA Cardiol* 2017;2:293–302.
13. Corrado D, Link MS, Calkins H. Arrhythmogenic right ventricular cardiomyopathy. *N Engl J Med* 2017;376:61–72.
14. Roberts WC, Podolak MJ. The king of hearts: analysis of 23 patients with hearts weighing 1000 grams or more. *Am J Cardiol* 1985;55:485–494.
15. Siegel RJ, Roberts WC. Electrocardiographic observations in severe aortic valve stenosis: correlative necropsy study to clinical, hemodynamic, and ECG variables demonstrating relation of 12-lead QRS amplitude to peak systolic transaortic pressure gradient. *Am Heart J* 1982;103:210–221.
16. Roberts WC, Day PJ. Electrocardiographic observations in clinically isolated, pure, chronic, severe aortic regurgitation: analysis of 30 necropsy patients aged 19 to 65 years. *Am J Cardiol* 1985;55:432–438.
17. Glick BN, Roberts WC. Usefulness of total 12-lead QRS voltage in diagnosing left ventricular hypertrophy in clinically isolated, pure, chronic, severe mitral regurgitation. *Am J Cardiol* 1992;70:1088–1092.
18. Dollar AL, Roberts WC. Usefulness of total 12-lead QRS voltage compared with other criteria for determining left ventricular hypertrophy in hypertrophic cardiomyopathy: analysis of 57 patients studied at necropsy. *Am J Med* 1989;87:377–381.
19. Shirani J, Maron BJ, Cannon RO III, Sheyda S, Roberts WC. Clinicopathologic features of hypertrophic cardiomyopathy managed by cardiac transplantation. *Am J Cardiol* 1993;72:434–440.

20. Roberts WC, Siegel RJ, McManus BM. Idiopathic dilated cardiomyopathy: analysis of 152 necropsy patients. *Am J Cardiol* 1987;60:1340–1355.
21. Shirani J, Roberts WC. Clinical electrocardiographic and morphologic features of massive fatty deposits ("lipomatous hypertrophy") in the atrial septum. *J Am Coll Cardiol* 1993;22:226–238.
22. Ross EM, Roberts WC. The carcinoid syndrome: comparison of 21 necropsy subjects with carcinoid heart disease to 15 necropsy subjects without carcinoid heart disease. *Am J Med* 1985;79:339–354.
23. Roberts WC, Barbin CM, Weissenborn MR, Ko JM. Electrocardiographic total 12-lead QRS voltage in patients having operative resection of syphilitic aortic aneurysm. *Am J Cardiol* 2015;116:973–976.
24. Shirani J, Berezowski K, Roberts WC. Quantitative measurement of normal and excessive (cor adiposum) subepicardial adipose tissue, its clinical significance, and its effect on electrocardiographic QRS voltage. *Am J Cardiol* 1995;76:414–418.
25. Roberts WC, Waller BF. Cardiac amyloidosis causing cardiac dysfunction: analysis of 54 necropsy patients. *Am J Cardiol* 1983;52:137–146.
26. Roberts WC, Becker TM, Hall SA. Usefulness of total 12-lead QRS voltage as a clue to diagnosis of patients with cardiac sarcoidosis severe enough to warrant orthotopic heart transplant. *JAMA Cardiol* 2018;3:64–68.
27. Wilensky RL, Yudelman P, Cohen AI, Fletcher RD, Atkinson J, Virmani R, Roberts WC. Serial electrocardiographic changes in idiopathic dilated cardiomyopathy confirmed at necropsy. *Am J Cardiol* 1988;62:276–283.

# Total 12-Lead QRS Voltage in Patients Having Orthotopic Heart Transplantation for Heart Failure Caused by Adriamycin-Induced Cardiomyopathy

William C. Roberts[a, b] Sarah Haque[c] Shelley A. Hall[b]

[a]Baylor Scott and White Heart and Vascular Institute, Baylor University Medical Center, Dallas, TX, USA; [b]Division of Cardiology, Departments of Pathology and Internal Medicine, Baylor University Medical Center, Dallas, TX, USA; [c]Austin College, Sherman, TX, USA

**Keywords**

Adriamycin cardiomyopathy · Cardiotoxicity · Orthotopic heart transplantation

**Abstract**

***Objective:*** Although several studies have described the effects of adriamycin on the heart, electrocardiographic total 12-lead QRS voltage (distance in millimeters from the peak of the R wave to the nadir of either the Q or S wave, whichever was deeper, with 10 mm [1 mV] being standard) both before and after orthotopic heart transplantation (OHT) has not been reported. This study describes the total 12-lead QRS voltage in 8 patients studied at Baylor University Medical Center at Dallas, from 1994 to June 2018, who underwent OHT for severe heart failure caused by anthracycline-induced cardiomyopathy. ***Method:*** Prior to OHT, the total 12-lead non-paced QRS voltages ranged from 86 to 189 mm (mean 125 ± 56) and for paced QRS voltages from 82 to 113 mm (mean 97 ± 15). The total 12-lead QRS voltages post-OHT ranged from 100 to 190 mm (mean 130 ± 30). Total 12-lead QRS voltages were lower in patients with a pacemaker than without. ***Results/Conclusion:*** These low voltages are like those found in patients with carcinoid syndrome, severe cardiac adiposity, cardiac amyloidosis, and cardiac sarcoidosis.



## Introduction

Orthotopic heart transplantation (OHT) has proven to be a useful therapy for patients with heart failure (HF) secondary to adriamycin cardiotoxicity [1]. Little electrocardiographic data are available in patients with HF secondary to adriamycin toxicity severe enough to warrant OHT. To fill this void, we measured the total 12-lead QRS voltage in 8 patients who underwent OHT for severe HF secondary to adriamycin cardiotoxicity.

## Materials and Methods

Review of all OHT cases performed at Baylor University Medical Center at Dallas from 1994 through June 2018, a 24-year period, yielded 8 patients who had received anthracycline therapy. The native hearts for all 8 patients were examined and described by one of us (W.C.R.). The clinical records and all available electrocardiograms recorded between the onset of HF and OTH for each patient were reviewed. The total 12-lead QRS voltage was measured by S.H. and confirmed by W.C.R.

## Results

The pertinent clinical, electrocardiographic, and morphologic findings are summarized in Table 1. Three patients had non-Hodgkin lymphoma, 3 had breast cancer, and 2 had leukemia. At the time of cancer diagnosis and treatment, the patients ranged in age from 6 to 64 years (mean 36 ± 20),

**Table 1.** Pertinent clinical and morphological findings in 8 patients with adriamycin-induced cardiomyopathy

| Case No. | Age at cancer Dx and Rx, years | Age at OHT, years | Year of OHT | Type of cancer | Rad Rx | Height, in | Body weight, lb | BMI | EF, % | Paced | QRS amplitude in each electrocardiographic lead | | | | | | | | | | | | Total 12-lead QRS voltage, mm | HW, g | Floating heart | Alive in 6/2018 | Intervals, days | |
|---|---|---|---|---|---|---|---|---|---|---|---|---|---|---|---|---|---|---|---|---|---|---|---|---|---|---|---|---|
| | | | | | | | | | | | I | II | III | aVR | aVL | aVF | V1 | V2 | V3 | V4 | V5 | V6 | | | | | P or NP ECG to OHT | OHT to PHT ECG |
| Men | | | | | | | | | | | | | | | | | | | | | | | | | | | | |
| 1 | 8 | 26 | 4/2015 | Leukemia | no | 70 | 183 | 26 | 10 | NP | 11 | 7 | 10 | 7 | 9 | 9 | 20 | 36 | 24 | 15 | 19 | 22 | | | | | | |
| | | | | | | | | | | PHT | 12 | 9 | 13 | 8 | 11 | 9 | 6 | 13 | 14 | 8 | 9 | 9 | 121 | | | | | |
| 2 | 6 | 30 | 9/2008 | Leukemia | no | 71 | 185 | 27 | 15 | P | 2 | 5 | 5 | 2 | 5 | 4 | 11 | 14 | 18 | 6 | 5 | 5 | 82 | 365 | no | no | 109 | 14 |
| | | | | | | | | | | PHT | 7 | 7 | 7 | 6 | 6 | 5 | 16 | 35 | 49 | 32 | 12 | 8 | 190 | | | | | |
| 3 | 50 | 55 | 5/2011 | Lymphoma[1] | no | 68 | 220 | 33 | 15 | P | 4 | 12 | 10 | 5 | 5 | 8 | 5 | 5 | 5 | 7 | 10 | 8 | 84 | 525 | yes | yes | 46 | 135 |
| | | | | | | | | | | PHT | 11 | 7 | 5 | 9 | 8 | 3 | 9 | 16 | 15 | 16 | 15 | 10 | 124 | | | | | |
| Women | | | | | | | | | | | | | | | | | | | | | | | | | | | | |
| 4 | 30 | 37 | 5/2017 | Lymphoma[1] | yes | 62 | 180 | 33 | 15 | NP | 4 | 7 | 12 | 4 | 8 | 10 | 9 | 14 | 10 | 8 | 7 | 6 | 99 | 260 | yes | yes | 252 | 32 |
| | | | | | | | | | | PHT | 9 | 1 | 9 | 5 | 10 | 5 | 8 | 23 | 7 | 8 | 8 | 7 | 100 | | | | | |
| 5 | 38 | 50 | 5/2007 | Breast | yes | 64 | 180 | 31 | 10 | NP | 5 | 3 | 5 | 2 | 4 | 4 | 5 | 9 | 18 | 12 | 11 | 8 | 86 | 405 | yes | yes | 16 | 27 |
| | | | | | | | | | | PHT | 12 | 5 | 11 | 7 | 11 | 4 | 8 | 9 | 10 | 10 | 12 | 10 | 109 | | | | | |
| 6 | 41 | 64 | 5/2004 | Breast | yes | 63 | 135 | 24 | 10 | P | 7 | 6 | 7 | 6 | 6 | 6 | 5 | 2 | 28 | 18 | 11 | 9 | 111 | 325 | no | no | 47 | 14 |
| | | | | | | | | | | PHT | 9 | 10 | 8 | 10 | 6 | 6 | 9 | 20 | 24 | 21 | 17 | 11 | 151 | | | | | |
| 7 | 49 | 65 | 3/2011 | Lymphoma[1] | yes | 61 | 146 | 28 | – | P | 8 | 10 | 16 | 8 | 4 | 16 | 6 | 6 | 13 | 5 | 14 | 7 | 113 | 560 | yes | yes | 74 | 184 |
| | | | | | | | | | | PHT | 12 | 8 | 11 | 10 | 14 | 6 | 8 | 7 | 8 | 8 | 9 | 12 | 113 | | | | | |
| 8 | 64 | 68 | 9/2011 | Breast | no | 64 | 155 | 27 | 15 | P | 4 | 5 | 8 | 2 | 6 | 5 | 3 | 5 | 20 | 18 | 11 | 8 | 95 | 500 | yes | yes | 98 | 14 |
| | | | | | | | | | | PHT | 10 | 5 | 7 | 7 | 9 | 3 | 5 | 14 | 18 | 23 | 20 | 14 | 135 | | | | | |

AF, atrial fibrillation; BMI, body mass index; CI, cardiac index; Dx, diagnosis; ECG, electrocardiogram; EF, ejection fraction; HW, heart weight; LV, left ventricular; NP, non-paced; OHT, orthotopic heart transplant; P, paced; PHT, post-OHT; Rad, radiation; Rx, treatment; –, no information available. [1] Non-Hodgkin lymphoma.

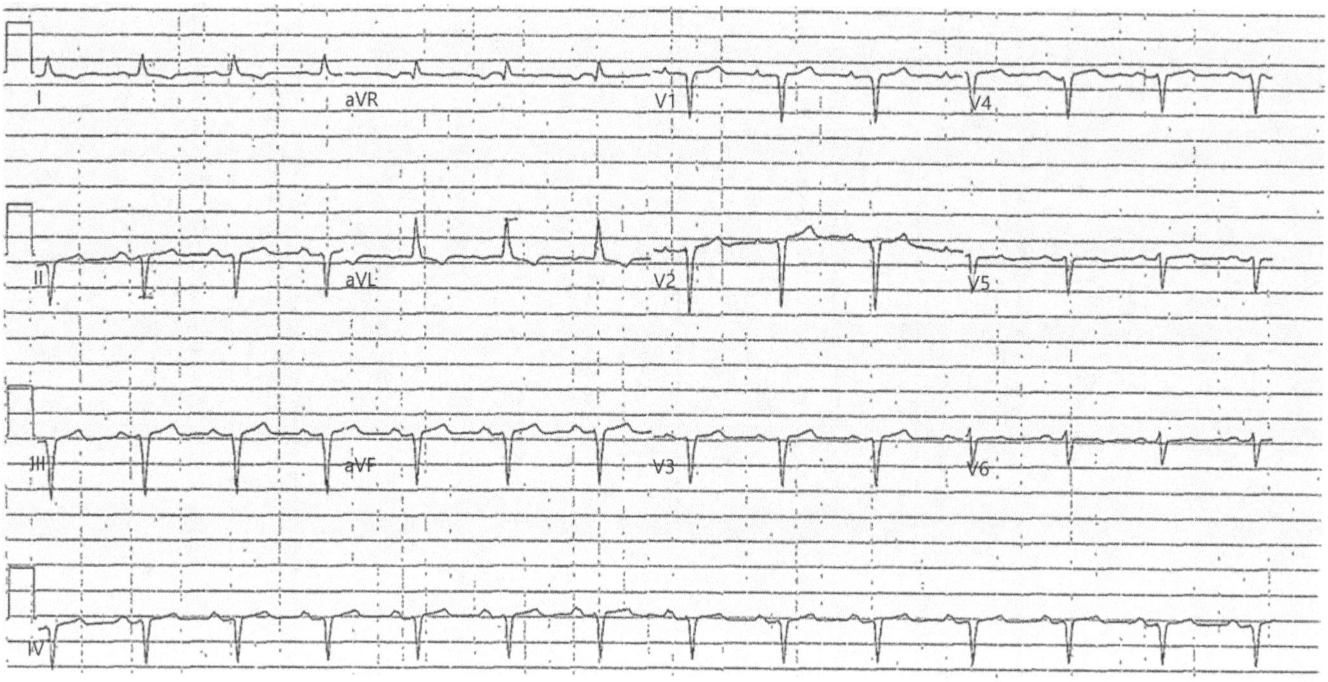


**Fig. 1.** Case No. 4. Pre-OHT non-paced electrocardiogram. The total 12-lead QRS voltage was 99 mm.

and at OHT from 26 to 68 years (mean 49 ± 17). The interval from the start of anthracycline treatment to OHT ranged from 4 to 24 years (mean 14 ± 8). Of the 8 patients, 3 were men and 5 were women. The body mass index ranged from 24 to 33 (mean 29 ± 3). The heart weights ranged from 260 to 558 g (mean 414 ± 105). Four patients were known to have received mediastinal irradiation at some point during chemotherapy. Adriamycin-induced cardiomyopathy was diagnosed prior to OHT in all 8 patients.

We obtained 3 non-paced and 5 paced pre-OHT electrocardiographic tracings and all 8 post-transplant tracings (Fig. 1). The total 12-lead QRS voltages prior to OHT ranged from 82 to 189 mm (mean 107 ± 49). Tracings for pre-OHT non-paced patients ranged from 86 to 189 mm (mean 125 ± 56), while pre-OHT paced voltages ranged from 82 to 113 mm (mean 97 ± 15). The total 12-lead QRS voltage post-OHT ranged from 100 to 190 mm (mean 130 ± 30). The basal portions of the cardiac ventricles in 4 of the 8 patients are shown in Figure 2.

## Discussion and Conclusion

Described herein are total 12-lead electrographic QRS voltages and characteristics of the native hearts of 8 patients who underwent OHT for HF caused by adriamycin-induced cardiomyopathy. The total paced and non-paced (means 97 ± 15 and 125 ± 56 mm, respectively) 12-lead QRS voltages seen in these 8 patients are similar to those found in carcinoid syndrome (mean 117 mm), cardiac adiposity (mean 120 mm), cardiac amyloidosis (mean 104 mm), and cardiac sarcoidosis (mean 117 mm) [2]. The native hearts had no grossly visible myocardial lesions in any of the 8 patients [3, 4].

A positive feature of this report is that it is the first to describe total 12-lead electrocardiographic QRS voltages in patients with HF secondary to adriamycin-induced cardiomyopathy severe enough to warrant OHT. A limitation of the present report is the small number of patients studied and particularly the small number of electrocardiograms available before pacemaker insertion. Also, the amount of adriamycin administered years before the OHT is not known.

## Acknowledgements

We thank Saba Ilyas for her excellent photographic work.

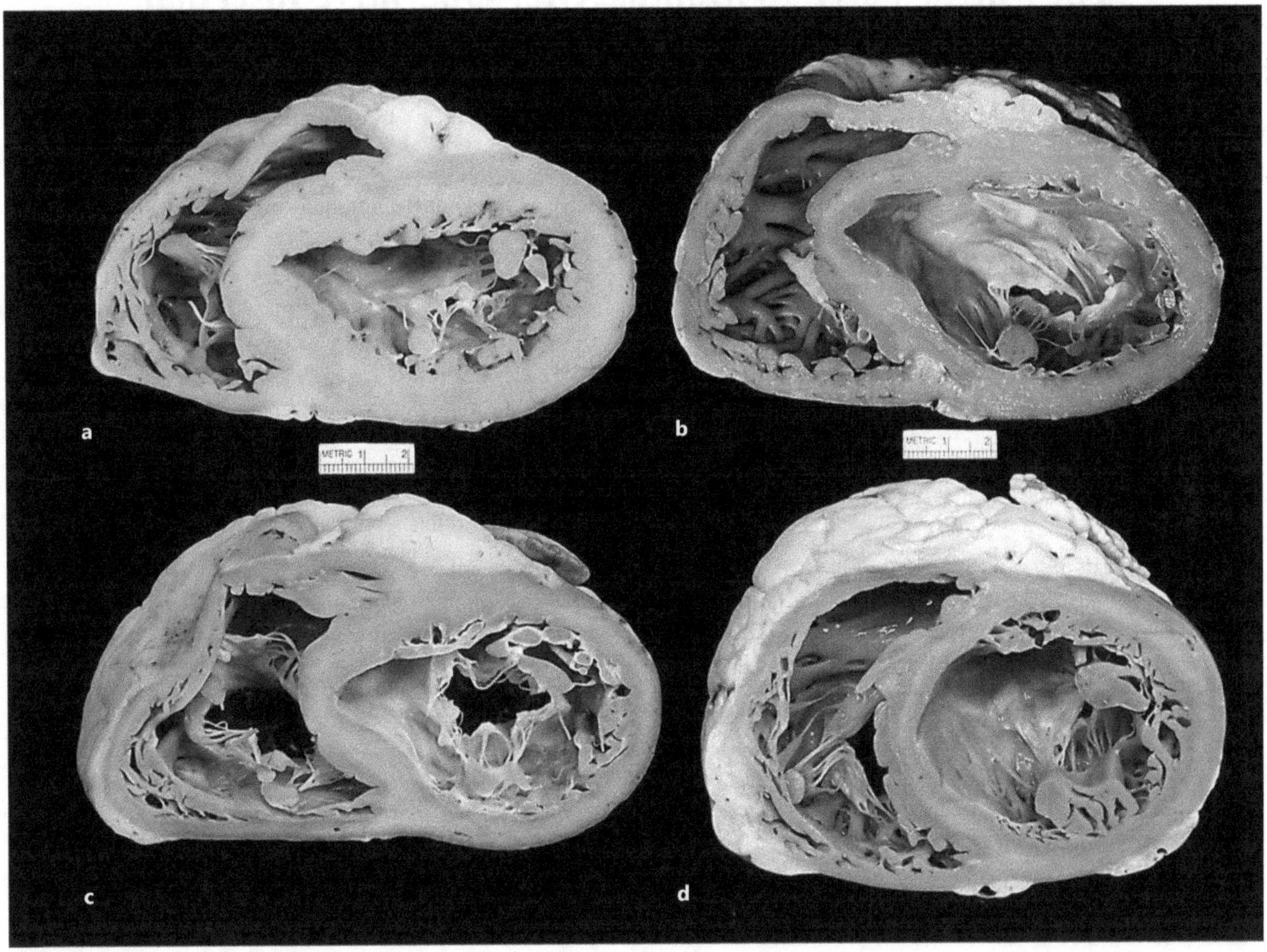

**Fig. 2.** Views of the basal portion of the ventricles in 4 patients having OHT for adriamycin cardiotoxicity. **a** Case No. 1. The total non-paced 12-lead QRS voltage prior to OHT was 189 mm and the heart weighed 370 g. **b** Case No. 2. The total non-paced 12-lead QRS voltage prior to OHT was 82 mm and the heart weighed 365 g. **c** Case No. 4. The total non-paced 12-lead QRS voltage prior to OHT was 99 mm and the heart weighed 260 g. **d** Case No. 5. The total non-paced 12-lead QRS voltage prior to OHT was 86 mm and the heart weighed 405 g.

## Statement of Ethics

The authors have no ethical conflicts to disclose.

## Disclosure Statement

The authors have no conflicts of interest to declare.

## References


1 Lenneman AJ, Wang L, Wigger M, Frangoul H, Harrell FE, Silverstein C, et al. Heart transplant survival outcomes for adriamycin-dilated cardiomyopathy. Am J Cardiol. 2013 Feb; 111(4):609–12.

2 Roberts WC, Filardo G, Ko JM, Siegel RJ, Dollar AL, Ross EM, et al. Comparison of total 12-lead QRS voltage in a variety of cardiac conditions and its usefulness in predicting increased cardiac mass. Am J Cardiol. 2013 Sep; 112(6):904–9.

3 Lefrak EA, Pitha J, Rosenheim S, Gottlieb JA. A clinicopathologic analysis of adriamycin cardiotoxicity. Cancer. 1973 Aug;32(2):302–14.

4 Isner JM, Ferrans VJ, Cohen SR, Witkind BG, Virmani R, Gottdiener JS, et al. Clinical and morphologic cardiac findings after anthracycline chemotherapy. Analysis of 64 patients studied at necropsy. Am J Cardiol. 1983 Apr; 51(7):1167–74.

# The Mitral Valve 16 Months After Operative Insertion of the Alfieri Stitch

Samreen Fathima, MD, Shelley A. Hall, MD, Paul A. Grayburn, MD, and William C. Roberts, MD*

**We describe considerable fibrous thickening of the mitral leaflets 16 months after insertion of an Alfieri stitch in a previously anatomically normal but functionally regurgitant mitral valve. Whether this type of mitral thickening will occur after percutaneous insertion of the mitral clip for pure mitral regurgitation remains to be determined.**  **(Am J Cardiol 2019;123:695−696)**

In the early 1990s, Alfieri et al[1] introduced what became known as "The Alfieri Stitch," a bowtie procedure or edge-to-edge mitral valve repair for patients with pure mitral regurgitation. The operation usually decreased the severity of the mitral regurgitation and it usually reduced the pulmonary arterial pressure. The procedure, however, was not without complications, a major one being the conversion of the previous mitral regurgitation to mitral stenosis. Subsequently, of course, percutaneous transcatheter mitral valve repair has proved to be effective and has replaced the operative approach.[2–5] Only 1 published photo late after insertion of "the stitch" has been found.[6] The present report describes another patient who had "the stitch" operatively inserted months earlier.

## Case Description

A 19-year-old man, who was born in January 1998, had heart failure (HF) shortly after birth. The degree of HF waxed and waned during the next 15 or so years. By June 2016 (age 17), the HF had reached the point that a left ventricular assist device was inserted and at the same procedure an Alfieri stitch was placed on the mitral leaflets to decrease the degree of functional mitral regurgitation. Neither the left ventricular assist device nor the Alfieri stitch proved to be beneficial. The patient gained 40 pounds during the next several months because of worsening HF. An echocardiogram 6 months before the heart transplant showed mild mitral regurgitation, thickening of the distal third of the mitral leaflets, severe dilatation of both ventricular cavities, and severe tricuspid valve regurgitation (Figure 1). Echocardiographic findings before and after placement of the Alfieri stitch are summarized in Table 1. In October 2017 (age 18), heart transplantation was performed. Examination of the native heart showed it to be typical of idiopathic dilated cardiomyopathy. It weighed 330 g. The mitral leaflets, which had been anatomically normal at the time of insertion of the Alfieri stitch, were now quite thickened by fibrous tissue, particularly in their distal halves (Figure 2). When contacted in November 2018, 13 months after the heart transplant, the patient was asymptomatic and working.

## Discussion

Described in this report is considerable fibrous thickening of the mitral leaflets after insertion of an Alfieri stitch 16 months earlier. Today, the Alfieri stitch operation is infrequently performed but the insertion of the mitral clip by the percutaneous route is now frequently performed.[2–4] Whether the percutaneous approach will also cause the leaflets to thicken and potentially convert an occasional patient from pure mitral regurgitation to mitral stenosis remains to be seen.

## Disclosures

The investigators have no conflicts of interest to disclose.

1. Alfieri O, Maisano F, De Bonis M, Stefano PL, Torracca L, Oppizzi M, La Canna G. The double-orifice technique in mitral valve repair: a simple solution for complex problems. *J Thorac Cardiovasc Surg* 2001;122:674–681.
2. Feldman T, Kar S, Rinaldi M, Fail P, Hermiller J, Smalling R. Percutaneous mitral repair with the MitraClip system: safety and midterm durability in the initial EVEREST (endovascular valve edge-to-edge repair study) cohort. *J Am Coll Cardiol* 2009;54:686–694.
3. Maisano F, La Canna G, Colombo A, Alfieri O. The evolution from surgery to percutaneous mitral valve interventions: the role of the edge-to-edge technique. *J Am Coll Cardiol* 2011;58:2174–2182.
4. Feldman T, Foster E, Glower DD, Glower DG, Kar S, Rinaldi MJ, Fail PS, Smalling RW, Siegel R, Rose GA, Engeron E, Loghin C, Trento A, Skipper ER, Fudge T, Letsou GV, Massaro JM, Mauri L. EVEREST II Investigators. Percutaneous repair or surgery for mitral regurgitation. *N Engl J Med* 2011;364:1395–1406.
5. Stone GW, Lindenfeld JA, Abraham WT, Kar S, Lim DS, Mishell JM, Whisenant B, Grayburn PA, Rinaldi M, Kapadia SR, Rajagopal V, Sarembock IJ, Brieke A, Marx SO, Cohen DJ, Weissman NJ, Mack MJ. for the COAPT Investigators. Transcatheter mitral-valve repair in patients with heart failure. *N Engl J Med* 2018;379:2307–2318.
6. Privitera S, Butany J, Cusimano RJ, Silversides C, Ross H, Leask R. Alfieri mitral valve repair clinical outcome and pathology. *Circulation* 2002;106:173–174.

Baylor Scott & White Heart and Vascular Institute, the Departments of Pathology and Internal Medicine (Division of Cardiology), Baylor University Medical Center, Dallas, Texas. Manuscript received August 7, 2018; revised manuscript received and accepted November 12, 2018.

See page 695 for disclosure information.

*Corresponding author: Tel: (214) 820-7911; fax: (214) 820-7533.
*E-mail address:* William.Roberts1@bswhealth.org (W.C. Roberts).

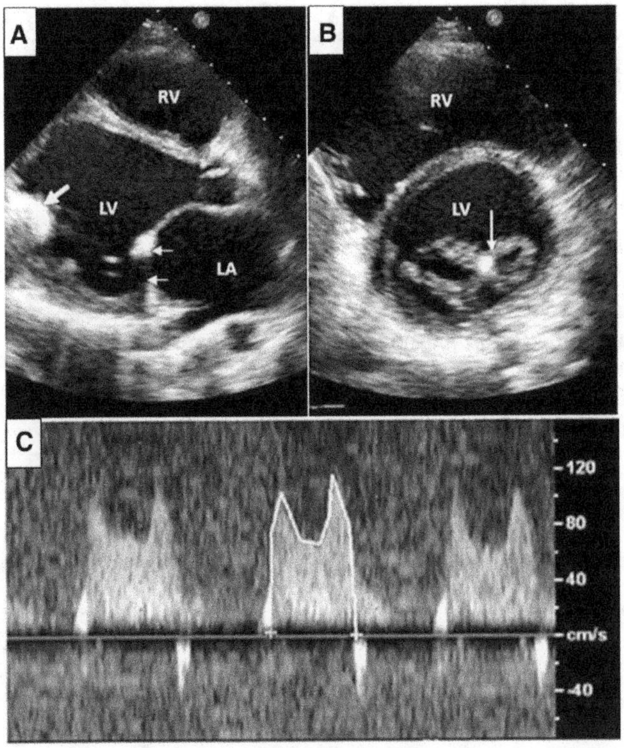


Figure 1. Echocardiographic images after insertion of a left ventricular assist device (LVAD) and Alfieri stitch. (*A*) Parasternal long-axis view showing thickened mitral leaflets with restricted diastolic excursion (*small arrows*). Both ventricular cavities and the left atrium are dilated (left ventricle at end-diastole = 6.2 cm, and at peak systole = 5.9 cm). The LVAD cannula is seen at lower left (*large arrow*). (*B*) Parasternal short-axis view showing Alfieri stitch (*arrow*) with double orifice mitral valve. (*C*) Mean transmitral gradient is 3 mm Hg by continuous wave Doppler.

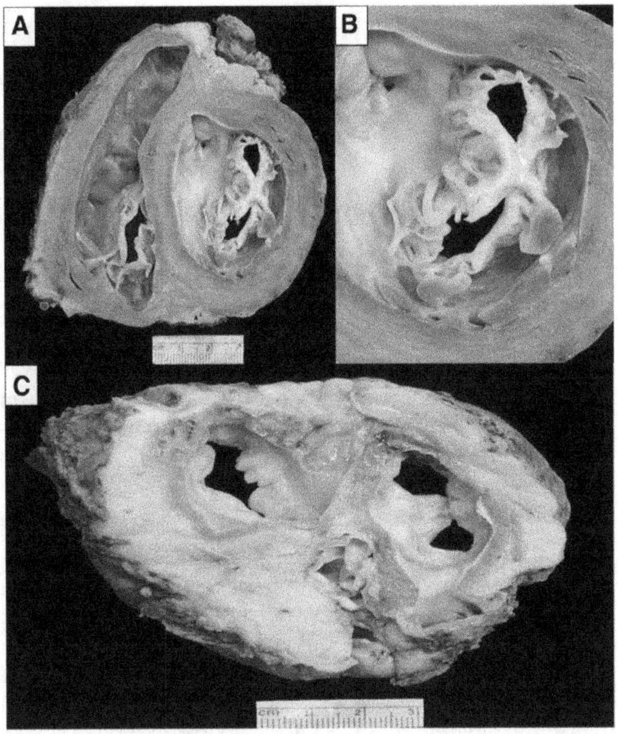


Figure 2. Photographs of the heart of patient described. (*A*). Cross section of the ventricles at the level of tricuspid and mitral valves showing the ventricular aspect of the Alfieri stitch. (*B*) A close-up of the mitral valves from the ventricular aspect. (*C*) View of the tricuspid and mitral valves after "deroofing" the atrial walls. The quantity of adipose tissue in the atrioventricular sulci is excessive.

Table 1
Echocardiographic data before and after placement of the Alfieri stitch

| Variable | Pre-OP (days) | Post-OP (days) | |
|---|---|---|---|
| | −10 | +1 | +330 |
| Peak velocity in early diastolic transmitral flow (m/s) | 1.8 | 1.1 | 1.0 |
| Decel time (m/s) | 230 | 89 | 282 |
| Mean gradient (mm Hg) | 0 | 6 | 3 |
| Mitral regurgitation (0-3+) | 3+ | 1+ | 3+ |
| Left ventricular internal diameter end diastole (mm) | 83 | 74 | 62 |
| Left ventricular posterior wall, peak systole (mm) | 69 | – | 59 |
| Left ventricular posterior wall, end diastole (mm) | 7 | 8 | 6 |
| Left ventricular ejection fraction (%) | 37 | 34 | 10 |

# Orthotopic Heart Transplantation for Ankylosing Spondylitis Masquerading as Nonischemic Cardiomyopathy

Samarthkumar J. Thakkar, MD[a], Paul A. Grayburn, MD[a,b], Shelley Anne Hall, MD[a,b], and William C. Roberts, MD[a,b,c,*]

**Described herein is a 48-year-old man who underwent orthotopic heart transplantation because of severe heart failure considered clinically due to idiopathic dilated cardiomyopathy, but examination of the operatively excised native heart disclosed classic features of ankylosing spondylitis. Orthotopic heart transplantation for this condition has not been reported previously.**  **(Am J Cardiol 2019;123:1732–1735)**

We recently studied the heart of a patient who had undergone orthotopic heart transplantation (OHT) for presumed idiopathic dilated cardiomyopathy and examination of the operatively excised heart disclosed it to have classic morphologic features of ankylosing spondylitis.[1,2] The patient clinically had aortic regurgitation, complete heart block, and periodic low back pain. Search of PubMed failed to disclose any report of OHT for ankylosing spondylitis. A description of this patient is the purpose of this report.

## Case Description

A 48-year-old male roofer, who was born in March 1970, had been well until May 2011 (age 41) when he developed the sudden onset of dyspnea and was hospitalized. His systolic blood pressure was about 200 mm Hg, his coronary arteries were free of obstructive lesions, and his left ventricular ejection fraction was about 15%. He was started on valsartan, carvedilol, isosorbide dinitrate, and amlodipine, but despite these medicines, he had frequent episodes of acute heart failure. During one episode in March 2015, he was found to have abnormal kidney function and an atrophic left kidney (cause unknown) that was excised. The main artery to the right kidney was found to be stenotic and a stent was inserted. At that time, he developed complete heart block and a dual chamber pacemaker was inserted. In July 2016, he was started on peritoneal dialysis and 2 months later, hemodialysis. In July 2017, cardiac resynchronization therapy defibrillator was inserted.

In April 2018, he developed cardiogenic shock and pulmonary edema and was transferred to Baylor University Medical Center at Dallas. On arrival, his blood pressure was 160/80 mm Hg. A precordial murmur was not heard but his respirations were extremely rapid. The electrocardiogram (Figure 1) showed atrial-sensed ventricular-paced rhythm and total 12-lead QRS voltage of 152 mm (10-mm standard).[3] The echocardiogram (Figure 2) showed the left ventricular chamber to be severely dilated, the ejection fraction to be about 20%, and severe aortic regurgitation to be present. At cardiac catheterization, the cardiac index was 1.5 L/min/m$^2$. Certain laboratory findings are listed in Table 1.

He underwent combined heart and kidney transplant in May 2018. The native heart weighed 675 g (Figures 3 and 4). The left ventricular cavity was considerably dilated longitudinally: the distance from the base of the right aortic valve cusp to the apex was 9.5 cm. The anterior mitral leaflet was severely thickened by dense fibrous tissue, and the posterior mitral leaflet was normal. The bases of each aortic cusp were thickened by similar fibrous tissue which extended cephalad onto the aorta in the areas of the commissures. The epicardial coronary arteries were free of atherosclerotic plaques.

## Discussion

Described herein is a 48-year-old man who underwent OHT because of severe heart failure attributed clinically to idiopathic dilated cardiomyopathy. Study of his explanted native heart, however, disclosed classic (specific) morphologic findings of ankylosing spondylitis,[1,2] distinctive and different from other cardiac conditions (Figure 5). Before OHT, echocardiogram disclosed severe aortic regurgitation. Although the degree of aortic regurgitation in our patient was severe by echocardiogram, a precordial murmur was not detected while in severe heart failure, probably the result of his rapid respiratory rate and his obesity (body mass index 33 kg/m$^2$). A precordial murmur had been present earlier when he was not in heart failure. His pulse pressure when hospitalized at our institution was 80 mm Hg.

Aortic regurgitation appears to occur in about 20% of patients with ankylosing spondylitis[4] and it usually appears after the appearance of the orthopedic consequences, although the reverse occurs, as in the present patient, on occasion. The severe thickening of the anterior mitral leaflet in ankylosing spondylitis in the

[a]Baylor Scott and White Heart and Vascular Institute, Baylor University Medical Center, Dallas, Texas; [b]Department of Internal Medicine (Division of Cardiology), Baylor University Medical Center, Dallas, Texas; and [c]Department of Pathology, Baylor University Medical Center, Dallas, Texas. Manuscript received November 1, 2018; revised manuscript received February 11, 2019; revised manuscript received and accepted February 11, 2019.

See page 1734 for disclosure information.

*Corresponding author: Tel: (214) 820-7911; fax: (214) 820-7533.

*E-mail address:* william.roberts1@BSWHealth.org (W.C. Roberts).

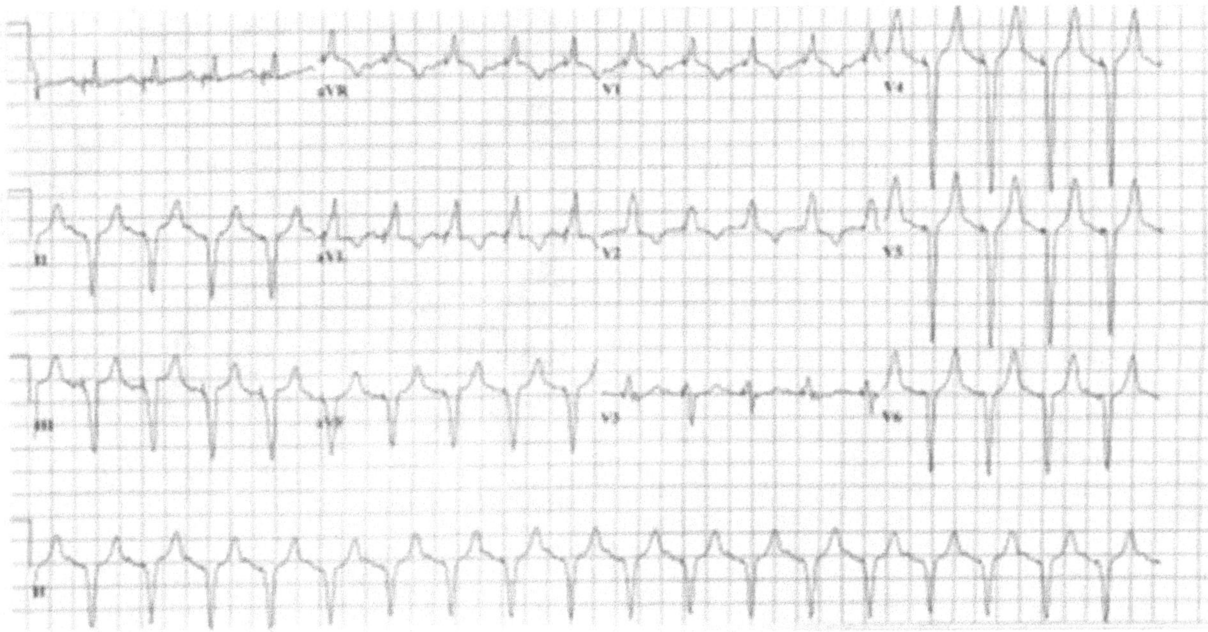

Figure 1. Electrocardiogram, recorded at the time of presentation, showing atrial-sensed ventricular-paced rhythm, biventricular pacemaker, and the total 12-lead QRS voltage of 152 mm.

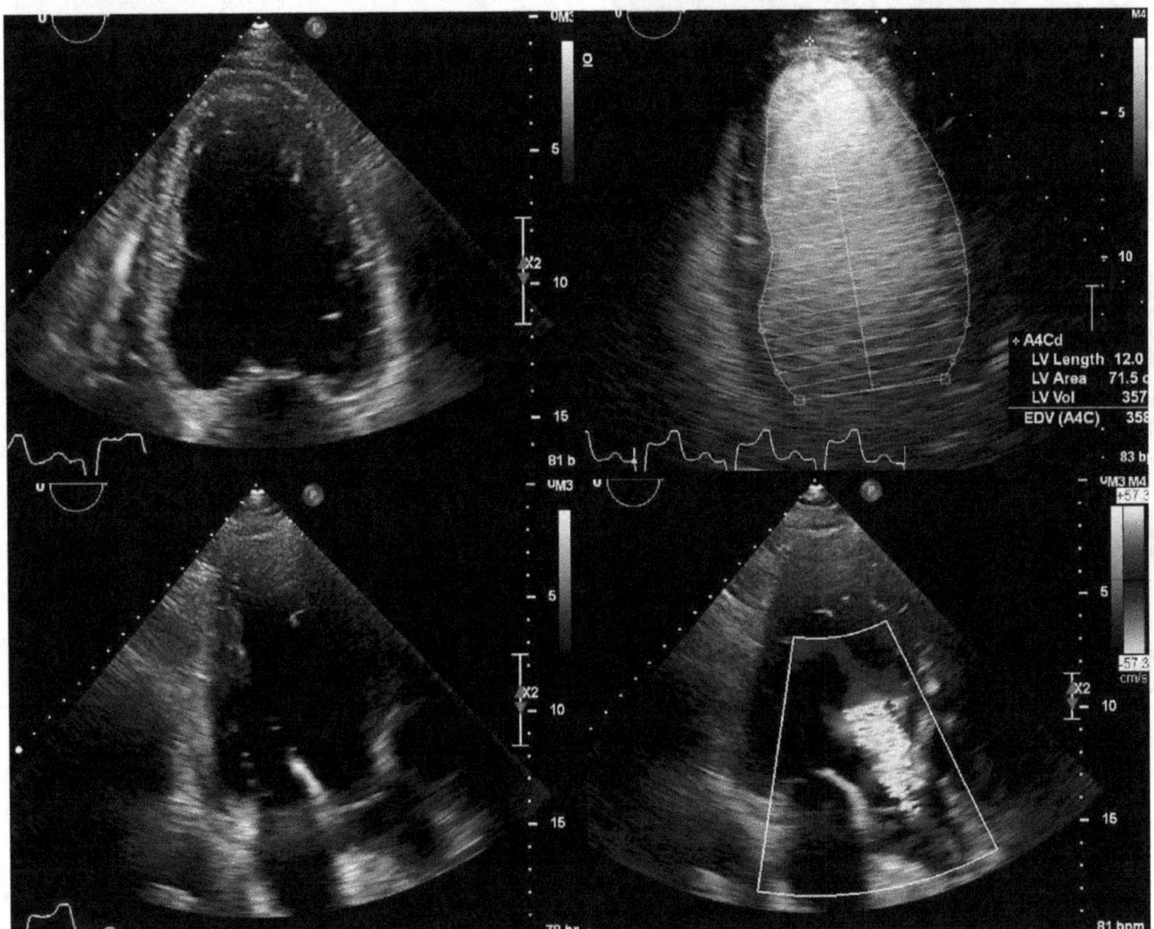


Figure 2. *Top left*: Apical 4-chamber view showing severely dilated, elongated left ventricle (LV) with normal right ventricular (RV) size and systolic function. An ICD lead is seen in the RV (arrow). *Top right*: Apical 4-chamber end-diastolic frame with ultrasound contrast. LV end-diastolic volume was 358 ml with LVEF 19% by biplane Simpson's method. *Bottom left*: Apical long-axis view showing severely thickened, restricted anterior mitral leaflet (yellow arrow). The posterior leaflet (white arrow) was of normal thickness and motion. *Bottom right*: Apical long-axis view with color Doppler imaging showing severe aortic regurgitation (AR).

Table 1
Pertinent admission laboratory findings in the patient described

| | |
|---|---|
| B-type natriuretic peptide (pg/ml) | 1895 |
| Creatinine (mg/dl) | 18 |
| Blood urea nitrogen (mg/dl) | 77 |
| Estimated GFR (ml/min/1.73 $m^2$) | 3 |
| Sodium (meq/L) | 136 |
| Potassium (meq/L) | 5.2 |
| Calcium (mg/dl) | 8.7 |
| Magnesium (mg/dl) | 2.2 |
| Phosphorous (mg/dl) | 2.0 |
| Total cholesterol (mg/dl) | 219 |
| Low density lipoprotein cholesterol (mg/dl) | 151 |
| High density lipoprotein cholesterol (mg/dl) | 35 |
| Triglyceride (mg/dl) | 241 |
| Hemoglobin A1c (%) | 5.8 |
| Rheumatic factor ([IU]/ml)* | 8 |
| ANA* | Negative |
| HLA-B 27* | Negative |
| C-reactive protein (mg/dl)* | 0.5 |

GFR = glomerular filtration rate.
* Test performed 6 months after the orthotopic heart transplant.

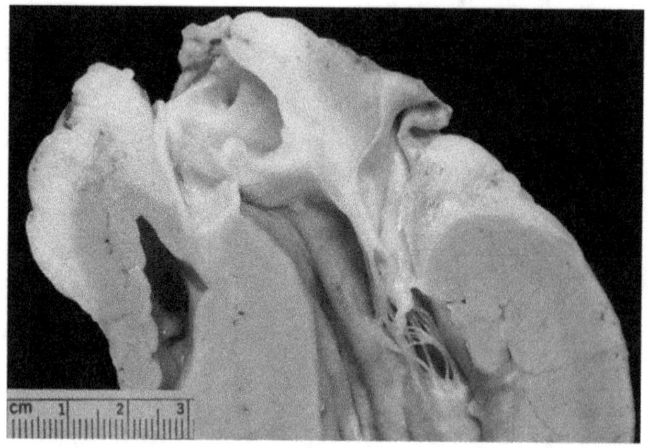

Figure 4. Shown here is a closer view of the mitral and aortic valve showing the remarkably thickened anterior mitral leaflet which is extending into the base of the posterior aortic valve cusp. The posterior mitral leaflet is normal.

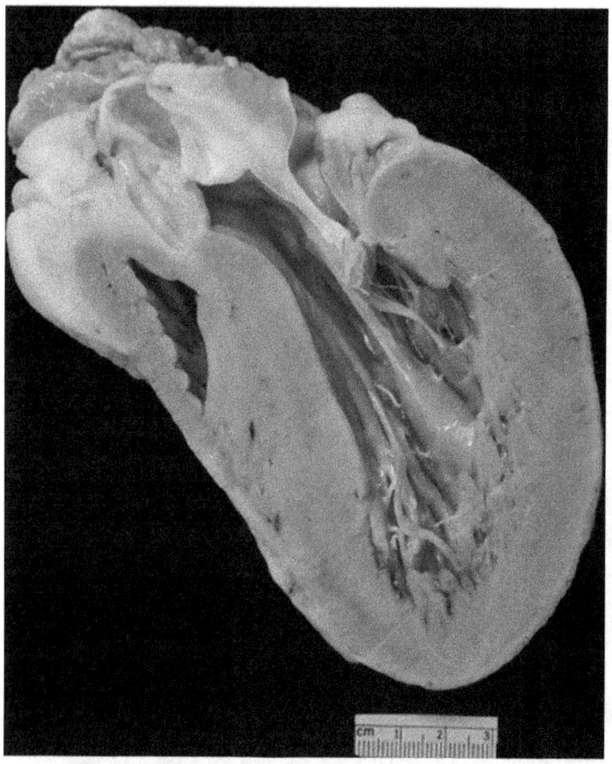

Figure 3. Shown here is the heart of a 48-year-old man showing a dilated left ventricular cavity with thickened left ventricular walls, enlarged papillary muscles, and thickened anterior mitral leaflet. The posterior mitral leaflet is normal (not thickened).

absence of thickening of the posterior mitral leaflet as shown in the present patient is diagnostic (Figure 5). Although all 8 patients (all men) with ankylosing spondylitis studied by Buckley and Roberts[1] at necropsy had extremely severe aortic regurgitation, only one of the 187 patients with ankylosing spondylitis studied clinically by Klingberg et al[4] had "severe" aortic regurgitation; 24 others had "mild", and 9 had "moderate" aortic regurgitation.

Interview of the patient and his wife 3 months after the OHT revealed that the patient indeed had had low back pain periodically for years, but he attributed it to his kidney disease rather than to the arthritic problem. Thus, the cardiac features of ankylosing spondylitis in this patient probably appeared after the clinical onset of his orthopedic back problem. Lateral chest radiograph, however, did not show changes of ankylosing spondylitis.

The dense fibrous tissue – characteristic of ankylosing spondylitis – was present in the membranous ventricular septum just above the location of the atrioventricular node and its presence in that location appears to be the cause of the patient's complete heart block diagnosed initially about 2 years before the OHT.

We were unable to find a previous publication of a patient with ankylosing spondylitis having an OHT.

## Disclosures

The authors have no conflicts of interest to disclose.

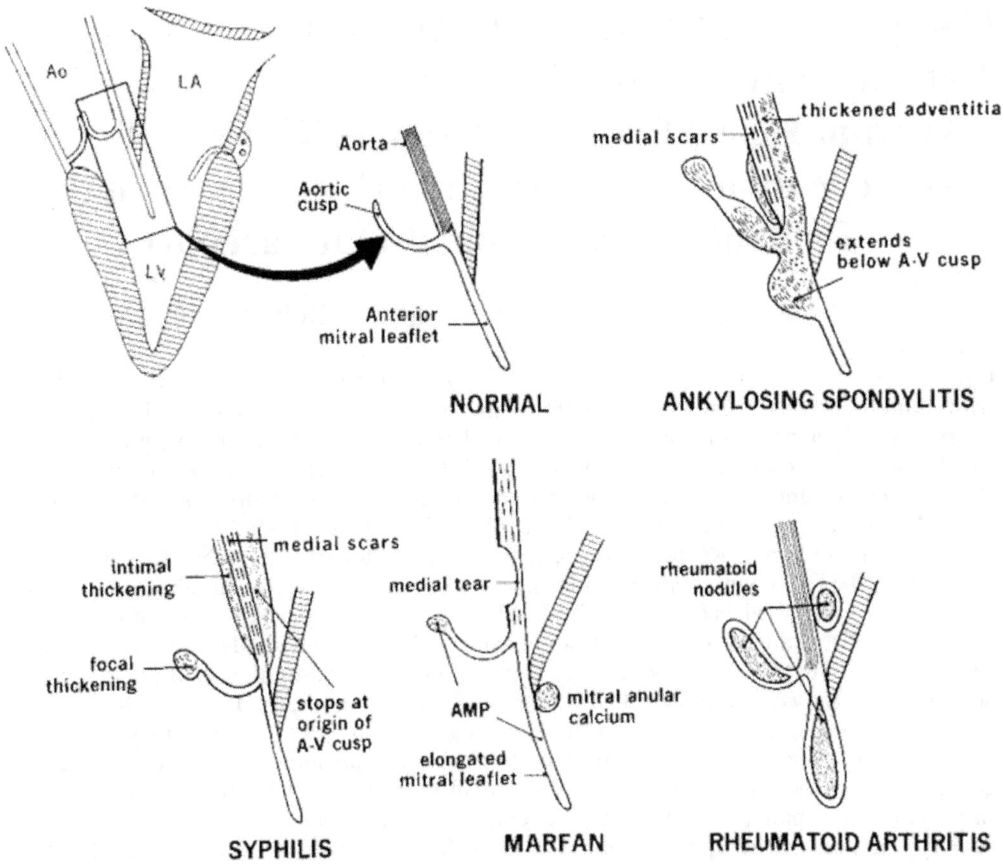


Figure 5. Diagram showing the distinctive morphologic features of 4 different cardiac conditions including *ankylosing spondylitis*. In *cardiovascular syphilis*, the aortic wall behind the sinuses of Valsalva is spared and the adventitial scar tissue does not extend below the aortic valve or involve mitral valve or ventricular septum. Only the distal margins of the aortic valve cusps are thickened in syphilis, not the proximal portions which are always involved in ankylosing spondylitis. In *rheumatoid arthritis*, the distinctive nodules similar to subcutaneous nodules, may infiltrate pericardium, myocardium and mural and valvular endocardium. If the valvular tissue is involved, regurgitation usually of only mild degree results. In the *Marfan syndrome*, aortic regurgitation is a consequence of disease of aortic wall, not of aortic valve; the aorta is thinner, and usually contains intimal-medial tears. The ascending aorta is diffusely involved, and dilatation of the aortic root causes the aortic regurgitation, which is usually severe. The mitral and rarely the aortic valve cusps may be redundant in patients with the Marfan syndrome.
Abbreviations: Ao = aorta; A-V = atrioventricular; LA = left atrium; LV = left ventricle.
*Reproduced with permission from the authors and the publisher.*[1]


1. Bulkley BH, Roberts WC. Ankylosing spondylitis and aortic regurgitation. Description of the characteristic cardiovascular lesion from study of eight necropsy patients. *Circulation* 1973;48:1014–1027.
2. Roberts WC, Hollingsworth JF, Bulkley BH, Jaffe RB, Epstein SE, Stinson EB. Combined mitral and aortic regurgitation in ankylosing spondylitis. Angiographic and anatomic features. *Am J Med* 1974;56:237–243.
3. Roberts WC, Filardo G, Ko JM. Comparison of total 12-lead QRS voltage in a variety of cardiac conditions and its usefulness in predicting increased cardiac mass. *Am J Cardiol* 2013;112:904–909.
4. Klingberg E, Sveälv BG, Täng MS, Bech-Hanssen O, Forsblad-D'Elia H, Bergfeldt L. Aortic regurgitation is common in ankylosing spondylitis: Time for routine echocardiography evaluation? *Am J Med* 2015;128:1244–1250.

# Comparison of Clinical and Morphologic Findings in Patients With Cardiac Sarcoidosis Severe Enough to Warrant Heart Transplantation in Those With -vs- Those Without Non-Caseating Granulomas in the Explanted Heart (Burnt-Out Sarcoid)

Samreen Fathima, MBBS[a,b], and William C. Roberts, MD[a,b,*]

**Can cardiac sarcoidosis with heart failure severe enough to warrant orthotopic heart transplantation (OHT) be present without non-caseating granulomas in the explanted heart? The objective is to compare clinical and morphological features in patients with cardiac sarcoidosis severe enough to warrant OHT with -vs-without non-caseating granulomas in the explanted heart. The study was conducted at Baylor University Medical Center in Dallas, Texas. From a total of 671 explanted hearts examined from 1993 to 2018, twenty-five (4%) had gross morphologic features characteristic of cardiac sarcoidosis. At the time of OHT, the patients ranged in age from 50 to 69 years [mean 57]. Cardiac sarcoidosis was diagnosed before OHT in 3 (12%) patients, by percutaneous biopsy of the heart in 2 patients and by histologic examination of the "left ventricular core" in 1 patient who had a left ventricular assist device inserted, and, by examination of the native heart after OHT in the remaining 22 (88%) patients. Of the 25 patients, 16 (64%) had typical sarcoid non-caseating granulomas in the explanted heart, and 9 (36%) had no granulomas in the explanted heart. Comparison of certain clinical and morphologic features in the group with -vs- the group without cardiac granulomas showed no significant differences. In conclusion, of patients with cardiac sarcoidosis severe enough to warrant OHT, some have typical non-caseating granulomas in the explanted heart and some do not. The clinical and gross morphologic features of those with and those without cardiac granulomas are similar.**  **(Am J Cardiol 2019;124:599−603)**

Sarcoidosis has usually been defined by the presence of non-caseating granulomas containing multinucleated giant cells, epithelioid cells and lymphocytes in one or more body organs. When sarcoidosis attacks an organ, scar tissue develops in the areas of the granulomas and eventually it appears that the scar tissue can obliterate all evidence of previous inflammation, including the giant cells. This scenario appears to occur in cardiac sarcoidosis. Herein, we describe certain clinical and cardiac morphologic findings in 25 patients who had orthotopic heart transplant (OHT) for what proved to be cardiac sarcoidosis. We compared clinical and morphologic features of the cases with to those without non-caseating granulomas in the explanted hearts.

## Methods

Since March 1993 one of us (WCR) has examined all specimens excised by cardiac surgeons at Baylor University Medical Center (BUMC) and submitted the report on each. From March 1993 through December 2018, we examined 671 native hearts excised at the time of OHT at BUMC. All hearts were opened and sections made by WCR. The weights of the hearts were all done by the same investigator after opening the chambers, removing any excess tissue (parietal pericardium for example), and incising the aorta and pulmonary trunk about 2 cm cephalad to the sino-tubular junction. The hearts were weighed within one week after their fixation in formaldehyde. Photographs were prepared on virtually all the explanted hearts, all of which have been retained. Of these 671 native hearts examined since 1993, twenty-five (4%) had gross morphologic features characteristic of cardiac sarcoidosis. Histologic sections were prepared in each heart, and stained by both hematoxylin/eosin and trichrome. At least 5 sections of myocardium were prepared in each case: 4 from the ventricles and 1 from the atria. All sections were examined by WCR. Photomicrographs were prepared from many of the cases. After examination of the heart and before submitting the final pathology report, the medical records in each case were examined.

## Results

Of the 25 cases, 16 (64%) had typical sarcoid non-caseating granulomas in the explanted heart, and 9 (36%) had no granulomas in the explanted heart. Comparison of

[a]Division of Cardiology, Departments of Internal Medicine, Baylor Scott & White Heart and Vascular Institute, Baylor University Medical Center, Baylor Scott & White Health, Dallas, Texas; and [b]Department of Pathology, Baylor Scott & White Heart and Vascular Institute, Baylor University Medical Center, Baylor Scott & White Health, Dallas, Texas. Manuscript received April 19, 2019; revised manuscript received and accepted May 7, 2019.

*Corresponding author: Tel: (214) 820-7911.

*E-mail address:* William.Roberts1@bswhealth.org (W.C. Roberts).

certain clinical and gross morphologic features in the group with -vs- the group without cardiac granulomas showed no significant differences (Table 1). Pertinent data in each of the 25 patients is tabulated in Table 2. Three patients (cases #2, #11 and #18 Table 2) had left ventricular assist devices inserted before OHT and all 3 had granulomas in the excised "left ventricular core", including one (case #18, Table 2) who did not have granulomas in the explanted heart. Of the 9 patients without granulomas in the explanted heart, 3 previously had morphologic proof of cardiac sarcoidosis (2 by percutaneous biopsies of the heart [cases #19 and #22, Table 2] and one by examination of the portion of left ventricular free wall excised to insert a left ventricular assist device [case #18, Table 2].) Each of these 3 patients in whom cardiac sarcoidosis was proven by tissue examination before OHT were treated with corticosteroid therapy (cases #18, #19, and #22, Table 2). Additionally, two of the remaining 22 patients in whom the diagnosis of cardiac sarcoidosis was not proven before OHT also were treated with corticosteroid drugs because of biopsy proved pulmonary sarcoidosis (Cases #2 and #24, Table 2). Two patients (case #4 and #7, Table 2) had significant coronary narrowing, one (case #4, Table 2) of whom had coronary artery bypass grafting. Electrocardiographic features before OHT in each of the 25 patients are tabulated in table 3.

Table 1
Comparison in patients with clinical and morphologic findings of cardiac sarcoidosis severe enough to warrant heart transplantation in those with -vs- those without non-caseating granulomas in the explanted heart

| Variable | Total (n = 25) | Cardiac granulomas | | p Value |
|---|---|---|---|---|
| | | No (n = 9) | Yes (n = 16) | |
| Age (years) | 57 ± 6 | 56 ± 9 | 57 ± 5 | 0.81 |
| Men | 13 (52%) | 6 (67%) | 7 (44%) | 0.41 |
| Women | 12 (48%) | 3 (33%) | 9 (56%) | |
| White | 19 (76%) | 6 (67%) | 13 (81%) | 0.63 |
| Black | 6 (24%) | 3 (33%) | 3 (19%) | |
| Duration (months), symptoms | 72 ± 53 | 76 ± 65 | 70 ± 48 | 0.79 |
| Atrial arrhythmias | 7 (28%) | 4 (44%) | 3 (20%) | 0.36 |
| Ventricular arrhythmias | 8 (32%) | 1 (11%) | 7 (47%) | 0.18 |
| Bundle branch block | | | | 0.28 |
| Left | 4 (16%) | 1 (11%) | 3 (19%) | |
| Right | 10 (40%) | 3 (33%) | 7 (44%) | |
| Indeterminate | 3 (12%) | 0 | 3 (19%) | |
| Total 12-lead QRS Voltage (mm) | 88 ± 36 | 99 ± 20 | 82 ± 41 | 0.30 |
| Total cholesterol (mg/dl) | 150 ± 42 | 160 ± 47 | 145 ± 40 | 0.44 |
| LDL cholesterol (mg/dl) | 90 ± 29 | 96 ± 27 | 87 ± 30 | 0.48 |
| Body mass index (Kg/m$^2$) | 28 ± 5 | 29 ± 7 | 28 ± 3 | 0.70 |
| Prior LVAD | 3 (12%) | 2 (22%) | 1 (6%) | 0.60 |
| Corticosteroid therapy | 5 (24%) | 4 (44%) | 1 (6%) | 0.097 |
| Heart weight (g) | | | | |
| Men | 490 ± 58 | 491 ± 80 | 492 ± 51 | 0.91 |
| Women | 423 ± 86 | 438 ± 141 | 418 ± 71 | 0.75 |
| Floating heart | 12 (48%) | 4 (44%) | 8 (53%) | 1.00 |

LDL = low density lipoprotein; LVAD =left ventricular assist device.

## Discussion

The present report describes 25 patients who underwent OHT because of chronic severe heart failure resulting from cardiac sarcoidosis: 16 of the patients had classic non-caseating granulomas in the operatively-excised native hearts and 9 had no granulomas in the explanted hearts, although 3 of them had typical granulomas in percutaneous biopsies of heart or in the "left ventricular core" excised at the time of insertion of left ventricular assist device. Comparison of various clinical and gross morphologic features of the 16 patients with granulomas in the explanted hearts to the 9 patients without disclosed no significant differences.

Typical gross and histologic features of cardiac sarcoidosis severe enough to warrant OHT include focal but extensive scars in the walls of both left and right ventricles and ventricular septum.[1–8] Scars in the atrial walls are infrequent.[5] The focal scars in the right ventricular wall are usually transmural; those involving the left ventricular wall may also be transmural but often they are only subepicardial, the opposite of what occurs in hearts of patients with coronary heart disease, which is subendocardial or transmural or both but not subepicardial.[9] The ventricular walls are more often thinner than normal rather than thicker than normal. The ventricular cavities are severely dilated (unless a left ventricular assist device had been inserted earlier). Histologically, the non-caseating granulomas are typically located within the scars and numerous ones are present in some scars. In most patients some ventricular wall scars contain granulomas and others do not. The numbers of nuclei present in the giant cells may exceed 50. Lymphocytes also are present.

How can we be certain that the 9 patients without non-caseating granulomas in the explanted hearts have cardiac sarcoidosis? In 3 of these 9 patients an earlier percutaneous biopsy (in 2) or examination of the portion of left ventricular wall excised to insert a left ventricular assist device (in 1) did indeed contain non-caseating granulomas. The interval from this tissue examination to the OHT in these 3 patients was 0.1, 7, and 53 months, respectively. Another supporting factor was that many of the ventricular wall scars in the 16 patients with granulomas present in the explanted heart also had ventricular-wall scars without any granulomas. The latter observation suggests it would not be a "stretch" for all the scars to eventually be devoid of granulomas. Three of the 9 patients without granulomas in the explanted hearts were treated with cortico-steroid therapy, a known cause of converting non-caseating granulomas into scars without granulomas.[1] (Each of the 3 patients in whom the diagnosis was made by examination of cardiac tissue some time before the OHT were treated with prednisone.)

The positive features of this report are the following: (1) no previous report has emphasized that cardiac sarcoidosis may be present without non-caseating granulomas being present in the heart. (2) No previous study has compared clinical and gross morphologic findings in the patients with to those without non-caseating granulomas in the heart.

Limitations of the present study include the following: (1) perhaps not enough histologic sections of myocardium were studied. (We examined at least 4 large

Table 2
Pertinent clinical and morphological findings in 25 patients who had orthotopic heart transplantation for cardiac sarcoidosis

| Case | Age (years) | Sex | Race | Duration of symptoms before OHT (months) | BMI ($Kg/m^2$) | TC (mg/dl) | LDL (mg/dl) | CI ($l/min/m^2$) | P-Rx | Clinical cardiac diagnosis | ICD | HW (g) | Heart floats | G | Location of granulomas | | |
|---|---|---|---|---|---|---|---|---|---|---|---|---|---|---|---|---|---|
| | | | | | | | | | | | | | | | RV | VS | LV |
| 1 | 50 | F | B | 132 | 25 | 124 | 74 | – | 0 | IDC | + | 440 | 0 | + | 1+ | 3+ | 3+ |
| 2 | 52 | M | W | 192 | 28 | 172 | 108 | 1.6 | + | IDC* | 0 | 440 | 0 | + | 1+ | 2+ | 1+ |
| 3 | 52 | F | B | 50 | 31 | 166 | 64 | 2.3 | 0 | IDC | + | 440 | 0 | + | 1+ | 3+ | 3+ |
| 4 | 53 | M | W | 12 | 27 | 188 | 112 | 1.6 | 0 | IDC | 0 | 555 | + | + | 3+ | 3+ | 3+ |
| 5 | 54 | F | W | 46 | 26 | 74 | 46 | 1.8 | 0 | IDC | 0 | 425 | 0 | + | 3+ | 3+ | 3+ |
| 6 | 54 | M | W | 108 | 30 | 210 | 134 | - | 0 | IDC | 0 | 511 | - | + | 3+ | 3+ | 3+ |
| 7 | 56 | F | W | 11 | 26 | 143 | 118 | – | 0 | IDC | 0 | 450 | + | + | 1+ | 3+ | 3+ |
| 8 | 57 | F | W | 46 | 30 | 138 | 94 | 1.4 | 0 | IDC | 0 | 380 | 0 | + | 3+ | 3+ | 3+ |
| 9 | 58 | F | W | 60 | 27 | 229 | 147 | 2.2 | 0 | IDC | + | 560 | + | + | 3+ | 3+ | 3+ |
| 10 | 58 | M | W | 48 | 25 | 114 | 64 | 1.2 | 0 | IDC | 0 | 420 | 0 | + | 3+ | 3+ | 3+ |
| 11 | 59 | F | B | 72 | 26 | 134 | 69 | 1.3 | 0 | IDC | + | 370 | 0 | + | 1+ | 2+ | 1+ |
| 12 | 60 | F | W | 36 | 28 | 130 | 93 | 1.2 | 0 | IDC | 0 | 401 | + | + | 1+ | 3+ | 3+ |
| 13 | 61 | F | W | 120 | 25 | 119 | 60 | 1.2 | 0 | IDC | 0 | 300 | + | + | 3+ | 3+ | 3+ |
| 14 | 63 | M | W | 84 | 33 | 109 | 52 | 1.6 | 0 | IDC | + | 470 | + | + | 3+ | 3+ | 3+ |
| 15 | 63 | M | W | 48 | 24 | 157 | 86 | 1.7 | 0 | IDC | 0 | 540 | + | + | 3+ | 3+ | 3+ |
| 16 | 67 | M | W | 48 | 30 | 116 | 70 | 1.6 | 0 | IDC | 0 | 510 | + | + | 3+ | 3+ | 3+ |
| 17 | 40 | F | W | 11 | 45 | 107 | 78 | 1.4 | 0 | IDC | 0 | 370 | 0 | 0 | 0 | 0 | 0 |
| 18 | 50 | M | W | 36 | 28 | 185 | 119 | 1.7 | + | CS | + | 605 | 0 | 0 | 0 | 0 | 0 |
| 19 | 53 | M | W | 60 | 31 | 233 | 120 | 1.9 | + | CS | 0 | 535 | 0 | 0 | 0 | 0 | 0 |
| 20 | 54 | F | B | 100 | 24 | 191 | 108 | 1.8 | 0 | IDC | 0 | 345 | 0 | 0 | 0 | 0 | 0 |
| 21 | 57 | M | W | 36 | 30 | 119 | 82 | 1.2 | 0 | IDC | 0 | 420 | + | 0 | 0 | 0 | 0 |
| 22 | 59 | M | W | 48 | 28 | – | – | – | + | CS | + | 420 | + | 0 | 0 | 0 | 0 |
| 23 | 62 | F | B | 216 | 19 | 182 | 129 | 1.5 | 0 | IDC | + | 600 | 0 | 0 | 0 | 0 | 0 |
| 24 | 65 | M | B | 139 | 29 | 160 | 82 | – | + | IDC | + | 475 | + | 0 | 0 | 0 | 0 |
| 25 | 69 | M | W | 36 | 23 | 101 | 50 | 1.3 | 0 | IDC | 0 | 475 | + | 0 | 0 | 0 | 0 |

AB = black; BMI = body mass index; CI = cardiac index; CS = cardiac sarcoidosis; F = female; G = granuloma; HW = heart weight; I = indirect; ICD = intracardiac defibrillator; IDC = ischemic dilated cardiomyopathy; L = left; LDL = low-density lipoprotein; LV = left ventricle; M = male; OHT = orthotopic heart transplant; P = prednisone Rx; R = right; RV = right ventricle; TC = total cholesterol; VS = ventricular septum; W = white.

* Because the patient had biopsy-proven pulmonary sarcoid, the patient clinically was considered to have cardiac sarcoid as well, but a cardiac biopsy done before the OHT was negative for sarcoid.

Table 3
Electrocardiographic findings before orthotopic heart transplantation in 25 patients with cardiac sarcoidosis

| Case | Paced | QRS amplitude in each electrocardiographic lead (mm) | | | | | | | | | | | | Total 12-lead QRS voltage (mm) | Arrhythmias | | BBB (Type) | CHB | Prolonged QT Interval |
|---|---|---|---|---|---|---|---|---|---|---|---|---|---|---|---|---|---|---|---|
| | | I | II | III | aVR | aVL | aVF | V1 | V2 | V3 | V4 | V5 | V6 | | A (Type) | V (Type) | | | |
| | 0 | 0 | 0 | 0 | 0 | 0 | 0 | 0 | 0 | 0 | 0 | 0 | 0 | 0 | 0 | 0 | | | |
| 1 | + | 2 | 23 | 13 | 6 | 7 | 28 | 4 | 12 | 16 | 20 | 18 | 12 | 161 | 0 | 0 | + (NS) | + | 0 |
| 2 | 0 | 14 | 12 | 8 | 13 | 11 | 7 | 12 | 8 | 8 | 18 | 22 | 22 | 155 | 0 | 0 | + (R) | 0 | 0 |
| 3 | + | 5 | 5 | 5 | 5 | 2 | 8 | 6 | 7 | 7 | 5 | 5 | 7 | 67 | 0 | + (VPC) | + (L) | 0 | 0 |
| 4 | + | 4 | 12 | 9 | 6 | 3 | 9 | 7 | 7 | 3 | 7 | 10 | 9 | 86 | 0 | + (VPC) | + (R) | + | 0 |
| 5 | + | 4 | 4 | 5 | 2 | 8 | 4 | – | – | – | – | – | – | – | 0 | 0 | 0 | + | 0 |
| 6 | – | – | – | – | – | – | – | – | – | – | – | – | – | – | – | – | – | - | - |
| 7 | + | 4 | 7 | 8 | 5 | 6 | 8 | 4 | 8 | 4 | 5 | 7 | 7 | 73 | 0 | + (VT) | 0 | 0 | 0 |
| 8 | 0 | 5 | 1 | 6 | 3 | 6 | 4 | 5 | 9 | 5 | 4 | 2 | 2 | 52 | + (AT) | 0 | + (R) | 0 | 0 |
| 9 | 0 | 8 | 8 | 15 | 3 | 11 | 12 | 5 | 7 | 4 | 4 | 6 | 6 | 89 | 0 | 0 | | | |
| | + | 3 | 3 | 4 | 2 | 3 | 3 | 3 | 7 | 3 | 3 | 4 | 4 | 69 | 0 | 0 | + (R) | 0 | 0 |
| 10 | + | 9 | 9 | 6 | 4 | 4 | 6 | 5 | 3 | 8 | 8 | 8 | 7 | 77 | 0 | 0 | + (L) | 0 | 0 |
| 11 | 0 | 11 | 11 | 17 | 8 | 14 | 13 | 9 | 5 | 9 | 12 | 16 | 19 | 144 | 0 | 0 | | | |
| | + | 10 | 12 | 19 | 8 | 14 | 15 | 8 | 9 | 10 | 13 | 15 | 14 | 147 | 0 | 0 | + (R) | + | 0 |
| 12 | 0 | 5 | 3 | 4 | 5 | 7 | 3 | 3 | 7 | 4 | 6 | 2 | 5 | 54 | + (AF) | + (VPC) | 0 | 0 | 0 |
| 13 | + | 4 | 4 | 5 | 3 | 6 | 4 | 4 | 10 | 5 | 7 | 7 | 8 | 72 | 0 | 0 | + (R) | + | + |
| 14 | + | 5 | 12 | 8 | 8 | 5 | 10 | 8 | 9 | 14 | 10 | 9 | 5 | 103 | 0 | + (VPC) | + (L) | + | 0 |
| 15 | 0 | 8 | 6 | 3 | 6 | 6 | 4 | 9 | 10 | 13 | 18 | 22 | 29 | 134 | | | | | |
| | + | 5 | 8 | 11 | 5 | 6 | 11 | 2 | 4 | 12 | 17 | 11 | 3 | 95 | + (AF) | + (VPC) | + (R) | 0 | 0 |
| 16 | + | 4 | 5 | 7 | 2 | 5 | 5 | 2 | 2 | 6 | 5 | 3 | 1 | 47 | 0 | + (VT) | + (NS) | + | 0 |
| 17 | 0 | 18 | 6 | 13 | 6 | 13 | 7 | 6 | 6 | 6 | 6 | 5 | 6 | 98 | + (APC) | + (VPC) | 0 | 0 | 0 |
| 18 | 0 | 7 | 11 | 14 | 5 | 9 | 12 | 6 | 14 | 19 | 7 | 10 | 7 | 121 | + (APC) | 0 | + (L) | 0 | 0 |
| 19 | + | 7 | 7 | 10 | 4 | 8 | 9 | 5 | 7 | 5 | 6 | 7 | 6 | 81 | 0 | 0 | 0 | + | 0 |
| 20 | 0 | 3 | 7 | 7 | 4 | 4 | 6 | 4 | 8 | 11 | 9 | 12 | 14 | 89 | 0 | 0 | 0 | 0 | + |
| 21 | 0 | 5 | 8 | 4 | 5 | 4 | 6 | 7 | 10 | 28 | 26 | 22 | 6 | 131 | + (APC) | 0 | + (R) | 0 | + |
| 22 | 0 | 4 | 1 | 5 | 4 | 3 | 4 | – | – | – | – | – | – | – | 0 | 0 | 0 | 0 | 0 |
| 23 | 0 | 10 | 11 | 10 | 7 | 7 | 7 | 10 | 9 | 7 | 9 | 10 | 10 | 107 | 0 | 0 | + (R) | 0 | 0 |
| 24 | 0 | 5 | 7 | 5 | 6 | 4 | 5 | 5 | 4 | 5 | 7 | 10 | 11 | 74 | + (AF) | 0 | + (R) | 0 | 0 |
| 25 | 0 | 10 | 5 | 6 | 6 | 11 | 12 | 11 | 6 | 4 | 4 | 12 | 4 | 91 | 0 | 0 | 0 | 0 | 0 |

A = atrial; AF = atrial fibrillation; APC = atrial premature complexes; AT= atrial tachycardia; BBB = bundle branch block; CHB = complete heart block; L = left; NS = non-specific; R = right; V= ventricular; VPC = ventricular premature complexes; VT = ventricular tachycardia.

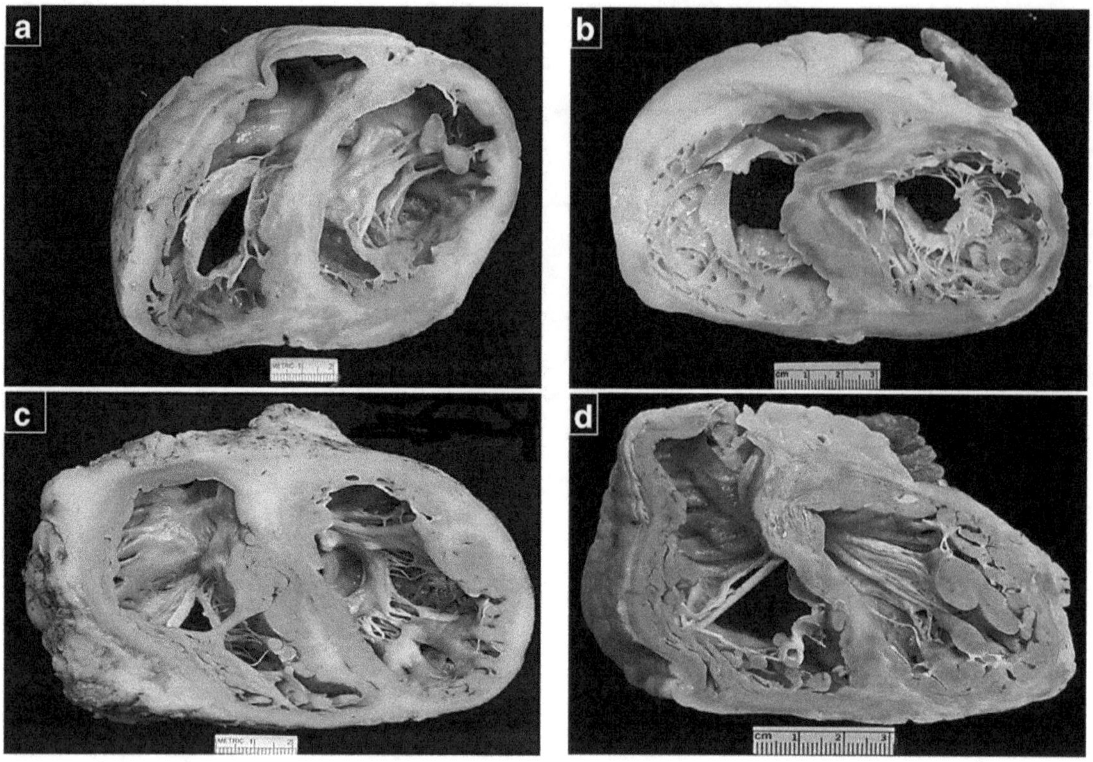


Figure 1. Shown here are basal portions of the heart in 4 patients, 2 of whom (*a* and *c*) had granulomas in the explanted heart and 2, (*b* and *d*) did not. (*a*) patient #5 (Table 2); (*b*) patient #23 (Table 2); (*c*) patient #12 (Table 2); *d*) patient #20 (Table 2). Both ventricles are dilated in each of these 4 patients. Portions of the tricuspid and mitral valves are visible in all 4 patients. The white areas of right ventricular free wall, ventricular septum and left ventricular free wall represent sites of scarring, some of which contained non-caseating granulomas and some of which did not.

[endocardium-to-epicardium] sections of the ventricular walls in all 25 patients and far more [up to 20] in a few patients.); (2) perhaps the 9 patients without tissue proof of cardiac sarcoidosis *in the explanted hearts*, namely the presence of non-caseating granulomas, did not have cardiac sarcoidosis. We believe this scenario to be highly unlikely because 3 of the 9 patients had earlier proof of cardiac sarcoidosis (biopsy or left ventricular "core" examination), and, additionally, we know of no other cardiac condition that even remotely resembles the full-blown morphologic features of cardiac sarcoidosis ( Figures 1 and 2).

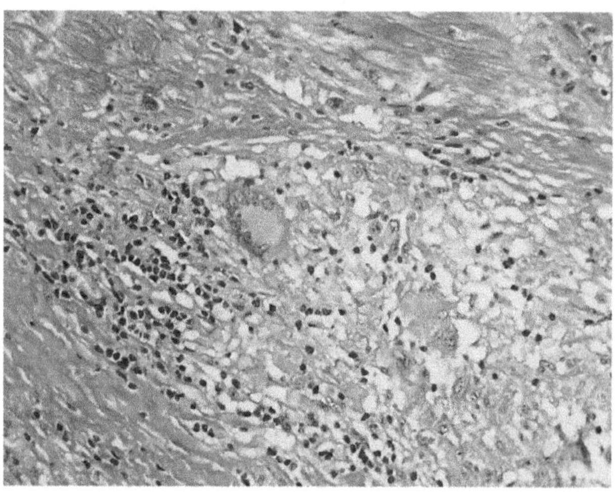

Figure 2. Photomicrograph of a portion of left ventricular free wall in patient #16 (Table 2). The myocardial wall is partially replaced by a dense fibrous tissue which stains blue within which is a sarcoid granuloma. Trichrome stain, original magnification × 40.

1. Roberts WC, McAllister HA Jr, Ferrans VJ. Sarcoidosis of the heart. A clinicopathologic study of 35 necropsy patients (Group I) and review of 78 previously described necropsy patients (Group II). *Am J Med* 1977;63:86–108.
2. Virmani R, Bures JC, Roberts WC. Cardiac sarcoidosis: a major cause of sudden death in young individuals. *Chest* 1980;77:423–428.
3. Donsky AS, Escobar J, Capehart J, Roberts WC. Heart transplantation for undiagnosed cardiac sarcoidosis. *Am J Cardiol* 2002;89:1447–1450.
4. Roberts WC, Vowels TJ, Ko JM, Capehart JE, Hall SA. Cardiac transplantation for cardiac sarcoidosis with initial diagnosis by examination of the left ventricular apical "core" excised for insertion of a left ventricular assist device for severe chronic heart failure. *Am J Cardiol* 2009;103:110–114.
5. Sharma PS, Lubahn JG, Donsky AS, Yoon ADH, Carry MM, Grayburn PA, Wood PB, Ko JM, Burton EC, Roberts WC. Diagnosing cardiac sarcoidosis clinically without tissue confirmation. *Proc (Bayl Univ Med Cent)* 2009;22:236–238.
6. Roberts WC, Chung MS, Ko JM, Capehart JE, Hall SA. Morphologic features of cardiac sarcoidosis in native hearts of patients having cardiac transplantation. *Am J Cardiol* 2014;113:706–712.
7. Armstrong D, Gonzalez-Stawinski GV, Ko JM, Hall SA, Roberts WC. The two extremes of cardiac sarcoidosis and the effect of prednisone therapy. *Am J Cardiol* 2015;115:150–153.
8. Roberts WC, Becker TM, Hall SA. Usefulness of total 12-lead QRS voltage as a clue to diagnosis of patients with cardiac sarcoidosis severe enough to warrant orthotopic heart transplant. *JAMA Cardiol* 2018;3:64–68.
9. Shirani J, Roberts WC. Subepicardial myocardial lesions. *Am Heart J* 1993;125:1346–1352.

# Examining Hearts Containing Left Ventricular Assist Devices at Necropsy

William C. Roberts, MD[a,b,c,*], Nuvaira Ather, MBBS[a], and Joseph M. Guileyardo, MD[b]

**There are no publications describing hearts at necropsy containing left ventricular assist devices (LVADs). The purpose was to study the relation of the LVAD cannula to the left ventricular (LV) cavity and wall. We studied the hearts at necropsy of 15 adults who had an LVAD inserted from 4 to 1,423 days (median 60) earlier. In 13 patients, the cannula had been inserted at an angle to the major longitudinal axis of the LV chamber, and in 11 patients, the orifice margin of the cannulas contacted the LV mural endocardium. In 3 patients, the LVAD cannula was inserted into the posterior wall, and, in another into the anterior wall. In the remaining 11 patients, the cannula had been inserted into the LV apex. Despite the insertion of the cannulas into the LV apex, the direction of the insertion was not into the longitudinal axis of the LV cavity in 9 patients. These unusual insertions in some patients may have altered flow into the orifice of the cannula; in others, based on their long postoperative survival, physiologic consequences were almost certainly absent. The presence of considerable quantities of subepicardial adipose tissue and pericardial adhesions from previous cardiac procedures (mainly coronary bypass) potentially interfered with achieving proper alignment of the LVAD cannula during its insertion. Misalignment of the cannulas of the LVAD in the LV cavity appears to be rather frequent.**
 **(Am J Cardiol 2020;125:244–250)**

The left ventricular assist device (LVAD) has been employed frequently during the past 20 years for treatment of patients with end-stage heart failure.[1–4] Most of these patients improve considerably following such implantation, but a few are not so fortunate. Described herein are cardiac necropsy findings in 15 patients who had received a LVAD at Baylor University Medical Center (BUMC) during a recent 5-year period. Our purpose was to examine the frequency of malalignment of the cannula of the LVAD in the left ventricular (LV) cavity. Such a study has not been published previously.

## Methods

From October 2012 to July 2017, a total of 193 patients received a LVAD at BUMC. Sixty-three were known to have died and autopsies were performed in 15 (24 %). These latter 15 patients are the subject of the present study. The autopsies were performed by one of us (JMG), and the hearts were opened, described, and the official report provided by another of us (WCR). After cleaning the hearts of extraneous tissue and removal of the LVAD cannula, the hearts were placed in a large container of 10% formaldehyde to determine, whether or not they floated. (Adipose tissue is lighter than myocardium so if the former is greatly increased, the heart usually arises to the surface.) The hearts were opened within a few days of the autopsy by 1 of 2 methods: cutting the ventricles into 1.0 to 1.5 cm thick slices parallel to the posterior atrioventricular sulcus or by cutting them by the left and right parasagittal method. Although the LVAD cannulas were in place, the hearts were photographed by Mrs. Saba Ilyas. The hearts were weighed after gently patting the surfaces with paper towels to remove excessive formaldehyde/water and by excising the aorta and pulmonary trunk by incisions about 1 cm above the respective sinotubular junctions. All the hearts were weighed within 1 week of the autopsy. At least 4 sections of each heart were prepared and submitted for histologic study and both hematoxylin/eosin and trichrome stains were prepared on all. The clinical records were examined in the 15 patients.

## Results

Certain clinical and morphologic findings in each of the 15 patients are displayed in Table 1. The 15 patients ranged in age at the time of the LVAD insertion from 44 to 73 years (mean 61); 11 were men and 4 were women; 13 were white and 2 were black. The body mass indexes just prior to the LVAD insertion ranged from 21 to 37 kg/m$^2$ (mean 31), and was >30 kg/m$^2$ in 8 (53%) of the 15 patients. The underlying cardiac disease was ischemic cardiomyopathy in 7 patients, idiopathic dilated cardiomyopathy in 6, adriamycin-induced cardiomyopathy in 1, and valvular heart disease (aortic stenosis with bicuspid valve) in 1 (case #6, Table 1). Seven different surgeons implanted the LVADs in the 15 patients, only 1 of whom is still on the BUMC staff. At the time of insertion of the LVAD, 4 patients who had tricuspid regurgitation also had a ring inserted into the tricuspid valve annulus. Two additional patients (case #2 and case #15, Table 1) also had replacement of the aortic valve

[a]Baylor Scott & White Heart and Vascular Institute, Baylor University Medical Center, Baylor Scott & White Health, Dallas, Texas; [b]Department of Pathology, Baylor University Medical Center, Baylor Scott & White Health, Dallas, Texas; and [c]Division of Cardiology, Department of Internal Medicine, Baylor University Medical Center, Baylor Scott & White Health, Dallas, Texas. Manuscript received August 28, 2019; revised manuscript received and accepted October 23, 2019.

See page 250 for disclosure information.

*Corresponding author: Tel: (214) 820-7911; fax: (214) 820-7533.

*E-mail address:* William.Roberts1@BSWHealth.org (W.C. Roberts).

Table 1
Pertinent clinical and morphologic findings in the 15 patients

| Case no. | Interval from LVAD insertion and death (days) | Age (years) at LVAD insertion | Age (years) at death | Race | Sex | BMI ($kg/m^2$) pre-LVAD | SH (Hx) | HW (g) | Heart float | CABG (pre-LVAD) | Diagnosis | Cause of death | Margin of LVAD cannula contacts mural endocardium | TV ring |
|---|---|---|---|---|---|---|---|---|---|---|---|---|---|---|
| 1 | 4 | 66 | 66 | White | M | 29 | + | 580 | 0 | 0 | IDC | LCOS | + | + |
| 2 | 10 | 67 | 67 | White | M | 37 | + | 900 | + | 0 | IDC* | Bleeding | 0 | 0 |
| 3 | 13 | 44 | 44 | White | F | 33 | + | 475 | + | + | IC | ICH | 0 (PML) | 0 |
| 4 | 18 | 64 | 64 | White | M | 37† | + | 795 | 0 | 0 | IDC | LCOS | 0 | 0 |
| 5 | 35 | 60 | 60 | White | M | 28 | 0 | 485 | 0 | + | IC | LCOS | + | + |
| 6 | 51 | 52 | 52 | White | M | 33 | + | 690 | + | 0 | VHD‡ | LCOS | + | + |
| 7 | 57 | 73 | 73 | White | M | 26 | + | 460 | 0 | + | IC | LCOS | + | 0 |
| 8 | 60 | 59 | 59 | White | F | 23 | 0 | 205 | + | + | IC | LCOS | + | 0 |
| 9 | 116 | 70 | 71 | Black | F | 21 | + | 515 | 0 | + | IC | LCOS | 0 | 0 |
| 10 | 177 | 57 | 58 | White | M | 27 | + | 480 | 0 | 0 | IDC | ICH | + | 0 |
| 11 | 204 | 64 | 65 | White | M | 28 | 0 | 490 | 0 | 0 | AC | ICH | + | 0 |
| 12 | 464 | 64 | 65 | Black | M | 34 | + | 485 | 0 | 0 | IC | LCOS | 0 | 0 |
| 13 | 578 | 67 | 69 | White | M | 35 | + | 465 | 0 | + | IC | Stroke | + | 0 |
| 14 | 984 | 55 | 57 | White | M | 37 | 0 | 740 | 0 | 0 | IDC | ICH | + | + |
| 15 | 1423 | 49 | 57 | White | F | 32 | + | 525 | + | 0 | IDC§ | ICH | + | 0 |

AC = adriamycin cardiomyopathy; BMI = body mass index; CABG = coronary artery bypass graft; F = female; g = grams; HW = heart weight; Hx = history; IC = ischemic cardiomyopathy; ICH = intracranial hemorrhage; IDC = idiopathic dilated cardiomyopathy; LCOS = low cardiac output syndrome; LVAD = left ventricular assist device; M = male; PML= posterior mitral leaflet; SH = systemic hypertension; TV = tricuspid valve; VHD = valvular heart disease.

* Operation was planned to insert only a LVAD but intraoperative echocardiogram showed moderate aortic regurgitation. Therefore, the anatomically normal aortic valve was replaced. The aortotomy could not close adequately, and then the 4.5 cm sized aorta, which proved to be histologically normal, was resected. Heavy postoperative bleeding lead to reoperation but bleeding persisted and was fatal.

† Five months earlier the BMI was 53 $kg/m^2$.

‡ Congenitally bicuspid stenotic aortic valve was replaced 7 years before the LVAD was inserted. Chronic heart failure persisted nevertheless.

§ Operation scheduled to insert an LVAD. When the impella was removed, moderate aortic regurgitation was apparent by intraoperative echocardiogram and then only the anatomically normal aortic valve was replaced followed then by insertion of the LVAD. She died 3.9 years later from intracerebral hemorrhage.

that was 3-cuspid and anatomically normal in each but was mildly to moderately regurgitant in each. Six of the 15 patients earlier had had coronary artery bypass grafting, including 2 patients (case #3 and case #8, Table 1) in whom coronary bypass was performed 10 and 30 days, respectively, before insertion of the LVAD. Three patients had cancer, 2 of whom earlier had received chemotherapy; 1 additional patient (case #15, Table 1) developed esophageal adenocarcinoma late after the LVAD insertion. Four patients developed infections after the LVAD insertion and it later healed: sternum infection in 2 (case #9 and case #14, Table 1) and "driveline" infection in 2 (case #12 and case #15, Table 1).

The interval between insertion of the LVAD and death varied from 4 to 1,423 days (mean: 280, median: 60); 8 patients (53%) died within 60 days of the LVAD insertion and 3 others within 204 days; 4 patients survived >1 year. Of the 8 patients who survived <60 days, 5 bled excessively and all 5 were returned to the operating room for control of bleeding. One of the 5 patients (case #2, Table 1) at the time of LVAD insertion also had aortic valve replacement for aortic regurgitation (anatomically normal valve) and resection of the mildly dilated ascending aorta (histologically normal) and postoperatively had horrendous uncontrolled bleeding. Of the other 3 patients who survived <60 days, 2 also had heavy bleeding postoperatively, 1 from the gastrointestinal tract (case #4, Table 1) and 1 from the thoracic cavity. All 8 patients who survived <60 days had evidence postoperatively of poor cardiac output. Of the 7 patients who survived >60 days, 5 had a stroke secondary to recognized intracerebral hemorrhage in 4 and unclear in 1. Of the remaining 2 patients (case #9 and #12, Table 1), each appeared to have died from progressive decrease in cardiac output. Of the 15 patients, 13 received warfarin postoperatively; the 2 who did not (cases #1 and #2, Table 1) did not because of heavy bleeding postoperatively.

After removal of the LVAD cannula, the hearts in the 4 women ranged in weight from 205 to 525 g (mean 430) and

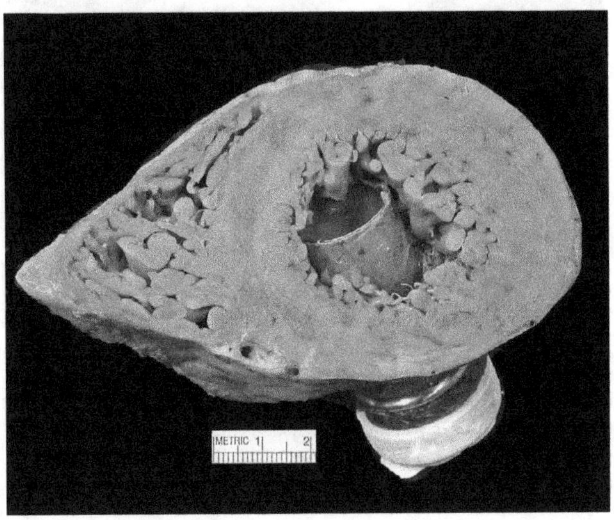


Figure 1. (Patient #1, Table 1). View of the cardiac ventricles showing the LVAD cannula pointing toward the anteroseptal wall. The interval from insertion of the LVAD to death was 4 days. Death resulted from progressive decrease of the cardiac output postoperatively.

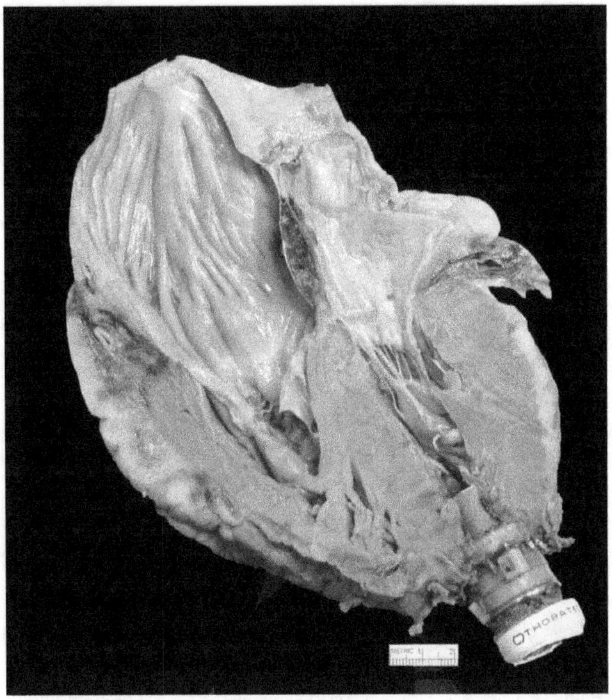

Figure 2. (Case #2, Table 1). Four-chamber view of the heart with the LVAD cannula pointing correctly. The patient at the time of insertion of the LVAD also had replacement of the aortic valve because of moderate aortic regurgitation and then replacement of the dilated (4.2 cm) ascending aorta. The patient died 10 days later because of uncontrollable bleeding.

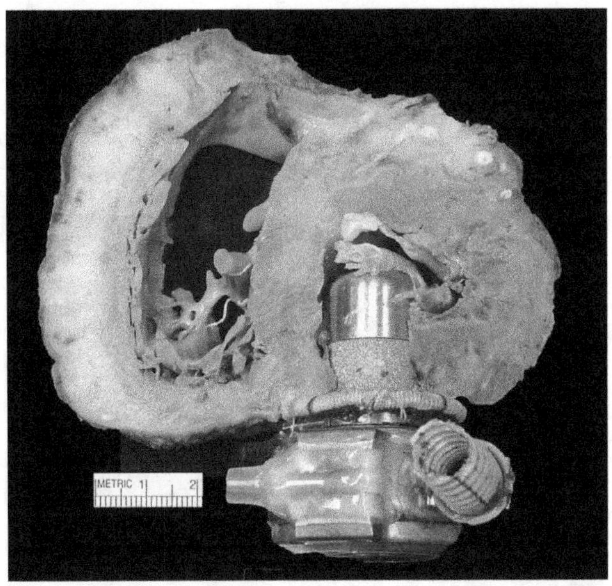


Figure 3. (Case #3, Table 1). View of the cardiac ventricles showing the cannula of the LVAD contacting the posterior mitral leaflet pushing it toward the anterior mitral leaflet. The patient, a 44-year-old woman, had an acute myocardial infarction with shock and underwent coronary artery bypass grafting within a few days of its onset. She could not be weaned from cardiopulmonary bypass and was transferred to BUMC for extracorporeal membrane oxygenation. Ten days after the coronary bypass, the LVAD was inserted into the left ventricle's posterior wall because of a thrombus in the left ventricular apex. The photo shows necrotic myocardium bordering the cannula. She died 13 days after insertion of the LVAD. The quantity of subepicardial adipose tissue is enormous.

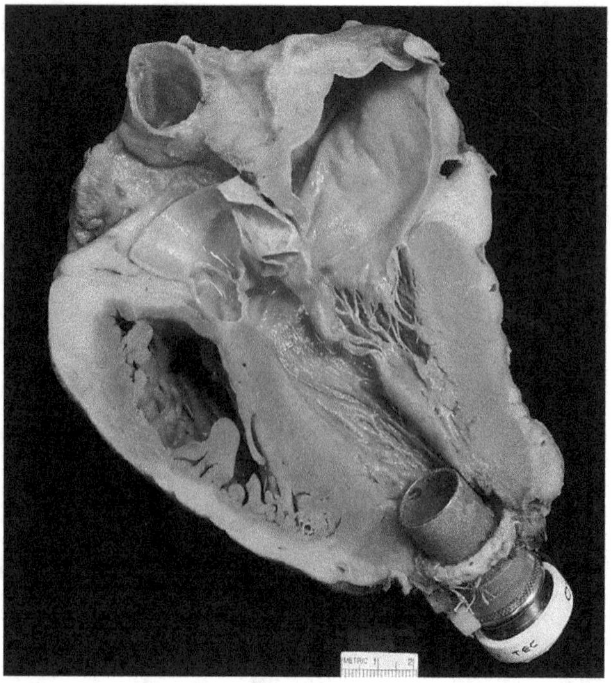

Figure 4. (Case # 4, Table 1). Heart showing the LVAD inserted into the LV apex appropriately. Nevertheless, flow into the LVAD was extremely low postoperatively. The LV ejection fraction postoperatively was about 10%. The LV cavity was not dilated postoperatively but the right ventricular cavity was greatly dilated. The aortic valve did not open after the LVAD was inserted. An impella was inserted to no avail.

in the 11 men, from 460 to 900 g (mean 597). Five (33%) of the 15 hearts examined floated in a container of formaldehyde. The cannulas plus pump in each patient weighed approximately 160 g. In 13 patients, the LVAD was Heartmate II and in 2 patients (case #3 and #7, Table 1) a Heartmate III. The cannulas were inserted into the LV cavities in 4 patients such that the margins of the cannulas did not contact the mural endocardium; in the remaining 11 patients, the margins of the cannulas contacted the mural endocardium or

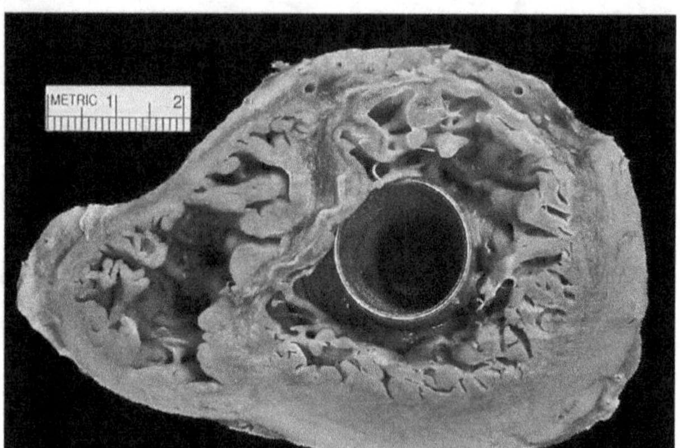


Figure 5. (Case #5, Table 1). Shown here is a cross section of the cardiac ventricles showing no interference with the orifice of the LVAD cannula in a 60-year-old man who had a "massive" acute myocardial infarction 10 years earlier followed shortly thereafter by coronary bypass. All 3 conduits were wide open at necropsy. A huge healed myocardial infarct involved the anterior wall and ventricular septum.

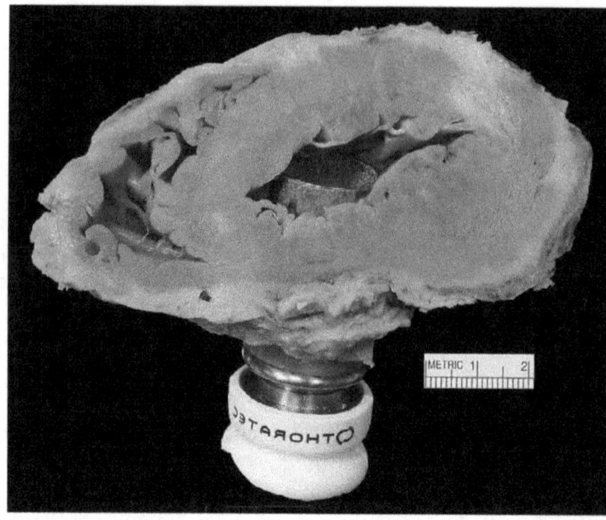


Figure 6. (Case #6, Table 1). This 52-year-old man had aortic valve replacement at age 45 because of a stenotic bicuspid aortic valve. The aortic valve was replaced with a mechanical prosthesis (St. Jude Medical device) and 5 years later evidence of heart failure appeared and progressed. The LVAD was inserted 51 days before death. The cannula points toward the anterior wall of the left ventricle.

the anterior mitral leaflet. The relations of the cannulas to the LV cavity are illustrated in Figures 1–15.

## Discussion

Described herein are necropsy findings in 15 patients who died at varying periods after insertion of a LVAD. The LVAD cannulas in 11 patients (73%) were inserted into the LV cavities at angles to the largest longitudinal dimensions of the cavities such that the margins of the cannulas contacted the mural endocardium, a manner that at least

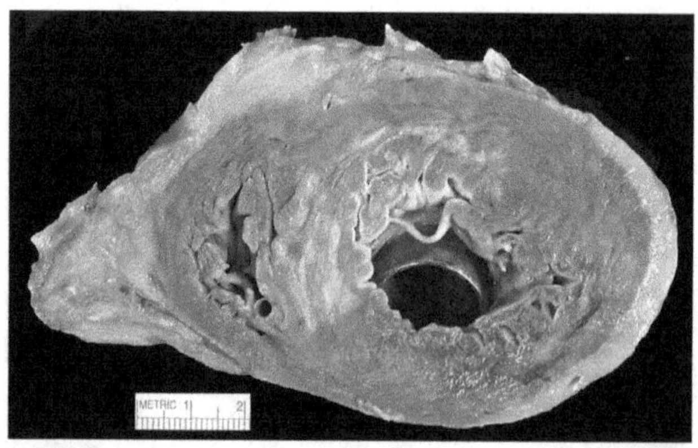

Figure 7. (Case #7, Table 1). Shown here are the more apical portions of the 2 ventricles showing the cannula of the LVAD pointing toward the posterior wall of left ventricle. Even though the orifice is partially obscured, the lumen of this cannula appears adequate. A large scar involves the anterior free wall and ventricular septum. The left ventricular cavity was mildly dilated. This 63-year-old man had an acute myocardial infarction at age 49 and at that time, underwent coronary artery bypass grafting. Years later, the heart failure appeared. He also underwent therapy for non-Hodgkin's lymphoma earlier. The LVAD was inserted 57 days before death. The postoperative period was characterized by features of the low cardiac output syndrome.

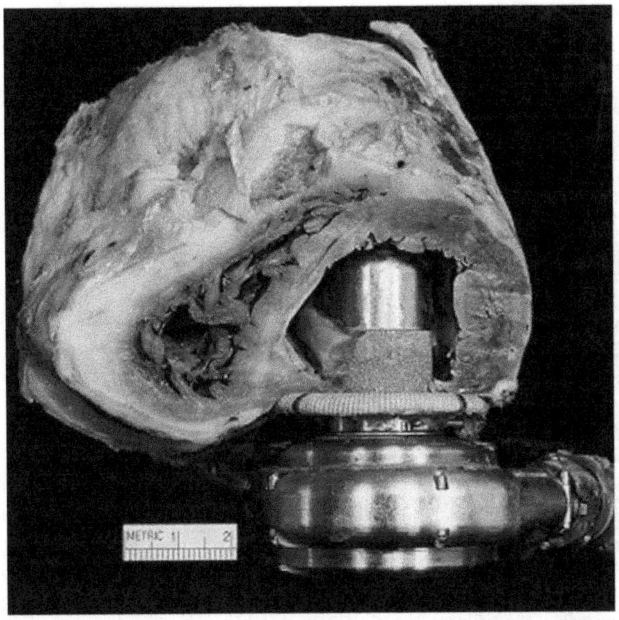


Figure 8. (Case #8, Table 1). Here, the cannula had been inserted into the posterior wall of left ventricle and it points directly to its anterior wall. The heart weighed only 205 g and the cannula and pump together weighed 160 g. The posterior wall and portions of the ventricular septum are scarred. This 59-year-old woman had diabetes mellitus diagnosed at age 31 and was on insulin thereafter. She had a posterior wall acute myocardial infarction several months before death and had a coronary artery bypass grafting 3 months before death. One month after the coronary bypass, the LVAD was inserted. Low cardiac output syndrome was present during the entire period after insertion of the LVAD.

potentially could partially obstruct the orifices of the cannulas. Of the 15 patients, 8 (53%) survived <60 days after insertion of the LVADs, and 3 others <6 months after the LVAD insertion.

Several findings may account for the nonlongitudinal positions of cannulas in the LV cavity. One is the large

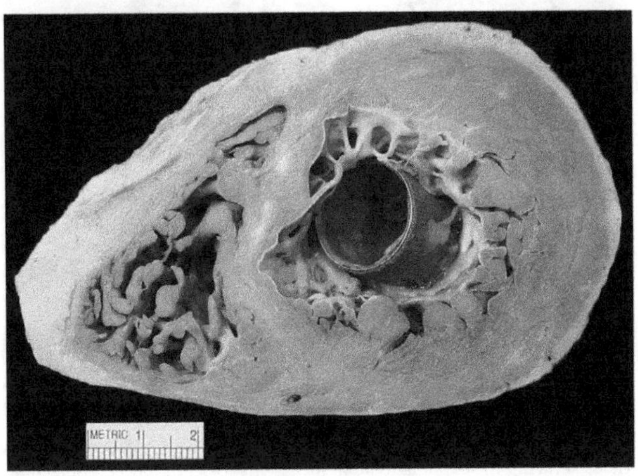


Figure 9. (Case #9, Table 1). Shown here are the 2 ventricles with the cannula pointing toward the ventricular septum. Although the margin of the cannula touches the anteroseptal mural endocardium, there is no interference to inlet into the cannula. This 71-year-old woman had an acute myocardial infarction 27 months before death and the LVAD was inserted 4.5 months before death. There was no apparent improvement from either the coronary bypass or the LVAD insertion.

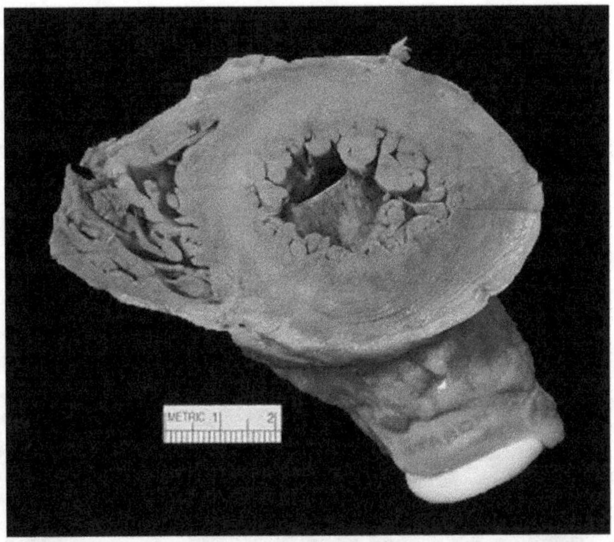


Figure 10. (Case #10, Table 1). The cannula here points toward the junction of anterior free wall and ventricular septum. The left ventricular cavity is relatively small. This 57-year-old man had evidence of idiopathic dilated cardiomyopathy for several years with chronic heart failure. The LVAD was inserted 177 days before death, which was due to sudden intracerebral hemorrhage.

quantity of adipose tissue covering the heart, particularly the LV apex, obscuring the ideal entrance, namely the LV apex, from perfect view for the surgeon. (Of the 15 patients, the body mass indexes were >30 kg/m$^2$ in 8 [53%].) At least 3 of the 15 patients had the LVAD cannulas inserted purposely into the LV posterior wall because the apical wall was calcified (case #12, Table 1) or the LV cavities were not dilated (cases #3 and #8, Table 1). Another patient (case #14, Table 1) had the cannula inserted into the

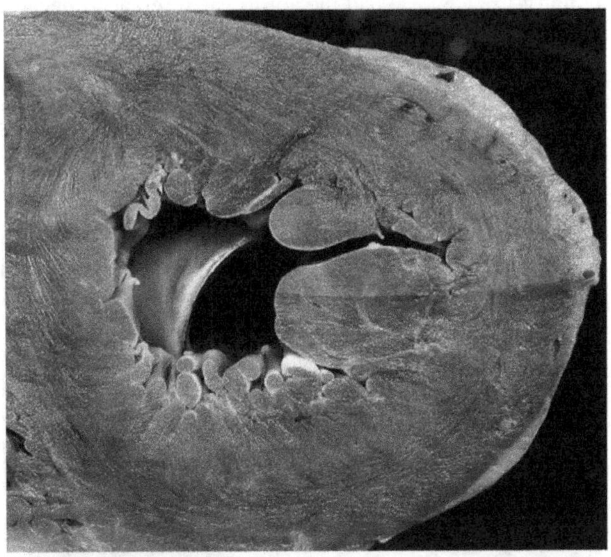

Figure 11. (Case #11, Table 1). Shown here is a cross section of the left ventricle showing the cannula pointing toward its lateral wall. Although this 65-year-old man had narrowed coronary arteries, there were no myocardial scars. At age 53, this patient had lymphoma diagnosed and was treated with adriamycin. The heart failure later was the result of the antilymphoma therapy. The LVAD was inserted 204 days before death, which was the result of sudden intracranial hemorrhage.

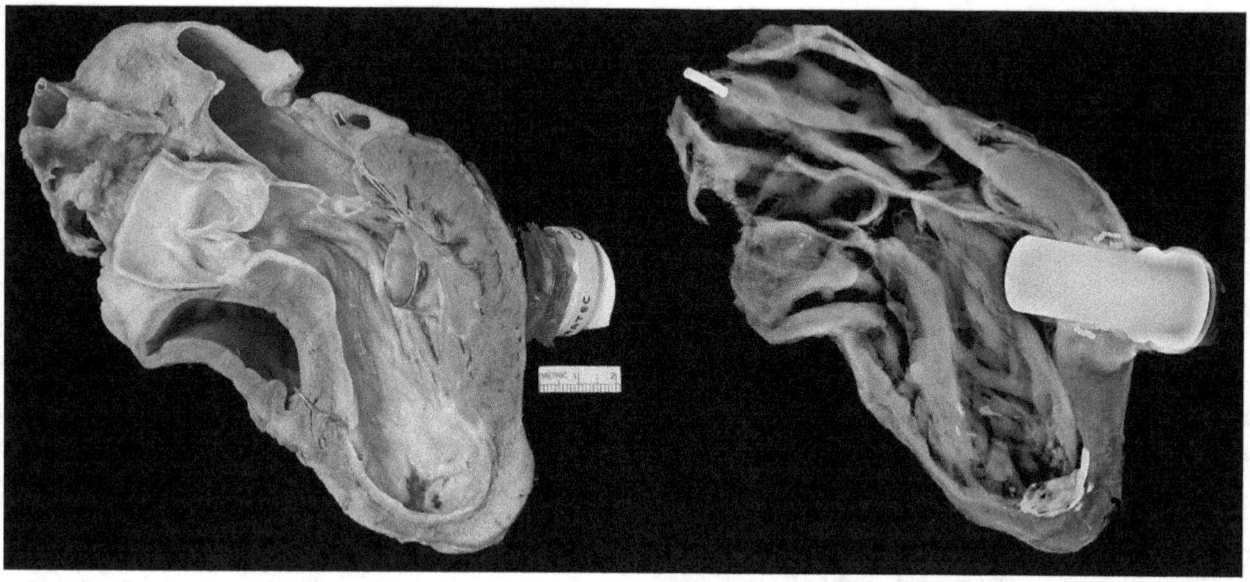

Figure 12. (Case #12, Table 1). Shown here is a left parasagittal view of the left side of the heart (*left*) and a radiograph of the heart (*right*). The cannula was inserted into the posterior wall of the ventricle and that route was chosen because the apex of the left ventricle was calcified. A large transmural scar is present in the apex and it involves much of the ventricular septum. It is possible that the cannula interfered with the function of the mitral valve. The patient died 464 days after the LVAD insertion.

anterior LV wall. Coronary bypass operations had been performed earlier in 6 patients (40%), producing pericardial adhesions, which potentially at least could play a role in obscuring the LV apex. Finally, inserting the cannula into a very small LV cavity of course can be hazardous. Patient #8 (Table 1) had a heart weighing only 205 g, whereas the inserted cannula and pump of the LVAD weighed 160 g.

Operating on one or more cardiac valves during the same operation where the LVAD is inserted appears to add significant complexity to the procedure. Two patients (cases #2 and #15, Table 1) had the aortic valve replaced because of aortic regurgitation, one of whom (case #2, Table 1) also had the ascending aorta replaced.[5,6] The latter patient died from excessive bleeding postoperatively. In addition, 4 (27%) patients had insertion of a ring in the tricuspid valve annulus because of associated tricuspid regurgitation, a procedure unproved to provide benefit when performed at the time of LVAD insertion.[7,8]

Of the 15 patients, 13 bled excessively postoperatively including 12 who were receiving warfarin. Of the 8 patients who survived <60 days, 7 bled excessively postoperatively, 6 of whom were receiving warfarin. Of the 7 patients who survived >60 days, all of whom were receiving warfarin, 6 bled excessively (intracerebral hemorrhage in 4, subarachnoid hemorrhage in 1 and gastrointestinal in 1); the remaining

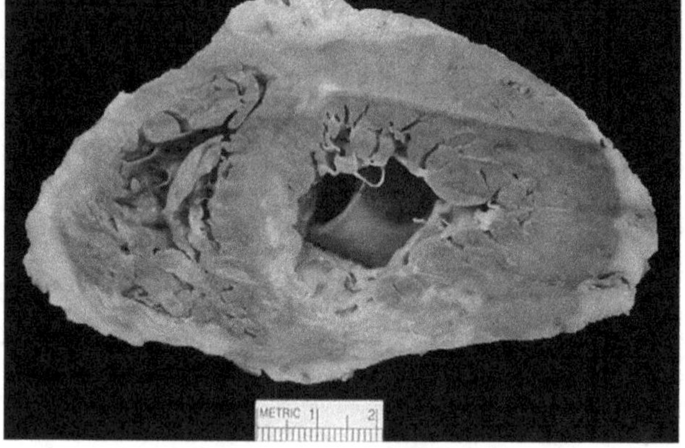

Figure 13. (Case #13, Table 1). The cannula here points toward the ventricular septum in an obese man (body mass index 37 kg/m$^2$). The LVAD was inserted 578 days earlier. Death was the consequence of a stroke. Because no autopsy was done, the type of stroke is unclear.

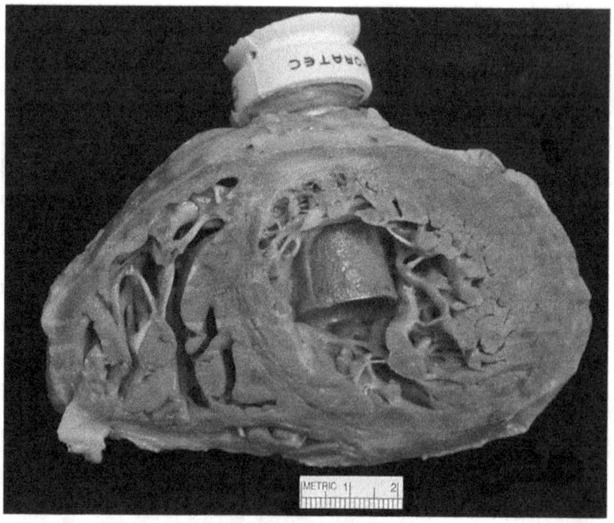

Figure 14. (Case #14, Table 1). Shown here is a cross section of the ventricles showing the cannula to be in the anterior wall of left ventricle and it points toward its posterior wall. A small scar is present in the anterior wall just anterior to the route of the cannula. Insertion of the cannula into the anterior wall of the left ventricle potentially could damage an epicardial coronary artery. Although the margin of the lumen of the cannula contacts the posterior left ventricular free wall, the orifice appears to be wide open. This 58-year-old man had idiopathic dilated cardiomyopathy and died from sudden intracerebral hemorrhage.

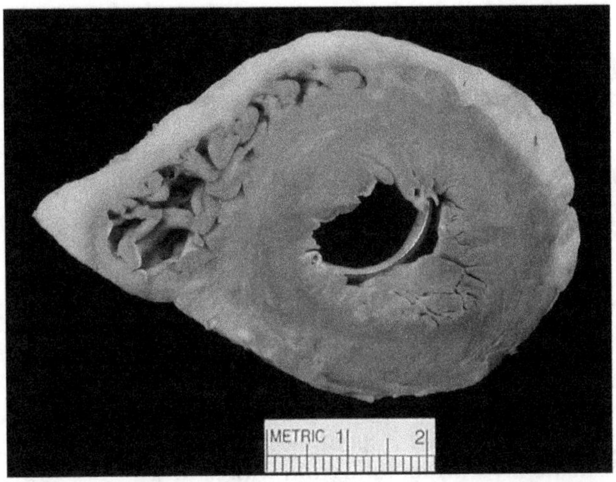

Figure 15. (Case #15, Table 1). Shown here is a cross section of the more apical portion of the ventricles. The LVAD occupies virtually the entire LV cavity. Although the myocardium obliterates about 40% of the cannula's lumen, its lumen appears adequate for proper inflow. This 52-year-old woman developed esophageal adenocarcinoma late after the LVAD insertion.

patient (case # 13, Table 1) had a stroke and autopsy did not include examination of the brain so the cause of the stroke is unclear.[9,10]

The positive feature of the present report is that it is the first to describe morphologic cardiac findings in hearts at necropsy in patients who earlier had had a LVAD inserted. A limitation of this report is that it does not describe imaging or hemodynamic findings postoperatively in these patients. Although the margins of the cannulas contacted the mural endocardium in most patients (11 of 15), we could not be certain from the morphologic studies whether this contact caused any inlet obstruction. Finally, death appears to occur in peak ventricular systole so that the relation of the cannulas to the LV walls during end-diastole is unclear.[11]

## Disclosures

None of the authors has any financial conflict of interest to disclose.

## Acknowledgment

The authors wish to acknowledge Saba Ilyas for her exceptional photography contribution.

1. Metra M, Ponikowski P, Dickstein K, McMurray JJV, Gavazzi A, Bergh C-H, Fraser AG, Jaarsma T, Pitsis A, Mohacsi P, Böhm M, Anker S, Dargie H, Brutsaert D, Komajda M on behalf of the Heart Failure Association of the European Society of Cardiology. Advanced chronic heart failure: a position statement from the Study Group on Advanced Heart Failure Association of the European Society of Cardiology. *Eur J Heart Fail* 2007;9:684–694.
2. Rose EA, Gelijns AC, Moskowitz AJ, Heitjan DF, Stevenson LW, Dembitsky W, Long JW, Ascheim DD, Tierney AR, Levitan RG, Watson JT, Meier P for the Randomized Evaluation of Mechanical Assistance for the Treatment of Congestive Heart Failure (REMATCH) Study Group. Long-term use of a left ventricular assist device for end-stage heart failure. *N Engl J Med* 2001;345:1435–1443.
3. Stewart GC, Givertz MM. Mechanical circulatory support for advanced heart failure: patients and technology in evolution. *Circulation* 2012;125:1304–1315.
4. Feldman D, Pamboukian SV, Teuteberg JJ, Birks E, Lietz K, Moore SA, Morgan JA, Arabia F, Bauman ME, Buchholz HW, Deng M, Dickstein ML, El-Banayosy A, Elliot T, Goldstein DJ, Grady KL, Jones K, Hryniewicz K, John R, Kaan A, Kusne S, Loebe M, Massicotte MP, Moazami N, Mohacsi P, Mooney M, Nelson T, Pagani F, Perry W, Potapov EV, Rame JE, Russell SD, Sorensen EN, Sun B, Strueber M, Mangi AA, Petty MG, Rogers J. The 2013 International Society for Heart and Lung Transplantation Guidelines for mechanical circulatory support: executive summary. *J Heart Lung Transpl* 2013;32:157–187.
5. Pal JD, Klodell CT, John R, Pagani FD, Rogers JG, Farrar DJ, Milano CA for the HeartMate II Clinical Investigators. Low operative mortality with implantation of a continuous-flow left ventricular assist device and impact of concurrent cardiac procedures. *Circulation* 2009;120 (suppl 1):S215–S219.
6. John R, Mantz K, Eckman P, Rose A, May-Newman K. Aortic valve pathophysiology during left ventricular assist device support. *J Heart Lung Transpl* 2010;29:1321–1329.
7. Oezpeker C, Zittermann A, Paluszkiewicz L, Piran M, Puehler T, Sayin AO, Ensminger S, Milting H, Morshuis M, Gummert JF. Tricuspid valve repair in patients with left-ventricular assist device implants and tricuspid valve regurgitation: propensity score-adjusted analysis of clinical outcome. *Interact Cardiovasc Thorac Surg* 2015;21:741–747.
8. Song HK, Gelow JM, Mudd J, Chien C, Tibayan FA, Hollifield K, Naftel D, Kirklin J. Limited utility of tricuspid valve repair at the time of left ventricular assist device implantation. *Ann Thorac Surg* 2016;101:2168–2175.
9. Wilson TJ, Stetler WR Jr, Al-Holou WN, Sullivan SE, Fletcher JJ. Management of intracranial hemorrhage in patients with left ventricular assist devices. *J Neurosurg* 2013;118:1063–1068.
10. Acharya D, Loyaga-Rendon R, Morgan CJ, Sands KA, Pamboukian SV, Rajapreyar I, Holman WL, Kirklin JK, Tallaj JA. INTERMACS analysis of stroke during support with continuous-flow left ventricular assist devices – risk factors and outcomes. *J Am Coll Cardiol* 2017;10:703–711.
11. Roberts WC. Two observations suggesting that we die in ventricular systole. *Am J Cardiol* 2012;110:915–917.

# Acute Isolated Coronary Artery Dissection Causing Massive Acute Myocardial Infarction and Leading to Unsuccessful Coronary Bypass, Extracorporeal Life Support, and Successful Cardiac Transplantation

Julie Cox, RN[a], William C. Roberts, MD[a], Faris G. Araj, MD[b], Jamie Jarzembowski, RN[a], Cesar Y. Guerrero-Miranda, MD[a], Andrea Cooley, DO[c], Charles S. Roberts, MD[a], and Dan M. Meyer, MD[a,*]

**Described herein is a 42-year-old woman who suddenly developed a spontaneous isolated coronary arterial dissection which led to massive acute myocardial infarction with shock, unsuccessful coronary artery bypass grafting, transiently successful extracorporeal life support, and finally successful heart transplant. Such a sequence of events is exceedingly rare for patients with coronary dissection and prompted this report.**  **(Am J Cardiol 2020;125:1446−1448)**

Isolated coronary arterial dissection is an unusual type of coronary disease. It primarily effects women, usually those <50 years of age, and is usually successfully managed without percutaneous coronary intervention or coronary bypass.[1-6] Recently, a 42-year-old woman presented with sudden isolated coronary dissection resulting in acute myocardial infarction with shock leading to coronary artery bypass grafting (CABG) and finally to cardiac transplantation. Such dramatic complications and therapy of coronary dissection prompted this report.

## Case description

A previously healthy 42-year-old woman was well until the sudden onset of left arm numbness while sitting. This event lead to an emergency room visit and hospitalization. She weighed 120 pounds; stood 67 inches in height, and her body mass index was 18.6 kg/m$^2$. Coronary angiography disclosed an acute dissection involving the left main and proximal left anterior descending and left circumflex coronary arteries (Figure 1). By echocardiogram, the left ventricular cavity was of normal size with generalized hypokinesis and the left ventricular ejection fraction was about 25%. Because of clear evidence of acute myocardial infarction with shock (blood pressure 80/60 mm Hg) a CABG was undertaken. A saphenous-vein conduit was placed in the left anterior descending and in first diagonal coronary artery. There was no apparent benefit from this procedure and she was transferred to Baylor University Medical Center (BUMC). Shortly after arrival at BUMC repeat sternotomy was performed because of the progressive lowering of the blood hematocrit (to 7 g/dl) and relatively low blood pressure (90/60 mm Hg). The bleeding was due to a tear in the right epigastric artery at the site of the venous cannula. Additionally, some bleeding was at the site of the anastomosis of the saphenous-vein conduit to the left anterior descending coronary artery. Thereafter, the left ventricular ejection fraction remained about 5%. Because of the continuing low cardiac output and low blood pressure, cardiac transplantation was performed (Eleven days after onset of the acute coronary event.). For the next week the ejection fraction remained low (about 25%) but by the third week postoperatively the ejection fraction had risen to about 45% and the patient was discharged. Routine surveillance endomyocardial biopsy showed no evidence of rejection, and the echocardiogram showed normal left ventricular function.

The native heart weighed 225 g. All coronary arteries were extremely small (Figure 2). Nearly all the left ventricular free wall and ventricular septum and a portion of the right ventricular wall posteriorly were acutely infarcted (Figure 3). The major epicardial coronary arteries were free of atherosclerotic plaque. The acute dissection involved the left main and proximal portions of the left anterior descending and left circumflex coronary arteries. The coronary anastomotic sites of the saphenous veins to both coronary arteries were severely narrowed. Only the tip of a clothes pin could traverse either anastomotic site.

## Discussion

The hitherto described patient with sudden onset of coronary arterial dissection is clearly an "outlier" among previously reported patients with this coronary event.[1-6] Most of these patients are managed conservatively (without percutaneous coronary intervention or coronary artery bypass grafting) with good results. Indeed, to subject any of these patients to either percutaneous coronary intervention or CABG is unusual, particularly the latter. The present patient developed

[a]Departments of Cardiac Transplantation, Internal Medicine (Division of Cardiology), Cardiac Surgery, and the Baylor Scott & White Heart and Vascular Institute, Baylor University Medical Center, Dallas, Texas; [b]Department of Medicine (Division of Cardiology), University of Texas Southwestern Medical Center, Dallas, Texas; and [c]Department of Surgery, UT Health Tyler, Tyler, Texas. Manuscript received December 30, 2019; revised manuscript received and accepted January 29, 2020.

See page 1447 for disclosure information.

*Corresponding author: Tel: (469) 800-7760; fax: (469) 800-7770.
*E-mail address:* Dan.Meyer@BSWHealth.org (D.M. Meyer).

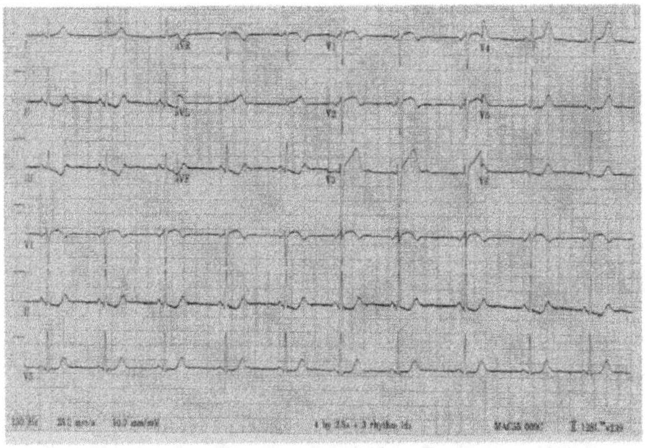

Figure 1. Twelve-lead electrocardiogram showing ST segment elevation in leads V1-V3, and ST segment depression in leads II, III, aVF, V5-V6 when she was initially hospitalized.

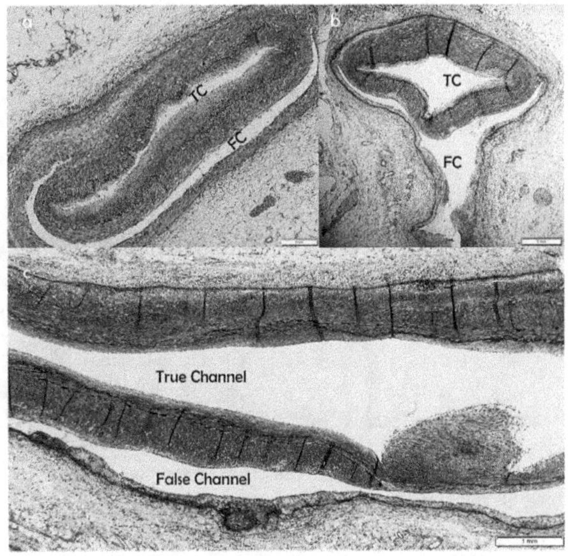



Figure 3. Photomicrograph of the let main (*A*), left circumflex (*B*), and proximal left anterior descending (*C*) coronary arteries in the patient described. Neither the true channel (TC) nor false channel (FC) are filled with blood. The luminal narrowing was due to the FC compressing the TC resulting in obstruction of the TC. Movat stains: ×100 (*a*); ×20 (*b*), and ×20 (*c*).

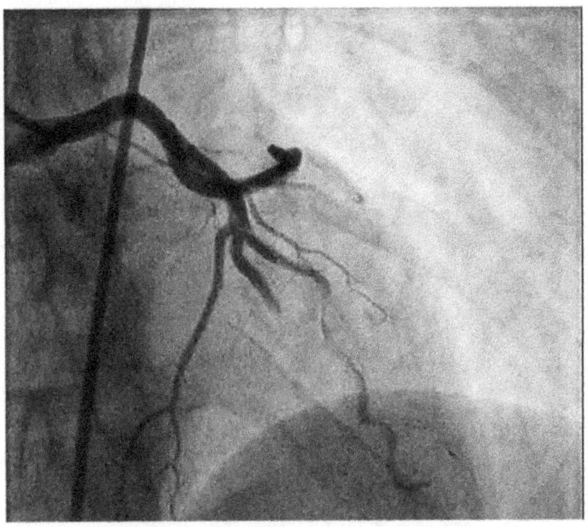

Figure 2. Coronary angiography when initially hospitalized showing a dissection of the left main coronary artery with extension into the left anterior descending and left circumflex arteries.

massive acute myocardial infarction leading to shock, and "bailout" CABG was performed. This procedure failed to improve the clinical picture. The failure of the CABG led to the use of veno-arterial ECMO which provided just enough survival time for successful orthotopic heart transplantation to be performed. Few published reports have described short-term mechanical circulatory support in patients with spontaneous coronary dissection who develop acute myocardial infarction with shock,[7-11] and few heart transplantations have been performed in these patients.[12-14]

Why did the patient described have a massive acute myocardial infarction leading to shock from the coronary dissection? The answer likely is the consequence of sudden severe narrowing of the true lumens by compression from the false lumens of not just one coronary artery but all 3 major left-sided coronary arteries, namely the left main, left anterior descending, and left circumflex, quite an unusual circumstance for spontaneous coronary dissection. Presumably, the dissection in the left main continued uninterrupted into the left anterior descending and into the left circumflex coronary arteries. Most commonly spontaneous coronary dissection involves just a single coronary artery and not always proximally.[1-5]

Why did the CAGB procedure in this patient produce nonbeneficial clinical improvement? The patient described weighed only 120 pounds and had a low body mass index (18.6 kg). The explanted heart weighed only 225 g, the expected heart size of a 10 year old. Consequently, the coronary arteries were quite small (The size of the epicardial coronary arteries is proportional to cardiac mass.[15]). Performing coronary bypass in patients with small epicardial coronary arteries, particularly those free of atherosclerotic plaque, generally lead to nonideal results. The anastomotic sites of the saphenous vein conduits to the left anterior descending and to the first diagonal coronary arteries were so tight that perfusion of the myocardium distal to these anastomotic sites must have been virtually nil (Figure 4).

Why the cardiogenic shock in the patient described? The reason, of course, was the massive extent of the acute infarct, which involved to some degree the entire left ventricular free wall and ventricular septum from apex to base.

Orthotopic heart transplantation is a rare event in patients with spontaneous coronary dissection, but it was a life-saving procedure for the present patient. In an analysis of 327 patients with spontaneous coronary dissection described by Saw et al,[5] only 6 (2%) underwent CABG and apparently none had heart transplantation. More than 80% of their patients were treated without either percutaneous coronary intervention or coronary bypass.

## Disclosures


The authors have no conflicts of interest to disclose.

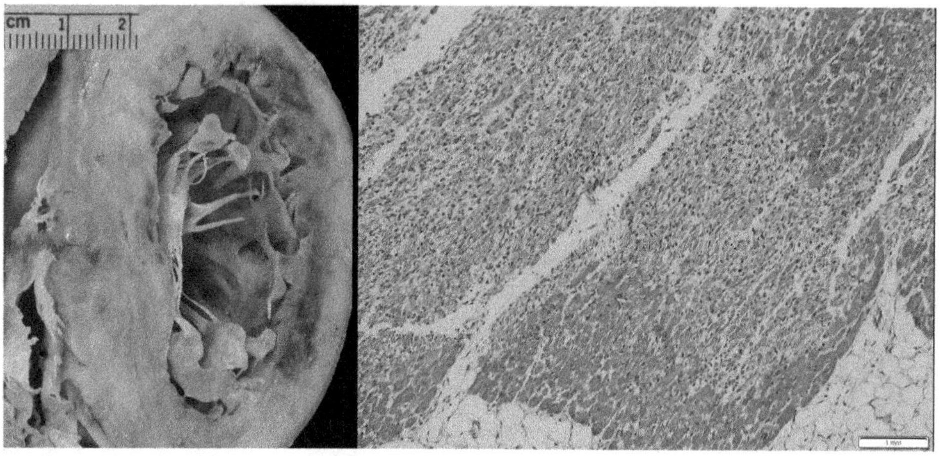

Figure 4. Photograph of the left ventricle (*left*) showing focal necrosis (infarct) of the entire wall, and photomicrograph (*right*) showing focal myocardial necrosis (Trichrome stain, ×100).


1. Vanzetto G, Berger-Coz E, Barone-Rochette G, Chavanon O, Bouvaist H, Hacini R, Blin D, Machecourt J. Prevalence, therapeutic management and medium-term prognosis of spontaneous coronary artery dissection: results from a database of 11,605 patients. *Eur J Cardiothorac Surg* 2009;35:250–254.
2. Tweet MS1, Hayes SN, Pitta SR, Simari RD, Lerman A, Lennon RJ, Gersh BJ, Khambatta S, Best PJ, Rihal CS, Gulati R. Clinical features, management, and prognosis of spontaneous coronary artery dissection. *Circulation* 2012;126:579–588.
3. Alfonso F1, M Paulo, Lennie V, Dutary J, Bernardo E, Jiménez-Quevedo P, Gonzalo N, Escaned J, Bañuelos C, Pérez-Vizcayno MJ, Hernández R, Macaya C. Spontaneous coronary artery dissection: long-term follow-up of a large series of patients prospectively managed with a "conservative" therapeutic strategy. *JACC Cardiovasc Interv* 2012;5:1062–1070.
4. Saw J, Mancini GBJ, Humphries KH. Contemporary review on spontaneous coronary artery dissection. *J Am Coll Cardiol* 2016;68:297–312.
5. Saw J, Humphries K, Aymong E, Sedlak T, Prakash R, Starovoytov A, Mancini GBJ. Spontaneous coronary artery dissection: clinical outcomes and risk of recurrence. *J Am Coll Cardiol* 2017;70:1148–1158.
6. Adlam D, Alfonso F, Maas A, Vrints C, Writing Committee, Al-Hussaini A, Bueno H, Capranzano P, Gevaert S, Hoole SP, Johnson T, Lettieri C, Maeder MT, Motreff P, Ong P, Persu A, Rickli H, Schiele F, Sheppard MN, Swahn E. European Society of Cardiology, acute cardiovascular care association, SCAD study group: a position paper on spontaneous coronary artery dissection. *Eur Heart J* 2018;39:3353–3368.
7. Padukone A, Sayeed AK, Marczin N, García Sáez D, Zych B, Mohite PN, Zeriouh M, Smith RD, Simon AR, Sabashnikov A, Popov AF. Salvage myocardial revascularization in spontaneous left main coronary artery dissection with cardiogenic shock - the role of mechanical circulatory support. *Perfusion* 2017;32:171–173.
8. Patanè F, Boffini M, Sansone F, Campanella A, Rinaldi M. ECMO as a bridge to transplantation in biventricular dysfunction due to primary spontaneous coronary artery dissection. *Transpl Int* 2009;22:500–502.
9. Evans R. Post-partum spontaneous coronary artery dissection and the use of veno-arterial extra-corporeal membrane oxygenation. *Nurs Crit Care* 2014;19:304–309.
10. Farhood M, Orasanu G, Deo S, Medaloin B, Zacharias M, Ginwalla M, Oliveria G, Park S, Sareyyupoglu B, Elamm C. Refractory cardiogenic shock secondary to postpartum multivessel spontaneous coronary artery dissection rescued with biventricular assist devices. *J Am Coll Cardiol* 2016;67:1198.. Supplement 1-2359.
11. Jorge-Pérez P, García-González MJ, Ávalos-Pinto RM, G-Cosio-Carmena MD, Renes-Carreño E, Delgado JF, Yanes-Bowden G, Ferrer-Hita JJ. Spontaneous coronary dissection and cardiogenic shock requiring mechanical circulatory support in a non-transplant center. *Int J Cardiol* 2016;221:629–630.
12. Curiel P, Spinelli G, Petrella A, Gori A, De Maria R, Bonacina E, Gronda E. Postpartum coronary artery dissection followed by heart transplantation. *Am J Obstet Gynecol* 1990;163:538–539.
13. Ferrari E, Tozzi P, von Segesser LK. Spontaneous coronary artery dissection in a young woman: from emergency coronary artery bypass grafting to heart transplantation. *Eur J Cardiothorac Surg* 2005;28: 349–351.
14. Bashir M, Mustafa H, Singh H, Bonser R. Cardiac transplantation for spontaneous coronary artery dissection. *Interact Cardiovasc Thorac Surg* 2013;16:91–92.
15. Roberts CS, Roberts WC. Cross-sectional area of he maximal portions of the three major epicardial coronary arteries in 98 necropsy patients with different coronary event. Relation to heart weight, age and sex. *Circulation* 1980;62:953–959.

# Examining One's Own Heart

William C. Roberts, MD[a,b,*], and Saba Ilyas, BS[a]

Although billions of people have inhabited planet Earth, few have examined their own heart. Cardiac transplantation, which began December 3, 1967, is the procedure that made self-examination possible.

At Baylor University Medical Center (BUMC) in Dallas, we began showing heart transplantation recipients their hearts in 2010. Since that time, we have shown 157 patients their own hearts (through March 2020). The exercise was initiated not by me or another physician but by a heart transplant recipient, Mr. Marvin Jones. I was walking in the corridor near the cardiac catheterization waiting room and next to me was Mr. Jones. He leaned over and asked if I was Dr. Roberts. "Yes," I answered. He said, "I understand that you have my heart." I invited him to our weekly cardiovascular pathology conference so that several physicians could observe a person examining their own heart.[1] Subsequently, the heart transplant cardiologists, surgeons, their nurses and coordinators have gotten on board to encourage their heart transplant patients to "Call Dr. Roberts" to make the arrangements to view their own hearts. Some of the patients had their heart transplants many years earlier. Fortunately, BUMC has provided us with a heart storage facility and all transplant and autopsy hearts have resided there since 1993. Thus, all heart transplant recipients who want to see their hearts since that time can have their requests fulfilled.

How does the procedure to view their own heart work? One of us (SI) meets the recipient at a designed location and brings him/her to the cardiovascular laboratory. Most recipients do not come alone. They bring their family – spouses, offspring, grandchildren and friends. We sit around a table and I ask the recipient a few questions. I usually begin by discussing their cardiac illness. When did the cardiac illness start? What were the initial symptoms and signs? What diagnosis did your physician indicate that you had? Did other family members have a similar cardiac condition? What type of work do (did) you do? Are you still working? How did you get to BUMC? Who told you that you could see your own heart? During this questioning section the heart is laid out before me on the table (covered by a towel) and the transplant recipient is sitting to my right. I usually ask if they are ready to see their own heart. I prewarn them that their heart is no longer reddish brown but tan because it has resided in formaldehyde for some time. The blue towel is then pulled away. I always look at their face as the towel is removed. Nearly always there is no change in facial expression. Of the 157 recipients to whom I have shown their heart, only one turned his head as the towel was being removed. Only one recipient cried. He, however, was the youngest (age 21) who only 2 months earlier had developed a fulminating myocarditis. The shock of suddenly becoming terribly ill from a previously healthy life and then confronted with his own heart certainly made his crying understandable.

The hearts, of course, had been incised before their showing and a few sections had been prepared for histologic study. We discuss the anatomic location of the cardiac chambers, the valves, and how the blood flows through the heart. The most striking finding to most recipients is the yellow covering of portions of the heart due to the subepicardial adipose tissue. The patients with ischemic cardiomyopathy, obviously, have one or more left ventricular scars and those are pointed out and their origins discussed. Nearly all of the patients who had heart transplants have dilated ventricles and the more dilated the ventricle the lower the ejection fraction. Nearly all recipients are familiar with the concept of ejection fraction. I show with my hand how poorly a dilated ventricle contracts in contrast to a normal-sized ventricle. The recipients are usually shocked by the size of the normal ventricle with an ejection fraction of 60% to 70% in contrast to their left ventricle with an ejection fraction of 10% to 15%. In contrast to the hearts with ischemic cardiomyopathy the recipients with idiopathic dilated cardiomyopathy are disappointed to learn that we have no idea what caused their condition.

After the viewing of the heart, I give the recipient and their families a little "sermon" on heart transplantation in general to help them understand how lucky they are to have received a new heart. With the use of a flip chart I point out the present US population (≈330 million), the number >20 years of age (≈240 million) and then ask how many of the latter 240 million have chronic heart failure. The response is usually in the multiple decades. The answer, of course, is approximately 6.5 million. Then we discuss the number of those 6.5 million who each year in the US have a heart transplant. Their answers are usually astronomical compared to the actual number (approximately 3,000). This revelation is usually a shock to the recipients and to their families. The point of this exercise is to emphasize how lucky they are and that now it is their responsibility to take care of the new heart. We discuss what they eat for breakfast, lunch and dinner and what snacks are eaten in between meals and at bedtime. The first food mentioned for all meals usually is the flesh consumed (bovine muscle [beef], porcine muscle [pork], chicken, etc.). Most of the transplant recipients are overweight (body mass index $\geq$30 kg/m$^2$) so we discuss reducing the number of calories consumed daily.[2] We discuss whether they exercise and if so, how much, and its importance for them. The nonrecipient family members also hear these discussions and I have heard later that some of them have changed "their ways."

A surprise for me has been how few of the transplant recipients know the actual name of their cardiac diagnosis. When I ask, "What cardiac diagnosis did your cardiologist say you had?" The answer is usually "heart failure." Whether ischemic cardiomyopathy or idiopathic cardiomyopathy is usually unclear. Those with cardiac amyloidosis or hypertrophic cardiomyopathy or cardiac sarcoidosis, or arrhythmogenic right

[a]Baylor Scott & White Heart and Vascular Institute, Dallas Texas; and [b]Division of Cardiology, Department of Internal Medicine, Baylor University Medical Center, Baylor Scott & White Health, Dallas Texas. Manuscript received March 20, 2020; revised manuscript received and accepted April 14, 2020.

See page 51 for disclosure information.

*Corresponding author: Tel: (214) 820-7911; fax: (214) 820-7933.

*E-mail address:* William.Roberts1@bswhealth.org (W.C. Roberts).

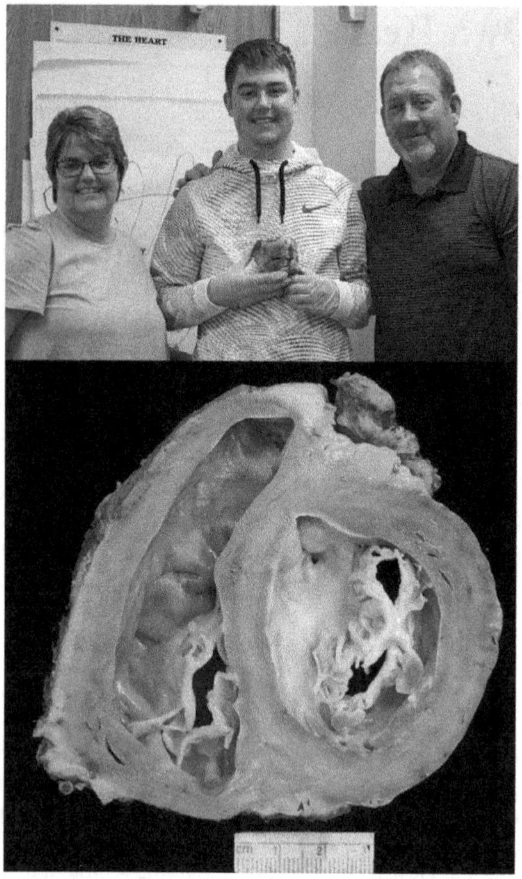


Figure 1. Grant J. Kepheart, a 19-year-old man, had a heart transplant in October 2017 for heart failure secondary to idiopathic dilated cardiomyopathy and the heart viewing was 75 days later. At age 16, a left ventricular assist device was inserted because of severe right sided heart failure, and an Alfieri stitch procedure was performed because of severe functional mitral regurgitation. Since the heart transplant he has been asymptomatic. His heart weighed 330 g.

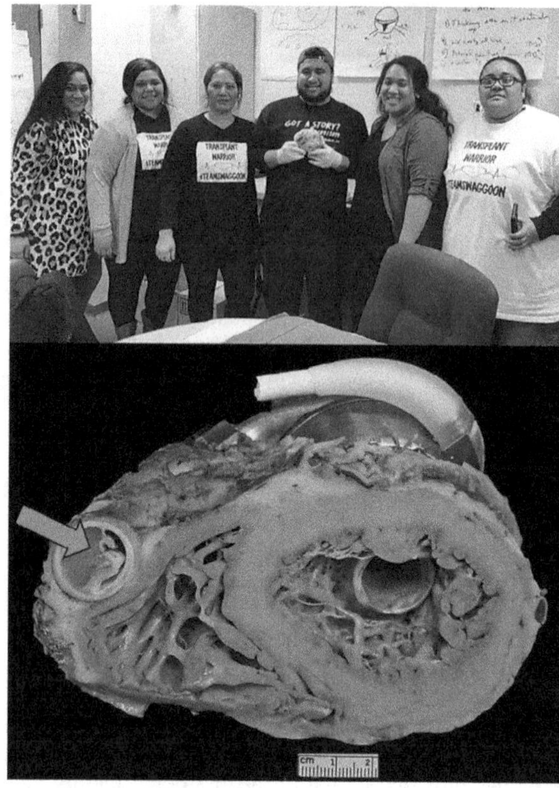


Figure 2. Kennedy Ngungutau, a 24-year-old Polynesian man, had a left ventricular assist device (LVAD) inserted in March 2018, and a heart transplant in April 2019, and his heart viewing was in February 2020. His excised heart weighed 420 g. His previous body weight was up to 290 lbs. His family came with him to observe the heart viewing. *Bottom:* The lumen of the canula from his LVAD is severely narrowed by thrombus (arrow). In his letter granting us permission to show the family picture, he wrote: "*...It was a great experience. I have lost 14 lbs. in the last month because I started to stay healthy with eating, and the times I eat and everything and I thank you all for it.*"

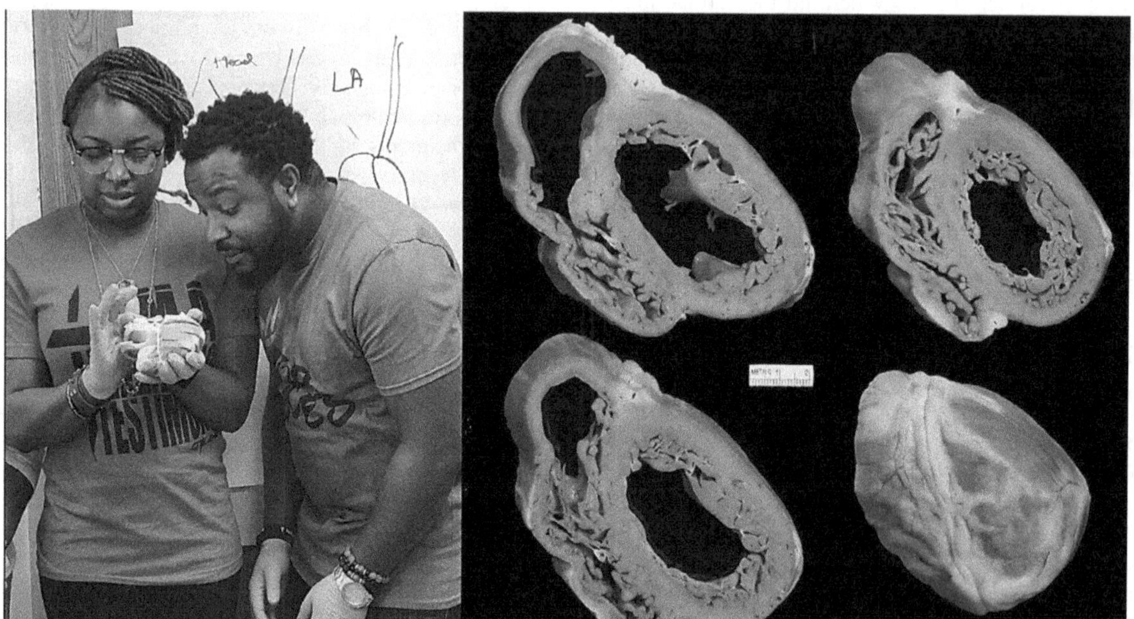


Figure 3. Erica P. Wilcox, a 33-year-old woman, had a heart transplant in May 2017 for heart failure secondary to idiopathic dilated cardiomyopathy and her heart viewing was in September 2019. At 25 years of age she weighed 260 pounds and subsequently lost to a body weight of 130 lbs. Her heart weighed 390 g. Her husband is quite curious about his wife's heart.

ventricular cardiomyopathy or valvular heart disease is usually known. I write their proper diagnosis in bold letters on the flip chart paper and give it to them to take home.

And finally, photos of the recipients standing up holding their hearts just in front of their sternum (Figures 1-21) are made routinely by SI. While the recipients continue to hold their hearts, they are photographed with their family members. Finally, while still holding their heart they are usually photographed with me. The pictures of their hearts and pictures holding their hearts are sent to the recipients. The exercise usually takes 45 to 60 minutes. My impression is that the activity is useful to both recipients and families.

A sidelight: The media, both television and print, have been fascinated by the idea of a person seeing his/her own heart. Consequently, several local and national networks have aired these activities. One recipient learned of the possibility of seeing her own heart by reading a piece in *Reader's Digest*, which described one of these Heart-to-Heart sessions at BUMC.

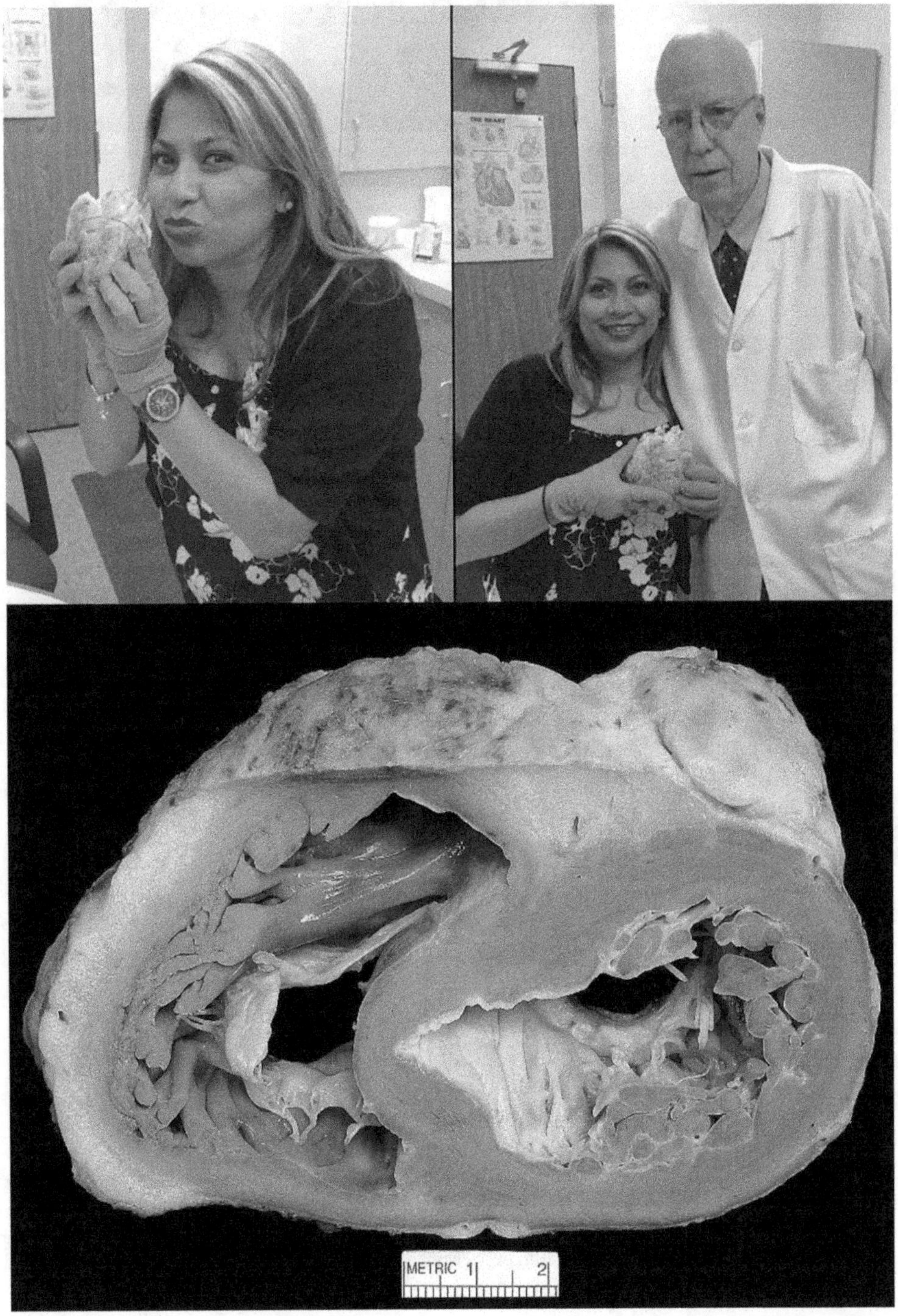


Figure 4. Manuela Arechiga, a 39-year-old woman, had a heart transplant in February 2015 and her heart viewing in July 2015. She had had a mitral valve replacement with a mechanical prosthesis in July 2014 for pure mitral regurgitation. In retrospect, the mitral valve replacement likely had been done for secondary mitral regurgitation, the consequence of idiopathic dilated cardiomyopathy. The cause of the endocardial thickening focally within the left ventricle is unclear. Her heart weighed 255 g.

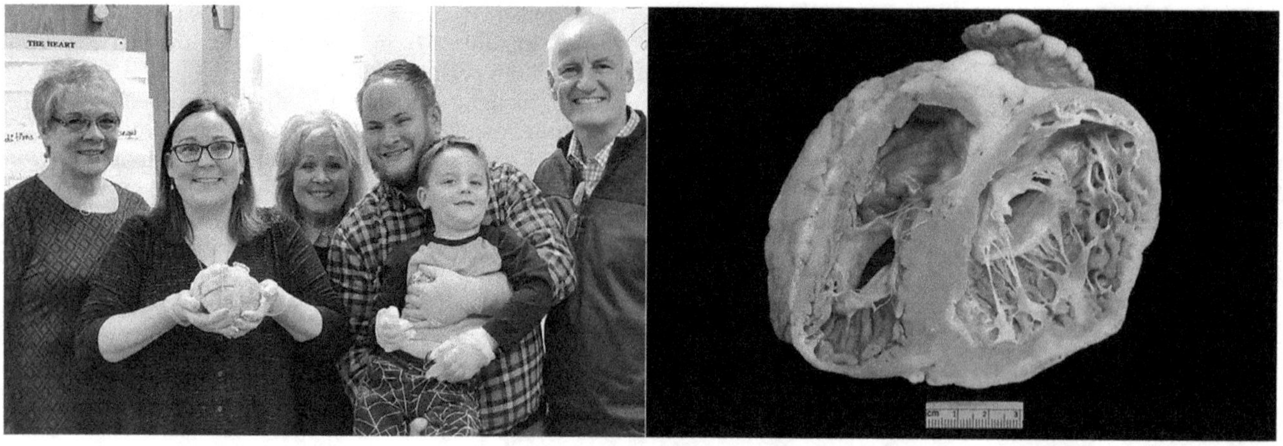

Figure 5. Marley Sterns, a 41-year-old woman, had a heart transplant in July 2019 because of severe heart failure from cardiac sarcoidosis and her heart viewing in October 2019. She developed heart failure about 8 years before her heart transplant. *Left*: Shown with her are members of her family. *Right*: The left ventricular wall is severely thin and typical sarcoid granulomas are present in the scarred areas. In her letter giving us permission to show the family picture, she wrote: *"...That experience meant so much to me and my family."*

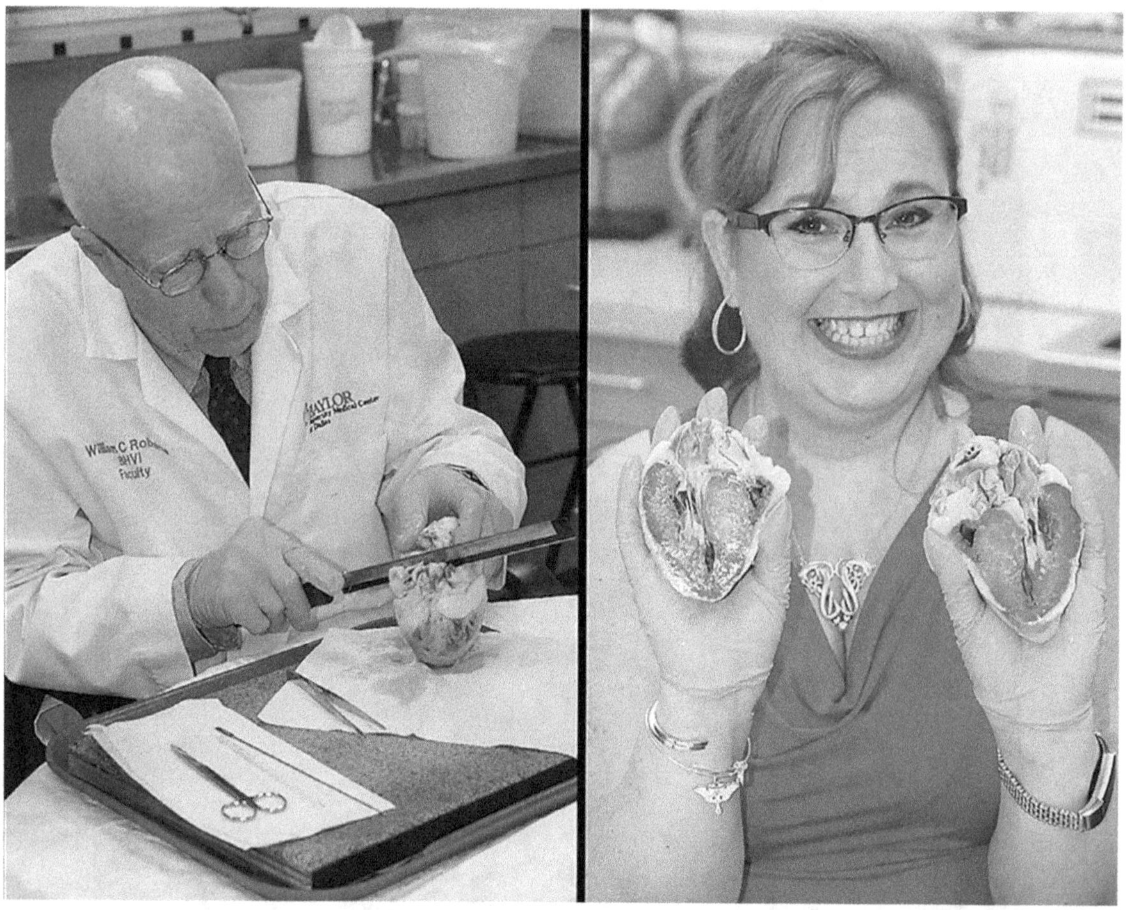


Figure 6. Lisa Salberg, a 48-year-old woman, had a heart transplant in April 2017 for hypertrophic cardiomyopathy and her heart viewing in August 2019. She brought her heart to WCR to open. She then had it plasticized so that she could keep it and show it to anyone interested. Her heart weighed 340 g. Ms. Salberg is the Founder and CEO of the Hypertrophic Cardiomyopathy Association located in Danville, New Jersey. She is a lovely lady who has done much for patients with hypertrophic cardiomyopathy.

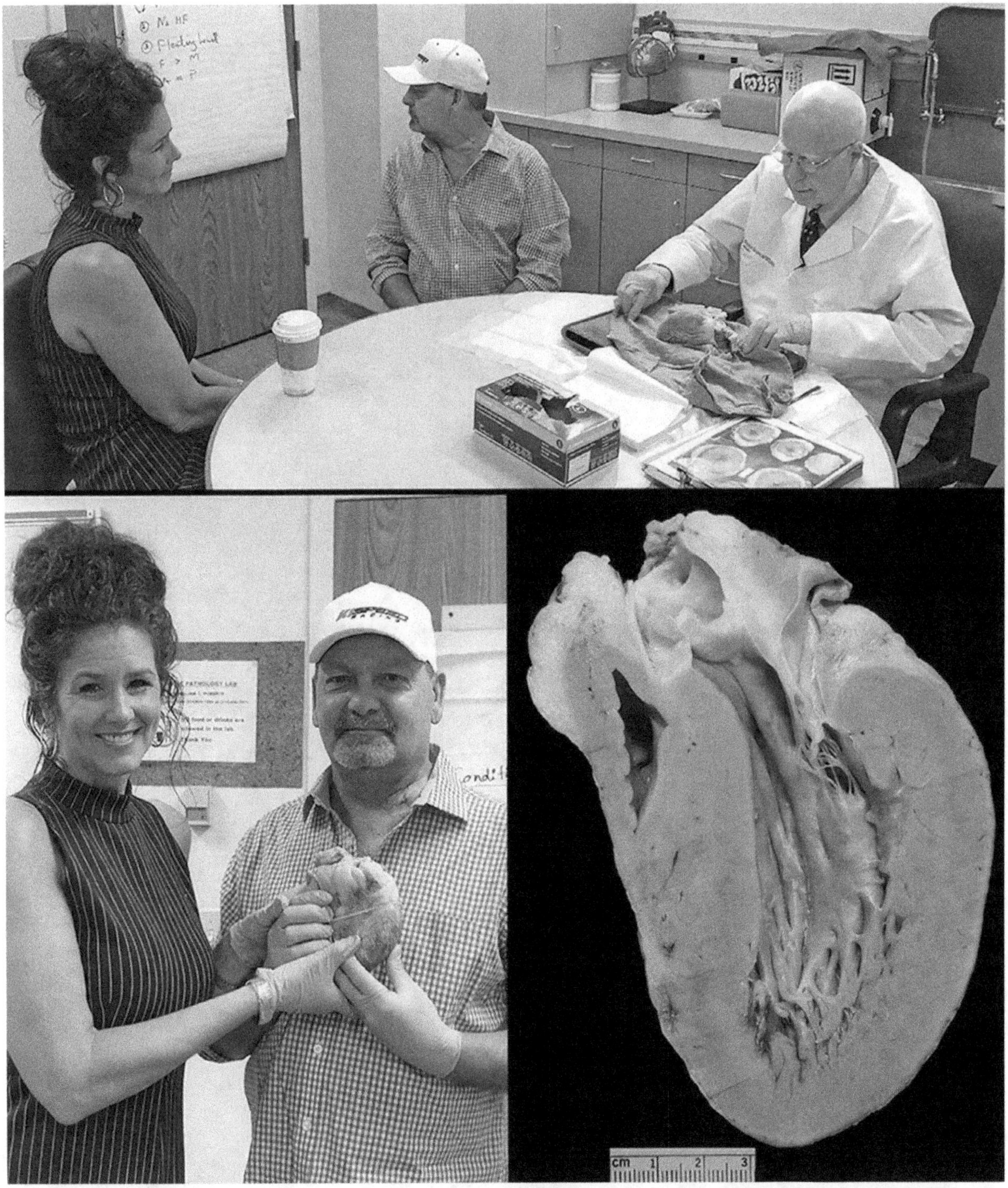

Figure 7. Jimmy Taylor, a 48-year-old man, had a combined heart and kidney transplant in May 2018 and his heart viewing in August 2019. The cause of the heart transplant was unclear clinically, but study of the actual heart showed classic features of ankylosing spondylitis. The heart weighed 675 g. While at the round table, I asked him if he was ready to see his heart? He replied, "Yes." But as I took the towel off his heart, he turned his head to the right and didn't look for a few minutes. Later he smiled. His wife Kelli is to his right. In his consent letter he wrote: *"We are so very blessed, and we hope that our journey is an inspiration to others who may have lost hope and a useful tool to those who help people like us."*

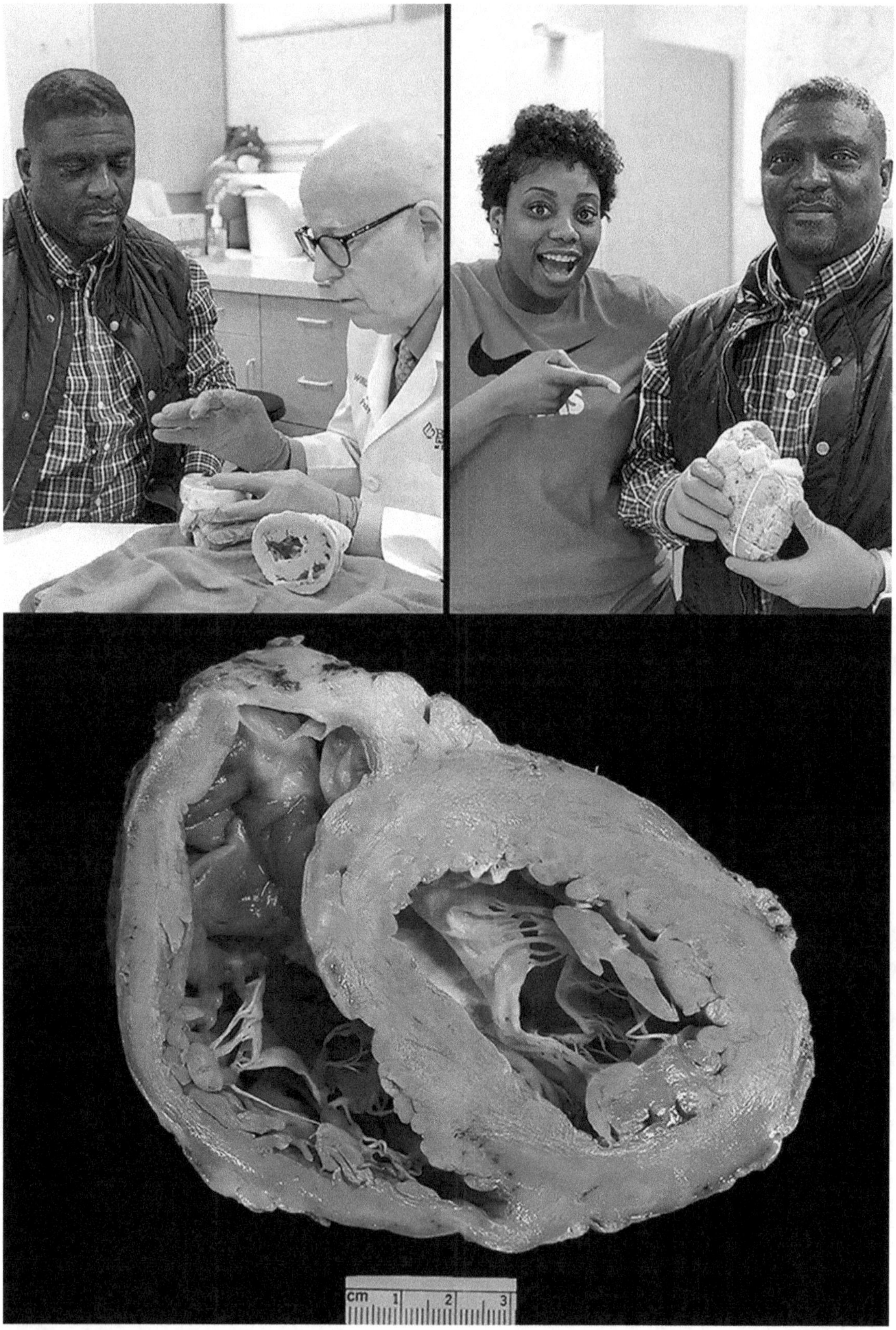


Figure 8. Todd Hickman, a 50-year-old man, had a heart transplant in December 2017 because of severe heart failure secondary to idiopathic dilated cardiomyopathy and his heart viewing in February 2020. At one time he weighed 290 lbs. He had had heart failure since age 41. Both of his paternal grandparents died of heart disease and a paternal uncle had a heart transplant at another hospital in 2016. *Top right*: His wife is obviously pointing at his heart. His heart weighed 565 g.

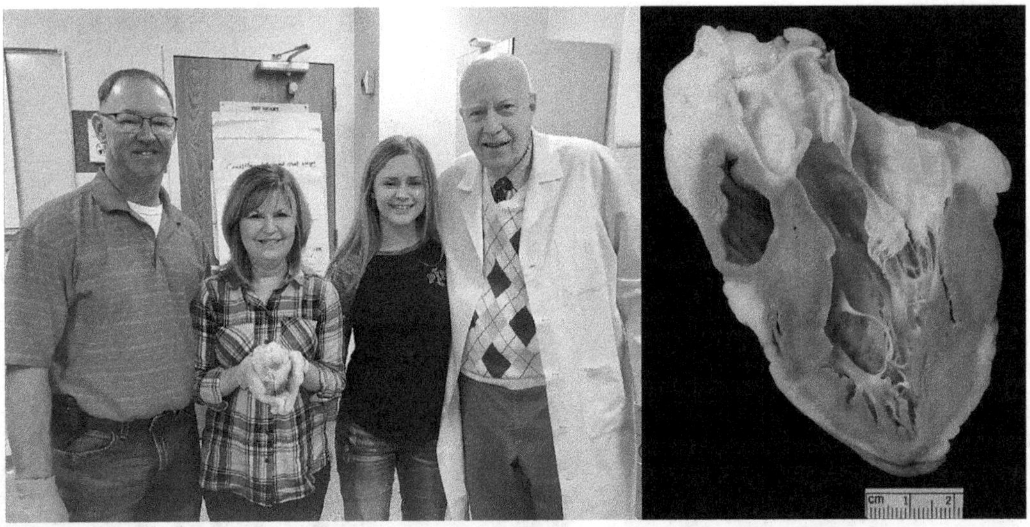

Figure 9. Vickie Coker, a 55-year-old, five-foot-tall woman, with her husband and 21-year-old daughter had a heart transplant for hypertrophic cardiomyopathy in January 2020 and the heart viewing in February 2020. Both mother and daughter had hypertrophic cardiomyopathy. The daughter (shown here) had a heart transplant at age 13. A son had died of hypertrophic cardiomyopathy in his teenage years. One of Mrs. Coker's sisters had ablation for atrial fibrillation at age 42, and later a heart transplant due to hypertrophic cardiomyopathy. The same sister had 2 daughters, both of whom had hypertrophic cardiomyopathy. Another sister died suddenly with heart failure and she too probably had the same condition. *Left*: Her husband and daughter with WCR. Ms. Coker's heart weighed only 255 g. The heart is unusual for hypertrophic cardiomyopathy in that there is no evidence of left ventricular outflow obstruction, no scarring in the ventricular walls, and the ventricular septum is only minimally thicker than the left ventricular free wall. In her consent letter she stated: *"I hope and pray that my story helps people see the importance of organ donation."*

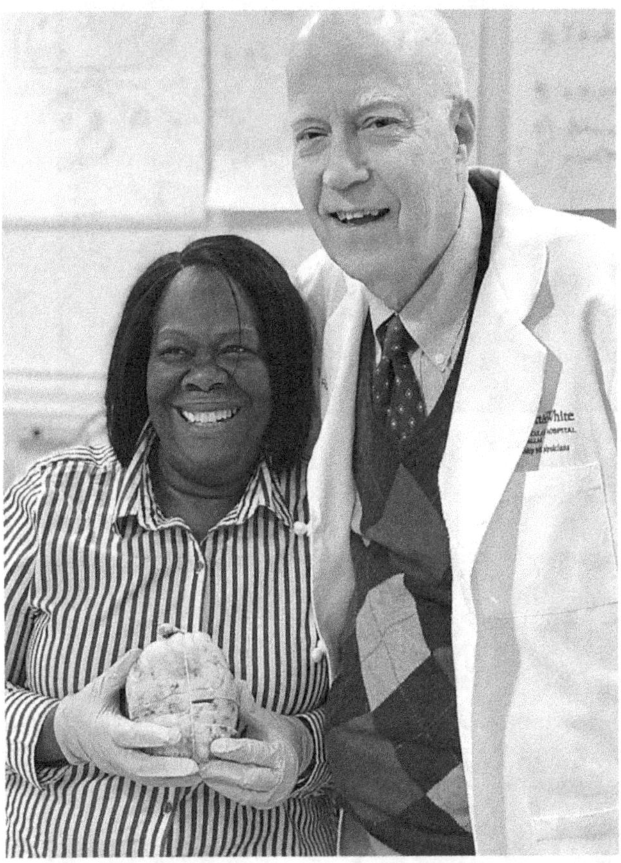

Figure 10. Debra R. Bruce, a 57-year-old woman, had a heart transplant in January 2018 because of severe heart failure secondary to idiopathic dilated cardiomyopathy and the heart viewing in January 2020. She had a son who had died of heart failure probably also from idiopathic dilated cardiomyopathy. Her heart weighed 425 g. In her consent letter she indicated that showing her heart was *"...one of the best days of my life."*

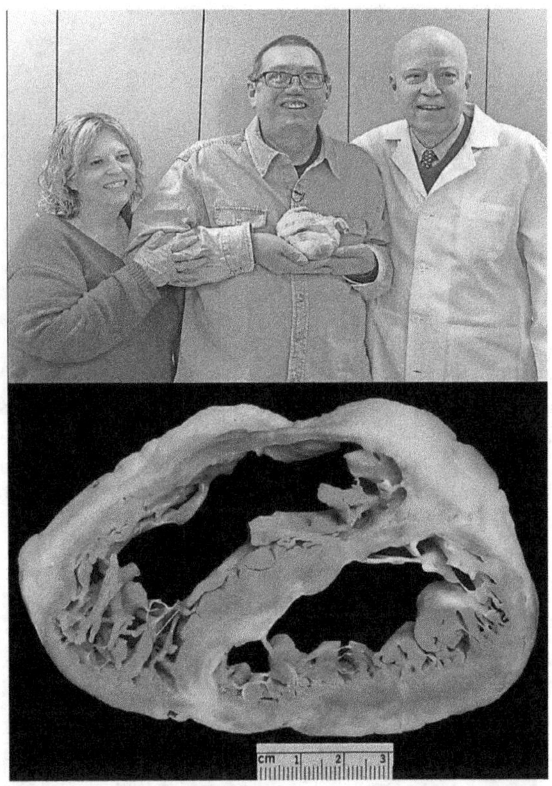

Figure 11. Darryl Glen Moore, a 58-year-old man, had a heart transplant in November 2019 for burnt-out cardiac sarcoidosis and the heart viewing in February 2020. He had classic gross features of cardiac sarcoidosis, but no granulomas were found in the heart. The white areas displayed in the photograph are scarred areas, but no granulomas were found within them. The coronary arteries were wide open. The heart weighed 440 g and he weighed 170 lbs. He had received immunosuppression with Imuran for 5 years prior to the transplant because of autoimmune hepatitis. Possibly this drug (Azathioprine) wiped out the granulomas.

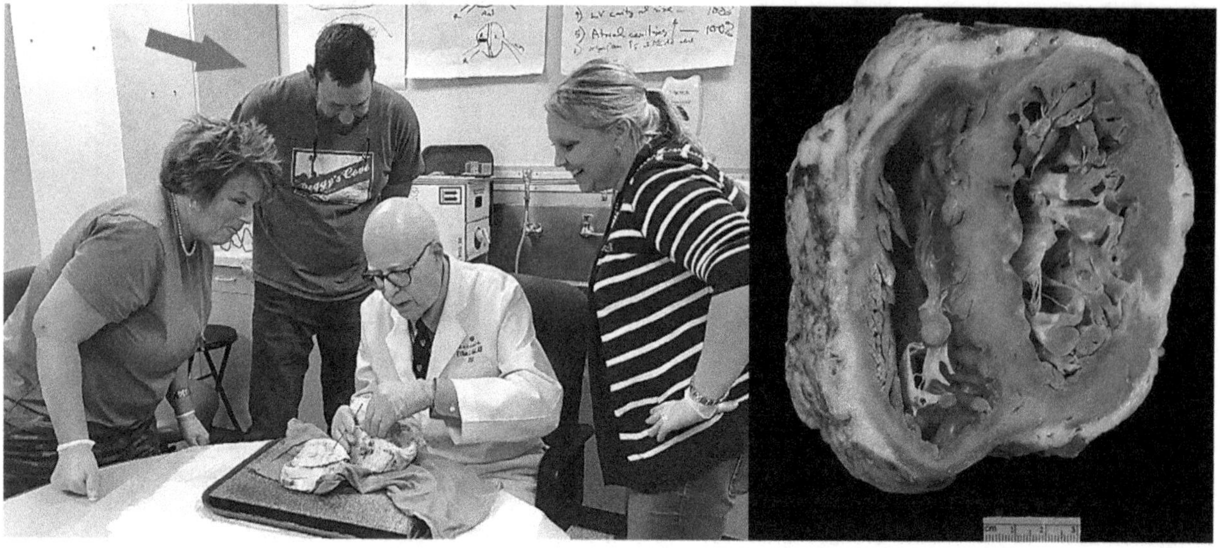

Figure 12. Robert J. Kraus (arrow), a 58-year-old man, had a heart transplant in March 2019 and the heart viewing in October 2019. His congenitally bicuspid aortic valve had been replaced when he was 21 years of age because of severe aortic regurgitation secondary to infective endocarditis. The mechanical prothesis worked well for 35 years. His resected heart weighed 915 g. Six years earlier he weighed 275 lbs. The heart is nearly surrounded by adipose tissue.

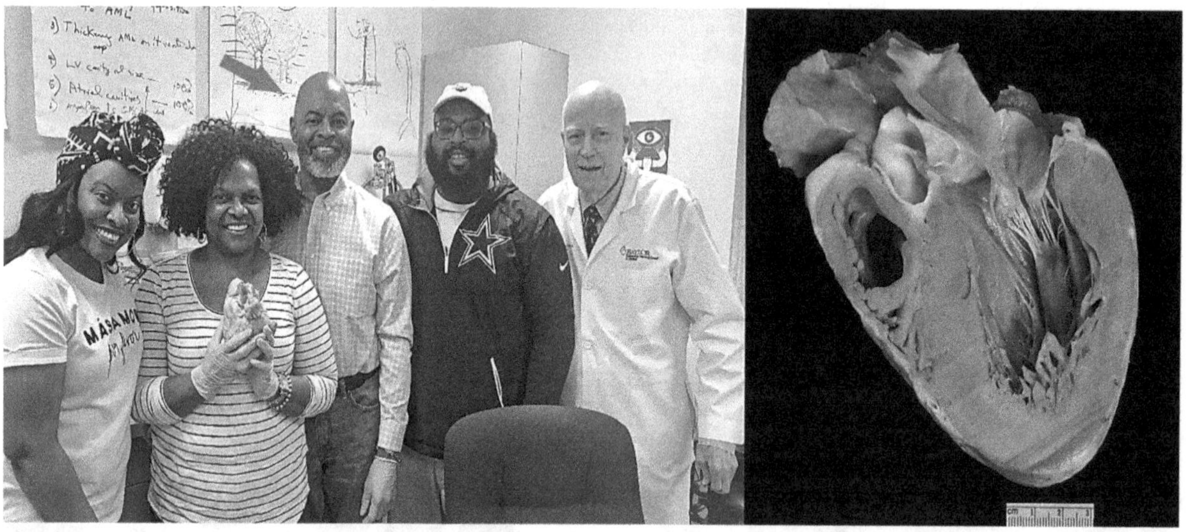

Figure 13. Ellis Robert Mayberry (arrow), a 61-year-old man, had a heart transplant in February 2019 because of amyloidosis and the heart viewing in February 2020. He has been asymptomatic subsequently. His wife, adjacent to her husband, is holding his heart. His amyloid-infiltrated heart is shown, and it weighed 580 g. He also had a renal transplant at the time of his heart transplant.

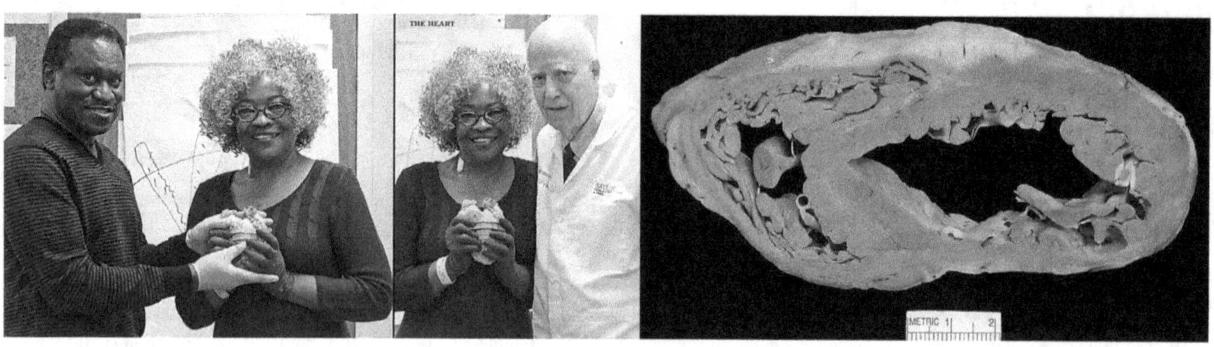

Figure 14. Sandra Jean Harvey, a 62-year-old woman, had a heart transplant in April 2017 because of idiopathic dilated cardiomyopathy and the heart viewing in January 2018. Her heart was relatively small (320 g) even though she had weighed 230 lbs. at one time. *Left*: Both she and her husband are holding her heart. *Center*: Photograph with WCR. *Right*: A cross-section of her cardiac ventricles. In her consent letter she wrote: *"I still talk about the conversation with Dr. Roberts and seeing my heart is still enlightening to me and other to do the right things for our health."*

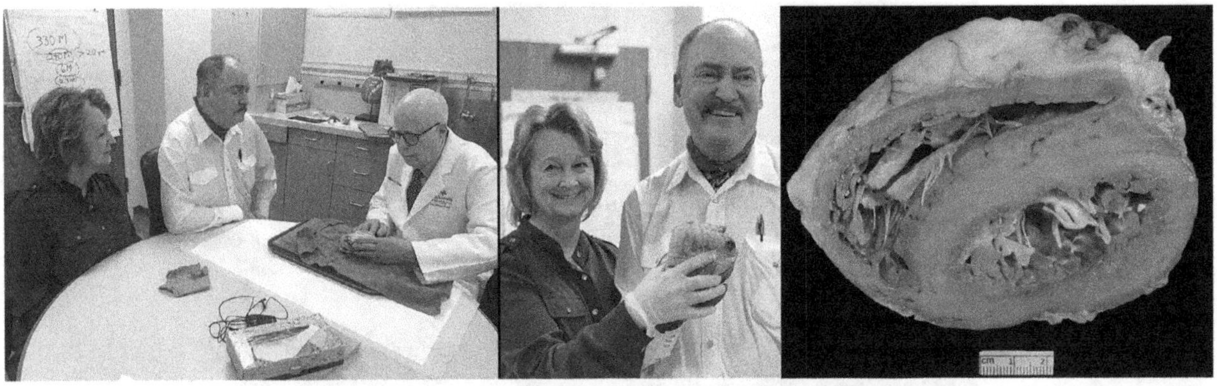

Figure 15. Mark Lehman, a 62-year-old man, had a heart transplant because of severe heart failure resulting from severe mitral regurgitation secondary to mitral valve prolapse in December 2019 and the heart viewing in January 2020. He also had severe coronary arterial narrowing but no myocardial lesions. His heart weighed 455 g.

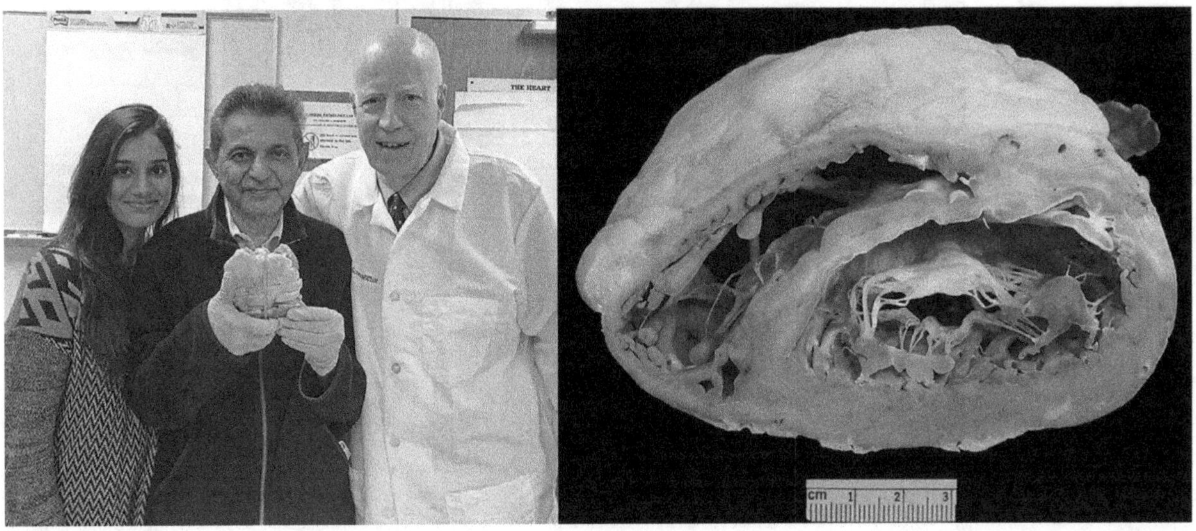

Figure 16. Habib Nooruddin, a 64-year-old man, had a heart transplant in September 2017 for ischemic cardiomyopathy and the heart viewing in November 2017. His heart weighed 302 g and he weighed 143 lbs. There is considerable scarring in the anteroseptal and anterolateral portions of his left ventricular wall. The cavity is quite dilated. The epicardial coronary arteries are severely narrowed by atherosclerotic plaque. In his consent letter he wrote: *"It's an honor to be included in your article, continuing to educate people about organ donation and how it impacts the lives of families. One donation can positively change the lives of so many individuals."*

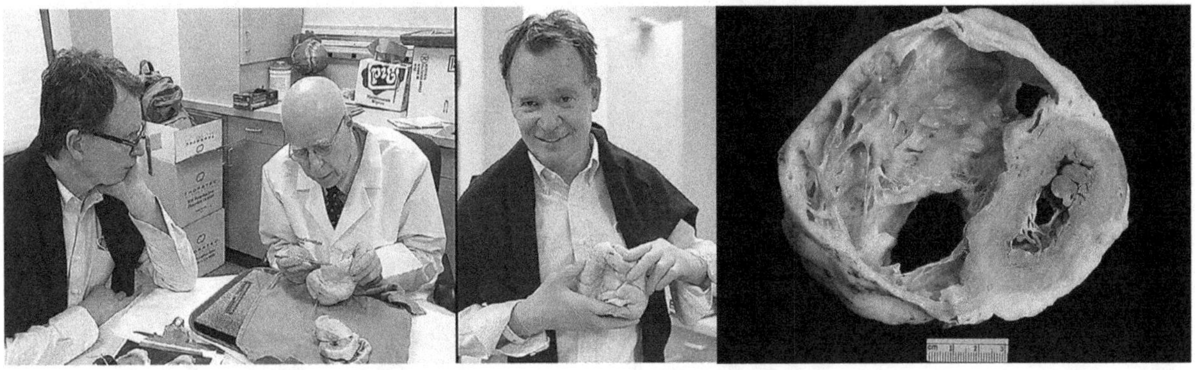

Figure 17. Zack Bacon, a 65-year-old man, had a heart transplant in July 2018 for heart failure secondary to arrhythmogenic right ventricular cardiomyopathy and the heart viewing in September 2018. *Left*: WCR explaining his heart disease to him. *Center*: Mr. Bacon is holding his own heart. *Right*: A picture of his heart showing a huge right ventricular cavity, a much smaller left ventricular cavity, and much of the right ventricular free wall replaced by adipose tissue. His heart weighed 485 g.

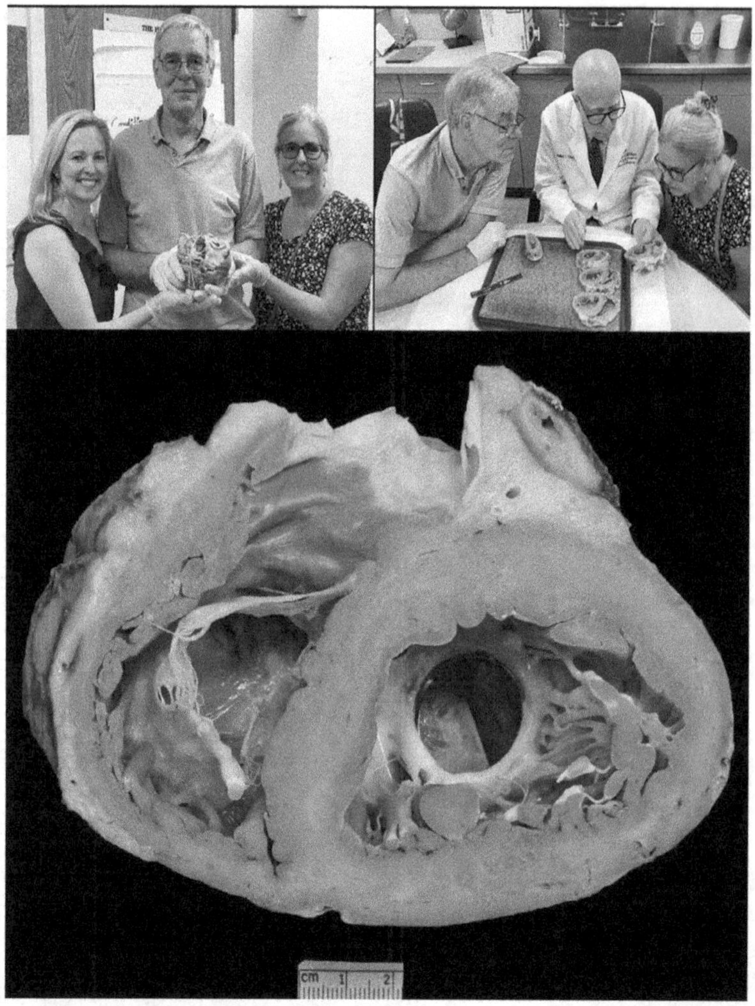

Figure 18. Mark Francis Gengler, a 66-year-old man, had a heart transplant in May 2019 for probable valvular heart disease and the heart viewing in September 2019. At age 46, both mitral and aortic valves were replaced, and his ascending aorta was resected and replaced. His heart weighed 620 g. He has done well since the transplant.

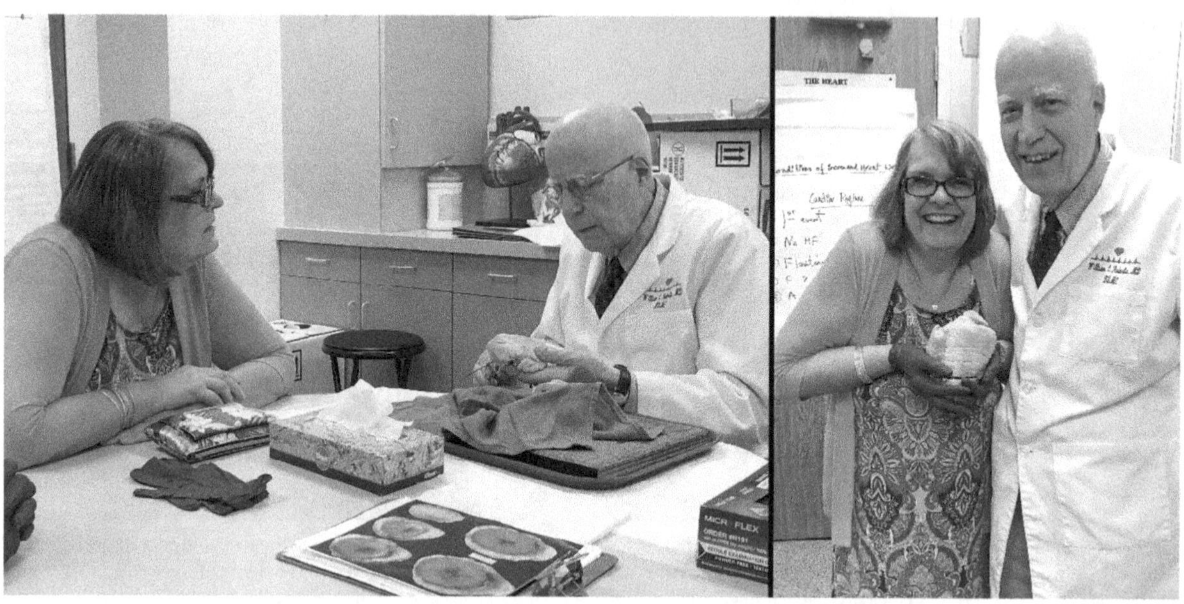

Figure 19. Karen Acheson, a 67-year-old woman, had a heart transplant in June 2016 because of severe heart failure secondary to idiopathic dilated cardiomyopathy and the heart viewing in August 2018. She has been asymptomatic ever since. Her heart weighed 460 g.

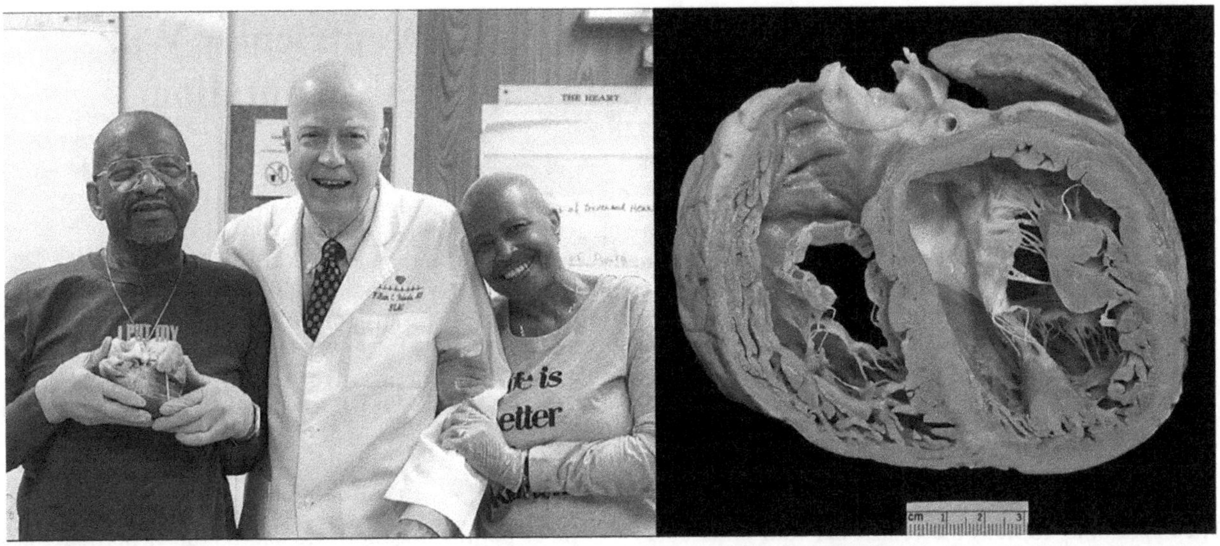

Figure 20. Harold Wilson, a 68-year-old man, had a heart transplant in April 2019 for heart failure secondary to idiopathic dilated cardiomyopathy and the heart viewing in September 2019. He has been asymptomatic subsequently. His heart weighed 385 g. At one time he weighed 270 lbs. He weighed 199 lbs. at the time of the transplant. In his consent letter he wrote: *"...thank you guys for all you've done in my life."*

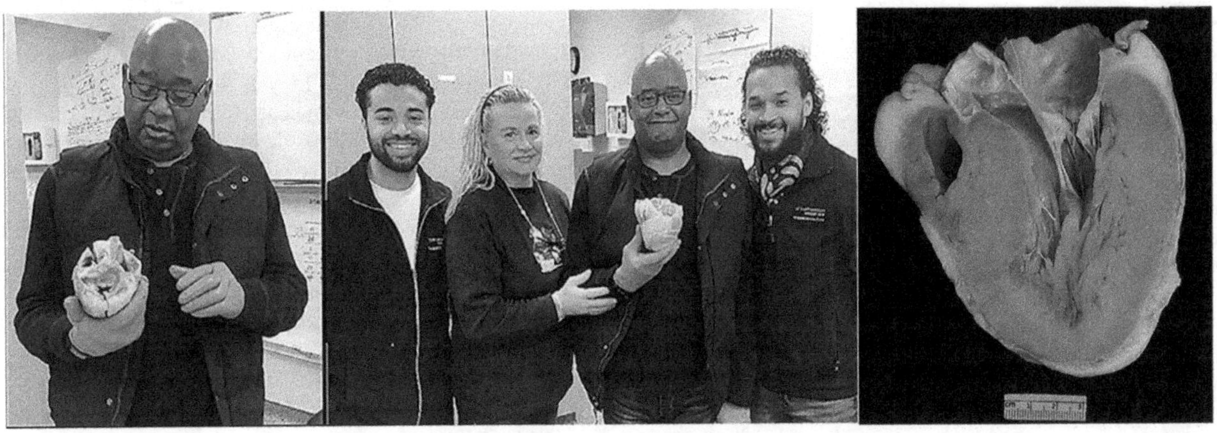

Figure 21. Alphonso Robinson, a 69-year-old man, had a heart transplant in August 2019 because of heart failure secondary to cardiac amyloidosis and the heart viewing in December 2019. He has been asymptomatic subsequently. *Left:* Mr. Robinson looking at his heart. *Center*: Mr. Robinson holding his heart with his wife and two children. *Right*: His amyloid-infiltrated heart weighed 580 g.

## Author credit statement

None.

## Disclosures

The authors have no conflicts of interest to disclose.


1. Roberts WC. So you want to see your heart. *Am J Cardiol* 2010;106:1520.
2. Roberts WC, Won VS, Vasudevan A, Kapoor P, Ko JM, Meyer DM, Hall SA, Gonzalez-Stawinski G. Comparison of characteristics of patients undergoing heart transplantation in the same hospital in two different time periods (1997 – 2012 and 2013-2015). *Am J Cardiol* 2016;118:288–291.

# Malignant Ventricular Tachycardia, Ventricular Wall Ablation, and Orthotopic Heart Transplantation

William C. Roberts, MD[a,b,c,*], Alexander T. Kietzman, BS[a,#], and Praveen K. Rao, MD[b]

**Described herein are three patients with refractory ventricular tachycardia and one or more unsuccessful ablation procedures finally leading to orthotropic heart transplantation (OHT). The latter procedure allowed examination of the ventricular ablation sites, an unusual opportunity reported previously in few patients (all case reports). The acute ablation lesions are unique, with necrosis of the myocardial fibers adjacent to the endocardium and encircled by layers of extravasated erythrocytes in the deeper myocardial wall. All 3 patients returned to normal activities following the OHT.**  **(Am J Cardiol 2021;149:150–154)**

The opportunity to study the ventricular walls after ablation procedures for episodes of ventricular tachycardia (VT) is infrequent. Such was the case in the three patients to be described herein. (Table 1).

## Case Descriptions

### *Case #1*

A 51-year-old obese, former truck driver, who was born in July 1963, had been well until age 49 (July 2012) when she had an acute myocardial infarct and received several coronary stents. Thereafter, she was in chronic heart failure and had several episodes of VT and an implantable cardioverter defibrillator (ICD) was inserted (2013). During the next several months she had a number of VT episodes and ICD shocks. As a consequence, an ablation procedure was done in August 2014. Nevertheless, the episodes of VT/ventricular fibrillation continued and the heart failure worsened leading to cardiogenic shock and the institution of extracorporeal membrane oxygenation in September 2014. Being unable to wean the patient from ECMO an orthotopic heart transplant (OHT) was performed 16 days later (September 2014). The post-transplant course was characterized by a number of complications requiring hospitalization for 5 continuous months following the OHT. Follow up in August 2020 (six years after the OHT) found the patient to be well and carrying out her many activities without difficulty.

The heart weighed 290 g and floated in a container of formaldehyde (due to the excessive subepicardial adipose tissue [fat is lighter than myocardium]). The left ventricular cavity was dilated. Scar, mainly subendocardial, was present in the anteroseptal wall. The ablation site was in the posterior (inferior) wall of the left ventricle (Figure 1.) The inner portion was necrotic and the outer portion consisted of collections of extravasated erythrocytes.

### *Case #2*

A 59-year-old, a metal fabricator and repairer of fire engines, had been well until age 40 (2,000) when he developed signs of heart failure and was medically treated. He did relatively well until age 55 (2015) when an episode of VT occurred and an ICD was inserted. During the next 4 years the symptoms of heart failure gradually worsened, and at age 59 (2019) episodes of VT became frequent and he experienced multiple ICD shocks. These episodes prompted an ablation procedure, the first, taking place 148 days before OHT. The VT was not hemodynamically tolerated, so a pacemapping strategy was used. The focus of the first VT ablation procedure was the anteroseptal right-ventricular outflow tract. A second VT was induced and believed to exit in the epicardium but it could not be isolated for ablation due to extensive epicardial fat.

Table 1
Certain features in each of the 3 obese patients having OHT because of recurring ventricular tachycardia and ventricular ablations

| Variable | Case 1 | Case 2 | Case 3* |
|---|---|---|---|
| Age at OHT (years) | 51 | 59 | 58 |
| Sex | Woman | Man | Man |
| Coronary narrowing >75% CSA | + (stents) | + | O |
| Body mass index (kg/m2) | 31 | 36 | 32 |
| Diabetes mellitus | + | 0 | 0 |
| Intracardiac defibrillator | + | + | + |
| Systemic hypertension | + | + | + |
| Total cholesterol (mg/dl) | 87* | 203 | 186 |
| LDL-cholesterol (mg/dl) | 42* | 124 | 88 |
| HDL-cholesterol (mg/dl) | 31* | 56 | 87 |
| Triglycerides (mg/dl) | 85* | 197 | 53 |
| Left ventricular assist device | 0 | + | 0 |
| Number of ablations performed | 1 | 3 | 1 |
| Interval between last ablation and OHT (days) | 15 | 2 | 362 |
| Heart weight (g) | 290 | 740 | 410 |
| Left ventricular Scar | + | 0 | + |
| Floating Heart (excess adiposity) | + | + | + |

*Abbreviations:* CSA=Cross sectional area; HDL=high-density lipoprotein; LDL=low-density lipoprotein; OHT= orthotopic heart transplant.
* Liver transplant at age 43.
***On statin

[a]Baylor Scott and White Heart and Vascular Institute, Baylor University Medical Center, Dallas, Texas; [b]Department of Medicine (Division of Cardiology), Dallas, Texas; and [c]Department of Pathology, Baylor University Medical Center, Dallas, Texas. Manuscript received September 22, 2020; revised manuscript received and accepted March 12, 2021.

[#]Present address: Baylor University, Waco Texas.

*Corresponding author: Tel: (214)-820-7911; fax: (214)-820-7533.

*E-mail address:* William.Roberts1@BSWHealth.org (W.C. Roberts).

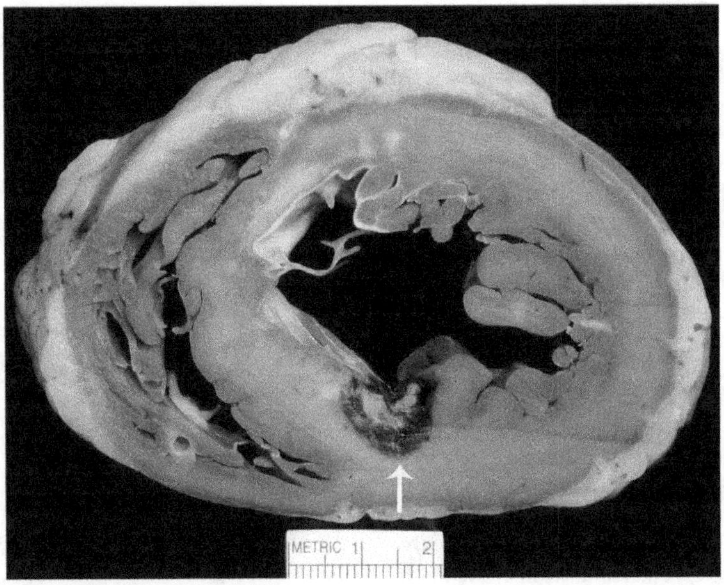

Figure 1. Case # 1. Cross-section of the cardiac ventricular showing the site of the ablation (arrow). A healed myocardial infarct is present in the anteroseptal wall.

Following this initial ablation procedure episodes of VT continued and the heart failure worsened prompting a second ablation procedure 73 days before OHT. On this occasion, the right ventricular outflow tract and right side of the ventricular septum were again ablated, and this time the aortic sinus of Valsalva also was ablated. At the end of the procedure, VT was still inducible causing hemodynamic instability. These were believed to be mid-septal in origin.

After the second ablation he had worsening low output heart failure and recurrent VT, leading to transfer to Baylor University Medical Center for insertion of a HeartMate 3 (Abbott Medical) left ventricular assist device 12 days before OHT. The episodes of VT continued prompting a third ablation 2 days before OHT. During this ablation several different VTs were mapped to the mid ventricular septum, which was very thick so half normal saline was used

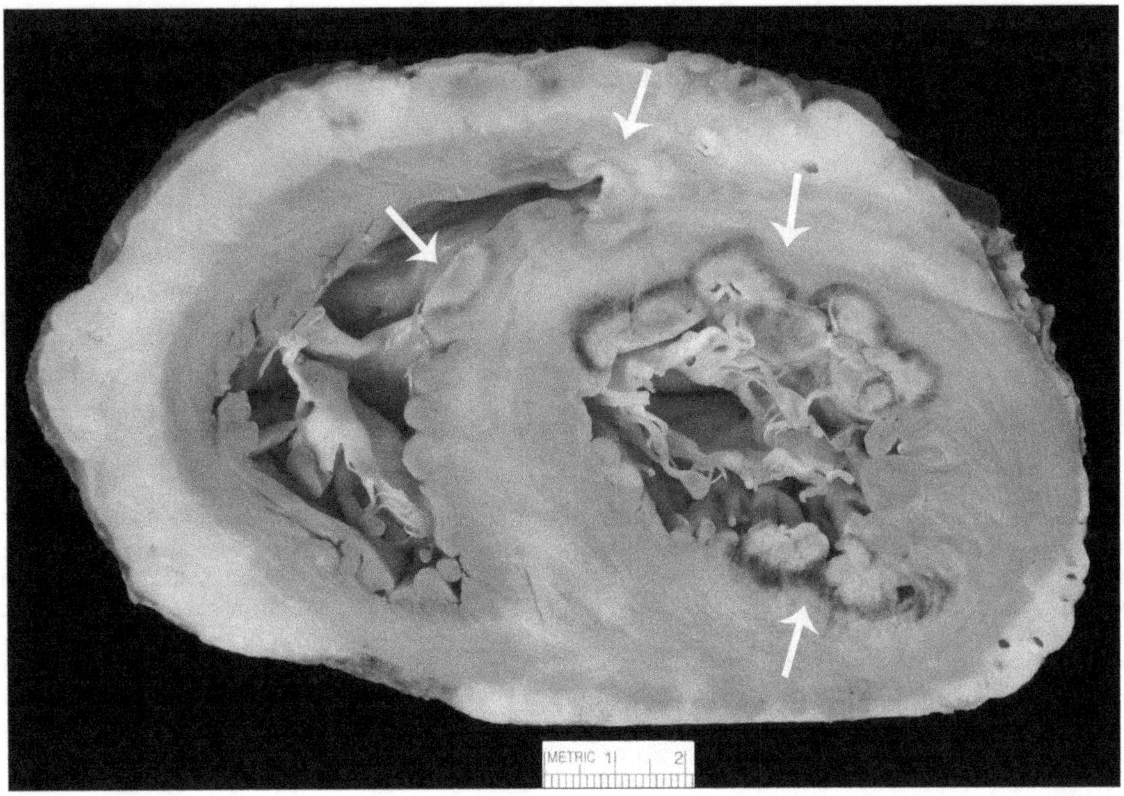

Figure 2. Case # 2. Cross-section of the cardiac ventricular showing at least 4 ablation sites. The quality of subepicardial adipose tissue is huge.

as the irrigant through a 4-mm Flex Ability F/J sensor enabled ablation catheter (Abbott Cardiovascular, Plymouth, MN) at up to 45 Watts to create larger and deeper lesions. (Half normal saline reduces the ionic concentration of the surrounding fluid, thereby drawing more radiofrequency energy into the tissue[1]). Overall, 10 different VT circuits were mapped and ablated between the anteroseptum and inferoseptum, both from the right ventricular and left ventricular sides of the septum. The lesions set was broad, extending off the septum to the anterior and inferior left ventricular walls. At the end of his third ablation the patient was no longer inducible to monomorphic VTs, but was still inducible into ventricular fibrillation. The night after ablation he had recurrent ventricular fibrillation requiring defibrillation. OHT was done the following day (November 2019).

The explanted heart weighed 740 g and floated in a container of formaldehyde because of the excessive adipose tissue. The 3 ablation sites are shown in Figure 2. No grossly-visible scars were seen in the ventricular walls, but histologically the quantity of fibrous tissue in the interstitium was focally increased. Also, as shown in Figure 2 the left anterior descending coronary artery was severely narrowed by atherosclerotic plaque. The left circumflex was narrowed 51-75% in cross-sectional area by plaque. (A diagnosis of coronary artery disease was not made during life.) Photomicrographs of the ablation lesion is shown in Figure 3.

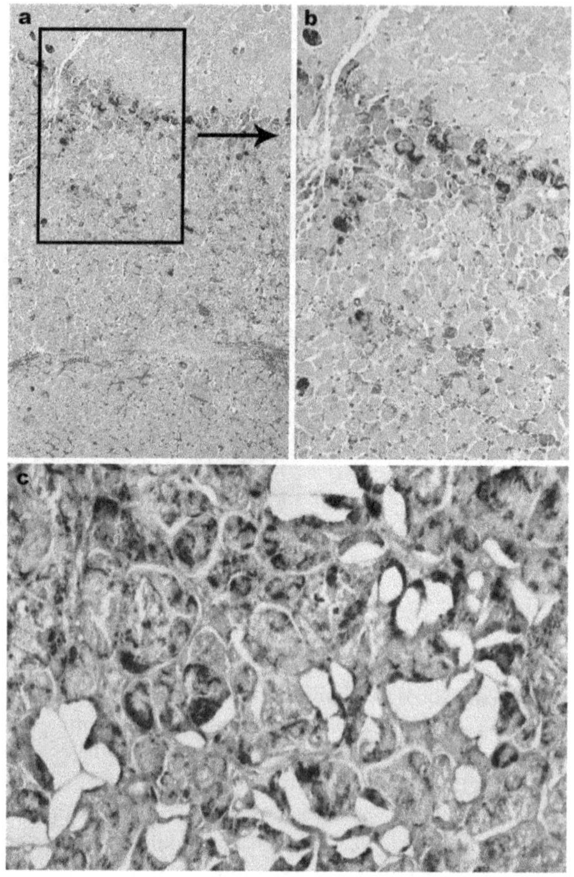

Figure 3. Case #2. Photomicrographs of the ablation lesion, all stained by trichrome. a The portion on the top in closest to the endocardium. The more centered portions show individual myocytes which are actually destroyed. The portion on the bottom are preserved myocytes with focal extravascular of erithocytes, x 100. b Higher power of the portion in brackets in a (x 200). c Close-up view of acutely destroyed myocytes, x 400, in another ablated area.

*Case #3*

A 58-year-old Hispanic man who was born in February 1961 had a liver transplant at age 42 (2004) because of hepatitis C-induced cirrhosis. Systemic hypertension developed thereafter followed later by deep vein thrombosis and pulmonary embolism leading to chronic warfarin therapy. At age 57 (June 2018) he had a syncopal episode and was found to have VT with a rate of 230 beats/minute.

After cardioversion he had periods of 2:1 atrioventricular block. His left ventricular ejection fraction was 35%. Cardiac magnetic resonance imaging disclosed a myocardial scar at the right ventricular insertion into the ventricular septum involving about 5% of the left ventricular wall. Angiography showed no obstructive coronary artery disease. He underwent cardiac resynchronization therapy defibrillator (CRT-D), followed by a sotalol load.

He subsequently presented with recurrent VT and underwent VT ablation. He had an infra-Hisian conduction system disease. Both ventricles were mapped for scar. Both the left and right ventricular bipolar voltage was normal. Unipolar voltage suggested deep ventricular septal scar. He was non-inducible to any sustained VT, and was only inducible into ventricular fibrillation. Empiric ablation was done across his right bundle branch about one-third of the way toward the apex. There was also frequent ventricular premature complexes of a left bundle left inferior axis, which mapped to the base of the right ventricular outflow tract. Ablation was done using a 4/mm FlexAbility catheter (Abbott Medical) using normal saline as the irrigant, at up to 45W. No further ventricular premature complexes were seen after ablation, and he remained non-inducible to any sustained VT.

A year later he again developed VT storm and presented after 20 ICD shocks. At redo VT ablation, both ventricles were mapped and this time he was inducible into a fast-monomorphic VT that was hemodynamically unstable. He was defibrillated. Ablation was once again carried out using a 4/mm FlexAbility catheter (Abbott Medical), this time using half normal saline as the irrigate to achieve a deeper lesion. This region was targeted using sequential unipolar ablation at up to 45W from both the right and left sides of the ventricular septum. These areas were ablated until there was loss of pace capture. He was then inducible into a different VT that mapped higher in the ventricular septum using half normal saline with sequential unipolar ablation at up to 45W. At this point VT was no longer inducible.

During the early follow up period he developed recurrent VT refractory to medical management and extracorporeal membrane support initiated leading to OHT 2 weeks later. The explanted heart is shown in Figure 4. It weighed 410g. The right ventricular free wall focally consisted entirely of adipose tissue. Both ventricular cavities were dilated. Ablation lesion were present in most of the ventricular septum. No scars were present. Genetic testing disclosed a lumin A/C mutation.

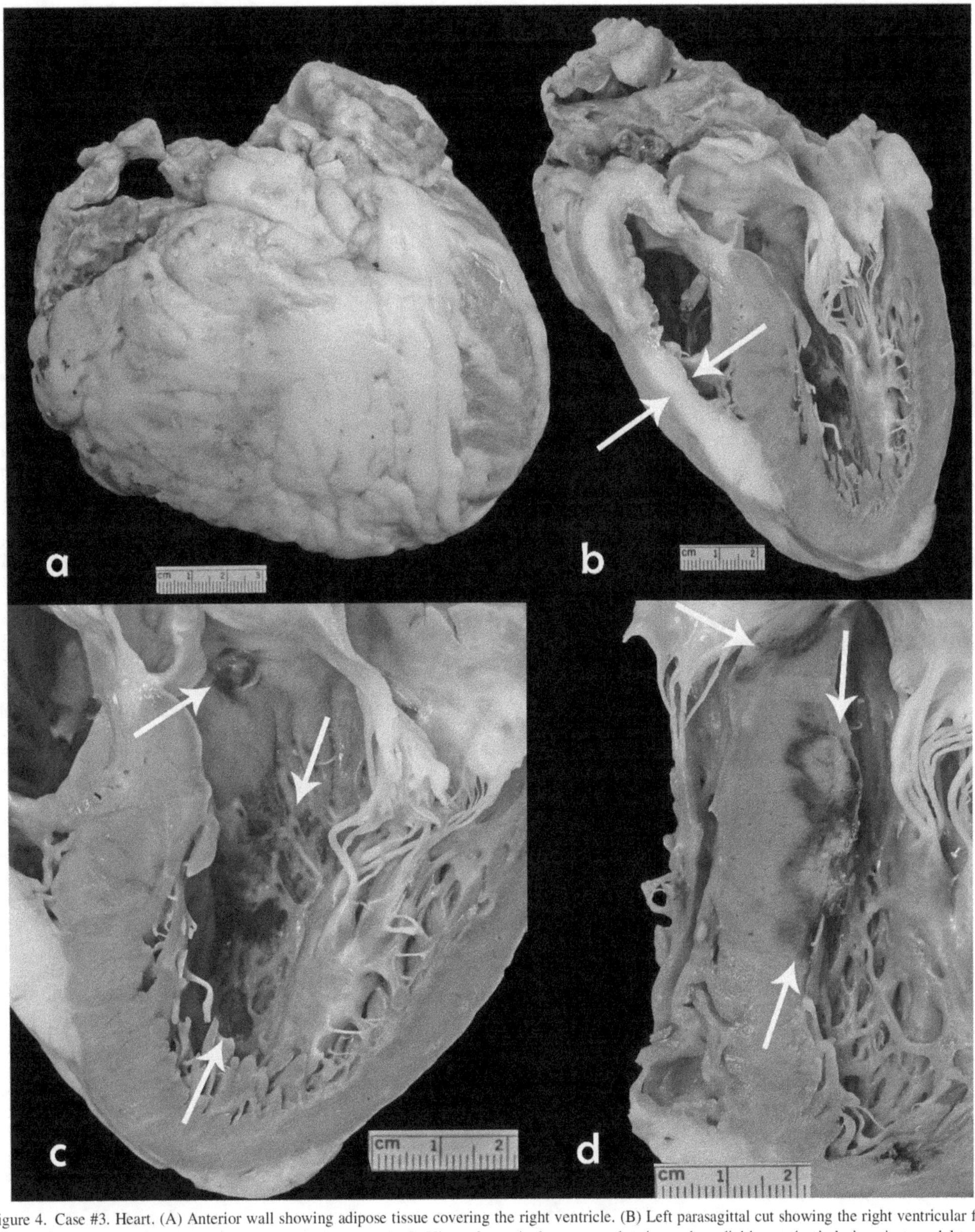


Figure 4. Case #3. Heart. (A) Anterior wall showing adipose tissue covering the right ventricle. (B) Left parasagittal cut showing the right ventricular free wall locally consisting of adipose tissue (between the arrows). (C) View of ventricular septum showing endocardial hemorrhagic lesions just caudal to the aortic valve and multiple lesions in the muscular ventricular septum(between the arrows). (D) Cross section of the ventricular septum showing the classic ablation lesions (between the arrows).

## Discussion

Described herein are 3 patients who had recurrent episodes of VT not eliminated by ablation procedures leading to OHT in each. The OHT provided the opportunity to study morphologically the cardiac ventricular ablation sites, something infrequently available in humans. In each patient the ablation sites were clearly distinguishable presumably because the intervals between the last ablation procedure and the OHT were short (15 days in case #1, 2 days in case # 2, and 14 days in case # 3). The area of myocardial necrosis was closest to the endocardium and these areas were surrounded by a semicircle of extravasated erythrocytes. Such lesions have been reproduced experimentally in dogs, sheep and pigs.[2-5] Such lesions have been reported in at least 7 other humans[6-12] (All case reports). These 7 previously reported cases had an assortment of conditions: coronary artery disease in 1[6]; idiopathic dilated cardiomyopathy in 2[7,10]; sarcoidosis in 2[8,11]; hypertrophic cardiomyopathy in 1,[9] and lamin AC / cardiomyopathy in 1.[12] The latter condition was present in our case #3. In each condition of these reports the myocardial lesions were illustrated grossly and usually histologically. Several reports indicate that the acute lesions (necrotic focus surrounded by collections of extravasated erythrocytes) heal by scarring.[5,6,7,8,11]

The unique feature of the patients reported is the description and clear illustration of the myocardial acute ablation lesion. Although these lesions have been described previously in nonhuman animals and in a few humans, exquisite illustrations, except for the report by Nakajma et al,[9] have not been provided. Details of the ablation procedure in case #1 are unavailable.

## Conflict of Interests

The authors declare that they have no known competing financial interests or personal relationships that could have appeared to influence the work reported in this paper.


1. Nguyen DT, Gerstenfeld EP, Tzou WS, Jurgens PT, Zheng L, Schuller J, Zipse M, Sauer WH. Radiofrequency ablation using an open irrigated electrode cooled with half-normal saline. *JACC Clin Electrophysiol* 2017;3:1103–1110.
2. Weber HP, Sagerer-Gerhardt M. *Laser-Based Approach to Cardiac Mapping and Arrhythmia Ablation*. Verlag London: Springer, Lasers in Cardiovascular Interventions; 2015:221–244. https://doi.org/10.1007/978-1-4471-5220-0_17.
3. Berte B, Cochet H, Magat J, Naulin J, Ghidoli D, Pillois X, Casassus F, Yamashita S, Saagar Mahida S, Nicolas Derval N, Méléze Hocini M, Quesson B, Bernus O, Weerasooriya R, Haïssaguerre M, Sacher F, Jaï P. Irrigated needle ablation creates larger and more transmural ventricular lesions compared with standard unipolar ablation in an bovine model. *Circ Arrhythmia Electrophysiol* 2015;8:1498–1506.
4. Krahn PRP, Singh SM, Ramanan V, Biswas L, Yak N, Anderson KJT, Barry J, Pop M, Wright GA. Cardiovascular magnetic resonance guided ablation and intra-procedural visualization of evolving radiofrequency lesions in the left ventricle. *J Cardiovasc Magn Reson* 2018;20:20. https://doi.org/10.1186/s12968-018-0437-z.
5. Tao S, Guttman MA, Fink S, Elahi H, Patil KD, Ashikaga H, Kolandaivelu AD, Berger RD, Halushka MK, Schmidt J, Herzka DA, Halperin HR. Ablation lesion characterization in scarred substrate assessed using cardiac magnetic resonance. *JACC Clin Electrophysiol* 2019;5:91–100. https://doi.org/10.1016/j.jacep.2018.11.001.
6. Knight BP, Bogner P, Wasmer K, Morady F. Human pathologic validation of left ventricular linear lesion formation guided by noncontact mapping. *J Cardiovasc Electrophysiol* 2002;13:79–82. https://doi.org/10.1046/j.1540-8167.2002.00079.x.
7. Sasaki T, Mudd J, Steenbergen C, Zviman MM, Miller CF, Nazarian S. Impact of scar, viable myocardium, and epicardial fat on substrate identification of ventricular tachycardia in a case with nonischemic cardiomyopathy. *Pacing Clin Electrophysiol* 2012;35:e345–e348. https://doi.org/10.1111/j.1540-8159.2011.03213.x.
8. Kaneko Y, Igawa O, Irie T, Adachi M, Nakajima T, Yokoo H, Nakazato Y, Kurabayashi M. Histopathological verification for successful ablation of mitral isthmus ventricular tachycardia complicated with cardiac sarcoidosis. *Intern Med* 2012;51:281–285. https://doi.org/10.2169/internalmedicine.51.6307.
9. Nakajima K, Miyamoto K, Matsuyama TA, Noda T, Ishibashi-Ueda H, Kusano K. Pathology after combined epicardial and endocardial ablation for ventricular tachycardia in a postmortem heart with hypertrophic cardiomyopathy. *HeartRhythm Case Rep* 2015;1:310–314. https://doi.org/10.1016/j.hrcr.2015.04.003.
10. Hori Y, Nakahara S, Mine S, Anjo N, Fujii A, Ueda Y, Isao T. Pathological autopsy of a patient that underwent a successful ablation of an electrical storm from the left ventricular summit. *Heart Vessels* 2016;31:2068–2073. https://doi.org/10.1007/s00380-016-0847-5.
11. Miyamoto K, Matsuyama TA, Noda T, Ishibashi-Ueda H, Kusano K. Pathology after a combination of sequential and simultaneous unipolar radiofrequency ablation of ventricular tachycardia in a postmortem heart with cardiac sarcoidosis. *Clin Case Rep* 2018;6:1219–1224. https://doi.org/10.1002/ccr3.1577.
12. Bhaskaran A, Bhat A, Trivil I, Muthiah K, Barrett W, Liang S, Kanthan A, Kumar S. Biventricular, endocardial, and epicardial substrate characterization for ventricular tachycardia and correlation with whole-heart macropathology and histopathology in a patient with lamin A/C cardiomyopathy. *HeartRhythm Case Rep* 2018;5:128–133. https://doi.org/10.1016/j.hrcr.2018.11.009.

# Huge right ventricular outflow tract aneurysm late following total repair of tetralogy of Fallot leading to orthotopic heart transplantation☆

William C. Roberts [1,2,3,*], Shaffin Siddiqui [1,#]

[1] Baylor Scott & White Heart and Vascular Institute, Baylor Scott & White Health, Dallas, Texas, USA
[2] Department of Internal Medicine (Cardiology), Baylor Scott & White Health, Dallas, Texas, USA
[3] Department of Pathology, Baylor University Medical Center, Baylor Scott & White Health, Dallas, Texas, USA

ARTICLE INFO

*Article history:*
Received 2 February 2021
Revised 24 February 2021
Accepted 25 February 2021

*Keywords:*
Tetralogy of Fallot, ventricular tachycardia
right-sided heart failure
bundle branch block

ABSTRACT

Described herein are 3 patients who underwent successful orthotopic heart transplantation (OHT) because of huge, calcified right ventricular outflow tract (RVOT) aneurysms after repair of tetralogy of Fallot 35, 43, and 59 years earlier. Two of the 3 patients developed recurring episodes of ventricular tachycardia simulating arrhythmogenic right ventricular cardiomyopathy.



## 1. Introduction

Operative correction of patients with tetralogy of Fallot (T of F) has been one of the seminal developments in medicine in the last century. Many such patients as a consequence have had entirely normal life spans compared to patients without operative intervention whose mean span is 5 years [1]. Despite these phenomenal operative results, some of the operative survivors develop debilitating right-sided heart failure, arrhythmias, right-ventricular outflow tract (RVOT) patch aneurysms, and other forms of cardiac dysfunction. We describe herein 3 men who developed huge RVOT aneurysms, a relatively infrequently described consequence of the corrective operation for patients with T of F, and right-sided heart failure; simultaneously, 2 of them developed refractory ventricular tachycardia (VT). All 3 patients subsequently underwent orthotopic heart transplantation (OHT).

### 1.1. Patients studied

Findings in the 3 men are summarized in Table 1. Each had successful OHT 35, 43, and 59 years, respectively, after the corrective operation at ages 6, 4, and 6 years, respectively. Two developed recurring episodes of VT, one of whom had multiple ventricular ablations without preventing the VT. All 3 had evidence of right-sided heart failure, worse in the patient without VT. The RVOT patch in all 3 patients was parietal pericardium. Follow-up after OHT (11 years in case #1; 7 years in case #2; and 5 months in case #3) disclosed that all 3 patients were asymptomatic and quite active.

## 2. Discussion

Each of the 3 patients described developed huge RVOT aneurysms involving the transannular patches decades after the operative correction of T of F. Calcific deposits developed in the parietal pericardial patches of all 3 patients, minimal in one and massive in 2. Confirmation of the presence of calcific deposits in the patches has been infrequent [2–7]. Calcific deposits in the patch can develop relatively early after its insertion. Seybold-Epting et al. [3] reported 10 patients among 252 patients with corrected T of F who had a parietal pericardium RVOT patch inserted, and 4 of them were confirmed to have developed microscopic-sized patch calcific deposits 6 to 36 months after the operation. This time span is too short to recognize patch calcific deposits by imaging studies or grossly. In contrast, the patients of this study accumulated the calcific deposits over the course of 35, 43, and 59 years. Ross et al. [8] reported a 16-year-old boy who developed massive calcific deposits in a parietal pericardial RVOT patch within 7 years after its insertion.

☆ Declaration of competing interest: The authors declare that they have no known competing financial interests or personal relationships that could have appeared to influence the work reported in this paper.

* Corresponding author.
*E-mail address:* william.roberts1@bswhealth.org (W.C. Roberts).
# Shaffin Siddiqui, Junior, Princeton University, Princeton, New Jersey.

**Table 1**
Comparison of findings in the 3 men having cardiac transplantation decades after total repair of tetralogy of Fallot.

| Variable | Case 1* | Case 2** | Case 3 |
|---|---|---|---|
| Age (years) | | | |
| At repair of tetralogy of Fallot | 6 | 4 | 6 |
| When RV outflow tract aneurysm first noted | 26 | 33 | 60 |
| At onset of heart failure | 26 | 33 | 60 |
| At onset of ventricular tachycardia | 26 | 33 | No VT |
| At orthotopic heart transplantation | 41 | 47 | 65 |
| At January 2021**** | 51 | 54 | 65 |
| Patch = Parietal pericardium | + | + | + |
| RV outflow patch calcified | +++ | + | +++ |
| Body mass index (kg/m^2) | 29 →25(OHT)→33 | 32 | 29 |
| Bundle branch block | +(Left) | +(Right) | +(Right) |
| Total 12-lead QRS voltage (mm) | 156 | 71 | 84 |
| Intracardiac defibrillator (age) | +(36) | +(33) | +(61) |
| Radiofrequency ablation | + | 0 | 0 |
| Pre-OHT Hemodynamics | | | |
| Left ventricle (s/d) (mm Hg) | 95/30 | – | – |
| Pulmonary artery (s/d) (mm Hg) | 35/15 | 45/20 | 45/5 |
| Right ventricle (s/d) (mm Hg) | 45/20 | 45/10 | 45/5 |
| Lowest LV ejection fraction (%) | 10 | 50 | 20 |
| Heart weight (g) | 655 | 505 | 590 |
| Cardiac adiposity (floating heart) | + | + | + |
| Coronary artery disease | 0 | 0 | 0 |

LV= left ventricular; RV = right ventricular; s/d = peak systolic/end diastolic; OHT = orthotropic heart transplant.

* From George BA, Jong MK, Lensing FD, Kuiper JJ, Roberts WC. "Repaired" tetralogy of Fallot mimicking arrhythmogenic right ventricular cardiomyopathy. *Am J Cardiol* 2011;108:326-329.

** From Donaldson EE, Jong MK, Gonzales-Stawinski G, Hall SA, Roberts WC. Secondary arrhythmogenic right ventricular cardiomyopathy decades after operative repair of tetralogy of Fallot. *Am J Cardiol* 2014;114;806-809.

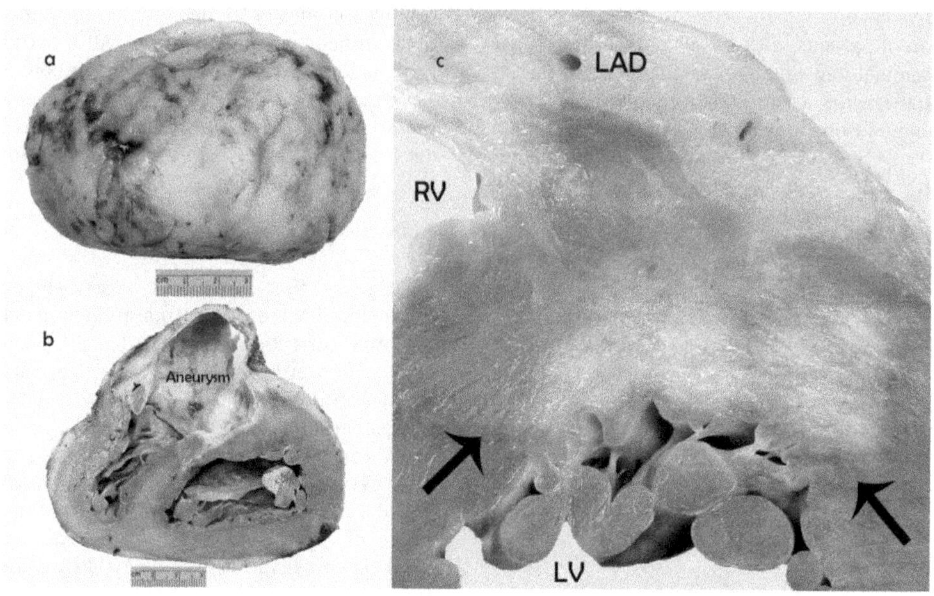


**Fig. 1.** Case#1. The heart. (a) Outside of the heart showing a huge quantity of adipose tissue covering both ventricles. (b) Opened right ventricle showing the huge aneurysm in the outflow tract. (c) Anterior wall of the left ventricle showing a healed ablation site, consisting of fibrous tissue and adipose tissue. The coronary arteries are free of plaque. The ablation had been performed 20 years earlier. LAD = left anterior descending; LV = left ventricular cavity; RV = right ventricular cavity.

Two of the 3 patients described had recurring VT, uncontrolled by either multiple antiarrhythmic agents or repeated ablation procedures. One of the 2 patients with VT had classic epsilon waves on the electrocardiogram, characteristic of arrhythmogenic right ventricular cardiomyopathy.

The occurrence of OHT after repair of T of F is an uncommon event (Table 2). Each of the 3 patients described herein returned to normal activities after their OHT. All 3 are asymptomatic as of January 2021.

**Table 2**
Previous publications of patients having repair for tetralogy of Fallot (T of F) with insertion of right ventricular outflow tract (RVOT) patch with follow-up thereafter.

| First author (reference) | Publication year | Patients with T of F | Patients receiving RVOT patch | Material of patch | Age (years) at total repair of T of F range (mean ± SD) [median] | Duration of follow-up (years)range (mean ± SD) [median] | Patients developing patch aneurysm | Patients develop-ing VT | Patients having OHT |
|---|---|---|---|---|---|---|---|---|---|
| Payne [9] | 1961 | 58 | 26 | Ivalon | – | 0.75-4 (1.9) | 3 | – | – |
| | | | 6 | Ivalon -Teflon | – | 0.66-2 (1.3) | 0 | – | – |
| | | | 26 | Teflon | – | 0.5-1.5 (0.6) | 0 | – | – |
| Rosenthal [10] | 1972 | – | 135 | Pericardial | – | – (0.5) | 8 | – | – |
| Kaplan [11] | 1973 | 150 | 54 | Pericardial | 0-26 | 0.5-14 | 16 | – | – |
| | | | 13 | Homograft | 0-26 | 0.5-14 | 1 | – | – |
| Rieker [12] | 1975 | 60 | | Teflon | 4-20 | – | 0 | – | – |
| Chiariello [2] | 1975 | 403 | 144 | Pericardial | 0.25-41 | – (1.25) | 7 | – | 0 |
| Seybold-Epting [3] | 1977 | 252 | 252 | Pericardial | – | 0.5-3 | 10 | – | – |
| Fuster [6] | 1980 | 396 | – | Ivalon or Teflon | 0-54 | 12-22 | 3 | 1 | 0 |
| Kirklin [13] | 1989 | 791 | 255 | Dacron | – [5] | >2-20 (9 ± 5) | 2 | – | 0 |
| Nollert [14] | 1993 | 490 | – | – | – (12 ± 9) | 1.06-35 (25 ± 13) | – | 0 | 0 |
| Knot-Craig [15] | 1997 | 193 | – | – | – (2 ± 0.2) | 0.1-26 (11 ± 7) | – | – | – |
| Nørgaard [16] | 1999 | 109 | 60 | Dacron or Pericardial | – [13] | 20-28 (26) | – | – | 1 |
| Gatzoulis [17] | 2000 | 793 | 274 | 274 | – (8 ± 8) [6] | 8-41 (21 ± 9) | – | 33 | 0 |
| Troost [18] | 2007 | 68 | – | – | – [24] | 1.3-18 (– ± 8) | – | – | 3 |
| Munkhammar [19] | 2013 | 31 | – | – | – [0.8] | 2-16 (9 ± 3) | – | 0 | 0 |
| Kotani [20] | 2013 | 41 | 11 | Dacron | 0.5-3.5 (0.9) | – [5.9] | – | 0 | 0 |
| Cuypers [21] | 2014 | 80 | 48 | – | 1.7-6.6 (4.3) | 31-43 | – | 26 | 0 |
| Galicia-Tornell [22] | 2015 | 52 | 52 | Dacron | – (4 ± 2) | – (6 ± 2) | 0 | 0 | 0 |
| Dłuzniewska [23] | 2018 | 83 | 54 | – | 0-30 [3] | – (30) | – | 13 | 0 |
| Simon [24] | 2019 | 38 | 27 | – | – (3.3 ± 1) | 19.5-35.8 (30.9) | – | 15 | – |
| Castilhos [25] | 2019 | 206 | 65 | – | 2-4 [3] | – (21 ± 8.2) | – | 15 | 0 |
| Padalino (26) | 2019 | 720 | 435 | Pericardial or homograft | 3.7-11.7 (5.7) | 1-21 | – | – | 0 |
| TOTALS | | 5014 | 1937 (2.58%) | | | | 50 (0.03%)* | 103 (0.06%)* | 4 (0.002%)* |

OHT = orthotopic heart transplant; VT = ventricular tachycardia; – = no information available.
* These percentages are out of the number of patients with RVOT patch (1,937 patients).

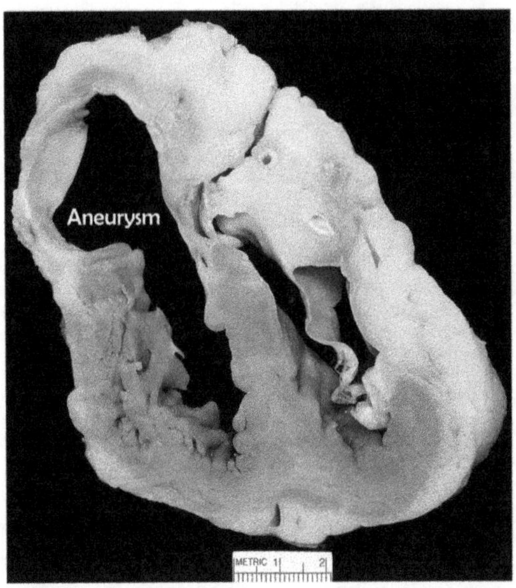


**Fig. 2.** Case #2. Opened right ventricle showing the huge aneurysm in the outflow tract. Both ventricles are nearly covered by adipose tissue. The coronary arteries are wide open.

A previously unreported finding in patients with repaired T of F is excessive cardiac adipose tissue. The hearts in all 3 patients described herein floated in a container of formaldehyde indicating excessive cardiac adipose tissue (adipose tissue is lighter than myocardium). The fat surrounding the left ventricle was especially extensive, an unusual feature. All 3 patients were overweight.

This manuscript, of course, has limitations: 1) Only 3 cases are described but OHT is, as Table 2 demonstrates, uncommon after total "correction" of T of F. Few other studies, however, have had such long intervals between the corrective operation and the OHT. 2) Although all 3 patients had huge RVOT aneurysms and right-sided heart failure, 2 patients had recurring VT prior to OHT (Figures 1–3).

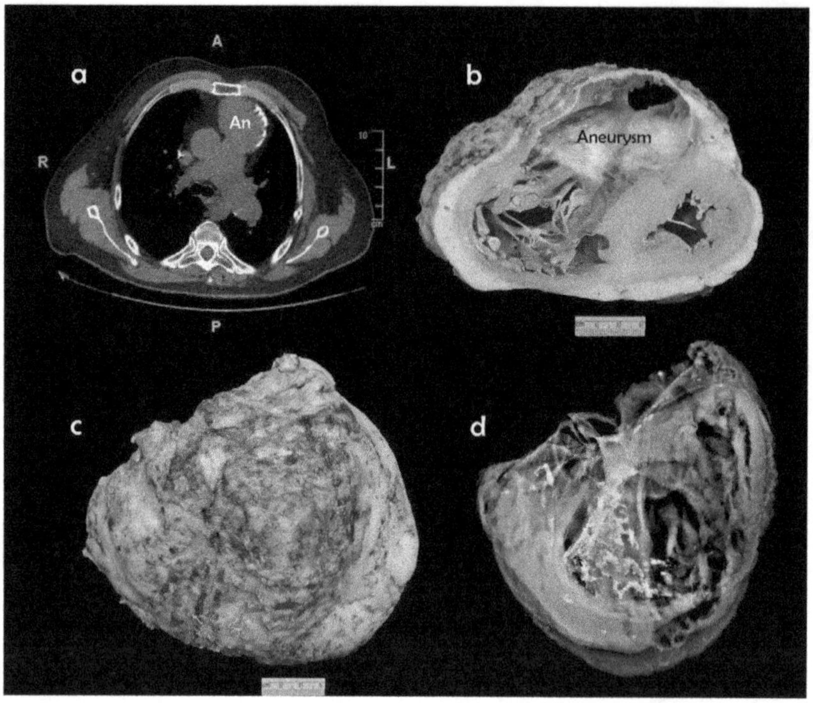


**Fig. 3.** Case #3. Heart. (a) Computed tomographic image showing the right ventricular outflow tract aneurysm (An) with calcium in its wall. (b) Opened right ventricle showing the outflow tract aneurysm. Adipose tissue nearly covers both ventricles. (c) Outside of the heart anteriorly showing the portion of the right ventricle that had been attached to the undersurface of the sternum. (d) Radiograph of the explanted heart displaying the calcium present in the outflow patch.

## References


[1] Campbell M. Natural history of cyanotic malformations and comparison of all common cardiac malformations. Br Heart J 1972;34:3–8 Chiariello L, Meyer J, Wukasch DC, Hallman GL, Cooley DA. Intracardiac repair of tetralogy of Fallot. Five-year review of 403 patients. *J Thorac Cardiovasc Surg* 1975;70:529-535.

[2] Seybold-Epting W, Chiariello L, Hallman GL, Cooley DA. Aneurysm of pericardial right ventricular outflow tract patches. Ann Thorac Surg 1977;24:237–40.

[3] Kirklin JW, Bargeron LM, Pacifico AD. The enlargement of small pulmonary arteries by preliminary palliative operations. Circ 1977;56:612–17.

[4] Arciniegas E, Farooki ZQ, Hakimi M, Perry BL, Green EW. Early and late results of total correction of tetralogy of Fallot. J Thorac Cardiovasc Surg 1980;80:770–8.

[5] Fuster V, McGoon DC, Kennedy MA, Ritter DG, Kirklin JW. Long-term evaluation (12 to 22 years) of open heart surgery for tetralogy of Fallot. Am J Cardiol 1980;46:635–42.

[6] Lane I, Treasure T, Leijala M, Shinebourne E, Lincoln C. Diminutive pulmonary artery growth following right ventricular outflow tract enlargement. Int J Cardiol 1983;3:175–85.

[7] Ross EM, McIntosh CL, Roberts WC. Massive" calcification of a right ventricular outflow parietal pericardial patch in tetralogy of Fallot. Am J Cardiol 1984;54:691–2.

[8] Payne WS, Kirklin JW. Late complications after plastic reconstruction of outflow tract in tetralogy of Fallot. Ann Surg 1961;154:53–7.

[9] Rosenthal A, Gross RE, Pasternac A. Aneurysms of right ventricular outflow patches. J Thorac Cardiovasc Surg 1972;63:735–40.

[10] Kaplan S, Helmsworth JA, McKinivan CE, Benzing G, Schwartz DC, Schreiber JT. The fate of reconstruction of the right ventricular outflow tract. J Thorac Cardiovasc Surg 1973;66:361–74.

[11] Rieker R, Berman M, Stansel HC. Postoperative studies in patients with tetralogy of Fallot. Ann Thorac Surg 1975;19:17–26.

[12] Kirklin JK, Kirklin JW, Blackstone EH, Milano A, Pacifico AD. Effect of transannular patching on outcome after repair of tetralogy of Fallot. Ann Thorac Surg 1989;48:783–91.

[13] Nollert G, Fischlein T, Bouterwek S, Böhmer C, Klinner W, Reichart B. Long-term survival in patients with repair of tetralogy of Fallot: 36-year follow-up of 490 survivors of the first year after surgical repair. JACC 1997;30:1374–83.

[14] Knott-Craig CJ, Elkins RC, Lane MM, Holz J, McCue C, Ward KE. A 26-year experience with surgical management of tetralogy of Fallot: risk analysis for mortality or late reintervention. Ann Thorac Surg 1998;66:506–11.

[15] Nørgaard MA, Lauridsen P, Helvind M, Pettersson G. Twenty-to-thirty-seven-year follow-up after repair for Tetralogy of Fallot. Eur J Cardiothorac Surg 1999;16:125–30.

[16] Gatzoulis MA, Balaji S, Webber SA, Siu SC, Hokanson JS, Poile C, et al. Risk factors for arrhythmia and sudden cardiac death late after repair of tetralogy of Fallot: a multicentre study. Lancet 2000;356:975–81.

[17] Troost E, Meyns B, Daenen W, Van de Werf F, Gewillig M, Van Deyk K, et al. Homograft survival after tetralogy of Fallot repair: determinants of accelerated homograft degeneration. Eur Heart J 2007;28:2503–9.

[18] Munkhammar P, Carlsson M, Arheden H, Pesonen E. Restrictive right ventricular physiology after tetralogy of Fallot repair is associated with fibrosis of the right ventricular outflow tract visualized on cardiac magnetic resonance imaging. Eur Heart Jl - Cardio Imag 2013;14:978–85.

[19] Kotani Y, Chetan D, Ono N, Mertens LL, Caldarone CA, Van Arsdell GS, et al. Late functional outcomes after repair of tetralogy of Fallot with atrioventricular septal defect: a double case-match control study. J Thorac Cardiovasc Surg 2013;145:1477–84.

[20] Cuypers JA, Menting ME, Konings EE, Opić P, Utens EM, Helbing WA, et al. Unnatural history of tetralogy of Fallot: prospective follow-up of 40 years after surgical correction. Circ 2014;130:1944–53.

[21] Galicia-Tornell M, Reyes-López A, Ruíz-González S, Bolio-Cerdán A, González-Ojeda A, Fuentes-Orozco C. Treatment of Fallot tetralogy with a transannular patch. Six years follow-up. Cir 2015;83:478–84.

[22] Dłużniewska N, Podolec P, Skubera M, Smaś-Suska M, Pająk J, Urbańczyk-Zawadzka M, et al. Long-term follow-up in adults after tetralogy of Fallot repair. Cardiovasc Ultrasound 2018;16:28.

[23] Simon BV, Subramanian S, Swartz MF, Wang H, Atallah-Yunes N, Alfieris GM. Serial follow-up of two surgical strategies for the repair of tetralogy of Fallot. Semin Thorac Cardiovasc Surg 2019;31:515–23.

[24] de Castilhos GM, Ley ALG, Daudt NS, Horowitz ESK, Leiria TLL. Routine detection of atrial fibrillation/flutter predicts a worse outcome in a cohort of tetralogy of Fallot patients during 23 years of follow-up. Pediatr Cardiol 2019;40:1009–16.

[25] Padalino MA, Pradegan N, Azzolina D, Galletti L, Pace Napoleone C, Agati S, et al. The role of primary surgical repair technique on late outcomes of Tetralogy of Fallot: a multicentre study. Eur J Cardiothorac Surg 2020;57:565–73.

# Frequency of Congruence and Incongruence Between the Clinical and Morphological Diagnoses in Patients Having Orthotopic Heart Transplantations at the Baylor University Medical Center at Dallas From 1993 to 2020

William C. Roberts, MD[a,b,c,*], and Yusuf M. Salam, BS[a]

**We studied the explanted hearts of 519 patients having Orthotopic Heart Transplant (OHT) at Baylor University Medical Center from 2013 to 2020 and compared the morphologic diagnoses to the clinical diagnoses before OHT. We then combined these findings with the findings from 314 patients who had been studied in the laboratory from 1993 to 2012. Thus, the total number of patients included in the overall study were 833. Among the 833 patients the morphologic and clinical diagnoses were congruent in 760 (91%) and incongruent in 73 (9%) cases. Most of the incongruity occurred among the patients with cardiac sarcoidosis (27/36 [75%]), arrhythmogenic right ventricular cardiomyopathy (11/19 [58%]), and hypertrophic cardiomyopathy (8/25 [32%]). The frequency of incongruence among 833 patients having OHT in an 27 year period was 9%, with no significant difference between the 314 patients studied from 1998 to 2012, and the 519 studied from 2013 to 2020.**  **(Am J Cardiol 2021;156:114−122)**

In 2014 we reported the frequency of congruence and incongruence between the clinical and morphologic diagnoses among 314 patients having OHT at the BUMC from 1993 to 2012.[1] The present report was prompted by examining the same question in the 519 patients who had OHT at BUMC from 2013 through 2020.

## Methods

During the last 27 years all hearts in patients having OHT at BUMC have been described and the official report issued by WCR and nearly all have been photographed (by Saba Ilyas). The morphologic diagnoses in all 833 cases described below were determined by WCR and all clinical records were examined by him near the time of examination of the heart. The coauthor of this manuscript (YMS) examined all morphologic and clinical reports in the 519 patients studied since the previous publication on this topic.

The hearts were fixed in formaldehyde, usually for 3 to 5 days. The hearts were opened by either left and right parasagittal cuts or the ventricles, by transverse cuts parallel to the atrioventricular sulcus posteriorly. If calcium was seen or palpated, radiographs usually were made of the gross specimens. The major coronary arteries were studied by sticking a long 2 mm wide probe into each coronary ostium and by examining periodic cross sections of the epicardial arteries. At least 4 sections of the walls of the cardiac ventricles were prepared in each case extending from endocardium to epicardium and the resulting histologic sections were stained by both hematoxyl-eosin and trichrome stains and examined by WCR.

Criteria for diagnosis of each of the cardiac conditions were presented and illustrated in our previous article on this topic.[1] Single gross photos of the major conditions are illustrated in Figures 2 to 9.

## Results

The major findings in this study are summarized in Figure 1 and in Tables 1 to 8 . The clinical and morphologic diagnoses were congruent in 760 (91%) and incongruent in 73 (9%) of the 833 patients studied at the BUMC from 1993 to 2020. The conditions with the largest degrees of incongruence between the clinical and morphologic diagnoses were cardiac sarcoidosis (75%), arrhythmogenic right ventricular cardiomyopathy (58%) and hypertrophic cardiomyopathy (32%). Illustrations of morphologic features in several conditions discussed are displayed in Figures 2-9.

## Discussion

The present study shows that the frequency of congruence between clinical and morphologic diagnosis at one large OHT center (BUMC) is high (89%) and that the frequency of incongruence between these diagnoses is low (11%). Excluding the previous study from this institution of 314 cases published in 2014,[1] at least 4 similar studies involving a total of 999 cases have asked a similar question.[2-5] The frequency of congruence between clinical and morphologic diagnoses ranged from 78% to 92% and the frequency of incongruence from 8% to 22%.

---

[a]Baylor Scott & White Heart and Vascular Institute, Baylor University Medical Center, Baylor Scott & White Health, Dallas, Texas; [b]The departments of Internal Medicine, Baylor University Medical Center, Baylor Scott & White Health, Dallas, Texas; and [c]The departments of Pathology, Baylor University Medical Center, Baylor Scott & White Health, Dallas, Texas. Manuscript received May 12, 2021; revised manuscript received and accepted June 18, 2021.

See page 122 for disclosure information.

*Corresponding author: Tel: (214) 820-7911; fax: (214) 820-7533.

*E-mail address:* william.roberts1@bswhealth.org (W.C. Roberts).

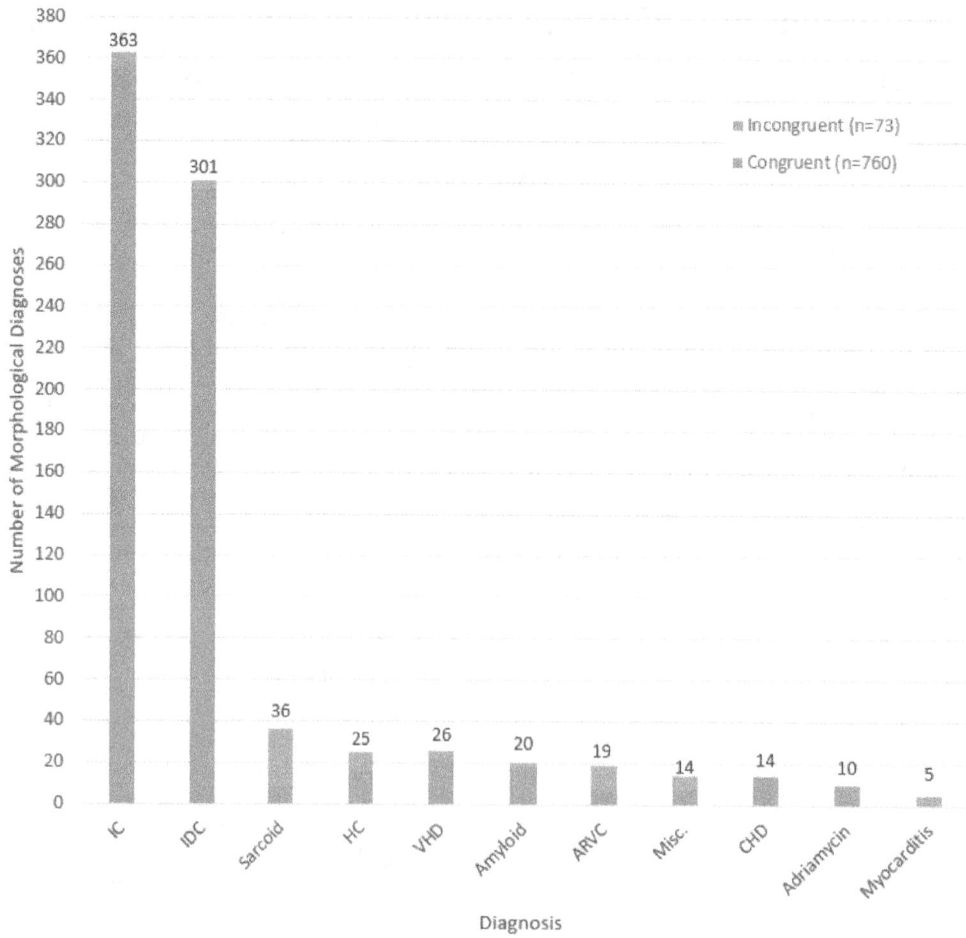


Figure 1. Bar graph showing frequency of congruence and incongruence among the various conditions leading to orthotopic cardiac transplantation among the 833 patients. ARVC = arrhythmogenic right ventricular cardiomyopathy; CHD = congenital heart disease; HC = hypertrophic cardiomyopathy; IC = ischemic cardiomyopathy; IDC = idiopathic dilated cardiomyopathy; Misc. = miscellaneous; VHD = valvular heart disease.

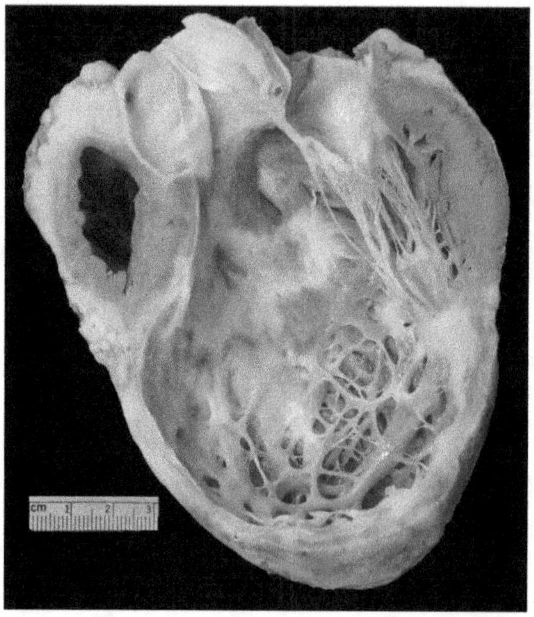

Figure 2. *Ischemic cardiomyopathy* (BDS 20-13794). This heart belonged to a 63 year-old man who had had heart failure since age 47. He underwent coronary artery bypass grafting at that time. In addition to the severe atherosclerosis of his epicardial coronary arteries, the left circumflex arose as the first branch of the right coronary artery and it coursed posterior to the aorta before it reached the left atrioventricular sulcus. The explanted heart weighed 540 grams. There was extensive left ventricular free wall scarring which also involved a portion of the ventricular septum and the mural endocardium over the scarred wall was thickened by fibrous tissue. The left ventricular cavity was severely dilated typical of ischemic cardiomyopathy.

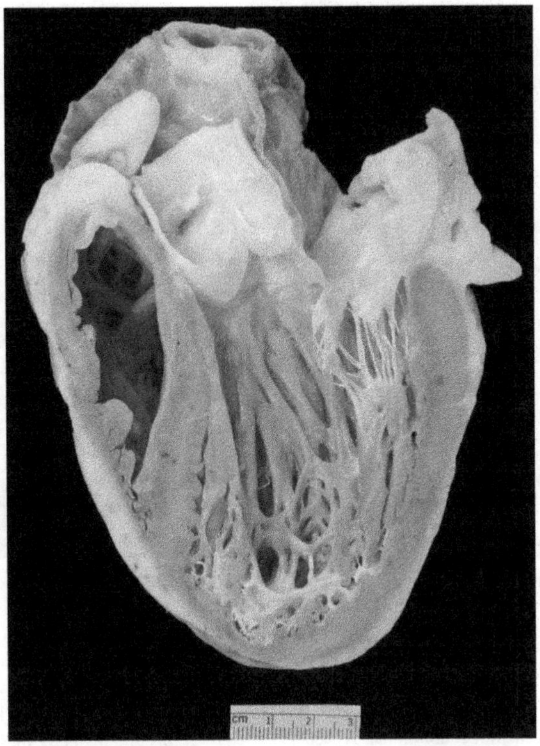

Figure 3. *Idiopathic dilated cardiomyopathy* (BDS 20-9936). Shown here is the heart of a 54 year-old man who had OHT in August 2020. He had evidence of heart failure for at least 4 years associated with periodic sustained ventricular tachycardia, permanent atrial fibrillation, and a left ventricular ejection fraction before OHT of 10%. The explanted heart weighed 520 grams. The coronary arteries were clean, and no grossly visible myocardial lesions were present. The mural endocardium in the left ventricular apex was thickened by fibrous tissue suggesting a previous thrombus at that site which had healed.

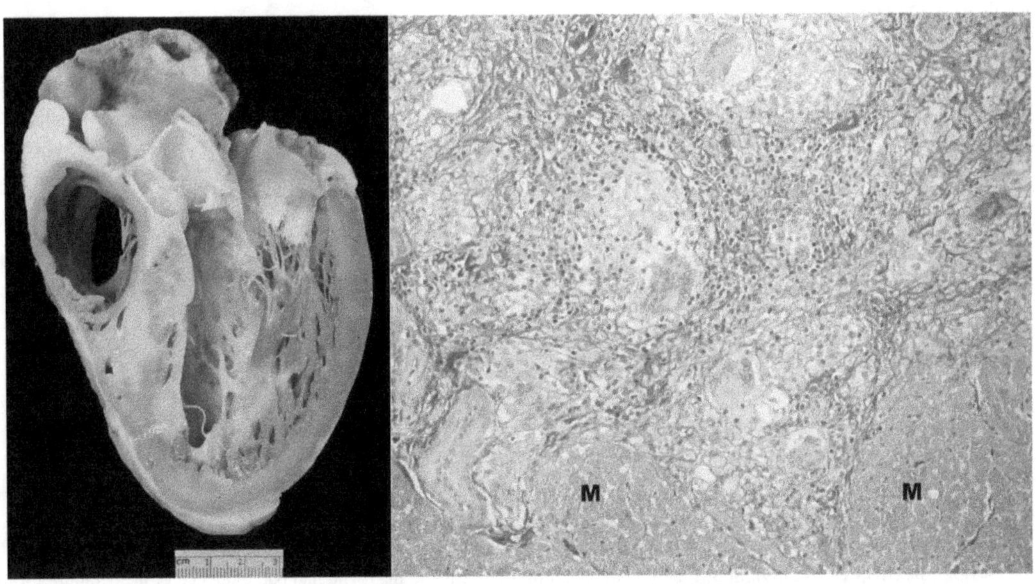


Figure 4. *Cardiac Sarcoidosis* (BDS20-4929). Shown here is the heart of a 39 year-old black man who was hospitalized with acute decomposition superimposed on chronic heart failure. He had frequent episodes of ventricular tachycardia. Cardiac sarcoidosis was not diagnosed clinically. The explanted heart weighed 405 grams and both ventricles were dilated. Left: The yellowish lesions in the ventricular walls represent scars containing numerous non-caseating granulomas. Right: Photomicrograph showing numerous granulomas in the scare tissue (blue). Trichrome stain, x 200. Left – M = Myocardium.

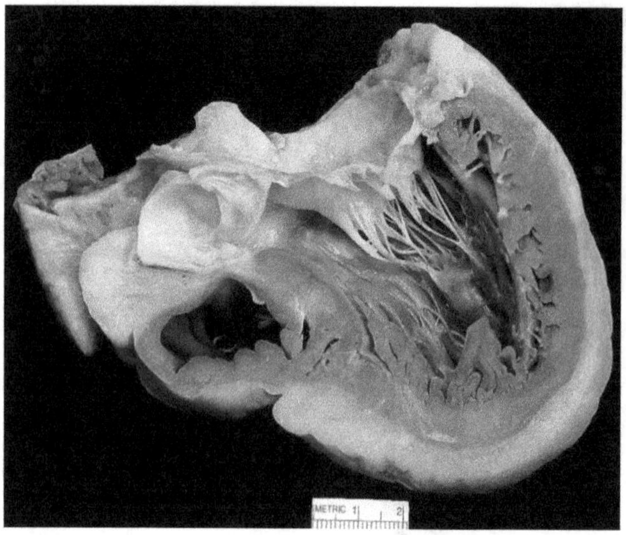

Figure 5. *Hypertrophic cardiomyopathy* (BDS 15-15951). The heart shown here belonged to a 43-year-old woman. She was diagnosed with hypertrophic cardiomyopathy at age 14 years after fainting while playing softball. She was otherwise asymptomatic until age 29 when she developed an arrhythmia and then exertional dyspnea. Both a transient ischemic attack and atrial fibrillation were diagnosed. Her left ventricular ejection fraction was said to be 40%. In the 5 years before OHT her episodes of atrial fibrillation increased, and she underwent three ablations. A year before OHT she developed evidence of heart failure. Hypertrophic cardiomyopathy was diagnosed in at least one other family member. The explanted heart weighed 345 grams and it floated in a container of formaldehyde due to the excessive subepicardial adipose tissue. Several scars were present in the ventricular septum and at the base of the left ventricular free wall and the left ventricular cavity was dilated. No mural endocardial plaque was present in the left ventricular outflow tract in apposition to the anterior mitral leaflet. The more basal portion of left ventricular free wall adjacent to the posterior mitral leaflet has a bird-shape, typical of non-obstructive hypertrophic cardiomyopathy. The quantity of subepicardial adipose tissue increased and the heart floated in a container of formaldehyde (Fat is lighter then myocardium).

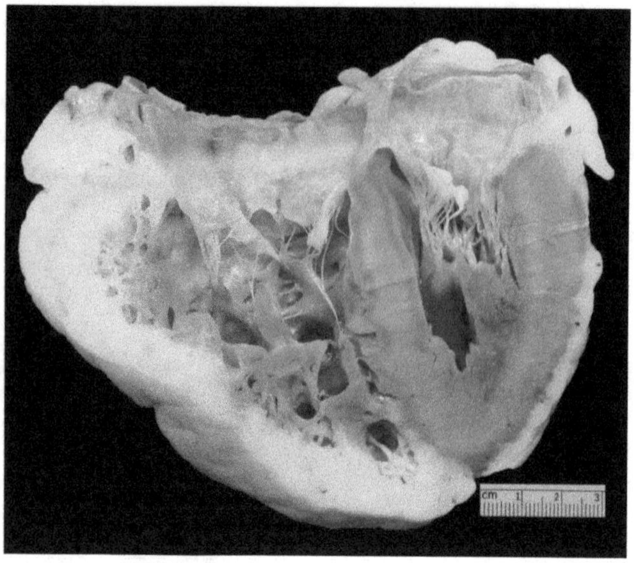

Figure 7. *Arrhythmogenic right ventricular cardiomyopathy* (BDS20-5438). Shown here is the heart of a 60-year-old man diagnosed with arrhythmogenic right ventricular cardiomyopathy when he was 46 years of age. Both atrial fibrillation and atrial tachycardia appeared two years later. The right ventricular free wall is replaced by adipose tissue. The left ventricular free wall and ventricular septum are normal. The heart weighed 470 grams and his body mass index was 36 kg/m$^2$ at the time of transplantation.

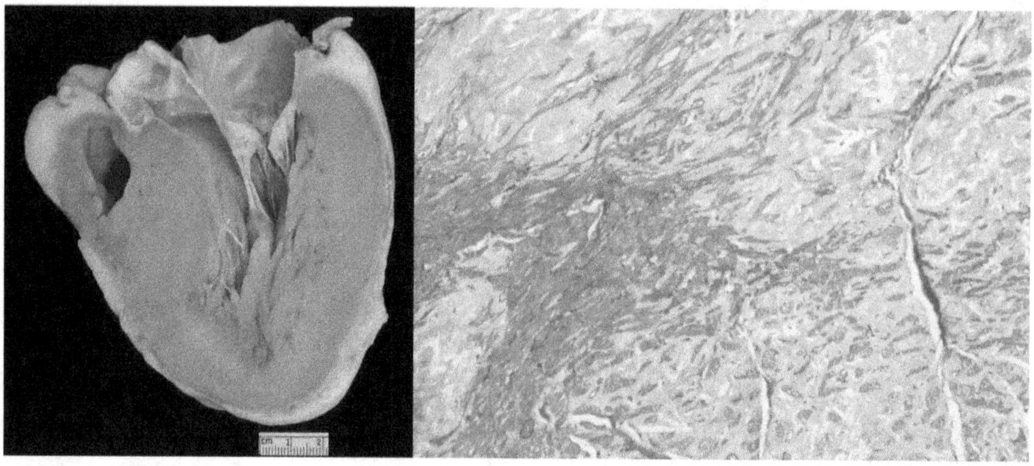

Figure 6. *Cardiac amyloidosis* (BDS 19-012189). Shown here is the heart of a 70-year-old man who had had evidence of heart failure for many years. Left: The heart was cut in a left parasagittal manner. The myocardium is uniform. The left ventricular cavity is not dilated. Amyloid was present throughout the myocardial walls. The quantity of subepicardial adipose tissue was also increased and the body mass index was 30 kg/m$^2$. The coronary arteries were wide open. The electrocardiogram showed extremely low voltage. He had had evidence of heart failure for a number of years. He also had obstructive sleep apnea. His body mass index was 31.5 kg/m$^2$. Right: Photomicrography showing extensive deposits in the left ventricular wall. The amyloid is blue and the myocytes are red. Trichrome stain, x 200.

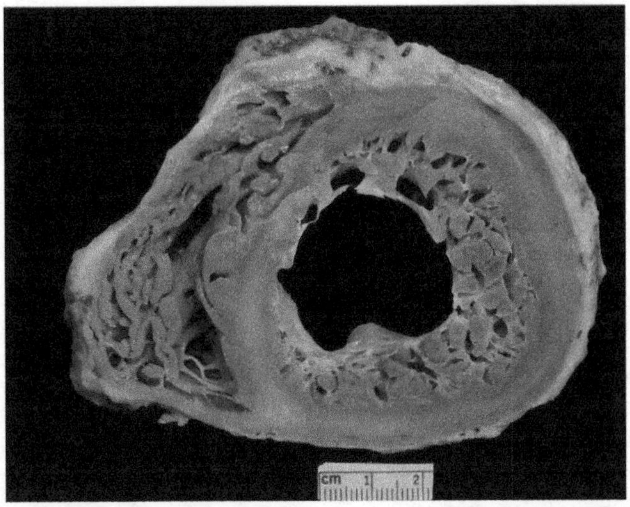

Figure 8. *Noncompaction cardiomyopathy* (BDS 18-16870). This 54-year-old woman whose heart is shown here, weighed 365 grams. The coronary arteries were not narrowed.

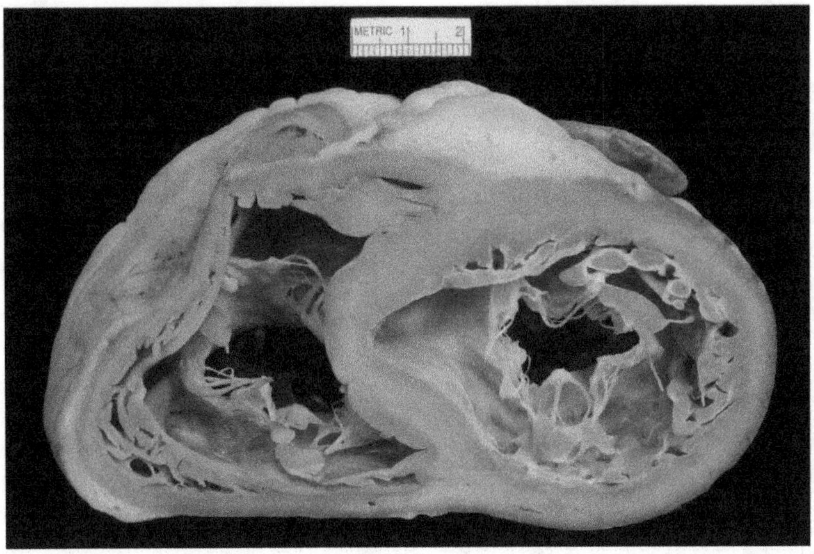

Figure 9. *Adriamycin cardiomyopathy* (BDS 17-06523). The heart in a 44-year-old woman who received adriamycin at age 37 for non-Hodgkin's lymphoma. By age 43 she was in severe heart failure (left ventricular ejection fraction, 15%). The explanted heart weighed only 260 grams and both ventricles were dilated. No grossly-visible lesions are present in the myocardial walls. The mural endocardium in focally thickened by fibrous tissue.

Table 1
Morphologic diagnoses in patients having cardiac transplantation at the BUMC 1993–2020 (n = 833)

| Variable | IC (n = 363) | IDC (n = 301) | CS (n = 36) | HC (n = 25) | VHD (n = 26) | CA (n = 20) | ARVC (n = 19) | Misc. (n = 14) | CHD (n = 14) | AC (n = 10) | M (n = 5) |
|---|---|---|---|---|---|---|---|---|---|---|---|
| Age (mean), (years) | | | | | | | | | | | |
| Men | 35–73 (59.8) | 19–76 (53.6) | 39–69 (53) | 19–68 (54.5) | 30–71 (56.5) | 42–74 (64) | 21–70 (50.9) | 52–68 (60.5) | 39–65 (49.4) | 27–55 (38) | 24–56 (36) |
| Women | 30–69 (57.9) | 26–70 (53.1) | 40–62 (56.3) | 19–56 (41.5) | 43–65 (55.4) | 0 | 44–57 (50) | 28.0–54.0 (40.4) | 44–56 (50) | 40–69 (55) | 46–60 (53) |
| Sex | | | | | | | | | | | |
| Men | 258 (73%) | 206 (66%) | 20 (56%) | 19 (76%) | 20 (80%) | 20 | 16 (84%) | 8 (57%) | 11 (77%) | 4 (40%) | 3 (60%) |
| Women | 52 (27%) | 104 (34%) | 16 (44%) | 6 (24%) | 5 (20%) | 0 | 3 (16%) | 6 (43%) | 3 (23%) | 6 (60%) | 2 (40%) |
| Heart Weight (mean), (grams) | | | | | | | | | | | |
| Men | 265–1000 (504) | 226–670 (430) | 405–670 (480) | 220–465 (349) | 480–770 (610) | 390–900 (607) | 314–686 (442) | 230–695 (523) | 495–880 (641) | 366–645 (477) | 415–545 (468) |
| Women | 255–726 (422) | 275–940 (528) | 287–562 (410) | 355–780 (555) | 258–484 (422) | – | 305–530 (418) | 225–470 (355) | 385–755 (510) | 260–558 (386) | 297–356 (326) |
| Morphological Features | | | | | | | | | | | |
| LV Cavity Size (mean), (cm) | 2.5–9.0 (5.5) | 2.0–10.0 (5.9) | 5.0–7.5 (6.0) | 2.5–7.5 (5.2) | 3.4–7.5 (4.1) | 3–8 (4.6) | 4.5–11 (5.6) | 2.0–7.2 (4.7) | 5.5–7 (6.1) | 5–8 (6.2) | 7.0–9.0 (8) |
| RV Cavity Size (mean), (cm) | 1.0–5.5 (3.0) | 0.9–9.0 (3.4) | 2.0–9.0 (4.2) | 1.0–4.5 (2.6) | 0.0–5.0 (2.3) | 2.0–9.0 (4.2) | 3.0–6.0 (5.0) | 2.0–5.5 (3.9) | 2.5–4 (3.2) | 2–3.5 (2.7) | 2.5–4.0 (3.2) |
| Grossly Visible LV Scarring | 325 (91%) | 61 (20%) | 32 (89%) | 20 (80%) | 11 (44%) | 0 | 15 (79%) | 6 (43%) | 6 (43%) | 0 | 4 (80%) |
| Grossly Visible Foci of Necrosis | 7 (9%) | 5 (2%) | 0 | 0 | 2 (8%) | 1 (5%) | 1 (5%) | 1 (7%) | 1 (7%) | 0 | 0 |
| Died Postoperatively | | | | | | | | | | | |
| ≤60 days | 11 (3%) | 2 (1%) | 0 | 0 | 1 (4%) | 1 (5%) | 0 | 0 | 0 | 1 (10%) | 0 |
| >60 days | 30 (8%) | 25 (8%) | 1 (3%) | 3 (12%) | 1 (4%) | 1 (5%) | 0 | 1 (7%) | 0 | 1 (10%) | 1 (20%) |
| Previous Major Cardiac Operation | | | | | | | | | | | |
| Coronary Artery Bypass Graft | 128 (36%) | 2 (1%) | 1 (3%) | 2 (8%) | 1 (4%) | 0 | 0 | 2 (14%) | 1 (7%) | 0 | 0 |
| LVAD Insertion | 77 (22%) | 69 (22%) | 4 (12%) | 11 (44%) | 1 (4%) | 1 (5%) | 1 (5%) | 2 (14%) | 1 (7%) | 1 (10%) | 1 (20%) |
| Valve Operation | 17 (5%) | 14 (4%) | 1 (3%) | 2 (8%) | 19 (76%) | 0 | 0 | 1 (7%) | 7 (50%) | 0 | 0 |
| BMI (kg/m^2) | | | | | | | | | | | |
| <25 | 87 (23%) | 75 (25%) | 11 (31%) | 8 (32%) | 7 (27%) | 6 (30%) | 6 (32%) | 6 (44%) | 5 (36%) | 2 (20%) | 4 (80%) |
| ≥25–30 | 148 (40%) | 111 (37%) | 18 (50%) | 11 (44%) | 10 (38%) | 10 (50%) | 8 (42%) | 3 (21%) | 6 (43%) | 4 (40%) | 0 |
| ≥30–35 | 85 (23%) | 54 (18%) | 2 (6%) | 6 (24%) | 6 (23%) | 4 (20%) | 3 (16%) | 1 (7%) | 2 (14%) | 4 (40%) | 0 |
| ≥35–40 | 16 (4%) | 34 (11%) | 0 | 0 | 1 (4%) | 0 | 2 (10%) | 1 (7%) | 1 (7%) | 0 | 1 (20%) |
| ≥40 | 8 (2%) | 6 (2%) | 0 | 0 | 0 | 0 | 0 | 0 | 0 | 0 | 0 |
| N/A | 29 (8%) | 21 (7%) | 5 (14%) | 0 | 2 (8%) | 0 | 0 | 3 (21%) | 0 | 0 | 0 |

AC = adriamycin cardiomyopathy; ARVC = arrhythmogenic right ventricular cardiomyopathy; BMI = body mass index; CA = cardiac amyloidosis; CHD = congenital heart disease; CS = cardiac sarcoidosis; HC = hypertrophic cardiomyopathy; IC = ischemic cardiomyopathy; IDC = idiopathic dilated cardiomyopathy; LV = left ventricular; LVAD = left ventricular assit device; Misc. = miscellaneous; M = myocarditis; RV = right ventricular; VHD = valvular heart disease

Table 2
Morphological and clinical diagnoses between then in patients having orthotopic heart transplantation at BUMC from 1998-2020

| Diagnosis | Diagnoses | | |
|---|---|---|---|
| | Morphological | Clinical | Incongruence |
| Ischemic Cardiomyopathy | 363 | 354 (97%) | 9 (3%) |
| Idiopathic Dilated Cardiomyopathy | 301 | 297 (99%) | 4 (1%) |
| Sarcoid | 36 | 9 (25%) | 27 (75%) |
| Hypertrophic Cardiomyopathy | 25 | 17 (68%) | 8 (32%) |
| Valvular Heart Disease | 26 | 23 (88%) | 3 (12%) |
| Amyloid | 20 | 19 (95%) | 1 (5%) |
| Arrhythmogenic RV Cardiomyopathy | 19 | 8 (42%) | 11 (58%) |
| Miscellaneous | 14 | 8 (57%) | 6 (43%) |
| Stab Wound | 1 | 1 | 0 |
| Unclear | 2 | 0 | 2 |
| Chagas' Disease | 2 | 1 | 1 |
| Noncompaction | 5 | 2 | 3 |
| Pericardial Heart Disease | 2 | 2 | 0 |
| Coronary Artery Dissection | 1 | 1 | 0 |
| Primary Pulmonary Hypertension | 1 | 1 | 0 |
| Congenital Heart Disease | 14 | 14 | 0 |
| Ventricular Septal Defect | 3 | 3 | 0 |
| Epstein's Anomaly | 1 | 1 | 0 |
| Discrete Subaortic Stenosis | 1 | 1 | 0 |
| RVOT Obstruction + ASD | 1 | 1 | 0 |
| Transposition (Complete) | 4 | 4 | 0 |
| Tetralogy of Fallot | 4 | 4 | 0 |
| Adriamycin | 10 | 10 | 0 |
| Myocarditis | 5 | 1 | 4 |
| Giant Cell | 1 | 1 | 0 |
| Mononuclear | 3 | 0 | 3 |
| Healed Lymphocytic | 1 | 0 | 1 |
| Total | 833 | 760 (91%) | 73 (9%) |

ASD = atrial septal defect; RV = right ventricular; RVOT = right ventricular outflow tract

Table 3
Clinical diagnosis in patients who have ischemic cardiomyopathy morphologically

| # | OHT date | Age (year) | Sex | Clinical diagnosis | BMI (Kg/m$^2$) | HW (g) | LV Scars | LVAD |
|---|---|---|---|---|---|---|---|---|
| 1 | 2000 | 46 | M | IDC | 27.1 | 610 | + | + |
| 2 | 1998 | 52 | M | IDC | 29.1 | 470 | + | 0 |
| 3 | 1998 | 57 | M | IDC | 20.3 | 505 | + | 0 |
| 4 | 2018 | 58 | M | IDC | 27.3 | 530 | + | 0 |
| 5 | 2016 | 59 | M | IDC | 25.3 | 340 | + | + |
| 6 | 2010 | 61 | F | IDC | 25.2 | 600 | + | 0 |
| 7 | 2014 | 63 | M | IDC | 28.2 | 515 | + | 0 |
| 8 | 2018 | 64 | F | IDC | 24.2 | 310 | + | 0 |
| 9 | 2010 | 67 | M | IDC | 25.9 | 530 | + | 0 |

BMI = Body Mass Index; F = Female; HW = Heart Weight; IDC = Idiopathic Dilated Cardiomyopathy; LV = Left Ventricular; LVAD = Left Ventricular Assist Device; M = Male; OHT = Orthotopic Heart Transplantation

Table 4
Clinical diagnosis in patients who have idiopathic dilated cardiomyopathy morphologically

| # | OHT date | Age (year) | Sex | Clinical diagnosis | BMI (Kg/m$^2$) | HW (g) | LV Scars | LVAD |
|---|---|---|---|---|---|---|---|---|
| 1 | 1998 | 47 | M | IC | 34 | 940 | 0 | 0 |
| 2 | 2003 | 61 | M | IC | 21 | 475 | 0 | 0 |
| 3 | 2017 | 62 | M | IC | 32.6 | 625 | 0 | 0 |
| 4 | 2015 | 66 | M | IC | 32.1 | - | 0 | + |

BMI = Body Mass Index; F = Female; HW=Heart Weight; IC = Ischemic Cardiomyopathy; LV = Left Ventricular; LVAS = Left Ventricular Assist Device; M = Male; OHT = Orthotopic Heart Transplantation

Table 5
Clinical diagnosis in patients who have cardiac sarcoidosis morphologically

| # | OHT date | Age (year) | Sex | Clinical diagnosis | BMI (Kg/m$^2$) | Lowest LVEF (%) | HW (g) | LV Scars | LVAD | CAD | SG |
|---|---|---|---|---|---|---|---|---|---|---|---|
| 1 | 2018 | 40 | F | IDC | 46.6 | 40 | 370 | + | 0 | 0 | 0 |
| 2 | 2019 | 41 | F | IDC | 29.7 | 10 | 480 | + | 0 | 0 | + |
| 3 | 2015 | 48 | F | IDC | 32.8 | 20 | 340 | + | 0 | 0 | + |
| 4 | 2019 | 48 | M | IDC | 26.0 | 60 | 440 | + | 0 | 0 | 0 |
| 5 | 2012 | 50 | F | IDC | 27.0 | 20 | 440 | + | 0 | 0 | + |
| 6 | 2005 | 50 | M | IDC | 24.7 | 10 | 605 | + | + | 0 | 0 |
| 7 | 2010 | 52 | F | IDC | 28.7 | 20 | 440 | + | 0 | 0 | + |
| 8 | 2005 | 52 | M | IDC | 21.6 | 20 | 440 | + | + | 0 | + |
| 9 | 2014 | 54 | F | IDC | 25.2 | 15 | 425 | + | 0 | 0 | + |
| 10 | 2015 | 54 | M | IC | 25.7 | 45 | 670 | + | + | + | 0 |
| 11 | 2017 | 54 | M | IDC | 23.4 | 15 | 355 | + | 0 | 0 | 0 |
| 12 | 2017 | 54 | F | IDC | 24.1 | 10 | 345 | + | 0 | 0 | 0 |
| 13 | 1999 | 54 | M | IDC | 27.5 | 10 | 510 | + | 0 | 0 | + |
| 14 | 2009 | 56 | F | IDC | 25.7 | 15 | 450 | + | 0 | 0 | + |
| 15 | 2013 | 57 | M | IDC | 26.0 | 15 | 420 | + | 0 | 0 | 0 |
| 16 | 2013 | 58 | M | IDC | 24.7 | 10 | 420 | + | 0 | 0 | + |
| 17 | 2012 | 58 | F | IDC | 26.4 | 20 | 560 | + | 0 | 0 | + |
| 18 | 2006 | 59 | F | IDC | 20.8 | 20 | 370 | + | + | + | + |
| 19 | 2015 | 60 | F | IDC | 28.4 | 15 | 400 | + | 0 | 0 | + |
| 20 | 2016 | 61 | F | IDC | 24.5 | 5 | 300 | + | 0 | 0 | + |
| 21 | 2013 | 62 | F | IDC | 22.2 | 10 | 600 | + | 0 | 0 | 0 |
| 22 | 2013 | 63 | M | IDC | 34.1 | 10 | 470 | + | 0 | 0 | + |
| 23 | 2017 | 63 | M | IDC | 23.3 | 10 | 540 | + | 0 | 0 | + |
| 24 | 2016 | 67 | M | IDC | 29.5 | 10 | 510 | + | 0 | 0 | + |
| 25 | 2018 | 69 | M | IDC | 23.7 | 10 | 475 | + | 0 | 0 | 0 |

BMI = Body Mass Index; CAD = Coronary Artery Disease; F = Female; HW = Heart Weight; IC = Ischemic Cardiomyopathy; IDC = Idiopathic Dilated Cardiomyopathy; LV = Left Ventricular; LVAD = Left Ventricular Assist Device; M = Male; OHT = Orthotopic Heart Transplantation; SG = Sarcoid Granuloma

Table 6
Clinical diagnosis in patients who have hypertrophic cardiomyopathy morphologically

| # | OHT date | Age (year) | Sex | Clinical diagnosis | BMI (Kg/m$^2$) | Lowest LVEF (%) | HW (g) | LV Scars | LVAD |
|---|---|---|---|---|---|---|---|---|---|
| 1 | 2010 | 25 | F | IDC | 26.9 | 15 | 370 | + | + |
| 2 | 2015 | 52 | M | IDC | 34.7 | 60 | 435 | + | 0 |
| 3 | 2012 | 54 | M | IDC | 28.2 | 10 | 570 | + | + |
| 4 | 1997 | 54 | M | IDC | 28.7 | 20 | 640 | + | 0 |
| 5 | 2012 | 61 | M | IDC | 23.6 | 10 | 530 | + | + |
| 6 | 2012 | 64 | M | IDC | 29.6 | 10 | 690 | 0 | + |
| 7 | 2009 | 68 | M | IDC | 32.4 | 10 | 780 | + | + |

BMI = Body Mass Index; F = Female; HW = Heart Weight; IDC = Idiopathic Dilated Cardiomyopathy; LV = Left Ventricular; LVAS = Left Ventricular Assist Device; M = Male; OHT = Orthotopic Heart Transplantation

Table 7
Clinical diagnosis in patients who have ARVC morphologically

| # | OHT date | Age (year) | Sex | Clinical diagnosis | BMI (Kg/m$^2$) | Lowest LVEF (%) | HW (g) | LV Scars | LVAD | CAD |
|---|---|---|---|---|---|---|---|---|---|---|
| 1 | 2012 | 21 | M | IDC | 26.5 | 10 | 490 | + | 0 | 0 |
| 2 | 2009 | 26 | M | IDC | 24.8 | 10 | 595 | + | 0 | 0 |
| 3 | 2008 | 30 | M | IDC | 27.6 | 10 | 685 | + | + | 0 |
| 4 | 2016 | 44 | F | IDC | 28.7 | 15 | 420 | 0 | 0 | 0 |
| 5 | 2008 | 44 | M | IDC | 22.5 | 25 | 315 | 0 | 0 | 0 |
| 6 | 2017 | 50 | M | IDC | 37.4 | 10 | 565 | + | 0 | 0 |
| 7 | 2020 | 55 | M | IDC | 23.2 | 15 | 350 | + | 0 | 0 |
| 8 | 2014 | 57 | F | IDC | 26.5 | 5 | 530 | + | + | 0 |
| 9 | 2019 | 58 | M | Unclear | 31.0 | 25 | 410 | + | 0 | 0 |
| 10 | 2019 | 59 | M | IC | 24.5 | 30 | 495 | + | 0 | + |
| 11 | 2020 | 60 | M | IDC | 35.8 | 50 | 470 | 0 | 0 | 0 |

ARVC = Arrhythmogenic Right Ventricular Cardiomyopathy; BMI = Body Mass Index; CAD = Coronary Artery Disease; F = Female; HW = Heart Weight; IC = Ischemic Cardiomyopathy; IDC = Idiopathic Dilated Cardiomyopathy; LV = Left Ventricular; LVAS = Left Ventricular Assist Device; M = Male; OHT = Orthotopic Heart Transplantation

Table 8
Previous publications on frequencies of congruence and incongruence of clinical & morphological diagnosis in patients having orthotopic heart transplantation

| First author (Reference) | Year of publication | Number of cases | Clinical & morphological diagnoses congruent | Clinical & morphological diagnoses incongruent |
|---|---|---|---|---|
| Bortman (2) | 1994 | 112 | 87 (78%) | 25 (22%) |
| Angelini (3) | 1999 | 257 | 237 (92%) | 20 (8%) |
| Luk (4) | 2009 | 296 | 245 (83%) | 51 (17%) |
| Roberts (1) | 2014 | 314 | 272 (87%) | 42 (13%) |
| Raeisi-Giglou (5) | 2017 | 334 | 274 (82%) | 60 (18%) |

Strengths of the present study are the following: (1) a large number of patients were included (nearly as many as all other similar studies put together); (2) all morphologic diagnoses were made by the same investigator (WCR who has specialized in cardiovascular pathology for 60 years); and (3) a large variety of data was examined in all 833 patients.

A possible limitation of the present report is the long period (27 years) in which the patients were studied and during that period the medical records where the clinical information was obtained changed on 3 different occasions. The changes required learning the new systems to obtain the required clinical information efficiently.

## Disclosures

The authors have no conflicts of interest to disclose.

## Acknowledgments

The initial data collection was started by Dr. Nuvaira Ather MD. Huzair Mehdi, Allan Zhang and Omar Khan all contributed significantly to the data collection. All specimens were catalogued and photographed by Saba Ilyas.

1. Roberts WC, Roberts CC, Ko JM, Filardo G, Capehart JE, Hall SA. Morphologic features of the recipient heart in patients having cardiac transplantation and analysis of the congruence or incongruence between the clinical and morphologic diagnoses. *Medicine* 2014;93:211–235.
2. Bortman G, Sellanes M, Odell DS, Ring WS, Olivari MT. Discrepancy between pre- and post-transplant diagnosis of end-stage dilated cardiomyopathy. *Am J Cardiol* 1994;74:921–924.
3. Angelini A, Boffa GM, Livi U, Barchitta A, Casarotto D, Thiene G. Discordance between pre and post cardiac transplant diagnosis: implications for pre- and postoperative decision making. *Cardiovasc Pathol* 1999;8:7–23.
4. Luk A, Metawee M, Ahn E, Gustafsson F, Ross H, Butany J. Do clinical diagnoses correlate with pathological diagnoses in cardiac transplant patients? The importance of endomyocardial biopsy. *Can J Cardiol* 2009;25:48–54.
5. Raeisi-Giglou P, Rodriguez ER, Blackstone EH, Tan CD, Hsich EM. Verification of heart disease: implications for a new heart transplantation allocation system. *JACC Heart Fail* 2017;5:904–913.

# Frequency of Peripartum Cardiomyopathy Among Women With Idiopathic Dilated Cardiomyopathy

William C. Roberts, MD[a,b,c,*], and Minseob Jeong, BS[a]

**Among women with idiopathic dilated cardiomyopathy (IDC), the percent who develop heart failure (HF) in the peripartum period (during pregnancy or within 6 months of parturition) compared with those women who develop HF outside the peripartum period is unclear. We studied 72 women with IDC who underwent orthotopic heart transplantation for severe HF, the onset of which was in the peripartum period in 8 (11%) and outside the period in 64 (89%). Comparison of many clinical and morphologic variables between these 2 groups showed significant differences only in the ages of onset of HF, age when orthotopic heart transplantation was performed, and the frequency of the presence of diabetes mellitus. Examination of the hearts in the 2 groups disclosed no significant differences. Thus, separation of the peripartum IDC cases from the nonperipartum IDC cases by either clinical or cardiac morphologic variables is difficult.**  **(Am J Cardiol 2021;157:101–106)**

Among women with idiopathic dilated cardiomyopathy (IDC) little information is available regarding the relation of the onset of heart failure (HF) to the peripartum period. We examined the hearts and clinical records of 72 women who had orthotropic heart transplantation (OHT) because of severe HF resulting from IDC to determine the number and percent of them who had the onset of HF in the peripartum period (onset of heart failure during pregnancy or within 6 months after parturition).

## Patients Studied

During a recent 11-year period (2010 to April 2021) we studied the hearts of 72 women who had undergone OHT for IDC. Each heart was opened, described, and the official report prepared by WCR. Each heart was photographed by Saba Ilyas. Most hearts were opened by left and right parasagittal cuts; some were opened by transverse cuts of the ventricles parallel to the posterior atrioventricular sulcus. At least 4 histologic sections were prepared extending from endocardium to epicardium. The prepared histologic sections were stained by both hematoxylin/eosin and trichrome and all sections were examined by WCR. The clinical records were reviewed by both MJ and WCR.

## Results

The major findings in the 2 groups of women are summarized in Table 1 and individual patient data are tabulated in Tables 2 and 3. Comparison of findings in the 8 women with peripartum cardiomyopathy to the 64 women with IDC with onset of HF not in the peripartum period disclosed significant differences in ages at onset of HF and ages at the time of OHT, and frequency of diabetes mellitus. The frequencies between the 2 groups were similar in frequencies of the other variables analyzed (Table 1).

## Discussion

An important feature of the present study is that all 72 patients underwent OHT. In past studies of peripartum cardiomyopathy, some patients were studied only clinically, some had myocardial biopsies via percutaneous catheter, and a few were studied at necropsy.[1–6] We found no previous studies of patients with peripartum cardiomyopathy where hearts were studied after OHT. Thus, all 72 patients had their hearts available for morphologic examination.

Comparison of morphologic features of the hearts in the 8 women with IDC in whom HF appeared during the peripartum period to those in the 64 women with IDC in whom the HF did not appear during the peripartum period showed no significant morphologic differences: all had very dilated ventricular cavities; insignificant narrowing of any of the major epicardial coronary arteries; dilated annuli of the tricuspid and mitral valves, and usually no grossly visible left ventricular scars. Histologic examination of the ventricular walls usually showed focal increase in interstitial fibrous tissue, enlargement of some and atrophy of other myocardial fibers, occasional small foci of replacement fibrous, and absence of any interstitial inflammatory cells in the ventricular walls.

[a]Baylor Scott & White Heart and Vascular Institute, Dallas, Texas; [b]Department of Internal Medicine, Baylor University Medical Center, Baylor Scott & White Health, Dallas, Texas; and [c]Department of Pathology, Baylor University Medical Center, Baylor Scott & White Health, Dallas, Texas. Manuscript received June 15, 2021; revised manuscript received and accepted July 16, 2021.

See page 103 for disclosure information.

*Corresponding author: Tel: (214) 820-7911; fax: (214) 820-7533.

*E-mail address:* william.roberts1@bswhealth.org (W.C. Roberts).

Table 1
Comparison of certain clinical and morphologic features in 72 women having orthotopic heart transplantation (OHT) for idiopathic dilated cardiomyopathy with onset of heart failure (HF) during the peripartum period versus not in the peripartum period

| Variable | Peripartum Cardiomyopathy | | p-value |
|---|---|---|---|
| | Yes (n = 8) | No (n = 64) | |
| Age at the onset of HF (mean) [years] | 23-33 (28) | 19-65 (45)[a] | <.0001 |
| Age at OHT (mean) [years] | 26-58 (41) | 20-70 (55) | 0.0009 |
| Interval from onset of HF to OHT (mean) [years] | 3-27 (13) | <1-20 (8)[a] | 0.1329 |
| Race | | | |
| Black | 5 (63%) | 23 (36%) | |
| White | 2 (25%) | 38 (59%) | 0.1745 |
| Hispanic | 1 (12%) | 3 (5%) | |
| Systemic hypertension | 4 (50%) | 32 (50%) | 1 |
| Diabetes mellitus | 0 | 24 (38%) | 0.0457 |
| Body mass index (mean) [Kg/m^2] | 22-32 (27) | 17-42 (29) | 0.2962 |
| Implantable cardioverter defibrillator placement | 7 (88%) | 48 (75%) | 0.673 |
| Left ventricular assist device placement | 2 (25%) | 14 (22%) | 1 |
| Electrocardiogram | | | |
| Atrial fibrillation | 3 (38%) | 25 (39%) | 1 |
| Ventricular tachycardia | 3 (38%) | 17 (27%) | 0.6784 |
| Ventricular premature complexes | 1 (13%) | 16 (25%) | 0.6699 |
| Morphology | | | |
| Heart weight (mean) [g] | 255-540 (416) | 235-660 (411) | 0.9341 |
| LV cavity size (mean) [cm] | 4.0-8.0 (5.9) | 2.5-8.0 (5.5) | 0.613 |
| Microscopic fibrosis | 5 (63%) | 54 (84%) | 0.1506 |
| Death within 30 days after OHT | 0 | 2 (3%)[b] | 1 |
| Death within 365 days after OHT | 0[d] | 2/59 (3%)[ce] | 1 |

HF = heart failure; LV = left ventricle; OHT = orthotopic heart transplant

a: Forty two patients

b: One died 1 day after OHT due to bleeding; 1 died 17 days after OHT due to low cardiac output syndrome during the entire postoperative period

c: One died 4 months after OHT due to stroke; 1 died 8 months after OHT due to non-healing surgical wound

d: Four patients had not reached 365 days after OHT as of April 2021

e: Two patients died within 30 days after the OHT; 2 patients died within 365 days but later than 30 days; 3 patients had not reached 365 days after OHT as of April 2021

Table 2
Clinical and morphologic features of 8 patients with idiopathic dilated cardiomyopathy having onset of heart failure in the peripartum period

| Patient number | Race | Age at OHT (years) | Interval (years) between onset of CHF to OHT | Number of offspring | SH | DM | S | BMI (kg/m$^2$) | ICD | LVAD | Electrocardiogram | | | Morphology | | 30 day survival | 1 year survival |
|---|---|---|---|---|---|---|---|---|---|---|---|---|---|---|---|---|---|
| | | | | | | | | | | | AF | VT | VPC | HW (g) | LVd (cm) | | |
| 1 | B | 26 | 3 | 1 | 0 | 0 | 0 | 36 | 0 | + | 0 | 0 | 0 | 430 | — | + | + |
| 2* | W | 28 | 5 | 2 | 0 | 0 | 0 | 30 | + | 0 | 0 | + | 0 | 350 | — | + | —‡ |
| 3 | W | 36 | 6 | — | 0 | 0 | 0 | 26† | + | 0 | 0 | 0 | 0 | 540 | — | + | + |
| 4 | H | 39 | 13 | 1 | 0 | 0 | 0 | 28 | + | + | + | 0 | 0 | 255 | 4.0 | + | + |
| 5 | B | 44 | 11 | — | + | 0 | 0 | 22 | + | 0 | 0 | + (VF) | 0 | 520 | 8.0 | + | —‡ |
| 6 | B | 46 | 22 | — | + | 0 | + | 25 | + | 0 | 0 | 0 | 0 | 375 | 6.0 | + | + |
| 7 | B | 52 | 20 | — | + | 0 | 0 | 24 | + | 0 | + | 0 | 0 | 420 | — | + | —‡ |
| 8 | B | 58 | 27 | — | + | 0 | 0 | 25 | + | 0 | + | + | + | 440 | 5.5 | + | —‡ |

AF = atrial fibrillation; B = black; BMI = body mass index; CHF = congestive heart failure; DM = diabetes mellitus; H = hispanic; HT = heart transplant; HW = heart weight; ICD = implantable cardioverter defibrillator; LVAD = left ventricle assist device; LVd = left ventricle diameter; S = stroke; SH = systemic hypertension; VF = ventricular fibrillation; VPC = ventricular premature contraction; VT = ventricular tachycardia; W = white.

* Familial IDC.

† Gastric bypass at age 31.

‡ Four patients had not reached 365 days after HT as of April 2021.

We found few previously reported articles comparing findings in peripartum cardiomyopathy to those in women with IDC where onset of HF was not in the peripartum period. O'Connell et al[1] reported in 1986 fourteen patients with peripartum cardiomyopathy and compared findings in them to 55 patients with IDC without the onset of HF in the peripartum period. All had *myocardial biopsies* via the percutaneous route. These authors found only 1 clinical or morphologic difference in these 2 groups, and that was in age of onset of HF. Roberts and associates[2] in 1987 reported *at necropsy* 13 women with IDC whose onset of HF was during the peripartum period and compared findings in them to those of 26 necropsy women with IDC but in whom the onset of HF was not in the peripartum period. Again, the only clinical or morphologic difference between the 2 groups was the age at onset of HF. And finally, van Hoeven et al[3] in 1993 reported 26 women with IDC, 13 of whom had the onset of HF in the peripartum period and 13 had the onset of HF outside that period. All had *myocardial biopsies* via the percutaneous route. Of the 13 patients with peripartum cardiomyopathy, 5 (38%) had a poor outcome (death or progressive HF) and of the 13 patients with HF appearing in the nonperipartum period, 11 (85%) had a poor outcome. Otherwise, there was no significant differences between the peripartum and nonperipartum groups. None of the patients had evidence morphologically of myocarditis.

The women included in the present study all had severe HF, severe enough to warrant OHT. At follow-up 1 year after OHT, only 4 (6%) of the 72 patients had died.

This study has limitations. No genetic studies were performed. The number of patients taking birth-control pills or having elevated pulmonary or systemic blood pressures is not known.

In conclusion, comparison of clinical and morphologic features of women with IDC usually show no significant differences between those in whom the HF appeared initially during the peripartum and the nonperipartum periods. Approximately, 11% (8 of 72) of the women with IDC had the onset of HF during the peripartum period (Figures 1−6).

## Disclosures

The authors declare that they have no known competing financial interests or personal relations that could have appeared to influence the work reported in this study.

Table 3
Clinical and morphologic features of 64 patients with idiopathic dilated cardiomyopathy having onset of heart failure in the nonperiparum period

| Patient number | Race | Age at the onset of CHF (years) | Age at OHT (years) | Interval between onset of CHF to OHT (years) | Number of offspring | SH | DM | S | BMI (kg/m^2) | ICD | LVAD | Electrocardiogram | | | Morphology | | 30 day survival | 1 year survival |
|---|---|---|---|---|---|---|---|---|---|---|---|---|---|---|---|---|---|---|
| | | | | | | | | | | | | AF | VT | VPC | HW (g) | LVd (cm) | | |
| 1 | W | 20 | 20 | 0 | 0 | 0 | 0 | 0 | 27 | 0 | + | + | + | + | 290 | - | + | + |
| 2 | B | 29 | 29 | 0 | 4 | 0 | 0 | 0 | 25 | 0 | 0 | 0 | 0 | 0 | 360 | 5.0 | + | + |
| 3 | B | 25 | 32 | 7 | 0 | 0 | 0 | + | 22 | 0 | 0 | 0 | 0 | + | 390 | 6.0 | + | + |
| 4 | B | 19 | 34 | 15 | 1 | 0 | 0 | 0 | 36 | + | 0 | 0 | + (VF) | 0 | 420 | 2.5 | + | + |
| 5 | W | 24 | 35 | 11 | - | + | 0 | 0 | 33 | + | 0 | 0 | 0 | 0 | 474 | 9.5 | + | + |
| 6 | W | - | 39 | - | - | 0 | 0 | + | 38 | + | + | 0 | + | 0 | 385 | 4.5 | + | 0 |
| 7 | B | - | 39 | - | - | 0 | 0 | 0 | 35 | 0 | + | 0 | 0 | 0 | 371 | 4.5 | 0 | 0 |
| 8 | W | 39 | 40 | 1 | 2 | 0 | 0 | 0 | 39 | 0 | 0 | + | 0 | 0 | 370 | - | + | + |
| 9 | B | 40 | 41 | 1 | - | + | 0 | 0 | 25 | + | 0 | 0 | 0 | + | 355 | - | + | + |
| 10 | W | 42 | 43 | 1 | 3 | 0 | 0 | 0 | 39 | + | 0 | + | + | 0 | 570 | 6.0 | + | + |
| 11 | W | 30 | 47 | 17 | 2 | 0 | 0 | 0 | 28 | + | 0 | 0 | 0 | 0 | - | 4.5 | + | + |
| 12[a] | B | 42 | 48 | 6 | - | 0 | 0 | + | 19 | + | 0 | + | 0 | 0 | 380 | 7.5 | + | + |
| 13 | B | 43 | 48 | 5 | - | 0 | 0 | 0 | 27 | + | 0 | 0 | 0 | 0 | 455 | 7.5 | + | + |
| 14 | B | 39 | 48 | 9 | 2 | + | + | 0 | 33 | + | + | + | 0 | 0 | 345 | 5.0 | + | + |
| 15 | H | - | 49 | - | - | 0 | 0 | + | 23 | + | 0 | 0 | 0 | 0 | 235 | 5.0 | + | + |
| 16[a] | B | - | 49 | - | - | + | 0 | 0 | 30[b] | + | 0 | + | + | 0 | 525 | 5.5 | + | + |
| 17 | B | - | 51 | - | - | + | 0 | 0 | 39 | + | 0 | + | 0 | 0 | 440 | - | + | + |
| 18 | W | 42 | 52 | 10 | - | + | 0 | 0 | 39 | + | 0 | + | 0 | 0 | 410 | 5.5 | + | + |
| 19 | W | - | 53 | - | 2 | + | 0 | + | 27 | + | + | 0 | 0 | 0 | 406 | 4.5 | + | + |
| 20 | W | 39 | 53 | 14 | - | + | 0 | 0 | 38 | + | + | + | 0 | + | 530 | 4.5 | + | + |
| 21 | B | 50 | 54 | 4 | 0 | + | + | 0 | 27 | + | 0 | 0 | 0 | 0 | 435 | 6.5 | + | + |
| 22 | W | 47 | 54 | 7 | 0 | + | 0 | 0 | 27 | 0 | 0 | 0 | 0 | 0 | 335 | 4.0 | + | + |
| 23 | W | 46 | 54 | 8 | 3 | 0 | 0 | 0 | 29 | + | + | + | + | + | 365 | 5.0 | + | + |
| 24 | B | 50 | 54 | 4 | - | + | + | 0 | 24 | + | + | + | + | + | 415 | 6.5 | + | + |
| 25 | W | 39 | 55 | 16 | - | + | 0 | 0 | 32 | - | - | - | - | - | 455 | - | + | + |
| 26 | W | 50 | 55 | 5 | 3 | 0 | 0 | 0 | 27 | + | 0 | 0 | 0 | 0 | 540 | 5.0 | + | + |
| 27 | W | 44 | 55 | 11 | 2 | + | + | 0 | 28 | 0 | 0 | 0 | 0 | 0 | 310 | 3.5 | + | + |
| 28 | W | - | 55 | - | 1 | + | 0 | 0 | 25 | 0 | 0 | 0 | 0 | + | 340 | 5.0 | + | + |
| 29[a] | W | - | 56 | - | - | 0 | + | 0 | 25 | + | 0 | 0 | + | 0 | 408 | 8.0 | + | + |
| 30 | W | - | 56 | - | - | 0 | 0 | 0 | 39[b] | + | 0 | + | 0 | 0 | 430 | 4.5 | + | + |
| 31 | W | 52 | 56 | 4 | 1 | 0 | 0 | 0 | 34 | + | 0 | 0 | 0 | + | 310 | - | + | + |
| 32 | H | 37 | 57 | 20 | - | + | + | 0 | 28 | + | 0 | 0 | + | 0 | 484 | 5.5 | + | + |
| 33 | W | - | 57 | - | - | + | 0 | 0 | 27 | + | + | + | 0 | 0 | 530 | - | + | + |
| 34 | W | 51 | 57 | 6 | - | + | + | 0 | 42 | + | 0 | + | + | 0 | 380 | - | + | -[c] |
| 35 | B | 42 | 58 | 16 | - | 0 | 0 | 0 | 30 | + | 0 | 0 | 0 | + | - | - | + | -[c] |
| 36 | W | 44 | 59 | 15 | 1 | 0 | + | 0 | 31 | + | 0 | 0 | 0 | 0 | 428 | 5.5 | + | + |
| 37 | W | 52 | 59 | 7 | 2 | 0 | 0 | + | 32 | + | + | 0 | + | 0 | 615 | 6.5 | + | + |
| 38 | W | 52 | 59 | 7 | - | + | 0 | 0 | 27 | 0 | + | 0 | 0 | 0 | 265 | - | + | -[c] |
| 39 | W | 54 | 60 | 6 | 1 | + | + | 0 | 31 | 0 | 0 | + | 0 | 0 | 355 | 4.0 | + | + |
| 40 | B | 59 | 60 | 1 | 3 | + | + | 0 | 25 | + | 0 | 0 | + | + | 360 | - | + | + |
| 41 | W | - | 60 | - | - | 0 | + | 0 | 36 | 0 | 0 | + | + | 0 | 295 | - | + | + |
| 42 | B | 50 | 61 | 11 | 5 | + | 0 | 0 | 26 | + | 0 | 0 | 0 | 0 | 597 | 7.5 | + | + |
| 43 | B | 53 | 61 | 8 | 5 | 0 | + | 0 | 31 | + | 0 | + | 0 | 0 | 495 | 7.0 | + | + |
| 44 | W | 55 | 62 | 7 | - | + | 0 | + | 17 | 0 | 0 | + | + | + | 660 | 7.5 | + | + |
| 45 | B | 49 | 62 | 13 | 3 | + | + | 0 | 38 | + | 0 | 0 | 0 | 0 | 520 | - | + | + |
| 46 | B | 55 | 62 | 7 | 2 | 0 | 0 | 0 | 33 | + | 0 | 0 | + | + | 320 | 4.0 | + | + |
| 47 | W | 49 | 63 | 14 | - | 0 | 0 | 0 | 27 | + | 0 | + | 0 | 0 | 430 | 6.5 | + | + |
| 48 | W | - | 63 | - | 2 | 0 | + | 0 | 24 | + | 0 | + | 0 | 0 | 325 | 7.0 | + | + |
| 49 | W | - | 64 | - | 0 | + | + | 0 | 33 | + | 0 | + | 0 | 0 | 442 | 4.0 | + | + |
| 50 | W | 56 | 64 | 8 | - | 0 | 0 | 0 | 20 | + | 0 | 0 | 0 | 0 | 320 | 6.5 | + | + |
| 51 | W | - | 64 | - | 2 | 0 | 0 | 0 | 22 | 0 | 0 | 0 | 0 | 0 | 335 | - | + | + |
| 52 | W | - | 65 | - | 3 | + | + | 0 | 30 | 0 | + | + | 0 | 0 | 415 | 5.0 | + | + |
| 53 | W | 63 | 65 | 2 | - | 0 | + | 0 | 24 | + | 0 | + | 0 | + | 460 | 7.0 | + | + |
| 54 | B | 57 | 65 | 8 | 0 | 0 | 0 | 0 | 23 | + | 0 | 0 | + | + | 365 | 5.0 | + | + |
| 55 | B | - | 67 | - | 5 | + | + | 0 | 32 | + | 0 | 0 | 0 | 0 | - | 7.0 | + | + |
| 56 | W | - | 67 | - | 6 | 0 | 0 | 0 | 35 | + | 0 | 0 | 0 | 0 | 535 | 6.5 | + | + |
| 57 | W | - | 67 | - | - | + | 0 | 0 | 23 | + | 0 | 0 | 0 | 0 | 410 | 5.0 | + | + |
| 58 | B | 65 | 67 | 2 | - | + | 0 | 0 | 23 | + | 0 | + | 0 | 0 | 310 | 5.0 | + | + |
| 59 | W | - | 67 | - | 2 | + | + | 0 | 22 | + | + | 0 | 0 | + | 460 | 4.0 | 0 | 0 |
| 60 | B | 58 | 68 | 10 | - | + | + | 0 | 20 | + | 0 | + | 0 | + | 290 | 6.0 | + | + |
| 61 | W | - | 69 | - | 3 | + | + | 0 | 25 | + | 0 | 0 | 0 | 0 | 552 | 6.5 | + | + |
| 62 | B | - | 69 | - | - | 0 | + | 0 | 25 | + | + | 0 | 0 | 0 | 315 | - | + | 0 |
| 63 | W | 58 | 70 | 12 | 3 | 0 | + | 0 | 37 | + | 0 | 0 | + | 0 | 460 | - | + | + |
| 64 | H | - | 70 | - | - | + | + | 0 | 39 | 0 | 0 | 0 | 0 | 0 | 435 | - | + | + |

AF = atrial fibrillation; B = black; BMI = body mass index; CHF = congestive heart failure; DM = diabetes mellitus; H = hispanic; HT = heart transplant; HW = heart weight; ICD = implantable cardioverter defibrillator; LVAD = left ventricle assist device; LVd = left ventricle diameter; S = stroke; SH = systemic hypertension; VF = ventricular fibrillation; VPC = ventricular premature contraction; VT = ventricular tachycardia; W = white

a: Familial IDC
b: Gastric bypass

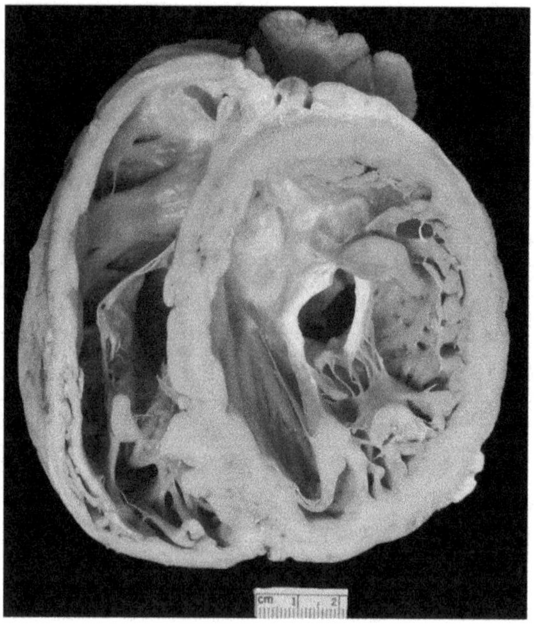

Figure 1. Case # 5, Table 2. Peripartum cardiomyopathy. The heart shown here has been opened by a cross-sectional cut parallel to posterior atrioventricular sulcus exposing both tricuspid and mitral valves and showing highly dilatated ventricular cavities. The walls of the ventricles are devoid of grossly visible lesions. The left anterior descending coronary artery is wide open. This patient was age 44 years at the time of OHT and 33 at the onset of heart failure.

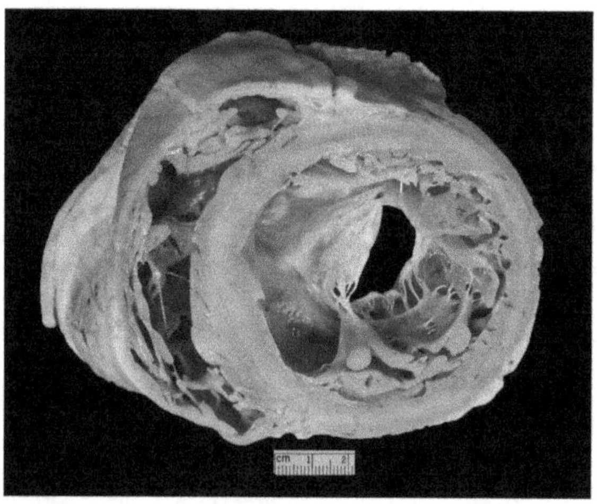

Figure 2. Case # 7, Table 2. Peripartum cardiomyopathy. Shown here is a hugely dilated left ventricle in a 52-year-old woman whose onset of heart failure was at age 32. No grossly visible lesions are noted in the ventriclular walls. The left anterior descending coronary artery is wide open. There was severe secondary mitral regurgitation.

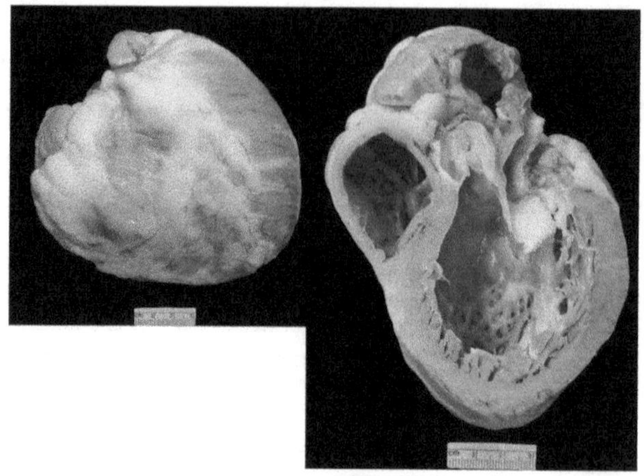

Figure 3. Case # 2, Table 2. Peripartum cardiomyopathy. Shown here on the left is the outside of the heart and on the right the very dilated ventricles. No lesions are noted in the ventricular walls. This patient had OHT at age 28 and the onset of heart failure when pregnant at age 23.

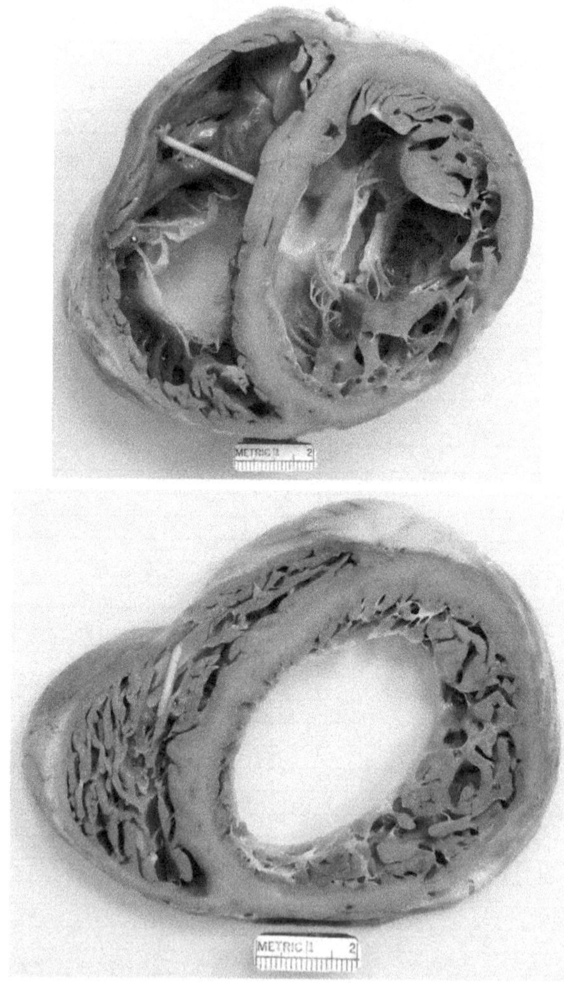

Figure 4. Case # 12, Table 3. Nonperipartum IDC. Shown here is the heart in a patient with IDC with onset of heart failure unassociated with pregnancy. Both ventricular cavities are greatly dilated. The left ventricular wall behind the posteromedial papillary muscle is thin due to scarring. Both tricuspid and mitral orifices are wide open. The bottom figure shows a cross sectional cut caudal to the upper photo showing noncompaction of both ventricles. An occasional patient with IDC also has noncompaction.

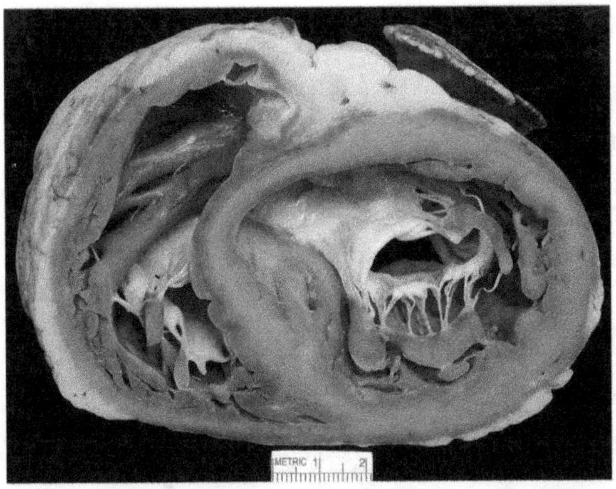

Figure 5. Case # 13, Table 3. Nonperipartum IDC. Shown here is a cross section of both ventricles showing both to be greatly dilated. No lesions are noted in the ventricular walls. The left anterior descending coronary artery is surrounded by adipose tissue, but its lumen is wide open. This woman was aged 48 at the time of OHT and 43 at the onset of heart failure.

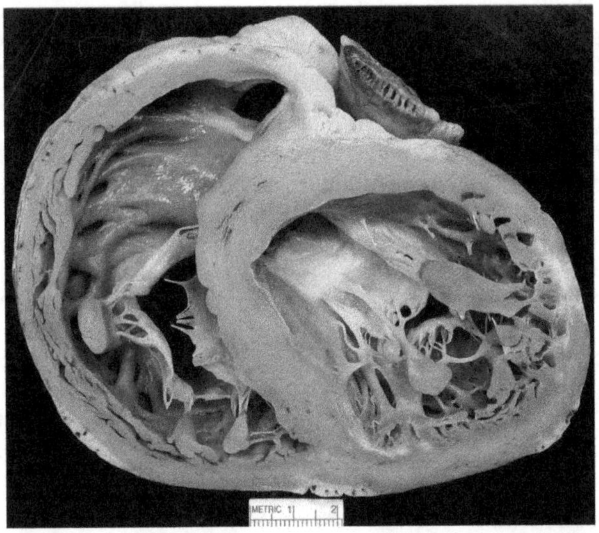

Figure 6. Case # 43, Table 3. Nonperipartum IDC. Shown here is a cross section of the heart in a 61-year-old woman who had onset of heart failure at age 53. Both ventricles are considerably dilated, and the wall of the left ventricle is transmurally scarred in its lateral portion and a small subendocardial scar is present at the junction of the posterior left ventricular free wall and ventricle septum. Again, the orifices of both atrioventricular valves are greatly dilated.


## Acknowledgment

Statistical analysis was done by Gelareh Rahimighazikalayeh. All specimens were cataloged and photographed by Saba Ilyas.



1. O'Connell JB, Costanzo-Nordin MR, Subramanian R, Robinson JA, Wallis DE, Scanlon PJ, Gunnar RM. Peripartum cardiomyopathy: clinical, hemodynamic, histologic and prognostic characteristics. *J Am Coll Cardiol* 1986;8:52–56.
2. Roberts WC, Siegel RJ, McManus BM. Idiopathic dilated cardiomyopathy: analysis of 152 necropsy patients. *Am J Cardiol* 1987;60:1340–1355.
3. Van Hoeven KH, Kitsis RN, Katz SD, Factor SM. Peripartum versus idiopathic dilated cardiomyopathy in young women—a comparison of clinical, pathologic and prognostic features. *Int J Cardiol* 1993;40:57–65.
4. Waller TA, Hiser WL, Capehart JE, Roberts WC. Comparison of clinical and morphologic cardiac findings in patients having cardiac transplantation for ischemic cardiomyopathy, idiopathic dilated cardiomyopathy, and dilated hypertrophic cardiomyopathy. *Am J Cardiol* 1998;81:884–894.
5. Zhang M, Tavora F, Huebner T, Heath J, Burke A. Allograft pathology in patients transplanted for idiopathic dilated cardiomyopathy. *Am J Surg Pathol* 2012;36:389–395.
6. Roberts WC, Roberts CC, Ko JM, Filardo G, Capehart JE, Hall SA. Morphologic features of the recipient heart in patients having cardiac transplantation and analysis of the congruence or incongruence between the clinical and morphologic diagnoses. *Medicine (Baltimore)* 2014;93:211–235.

# The Syndrome of Large Healed Single Discrete Myocardial Infarct with Severe Narrowing of Only One Major Epicardial Coronary Artery and Leading to Severe Chronic Heart Failure and Orthotopic Heart Transplantation

William C. Roberts, MD[a,*], and Omar S. Khan[b]

**Described herein are clinical and cardiac morphologic findings in 12 patients (age 43 to 70 years) (7 men) who underwent orthotopic heart transplantation (OHT) because of severe heart failure (HF) resulting from a single large discrete acute myocardial infarct that healed and was associated with severe narrowing of only one major epicardial coronary artery. Most myocardial infarcts are associated with severe narrowing of >1 major epicardial coronary artery and result in smaller myocardial infarcts. Another unusual feature was the total infarction of the ventricular septum in 3 of the 12 patients. Published by Elsevier Inc. (Am J Cardiol 2021;161:1−11)**

During a recent 4-year period we examined the hearts of 12 patients following orthotopic heart transplantation (OHT) and each had a very large single healed myocardial infarct and only a single severely narrowed epicardial coronary artery. Such a scenario we have not knowingly encountered previously. A description of certain clinical and cardiac morphologic features in these 12 patients is the purpose of this report.

## Methods

A list of the 12 patients with certain findings in them is displayed in Table 1. Since 1993 all hearts received in the surgical pathology division of the department of pathology in Baylor University Medical Center have been opened, described, and the official report prepared by WCR. Additionally, all tissues submitted for histologic examination were also prepared by WCR. All hearts were photographed by Saba Ilyas. The clinical records in all 12 patients were reviewed by both WCR and OSK.

## Results

The ages of the 12 patients ranged from 43 to 70 years (mean 57); four were women and 7 were men; 8 were white and 4 were black. The acute myocardial infarction occurred, determined in 9 patients, varied from 3 to 331 months (mean 73, median 73) before the OHT; the interval in 8 patients was >1 year. Systemic hypertension was present in 8 patients before their severe heart failure appeared. Diabetes mellitus was present in 6 patients; atrial fibrillation in 7; bundle branch block in 6; chronic renal disease in 4, two of whom had undergone a renal transplant. The body mass indices just before OHT ranged from 23 to 36 Kg/m$^2$ (mean 29). The transplanted recipient heart floated in a container of formaldehyde (due to excessive cardiac adipose tissue; fat is lighter than myocardium) in 4 patients. The explanted hearts ranged in weight from 310 to 550 g (mean 390): in the 5 women, from 310 to 445 g (mean 359) and in the 7 men, from 350 to 550 g (mean 413). The major epicardial coronary artery severely narrowed (determined by examining the recipient heart) was the left anterior descending in 7 and the right in 3; none of the major epicardial coronary arteries were severely narrowed in 2 of the operatively excised hearts (coronary angiogram at the time of the acute myocardial infarct showed severe narrowing of the infarct-related artery in 1 and in the other we simply do not have information at the time of the acute myocardial infarction). Non-paced electrocardiograms are illustrated in 2 patients in figures 1 and 2 and the explanted hearts in figures 3−14.

## Comments

Described herein are findings in 12 patients having OHT because of severe heart failure resulting from a large discrete acute myocardial infarction that healed and a single severely narrowed epicardial coronary artery. The heart failure appeared at the time of the acute infarct and lasted until the time of OHT. Each of the 12 patients had very dilated left ventricular cavities and extremely low left ventricular ejection fractions (10% to 20%). After healing of the acute myocardial infarction, none of the patients had angina pectoris. In 3 patients, the entire ventricular septum at some point was scarred transmurally. In all 12 patients the healed myocardial infarcts had sharp demarcations with the adjacent normal myocardium.

The occurrence of a single severely narrowed epicardial coronary artery associated with a large discrete healed myocardial infarct is unusual among patients with coronary artery disease studied after OHT or after autopsy. None of the major epicardial coronary arteries were free of

[a]Baylor Heart and Vascular Institute and the Departments of Internal Medicine and Pathology, Dallas, Texas; and [b]Baylor University Medical Center, Dallas, Texas. Manuscript received July 19, 2021; revised manuscript received and accepted September 10, 2021.

*Corresponding author: Tel: (214) 820 7911; fax: (214) 820 7533.

*E-mail address:* william.roberts1@bswhealth.org (W.C. Roberts).

Table 1
Clinical and Morphologic Findings in 12 Patients Whose Hearts at Time of Orthotopic Heart Transplant (OHT) Contained Severe Narrowing of One Major Coronary Artery and One Large Left Ventricular Scar

| Variable | Case Numbers | | | | | | | | | | | |
|---|---|---|---|---|---|---|---|---|---|---|---|---|
| | #1 | #2 | #3 | #4 | #5 | #6 | #7 | #8 | #9 | #10 | #11 | #12 |
| Age (years) | 43 | 45 | 46 | 51 | 54 | 57 | 61 | 64 | 64 | 64 | 69 | 71 |
| Age at AMI (years) | 31 | ? | 37 | ? | 29 | 51 | 49 | 54 | ? | 62 | 43 | 68 |
| Sex | M | F | M | F | F | M | M | F | M | F | M | M |
| Race | W | B | W | B | W | W | B | W | W | W | B | W |
| Body Weight (pounds) | 220 | 135 | 168 | 211 | 174 | 164 | 186 | 151 | 207 | 183 | 167 | 248 |
| Height (inches) | 66 | 64 | 64 | 65 | 68 | 69 | 73 | 66 | 61 | 66 | 65 | 73 |
| Body Mass Index (kg/m^2) | 36 | 23 | 29 | 35[a] | 27 | 24 | 25 | 24 | 29 | 30 | 27 | 33 |
| Systemic Hypertension | + | + | 0 | + | + | + | 0 | + | 0 | 0 | + | + |
| Bundle Branch Block (type) | + (R) | 0 | + (R) | 0 | 0 | + (R) | + (L) | + (R) | 0 | 0 | + (L) | 0 |
| Atrial Fibrillation | + | + | 0 | + | 0 | + | 0 | 0 | 0 | + | + | + |
| Diabetes Mellitus | + | 0 | 0 | + | 0 | 0 | + | + | 0 | + | + | 0 |
| Renal Disease | 0 | +[b] | 0 | 0 | 0 | + | +[b] | 0 | + | 0 | 0 | 0 |
| Percutaneous Coronary Intervention at Time of Acute MI | + | 0 | + | 0 | + | + | + | 0 | + | 0 | + | + |
| Total Cholesterol (mg/dL) | 96[c] | 164[c] | 127[c] | 114[c] | 117[c] | 139[c] | 62[c] | 107[c] | 208[d] | 175[c] | 175[c] | 156[c] |
| LDL Cholesterol (mg/dL) | 74[c] | 90[c] | 73[c] | 35[c] | 67[c] | 79[c] | 31[c] | 47[c] | 119[c] | 102[c] | 108[c] | 94[c] |
| HDL Cholesterol (mg/dL) | 12[c] | 59[c] | 49[c] | 69[c] | 38[c] | 41[c] | 26[c] | 54[c] | 29[c] | 37[c] | 47[c] | 42[c] |
| Triglycerides (mg/dL) | 174[c] | 127[c] | 96[c] | 103[c] | 86[c] | 93[c] | 26[c] | 47[c] | 296[c] | 269[c] | 107[c] | 168[c] |
| LV Diameter (cm) | 7.2 | 7.3 | - | 5.4 | 6.9 | - | 7.1 | - | 7.7 | - | 7.0 | - |
| Heart Weight (g) | 450 | 360 | 350 | 310 | 445 | 360 | 550 | 310 | 395 | 370 | 360 | 425 |
| Floating Heart | 0 | 0 | 0 | + | + | 0 | 0 | + | + | 0 | 0 | 0 |
| Location of LV Scarring | P-LAT | Apex | A-S-LAT | A-S | A-S | VS | A | VS | VS | LAT | P | Apex |
| Severely Narrowed CA | R | 0[e] | LAD | LAD | R | LAD | LAD | LAD | LAD | 0[f] | R | LAD |

*Abbreviations:* A = anterior; B = black; CA = coronary artery; D = diastole; F = female; HDL = high-density lipoprotein; HF = heart failure; LAD = left anterior descending; LAT = lateral; LDL = low-density lipoprotein; L = left; M = male; MI = myocardial infarction; P = posterior; R = right; S = septum; VS = ventricular septum; W = white

[a] Previous gastric banding operation
[b] Renal transplant
[c] Patient on statin
[d] Patient on ezetimibe
[e] Apparently acute MI never diagnosed. Thus, the status of the coronary arteries *at the time of the acute MI* is not known
[f] Patient's angiogram at the time of the acute MI disclosed severe narrowing of 1 major coronary artery. - = no information available

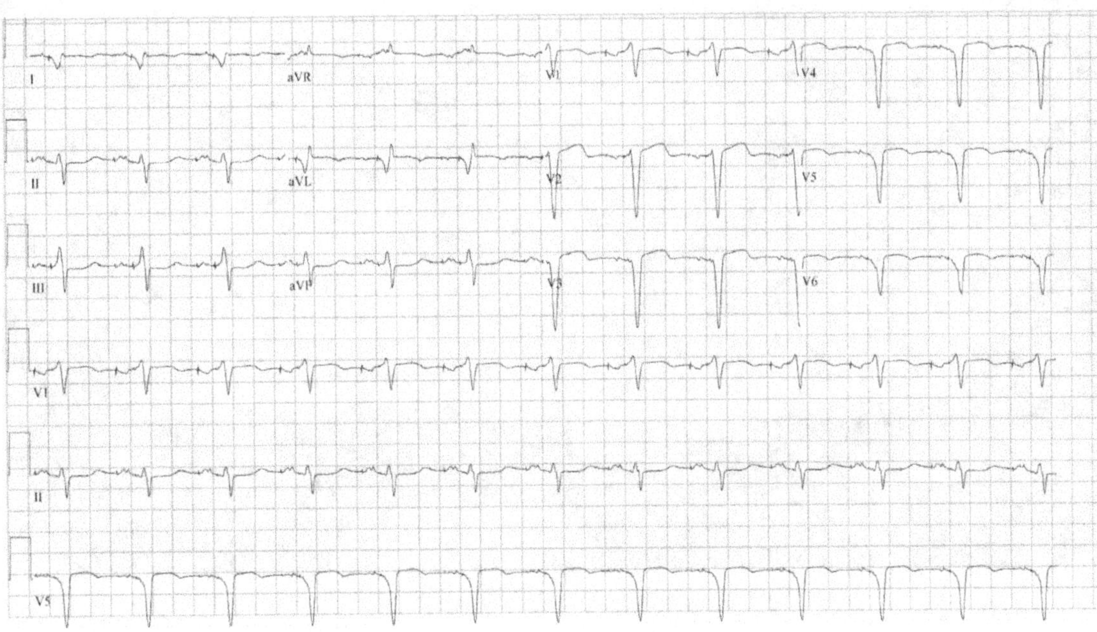


Figure 1. Case # 6, Table 1. This electrocardiogram is from the patient whose heart is shown in Figure 8. The entire ventricular septum and the wall at the apex is thin and completely scarred. The electrocardiogram shows deep Q or S waves throughout the precordium.

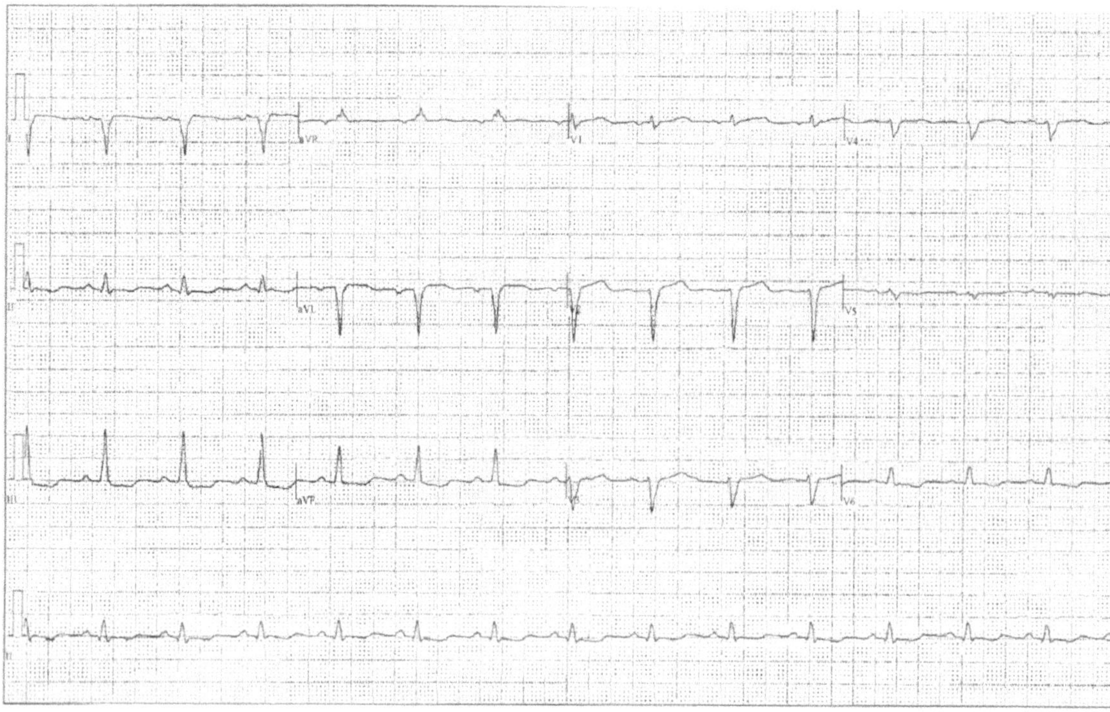

Figure 2. Case # 9, Table 1. Shown here is the electrocardiogram in case number 9 whose heart is shown in Figure 11. The ventricular septum is transmurally scarred. The electrocardiogram shows either Q or S waves across the precordium until V6 when there is an upright R wave.

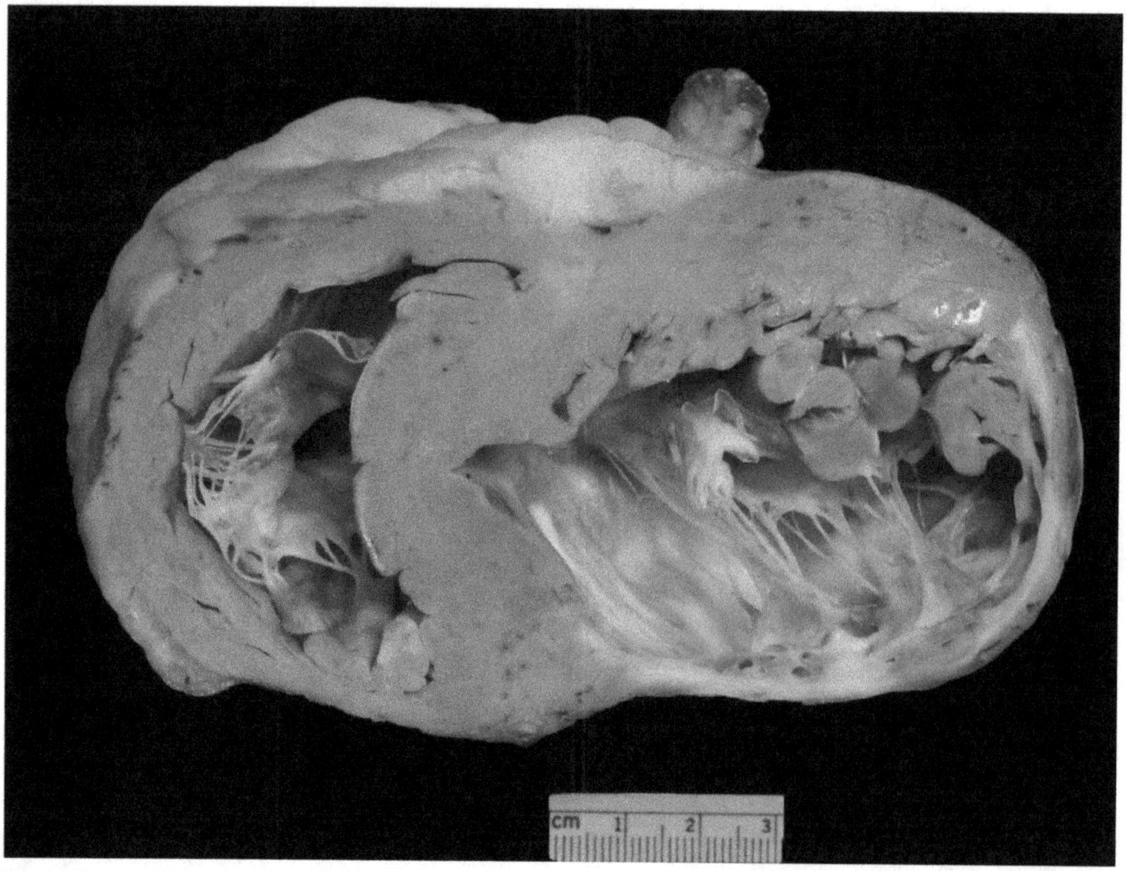

Figure 3. Case # 1, Table 1. Shown here is a cross sectional view of the heart of a 43-year-old man who had an acute myocardial infarction approximately 3 months before OHT. The entire lateral and posterior walls are scarred and if compared to the thickness of the ventricular septum and anterior left ventricular free wall, extremely thin. The lumen of the right coronary artery was severely narrowed by plaque whereas the left anterior descending and left circumflex had very adequate lumens.

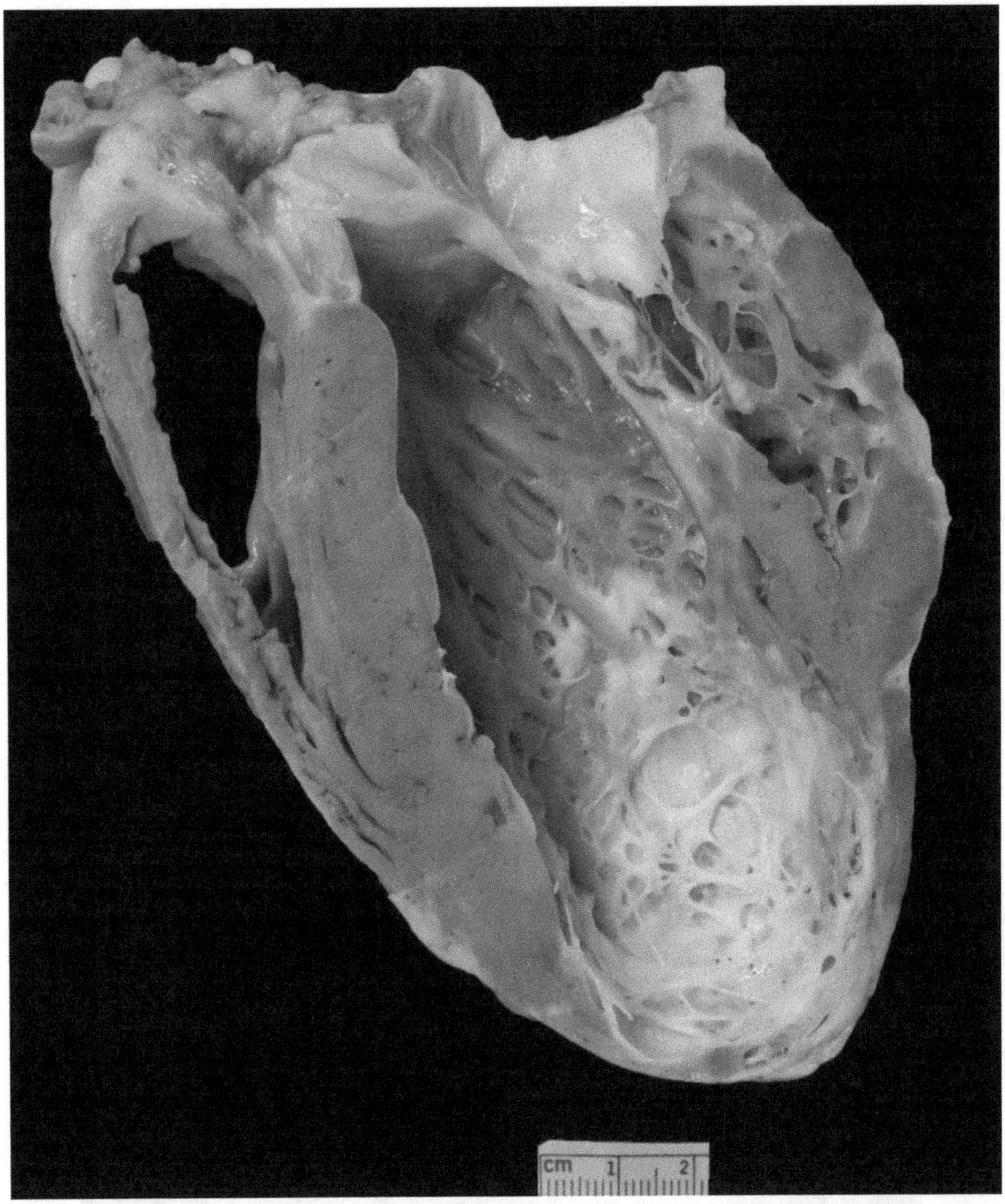


Figure 4. Case # 2. Shown here is a parasagittal cut of the left ventricle displaying its very dilated cavity and also the right ventricular outflow tract, the aortic valve, and portions of the mitral valve. The wall in the apical portion is scarred and the mural endocardium overlying the healed infarct consists of dense fibrous tissue. Both ventricular cavities are quite dilated. This heart belonged to a 44-year-old woman whose acute infarct occurred approximately six months before the heart transplant.

atherosclerotic plaques but only one major (left main, left artery descending left circumflex, and right) coronary artery was severely narrowed by plaque. We have studied numerous patients with coronary disease at autopsy and most with healed myocardial infarcts have >1 major epicardial coronary artery severely narrowed and much smaller infarcts than in the 12 patients described herein.[1–6] It appears that the size of a healed myocardial infarct is inversely related to the number of newly narrowed epicardial coronary arteries: severe narrowing of a single major epicardial coronary tends to result in a large myocardial infarct and severe dilation of the left ventricular cavity; severe narrowing of >1 major epicardial coronary artery tends to be associated with smaller myocardial infarcts and less left ventricular dilation and therefore less heart failure.

The presence of a single large infarct and a severely narrowed epicardial coronary artery raises the possibility of coronary embolism as the explanation for the unusual

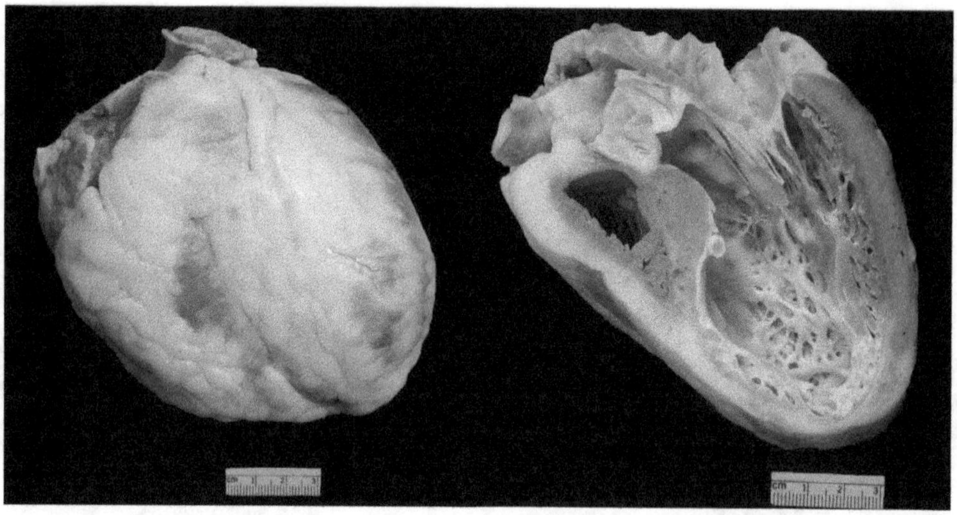

Figure 5. Case # 3. Shown here on the left is the anterior outside wall of the heart showing considerable increase of subepicardial adipose tissue. On the right is a large healed anterior, septal and apical myocardial infarct. The left ventricular cavity is quite dilated. The infarct has distinct junctions between the infarcted area and the normal area.

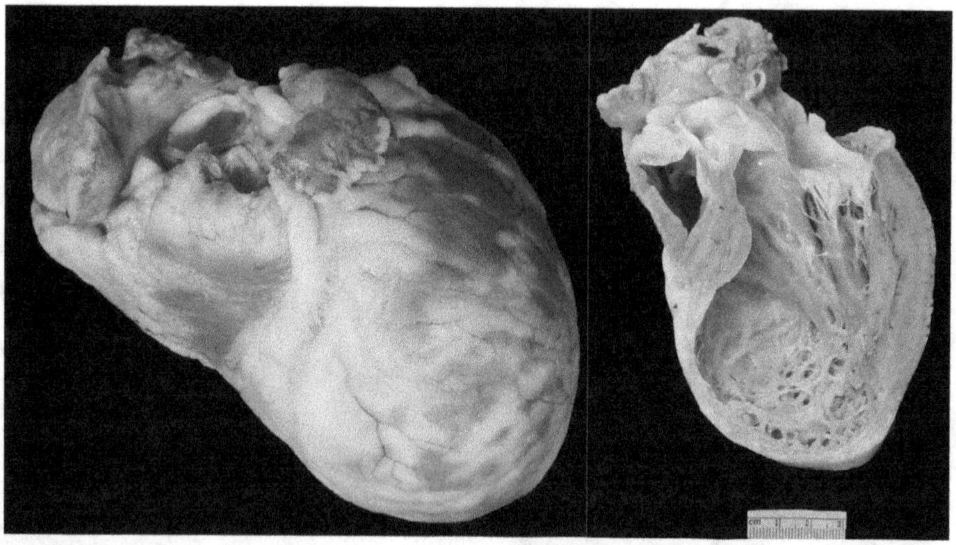

Figure 6. Case # 4, Table 1. Shown on the left is the outside of the heart showing transmural scarring in the anterior wall (whitish areas). The infarct occupies the apical half which is quite dilated. The acute infarct which healed occurred about 11 years before the heart transplant.

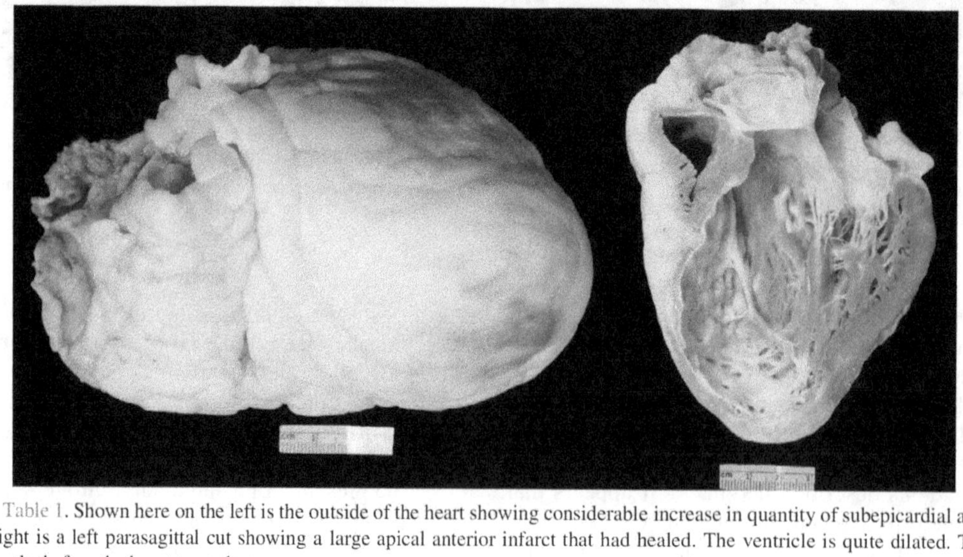

Figure 7. Case # 5, Table 1. Shown here on the left is the outside of the heart showing considerable increase in quantity of subepicardial adipose tissue and an apical bulge. The right is a left parasagittal cut showing a large apical anterior infarct that had healed. The ventricle is quite dilated. The infarct occurred approximately 3 months before the heart transplant.

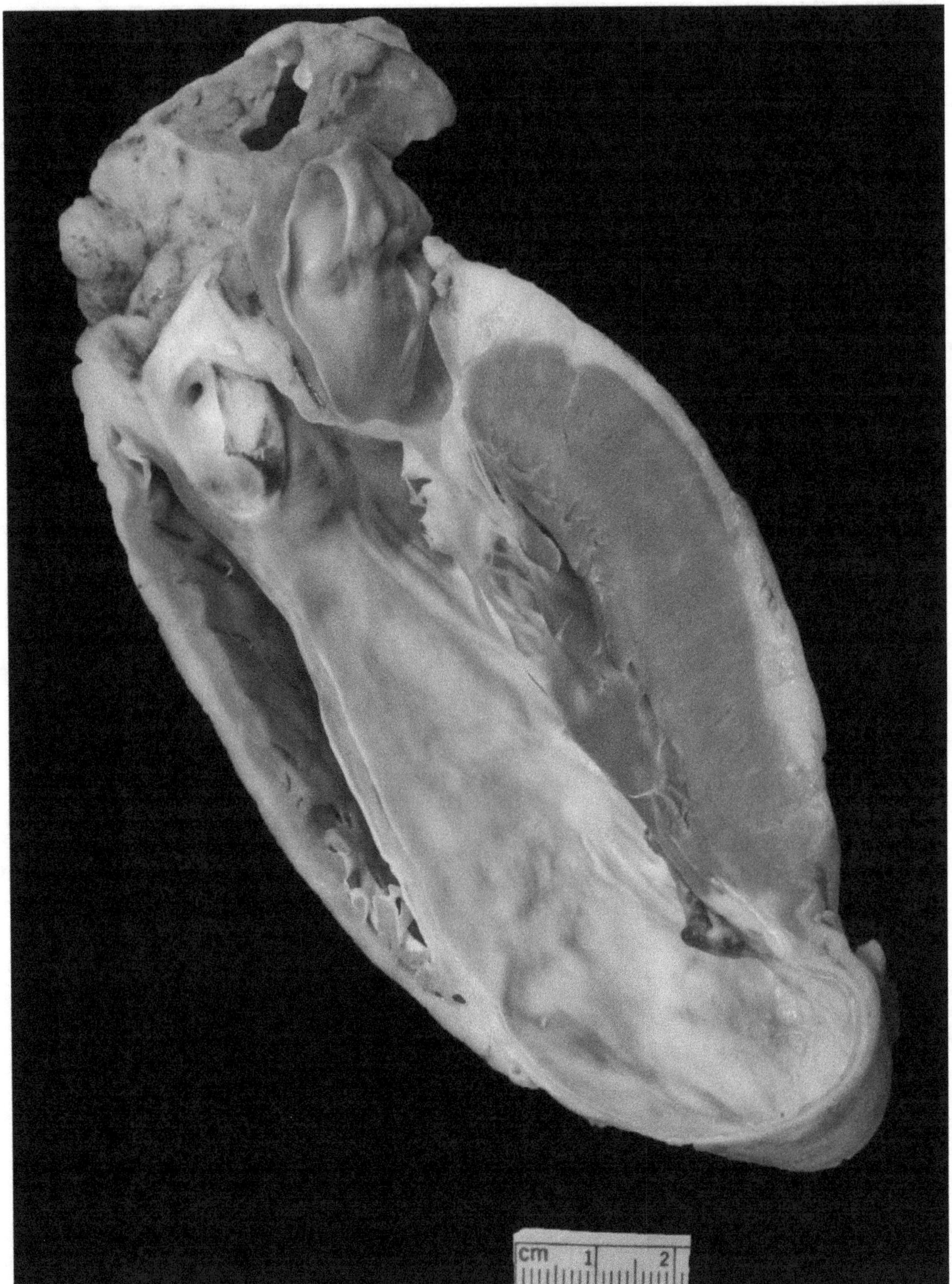


Figure 8. Case # 6, Table 1. Shown here is a left parasagittal cut of the left and right ventricles. The ventricular septum is totally transmurally scarred as is the apical wall which is aneurysmal. The non-infarcted wall is much thicker than normal. This patient is a 57-year-old man who had a myocardial infarct just over a year before the heart transplant. His electrocardiogram is shown in Figure 1.

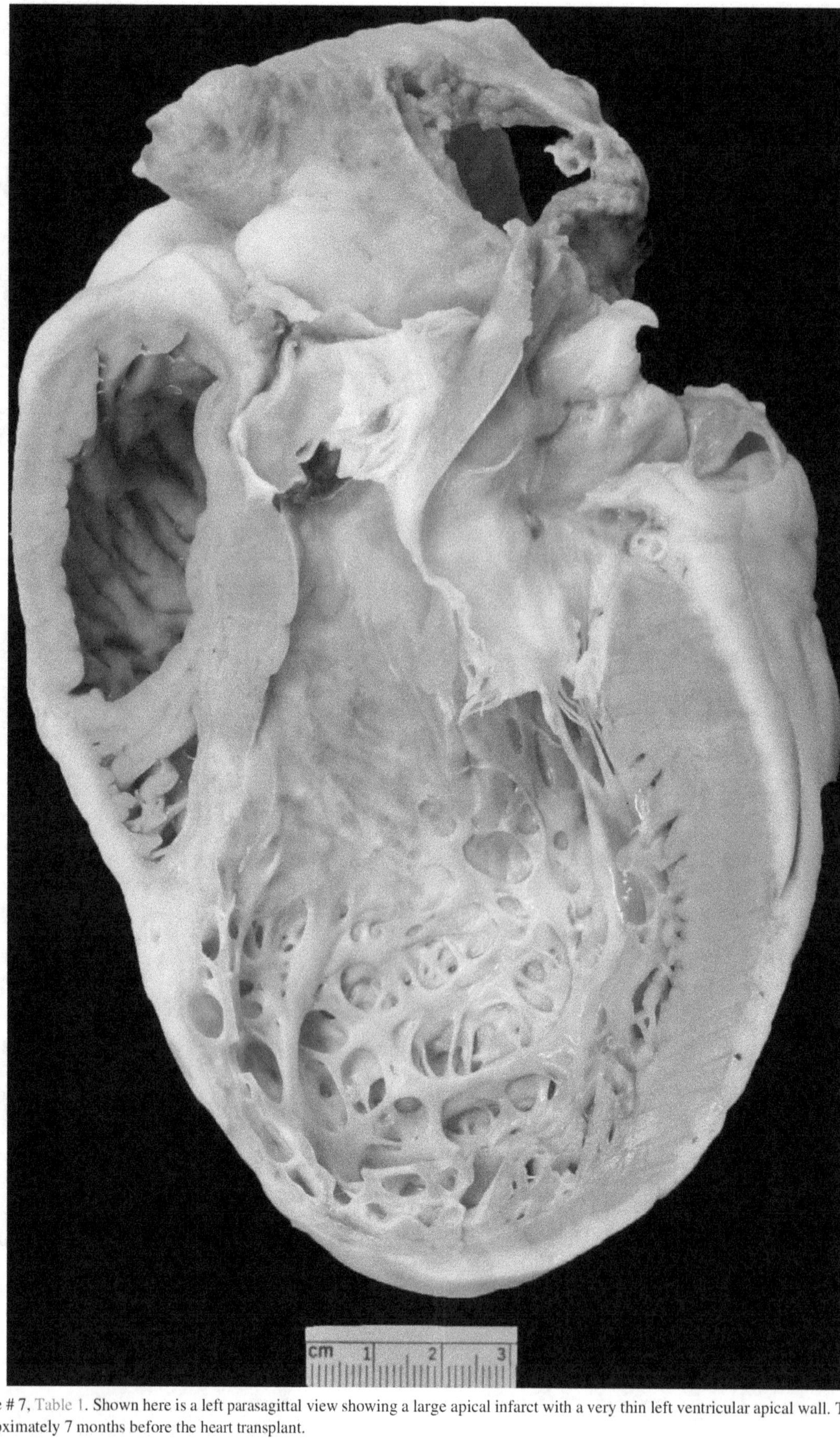


Figure 9. Case # 7, Table 1. Shown here is a left parasagittal view showing a large apical infarct with a very thin left ventricular apical wall. The acute infarct occurred approximately 7 months before the heart transplant.

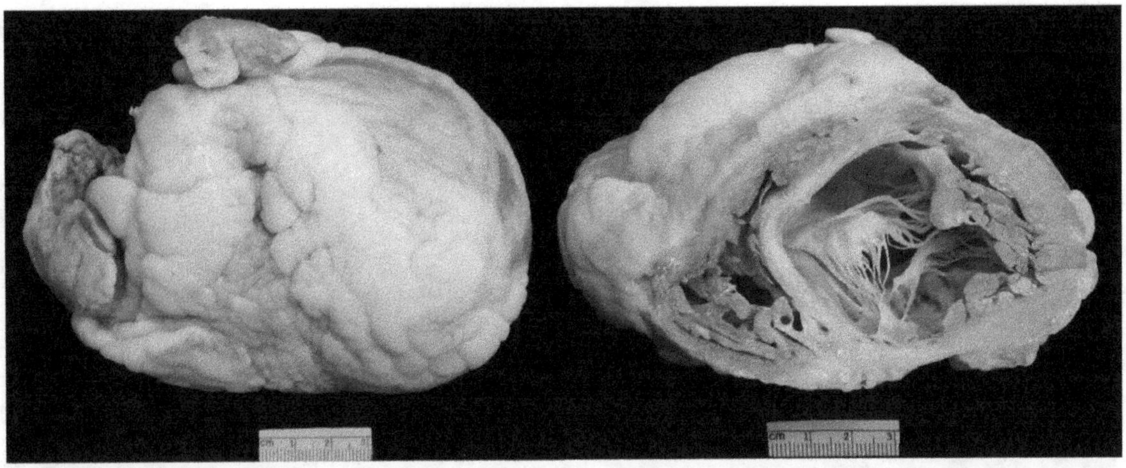

Figure 10. Case # 8, Table 1. Shown on the left is the outside of the heart showing a great deal of subepicardial adipose tissue which caused the heart to float in a container of formaldehyde. The right is a cross sectional view of the heart showing the ventricular septum and a portion of the posterior wall to be transmurally scarred. The left ventricular cavity is quite dilated.

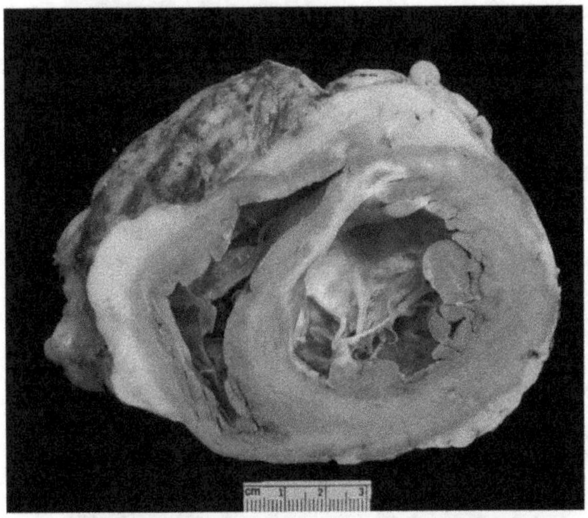

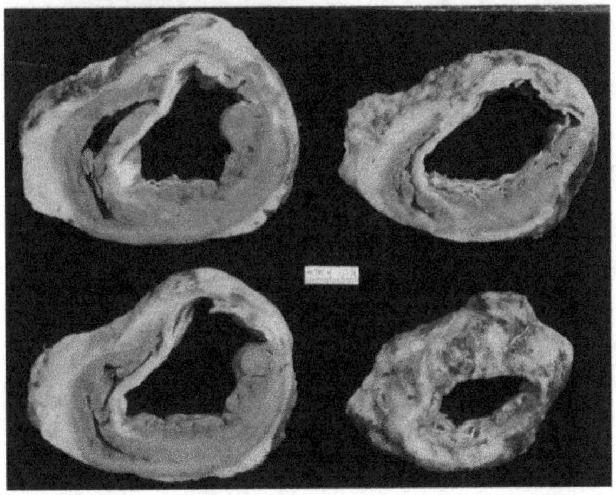

Figure 11. Case # 9, Table 1. Shown in the upper view is a cross-sectional cut of the ventricles just caudal to the atrioventricular valves. The ventricular septum and portions of the anterior wall of left ventricle are scarred. The quantity of subadipose tissue is huge. Shown in the bottom picture are cross-sections of the ventricles in more caudal sites. The ventricular septum is completely scarred in at least two of these sections. The bottom right is a picture of the apex where a left ventricular assist device had been inserted.

findings in our 12 patients.[7-9] The finding of chronic atrial fibrillation in 7 of the 12 patients also may support this thesis. The foramen ovale was closed in all 12 patients, and none had evidence of a vasculopathy. None of the 12 patients had evidence of valvular heart disease.

Another possibility to explain the relation between the large area of infarction (and later scarring) is the lack of collaterals between the infarct coronary arteries and the other major epicardial coronary artery. Lip and colleagues[10-17] have written extensively on this topic. Whether the lack of coronary collaterals accounts for the huge size of the infarcts or the finding of severe narrowing of only one major be epicardial coronary artery in the present study is unclear. Unfortunately, we are uncertain whether angiographic collaterals were seen at the time of the acute infarction in the patients.

The major limitation of the present study is the inability to establish the mechanism resulting in the large infarct and the severe narrowing limited to only one of the major coronary artery. The finding of healed infarction of nearly the entire ventricular septum in 3 of 12 patients is most unusual - unique in our experience - but again its mechanism of involvement is unclear.

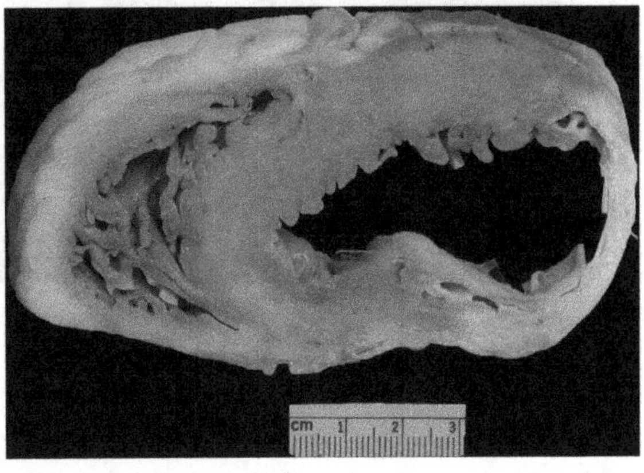

Figure 12. Case # 10, Table 1. Shown here is a cross-section of the ventricles midway between mitral anulus and left ventricular apex. The left ventricular free wall laterally has a thin wall and is covered on the epicardial surface by adipose tissue. The ventricular septum is quite thick.

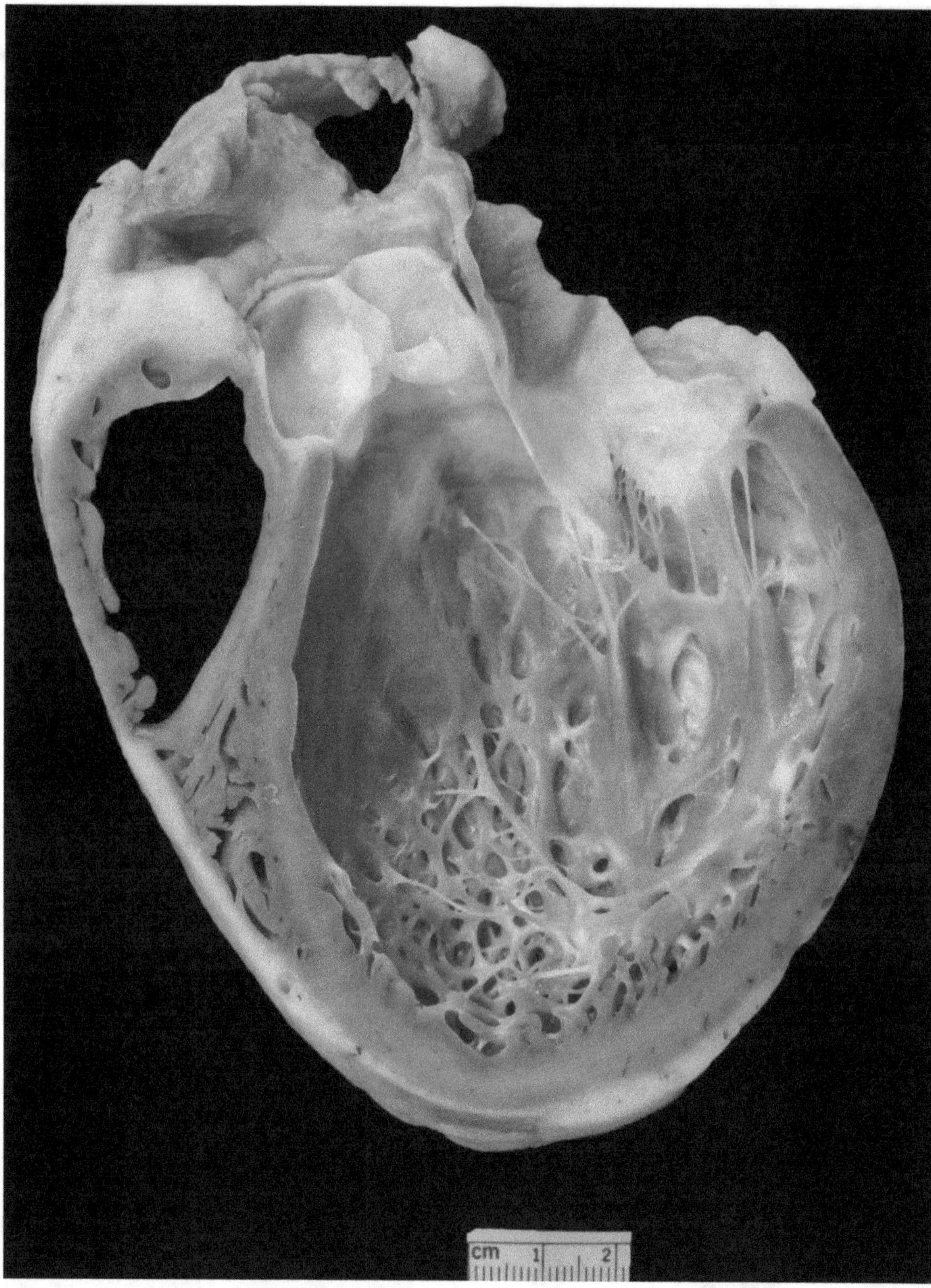


Figure 13. Case # 11, Table 1. Shown here is a left parasagittal cut showing the posterior wall scar extending from just below the mitral anulus to nearly the apex. Both ventricular cavities are quite dilated.

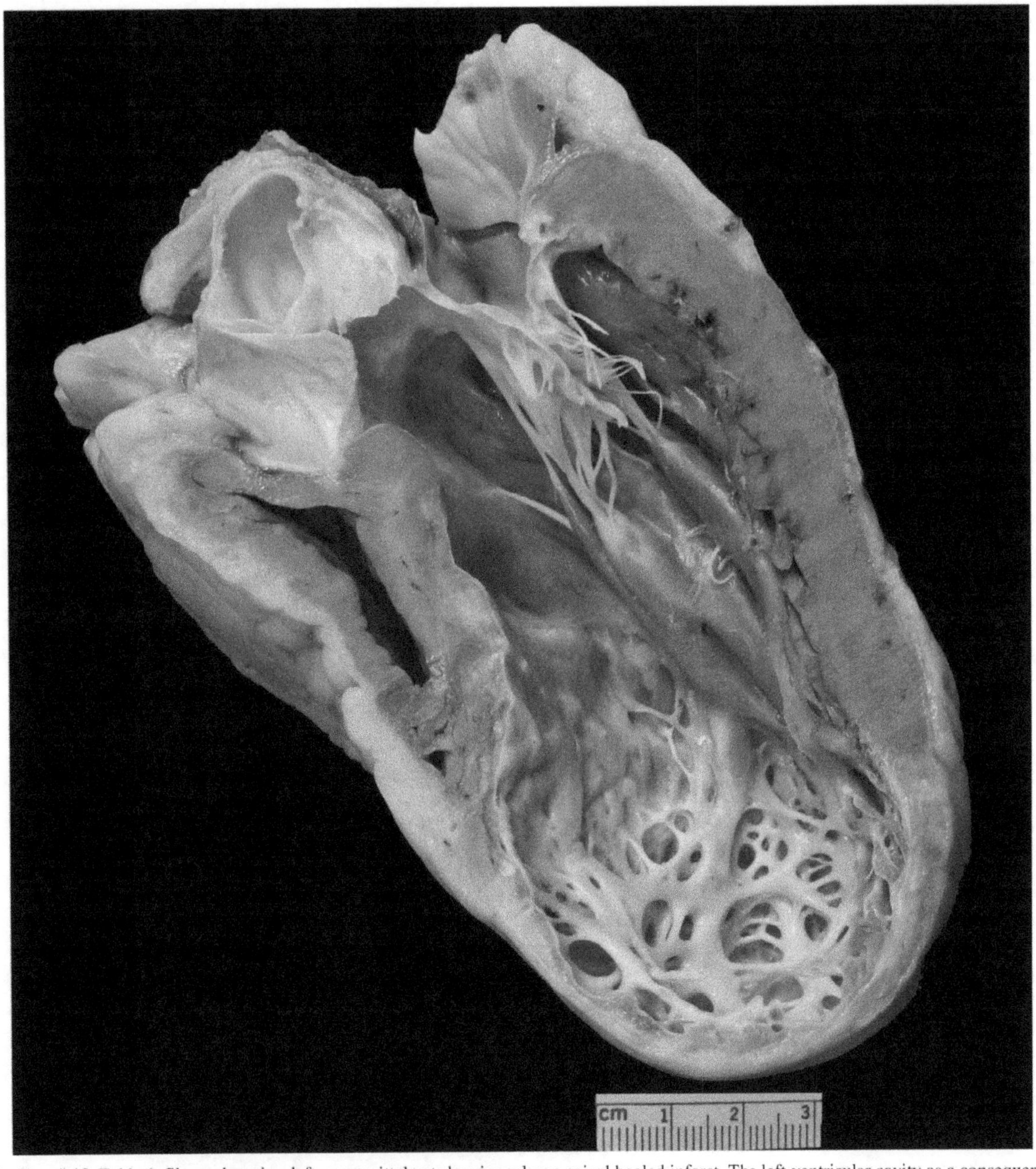


Figure 14. Case # 12. Table 1. Shown here is a left parasagittal cut showing a large apical healed infarct. The left ventricular cavity as a consequence is quite dilated. The acute infarct occurred about 9 months before the heart transplant.

## Declaration of interests

The authors declare that they have no known competing financial interests or personal relationships that could have appeared to influence the work reported in this paper.


1. Virmani R, Roberts WC. Non-fatal healed transmural myocardial infarction and fatal non-cardiac disease. Qualification and quantification of coronary arterial narrowing and of left ventricular scarring in 18 necropsy patients. *Br Heart J* 1981;45:434–441.
2. Cabin HS, Roberts WC. Relation of healed transmural myocardial infarct size to length of survival after acute myocardial infarction, age at death, and amount and extent of coronary arterial narrowing by atherosclerotic plaques: analysis of 70 necropsy patients. *Am Heart J* 1982;104:216–220.
3. Cabin HS, Roberts WC. Quantitative comparison of extent of coronary narrowing and size of healed myocardial infarct in 33 necropsy patients with clinically recognized and in 28 with clinically unrecognized ("silent") previous acute myocardial infarction. *Am J Cardiol* 1982;50:677–681.
4. Ross EM, Roberts WC. Severe atherosclerotic coronary artery disease healed myocardial infarction and chronic congestive heart failure, analysis of 81 patients studied at necropsy. *Am J Cardiol* 1986;57:44–50.
5. Roberts WC. Qualitative and quantitative comparison of amounts of narrowing by atherosclerotic plaques in the major epicardial coronary arteries at necropsy in sudden coronary death, transmural acute myocardial infarction, transmural healed myocardial infarction, and unstable angina pectoris. *Am J Cardiol* 1989;64:324–328.
6. Roberts WC, Potkin BN, Solus DE, Reddy SG. Mode of death, frequency of healed and acute myocardial infarction, number of major epicardial coronary arteries severely narrowed by atherosclerotic plaque, and heart weight in fatal atherosclerotic coronary artery disease: analysis of 889 patients studied at necropsy. *J Am Coll Cardiol* 1990;15:196–203.

7. Arnett EN, Roberts WC. Acute myocardial infarction and angiographically normal coronary arteries. An unproven combination. *Circulation* 1976;53:395–400.
8. Arnett EN, Roberts WC. Angiographically normal arteries after healing of acute myocardial infarction. *Practical Cardiol* 1976. July /August.
9. Roberts WC. Coronary embolism: a review of causes consequences and diagnostic considerations. *Cardiovasc Med* 1978;3:699–710.
10. Felmeden DC, Blann AD, Lip GY. Angiogenesis: basic pathophysiology and implications for disease. *Eur Heart J* 2003;24:586–603.
11. Tayebjee MH, Lip GYH, MacFadyen RJ. Collateralization and the response to obstruction of epicardial coronary arteries. *Quarterly J Med* 2004;97:259–272.
12. Lee KW, Lip GY, Blann AD. Plasma angiopoietin-1, angiopoietin-2, angiopoietin receptor tie-2, and vascular endothelial growth factor levels in acute coronary syndromes. *Circulation* 2004;19:2355–2360.
13. Tayebjee MH, Lip GY, Macfadyen RJ. Is there an association between hypertension and the development of coronary collateral flow? *J Hum Hypertens* 2005;19:757–759.
14. Tayebjee MH, Lip GY, Tan KT, Patel JV, Hughes EA, MacFadyen RJ. Plasma matrix metalloproteinase-9, tissue inhibitor of metalloproteinase-2, and CD40 ligand levels in patients with stable coronary artery disease. *Am J Cardiol* 2005;96:339–345.
15. Jaumdally R, Varma C, Macfadyen RJ, Lip GY. Coronary sinus blood sampling: an insight into local cardiac pathophysiology and treatment? *Eur Heart J* 2007;28:929–940.
16. Lim HS, Tayebjee MH, Tan KT, Patel JV, Macfadyen RJ, Lip GY. Is soluble CD40 ligand a mediator of angiogenesis in patients with coronary artery disease? *Thromb Res* 2008;122:307–313.
17. Bax JJ, Delgado V. Chronic total occlusion without collateral blood flow does not exclude myocardial viability and subsequent recovery after revascularization. *J* Nucl Cardiol 2019;26:1731–1733.

# Significance of myocardium within the inflow cannula of a left ventricular assist device

Minseob Jeong, MD[a], and William C. Roberts, MD[a,b,c]

[a]Baylor Scott & White Heart and Vascular Institute, Dallas, Texas; [b]Department of Internal Medicine, Baylor University Medical Center, Dallas, Texas; [c]Department of Pathology, Baylor University Medical Center, Dallas, Texas

**ABSTRACT**

Described herein is a 61-year-old man who underwent replacement of a left ventricular assist device that had been in place for 54 months. A small mass was attached to the margin of the excised metallic inflow cannula of the left ventricular assist device. Histologically, the mass was found to contain myocardium.

**KEYWORDS** Heartmate II; inflow cannula; left ventricular assist device; myocardium

Recently we encountered a fragment of myocardium attached to the margin of the inflow cannula of a Heartmate II that had been in place for 54 months. Such a surprising finding and its significance prompted this report.

## CASE DESCRIPTION

A 61-year-old man with known ischemic cardiomyopathy underwent replacement of a left ventricular assist device (LVAD) that had been in place for 54 months. The reason for its replacement was recurrent driveline fracture. A small

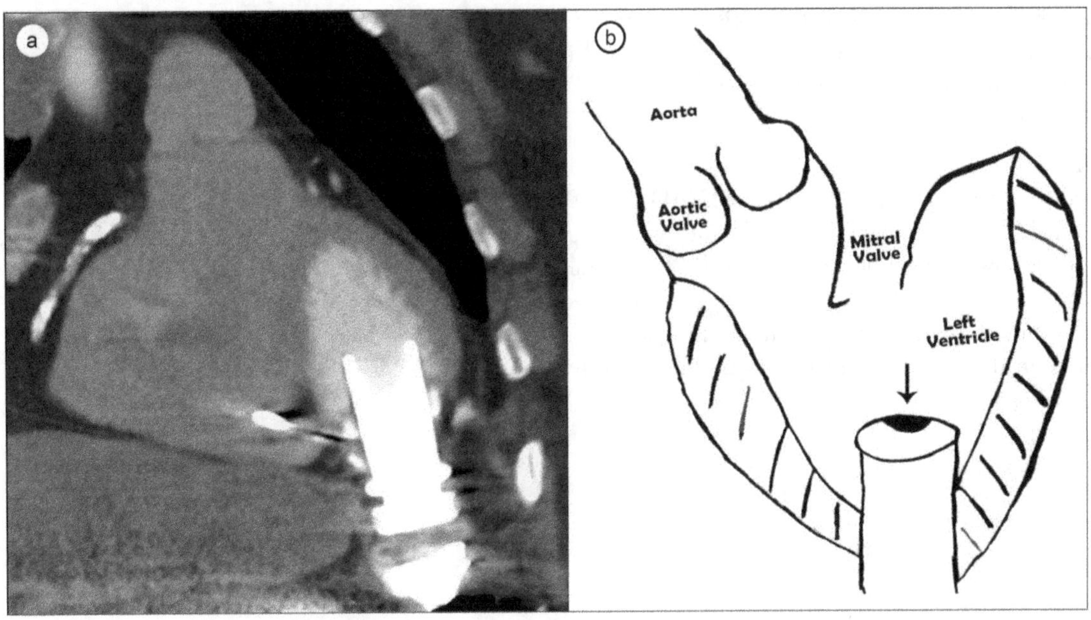


**Figure 1.** **(a)** Computed tomograph of the chest showing the location of the inflow cannula of the LVAD in the left ventricular cavity. **(b)** Diagram showing the myocardium (arrow) attached to the margin of the metallic inflow cannula of an LVAD that had burrowed into the posterior left ventricular free wall.

**Corresponding author**: William C. Roberts, MD, Baylor Scott & White Heart and Vascular Institute, 621 N. Hall Street, Suite H-030, Dallas, TX 75226 (e-mail: william.roberts1@bswhealth.org)

The authors report no funding or conflicts of interest.
Received January 31, 2022; Accepted February 2, 2022.

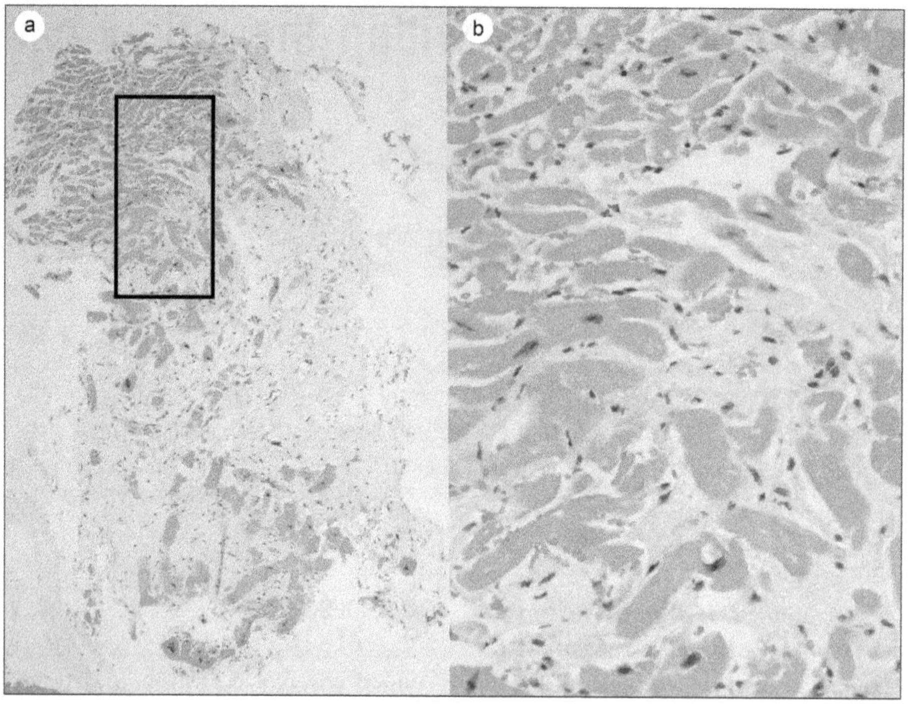



**Figure 2.** Photomicrographs of a portion of the excised mass from the LVAD inflow cannula that shows myocardium and fibrous tissue. Trichrome stains **(a)** 10×, **(b)** 100×.

mass was attached at the margin of the excised inflow cannula of the LVAD *(Figure 1)*. Study of the mass disclosed it to consist of myocardium and fibrous tissue *(Figure 2)*.

## DISCUSSION

Described herein is a patient who had an LVAD replacement with a fragment of myocardium attached to the margin of the metallic inflow cannula of a Heartmate II. The metallic orifice of the inflow cannula presumably had burrowed into the posterior left ventricular free wall, and myocardium was implanted on the inflow cannula. This finding indicates that the cannula was implanted into the left ventricular wall rather than entirely into the left ventricular cavity. Such implantation is not infrequent.[1,2]


1. Roberts WC, Ather N, Guileyardo JM. Examining hearts containing left ventricular assist devices at necropsy. *Am J Cardiol.* 2020;125(2): 244–250. doi:10.1016/j.amjcard.2019.10.013.
2. Ather N, Roberts WC. Location of the cannula of the left ventricular assist device in explanted hearts after orthotopic heart transplantation. *Am J Cardiol.* 2020;134:91–98. doi:10.1016/j.amjcard.2020.07.054.

www.ingramcontent.com/pod-product-compliance
Lightning Source LLC
LaVergne TN
LVHW062147200926
848484LV00007B/1873